Principles and Techniques of

Biochemistry and Molecular Biology

Edited by Keith Wilson and John Walker

Sixth edition

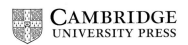
CAMBRIDGE
UNIVERSITY PRESS

CAMBRIDGE UNIVERSITY PRESS
Cambridge, New York, Melbourne, Madrid, Cape Town, Singapore, São Paulo

Cambridge University Press
40 West 20th Street, New York, NY 10011-4211, USA

www.cambridge.org
Information on this title: www.cambridge.org/9780521828895

First published by Edward Arnold 1975 as *A biologist's guide to principles
and techniques of practical biochemistry*
Second edition 1981; Third edition 1986
Third edition first published by Cambridge University Press 1992; Reprinted 1993
Fourth edition published by Cambridge University Press 1994 as
Principles and techniques of practical biochemistry; Reprinted 1995, 1997; Fifth edition 2000
Sixth edition first published by Cambridge University Press 2005
as *Principles and techniques of biochemistry and molecular biology*

Printed in Hong Kong

A catalogue record for this publication is available from the British Library.

Library of Congress Cataloguing in Publication data
Principles and techniques of biochemistry and molecular biology/edited by Keith Wilson,
  John Walker. – 6th ed.
      p.   cm.
   New & expanded ed. of: Principles and techniques of practical biochemistry. 5th ed. c2000.
   Includes bibliographical references and index.
   ISBN 0-521-82889-9 (alk. paper) – ISBN 0-521-53581-6 (pbk.: alk. paper)
     1. Biochemistry – Methodology.   2. Molecular biology – Methodology.   I. Wilson, Keith,
   1936–   . II. Walker, John M., 1948–   .   III. Principles and techniques of practical biochemistry.
   QP519.7.P75   2005
   572–dc22   2004054541   CIP

ISBN-13   978-0-521-82889-5 hardback
ISBN-10   0-521-82889-9 hardback

ISBN-13   978-0-521-53581-6 paperback
ISBN-10   0-521-53581-6 paperback

(Continued on p. xii)

Contents

The colour figure section is between pp. *142* and *143*.

Preface to the sixth edition

In the preface to previous editions of our book we set ourselves the task of producing an undergraduate text that covered the theoretical principles and practical details of the experimental techniques that are basic to an understanding of, and that support advances in, biochemistry. In the 30 years that have elapsed since the first edition was launched in 1975, there have been dramatic advances in our understanding of the biochemical processes that characterise living cells. Such advances are typified by the recent completion of the Human Genome Project and the emergence of numerous allied fields of study such as bioinformatics and proteomics. The new generic discipline of molecular biology embraces many of these areas of research and so we have felt it appropriate to broaden the title of the book to include molecular biology, as it clearly falls within our original objective. In the process of taking a decision on the content of this sixth edition of our book, we have also attempted to respond to the extremely constructive and encouraging feedback we have received to the survey we conducted of the many academic departments in UK and overseas universities and other institutions that routinely use our book and recommend it to their students. The outcome is that we have broadened the topics covered within the book by including two new chapters, one on cell culture, the other on microscopy. In addition we have considered it appropriate to include major new sections on the principles and practice of clinical biochemistry, including diagnostic enzymology and the statistical considerations underlying the assessment of the quality of quantitative analytical biochemical data and the role and operation of external quality assessment schemes such as the UK NEQAS. We have also taken the decision to modify our original aim of concentrating on those experimental techniques that undergraduates are most likely to encounter in their practical classes and, instead, to discuss all the techniques that now contribute to the rapid advances in our understanding of cellular function. Two specific examples of this new policy are, first, that we have felt it appropriate to place the emphasis of the chapter on mass spectrometry on its indispensable role in protein chemistry and proteomics and, secondly, within the chapter on membrane receptors to discuss in some detail the analytical techniques, such as plasmon-coupled resonance spectroscopy, that are central to modern approaches to the understanding of receptor function and cell signalling. Continuing chapters have been updated to cover recent developments and most include integrated text examples to support the principles discussed in the main text.

We welcome five new contributors: Alastair Aitken (mass spectrometry), Anwar Baydoun (cell culture), John Fyffe (clinical biochemistry), Kay Ohlendieck (centrifugation) and Stephen Paddock (microscopy). We would like to express our sincere thanks to all our contributors for their cooperation in producing this new edition. Sadly we must record the untimely death of Derek Gordon, the author of two chapters on spectroscopic techniques. Derek was an enthusiastic, dedicated and respected teacher of biochemistry, keen to emphasise to his students the chemical principles underlying many analytical techniques central to practical biochemistry.

We continue to welcome constructive comments from all students who use our book as part of their studies and academics who adopt the book to complement their teaching. Finally, we wish to express our gratitude to the authors and publishers who have granted us permission to reproduce their copyright figures and our thanks to Katrina Halliday and her colleagues at Cambridge University Press who have been so supportive in the production of this new edition.

John Walker and Keith Wilson
November 2004

Contributors

Professor A. Aitken
Division of Biomedical & Clinical Laboratory Sciences
University of Edinburgh
George Square
Edinburgh EH8 9XD
Scotland, UK

Dr A. R. Baydoun
School of Life Sciences
University of Hertfordshire
College Lane
Hatfield
Herts AL10 9AB, UK

Dr J. Fyffe
Consultant Clinical Biochemist
Department of Clinical Biochemistry
Royal Hospital for Sick Children
Yorkhill
Glasgow G3 8SF
Scotland, UK

Professor D. B. Gordon (Deceased)
Formerly
Department of Biological Sciences
Metropolitan University of Manchester
Chester Street
Manchester M15 6BH, UK

Professor K. Ohlendieck
Department of Biology
National University of Ireland
Maynooth
Co. Kildare
Ireland

Dr S. W. Paddock
Howard Hughes Medical Institute
Department of Molecular Biology
University of Wisconsin
1525 Linden Drive
Madison, WI 53706
USA

Dr R. Rapley
School of Life Sciences
University of Hertfordshire
College Lane
Hatfield
Herts AL10 9AB, UK

Professor R. J. Slater
School of Life Sciences
University of Hertfordshire
College Lane
Hatfield
Herts AL10 9AB, UK

Professor R. Thorpe
National Institute for Biological Standards and Control
Blanche Lane
South Mimms
Potters Bar
Herts EN6 3QG, UK

Dr S. Thorpe
National Institute for Biological Standards and Control
Blanche Lane
South Mimms
Potters Bar
Herts EN6 3QG, UK

Professor J. M. Walker
School of Life Sciences
University of Hertfordshire
College Lane
Hatfield
Herts AL10 9AB, UK

Professor K. Wilson
Emeritus Professor of Pharmacological Biochemistry
School of Life Sciences
University of Hertfordshire
College Lane
Hatfield
Herts AL10 9AB, UK

Abbreviations

The following abbreviations have been used throughout this book without definition.

AMP	adenosine 5′-monophosphate
ADP	adenosine 5′-diphosphate
ATP	adenosine 5′-triphosphate
bp	base-pairs
cAMP	cyclic AMP
CHAPS	3-[(3-chloroamidopropyl)dimethylamino]-1-propanesulphonic acid
c.p.m.	counts per minute
CTP	cytidine triphosphate
DDT	2,2-bis-(p-chlorophenyl)-1,1,1-trichloroethane
DMSO	dimethylsulphoxide
DNA	deoxyribonucleic acid
e^-	electron
EDTA	ethylenediaminotetra-acetate
FAD	flavin adenine dinucleotide (oxidised)
$FADH_2$	flavin adenine dinucleotide (reduced)
FMN	flavin mononucleotide (oxidised)
$FMNH_2$	flavin mononucleotide (reduced)
GTP	guanosine triphosphate
HAT	hypoxanthine, aminopterin, thymidine medium
Hepes	4(2-hydroxyethyl)-1-piperazine-ethanesulphonic acid
kb	kilobase-pairs
M_r	relative molecular mass
min	minute
NAD^+	nicotinamide adenine dinucleotide (oxidised)
NADH	nicotinamide adenine dinucleotide (reduced)
$NADP^+$	nicotinamide adenine dinucleotide phosphate (oxidised)
NADPH	nicotinamide adenine dinucleotide phosphate (reduced)
Pipes	1,4-piperazinebis(ethanesulphonic acid)
P_i	inorganic phosphate
p.p.m.	parts per million

p.p.b.	parts per billion
PP_i	inorganic pyrophosphate
RNA	ribonucleic acid
r.p.m.	revolutions per minute
SDS	sodium dodecyl sulphate
Tris	2-amino-2-hydroxymethylpropane-1,3-diol

Chapter 1

Basic principles

1.1 BIOCHEMICAL STUDIES

1.1.1 The aims of biochemical investigations

Biochemistry is concerned with the study of the chemical processes that occur in living organisms, with the ultimate aim of understanding cell function in molecular terms. Biochemists therefore undertake studies of topics such as:

- the structural, kinetic and thermodynamic characteristics of the molecules found in the whole range of living organisms;
- the function of these molecules and the mechanisms by which they recognise and interact with each other to produce ordered anabolic, catabolic, signalling, immunological and other pathways that characterise living processes;
- the pathways that operate for the synthesis and degradation of these molecules and the mechanisms responsible for errors in the pathways;
- the energetics of biological processes, including transport across cell membranes, the generation of cellular energy, energy conversion and exchange of energy with the surrounding environment;
- the storage, replication, expression, repair, recombination and control of genetic information and the development of cell specificity.

Pioneering biochemical investigations were carried out mainly on simple prokaryotic and eukaryotic organisms such as *Escherichia coli, Saccharomyces cerevisiae, Bacillus subtilis, Neurospora crassa* and *Chlorella pyrenoidosa*. As knowledge of the nature of cellular components and control mechanisms was gained from these studies and shown to have many similarities with comparable data being gained from multicellular organisms, so the whole spectrum of biologically diverse organisms was opened up as model systems for detailed biochemical studies. Biochemists have traditionally used *in vitro* model systems rather than whole cells or organisms because of their inherently greater biochemical simplicity for experimental study and interpretation of results. Nevertheless, *in vitro* studies have the potential danger that the disruption of cells or tissues may lead to artefacts that bear little resemblance to the *in vivo* situation.

In recent years, and particularly in the past decade, the growth of biochemical knowledge relating to cellular function has grown exponentially. This has come about largely through the development of techniques for the rapid sequencing of DNA fragments released by the action of restriction enzymes, of gene cloning and site-directed mutagenesis (Chapters 5 and 6) coupled with advances in protein sequencing by mass spectrometry (Chapter 9). These developments have given rise to numerous new disciplines such as genomics (the study of cell genomes), proteomics (the study of the whole protein complement of a cell) and molecular biology, all of which fall within the broad discipline of biochemistry.

1.1.2 The design of biochemical investigations

Advances in biochemistry, as in all the sciences, are based on the careful design, execution and data analysis of experiments designed to address specific questions or hypotheses. Such experimental design involves a discrete number of compulsory stages:

- the identification of the subject for experimental investigation;
- the critical evaluation of the current state of knowledge (the 'literature') of the chosen subject area, noting the strengths and weaknesses of the methodologies previously applied and the new hypotheses that emerged from the studies;
- the formulation of the question or hypothesis to be addressed by the planned experiment;
- the careful selection of the biological system (species, in vivo or in vitro) to be used for the study;
- the identification of the variable that is to be studied; the consideration of the other variables that will need to be controlled so that the selected variable is the only factor that will determine the experimental outcome;
- the design of the experiment, including the statistical analysis of the results, careful evaluation of the materials and apparatus to be used and the consequential potential safety aspects of the study;
- the execution of the experiment, including appropriate calibrations and controls, with a carefully written record of the outcomes;
- the replication of the experiment as necessary for the unambiguous analysis of the outcomes;
- the analyses of the outcomes, including the use of appropriate statistical tests;
- the formulation of the main conclusions that can be drawn from the results;
- the formulation of new hypotheses and of future experiments that emerge from the study.

Biochemical experiments usually have much experimental detail in common. For example, the control and measurement of pH, temperature and oxygen tension are essential considerations for many studies. They also involve common manipulations, notably the preparation of solutions of known concentration and the dispensation of small volumes of reagents. The aim of this chapter is to address many of these common issues of experimental design and data analysis.

Table 1.1 SI units – basic and derived units

Quantity	SI unit	Symbol (basic SI unit)	Definition of SI unit	Equivalent in SI units
Basic units				
Length	metre	m		
Mass	kilogram	kg		
Time	second	s		
Electric current	ampere	A		
Temperature	kelvin	K		
Luminous intensity	candela	cd		
Amount of substance	mole	mol		
Derived units				
Force	newton	N	$kg\,m\,s^{-2}$	$J\,m^{-1}$
Energy, work, heat	joule	J	$kg\,m^2\,s^{-2}$	$N\,m$
Power, radiant flux	watt	W	$kg\,m^2\,s^{-3}$	$J\,s^{-1}$
Electric charge, quantity	coulomb	C	$A\,s$	$J\,V^{-1}$
Electric potential difference	volt	V	$kg\,m^2\,s^{-3}\,A^{-1}$	$J\,C^{-1}$
Electric resistance	ohm	Ω	$kg\,m^2\,s^{-3}\,A^{-2}$	$V\,A^{-1}$
Pressure	pascal	Pa	$kg\,m^{-1}\,s^{-2}$	$N\,m^{-2}$
Frequency	hertz	Hz	s^{-1}	
Magnetic flux density	tesla	T	$kg\,s^{-2}\,A^{-1}$	$V\,s\,m^{-2}$
Other units based on SI				
Area	square metre	m^2		
Volume	cubic metre	m^3		
Density	kilogram per cubic metre	$kg\,m^{-3}$		
Concentration	mole per cubic metre	$mol\,m^{-3}$		

1.2 UNITS OF MEASUREMENTS

1.2.1 SI units

The French Système International d'Unités (the SI system) is the accepted convention for all units of measurement. Table 1.1 lists basic and derived SI units. Table 1.2 lists numerical values for some physical constants in SI units. Table 1.3 lists the commonly used prefixes associated with quantitative terms. Table 1.4 gives the interconversion of non-SI units of volume.

1.2.2 Solutions – the expression of concentration

A solution is a homogeneous mixture of one or more substances (solute(s)) in a major liquid component (solvent). The concentration of the solutes in the solution expresses the amount of each solute in a given amount (weight or volume) of the solvent. The simplest expression of concentration is in terms of

Table 1.2 SI units – conversion factors for non-SI units

Unit	Symbol	SI equivalent
Avogadro constant	L or N_A	$6.022 \times 10^{23}\,mol^{-1}$
Faraday constant	F	$9.648 \times 10^{4}\,C\,mol^{-1}$
Planck constant	h	$6.626 \times 10^{-34}\,J\,s$
Universal or molar gas constant	R	$8.314\,J\,K^{-1}\,mol^{-1}$
Molar volume of an ideal gas at s.t.p.		$22.41\,dm^3\,mol^{-1}$
Velocity of light in a vacuum	c	$2.997 \times 10^{8}\,m\,s^{-1}$
Energy		
Calorie	cal	$4.184\,J$
Erg	erg	$10^{-7}\,J$
Electron volt	eV	$1.602 \times 10^{-19}\,J$
Pressure		
Atmosphere	atm	$101\,325\,Pa$
Bar	bar	$10^5\,Pa$
Millimetres of Hg	mmHg	$133.322\,Pa$
Temperature		
Centigrade	°C	$(t°C + 273.15)\,K$
Fahrenheit	°F	$(t°F - 32)5/9 + 273.15\,K$
Length		
Ångström	Å	$10^{-10}\,m$
Inch	in.	$0.0254\,m$
Mass		
Pound	lb	$0.4536\,kg$

s.t.p., standard temperature and pressure.

Table 1.3 Common unit prefixes associated with quantitative terms

Multiple	Prefix	Symbol	Multiple	Prefix	Symbol
10^{24}	yotta	Y	10^{-1}	deci	d
10^{21}	zetta	Z	10^{-2}	centi	c
10^{18}	exa	E	10^{-3}	milli	m
10^{15}	peta	P	10^{-6}	micro	μ
10^{12}	tera	T	10^{-9}	nano	n
10^{9}	giga	G	10^{-12}	pico	p
10^{6}	mega	M	10^{-15}	femto	f
10^{3}	kilo	k	10^{-18}	atto	a
10^{2}	hecto	h	10^{-21}	zepto	z
10^{1}	deca	da	10^{-24}	yocto	y

weight per unit volume (w/v). Alternatives are v/v and w/w. Such expressions may also be in the form of a percentage in which case the w/v, w/w or v/v is multiplied by 100. Thus a 1% (w/v) sodium chloride solution contains $1\,g$ NaCl in $100\,cm^3$ water. Less commonly, solutions may be expressed as parts per million (p.p.m.) or parts per billion (p.p.b.) of total solution. Such units can mean grams per million (or billion) grams or cm^3 in a million (or billion) grams or cm^3. Thus

Table 1.4	Interconversion of non-SI and SI units of volume		
Non-SI unit	Non-SI subunit	SI subunit	SI unit
1 litre (l)	10^3 ml	$= 1 \, dm^3$	$= 10^{-3} \, m^3$
1 millilitre (ml)	1 ml	$= 1 \, cm^3$	$= 10^{-6} \, m^3$
1 micolitre (μl)	10^{-3} ml	$= 1 \, mm^3$	$= 10^{-9} \, m^3$
1 nanolitre (nl)	10^{-6} ml	$= 1 \, nm^3$	$= 10^{-12} \, m^3$

air contains approximately 8 p.p.m. carbon monoxide, where the units would be in volume. If the p.p.m relates to a solution in water, the approximation can be made that 1 g water is equivalent to $1 \, cm^3$. Hence 8 p.p.m. would be equivalent to 8 g in $1000 \, dm^3$ or 8 mg in $1 \, dm^3$ or $8 \, \mu g$ in $1 \, cm^3$ or 8 ng in $1 \, mm^3$ (see Table 1.4).

Molarity

The SI unit of the amount of any substance is the mole, defined as the amount that contains Avogadro's number (N_A) of molecules (6.022×10^{23}). It can also be defined as the amount of a substance in which the number of elementary entities is equal to Avagadro's constant. It is therefore possible to have a mole of molecules, of atoms, of ions or even of electrons. In practical terms, one mole of a substance is equal to its molecular mass expressed in grams, where the molecular mass is the sum of the atomic masses of the constituent atoms. Note that the term molecular mass is preferred to the older term molecular weight. The SI unit of concentration is expressed in terms of moles per cubic metre ($mol \, m^{-3}$) (see Table 1.1). In practice this is far too large for normal laboratory purposes and a unit based on a cubic decimetre (dm^3, 10^{-3} m) is preferred. However, some textbooks and journals, especially those of North American origin, tend to use the older unit of volume, namely the litre and its subunits (see Table 1.4) rather than cubic decimetres. In this book, volumes will be expressed in cubic decimetres or its smaller counterparts (Table 1.4). The molarity of a solution of a substance expresses the number of moles of the substance in $1 \, dm^3$ of solution. Molarity is expressed by the symbol M, but, since this has another use in the SI system (mega = M), $mol \, dm^{-3}$ is recommended instead. Nevertheless, molarity continues to be expressed as M in many textbooks and international journals as well as in conversation and will be used in this book.

It should be noted that atomic and molecular masses are both expressed in daltons (Da) or kilodaltons (kDa), where one dalton is an atomic mass unit equal to one-twelfth of the mass of one atom of the ^{12}C isotope. However, biochemists prefer to use the term relative molecular mass (M_r). This is defined as the molecular mass of a substance relative to one-twelfth of the atomic mass of the ^{12}C isotope. M_r therefore has no units. Thus the relative molecular mass of sodium chloride is 23 (Na) plus 35.5 (Cl), i.e. 58.5, so that one mole is 58.5 g. If this was dissolved in water and adjusted to a total volume of $1 \, dm^3$, the solution would be one molar (1 M).

Table 1.5 Interconversion of mol, mmol and μmol in different volumes to give different concentrations

Molar (M)	Millimolar (mM)	Micromolar (μM)
$1\ mol\ dm^{-3}$	$1\ mmol\ dm^{-3}$	$1\ \mu mol\ dm^{-3}$
$1\ mmol\ cm^{-3}$	$1\ \mu mol\ cm^{-3}$	$1\ nmol\ cm^{-3}$
$1\ \mu mol\ mm^{-3}$	$1\ nmol\ mm^{-3}$	$1\ pmol\ mm^{-3}$

Biological substances are most frequently found at relatively low concentrations and in *in vitro* model systems the volumes of stock solutions regularly used for experimental purposes are also small. The consequence is that experimental solutions are usually in the $mmol\ dm^{-3}$, $\mu mol\ dm^{-3}$ and $nmol\ dm^{-3}$ range rather than molar. Table 1.5 shows the interconversion of these units.

Example 1 CALCULATION OF MOLARITY

Question 1

How would you prepare $250\ cm^3$ of 0.1 M glucose?

Answer

The molecular formula of glucose is $C_6H_{12}O_6$ so its molecular mass is $(6 \times 12) + (12 \times 1) + (6 \times 16)$, i.e. 180 daltons. Hence, 180 g dissolved in $1\ dm^3$ would give a 1 M solution, so that 18 g dissolved in $1\ dm^3$ would give a 0.1 M solution. Hence to prepare $250\ cm^3$ of 0.1 M solution, 4.5 g of glucose would be dissolved in water and the total volume adjusted to $250\ cm^3$ in a volumetric flask.

Question 2

How would you prepare $10\ cm^3$ of 0.01 M glucose from a 0.1 M stock solution?

Answer

Applying the dilution formula, $M_1 V_1 = M_2 V_2$, $M_1 = 0.1$, V_1 is unknown, $M_2 = 0.01$, $V_2 = 10\ cm^3$. Hence $0.1 \times V_1 = 0.01 \times 10$, so V_1 must be $1.0\ cm^3$. Hence $1.0\ cm^3$ stock solution (dispensed via an accurate automatic pipette) would be diluted to $10\ cm^3$ in a volumetric flask.

Question 3

What is the approximate molarity of a solution of glucose that contains 20 p.p.m.?

Answer

A 20 p.p.m. solution contains 20 g in one million grams or 20 mg in one kilogram. Assuming that the density of the solution is $1\ g\ cm^{-3}$, this is equivalent to $20\ mg\ dm^{-3}$. Hence the molarity of the solution is $20 \times 10^{-3}/180$ M, i.e. 0.11×10^{-3} M or 0.11 M.

Question 4

What is the molarity of pure water?

Answer

Water has a molecular mass of $2 + 16 = 18$ daltons. The molarity of $1\ dm^3$ of water (equivalent to 1000 g if the density is assumed to be $1\ g\ cm^{-3}$) is therefore equal to 1000/18, i.e. 55.6 M.

Dilution

In the preparation of experimental solutions it is common practice to prepare dilute solutions from more concentrated stock solutions. This dilution is easily achieved using the formula $M_1 V_1 = M_2 V_2$, where M_1 and M_2 represent the initial and final molarities and V_1 and V_2 represent the initial and final volumes. For the preparation of a given dilution, three of the variables will be known and the fourth can be calculated.

1.2.3 **Concentration or activity?**

Ionisation and ionic strength

A solution of sodium chloride in water does not contain molecules of NaCl but rather individual sodium (Na^+) and chloride (Cl^{-1}) ions due to the process of ionisation. Ionisation is possible in this case because sodium chloride forms a crystal lattice in which the sodium and chloride ions are held together by purely ionic attraction, i.e. there is no covalent bond formation. Sodium chloride is typical of the majority of inorganic salts, all of which ionise more or less completely in solution. The process of ionisation in such cases is therefore shown as being irreversible. Collectively these salts are said to be strong electrolytes and contrast with many other compounds, mainly organic acids and bases, which are only partially ionised in solution and are therefore said to be weak electrolytes. The process of ionisation of weak electrolytes is shown as being reversible. Ionisation of weak electrolytes, such as the carboxylic acids, is possible because, although there is a covalent bond between the oxygen and hydrogen atoms in the carboxyl group, the bond is highly polarised so that there pre-exists a partial positive charge on the hydrogen atom. Ionisation to release a proton places a negative charge on the oxygen atom that can be delocalised over the other oxygen atom in the carboxyl group. This stabilises the carboxyl anion (COO^-) relative to the carboxyl group and encourages ionisation. The relative ease with which the ionisation of weak electrolytes occurs is discussed in Section 1.3. Yet other organic compounds, for example alcohols including simple sugars such as glucose, do not ionise at all in solution and are therefore said to be non-electrolytes.

For some biochemical studies involving the use of both strong and weak electrolytes it is more important to measure the amount of individual ions present in solution than to know the concentration of the compound from which they arise. Ionic strength (μ) is a measure of the total ion charge in solution and is determined by both the concentration of all the individual ions present and their charge. Its value is calculated by use of equation 1.1:

$$\mu = \frac{1}{2}(c_1 z_1^2 + c_2 z_2^2 \cdots c_n z_n^2)$$

$$= \frac{1}{2}\Sigma cz^2 \tag{1.1}$$

where Σ indicates the sum of all the terms of the following type, $c_1, c_2 \ldots c_n$ is the concentration of each individual ion in molarity, and $z_1, z_2 \ldots z_n$ is the charge on the individual ions (thus for Na^+ and K^+ $z = +1$, for Cl^- and NO_3^- $z = -1$, for Ca^{2+} $z = +2$, and for $SO_4^{2-} = -2$).

Whilst salts such as NaCl and KNO_3, which consist of monovalent ions, ionise almost completely in aqueous solution, those that consist of divalent ions, such as $MgSO_4$, ionise to a smaller extent owing to the process of ion-pairing. In this process, ions of opposite charge are attracted to each other in aqueous solution to form a tightly bound ion-pair that behaves as a single particle. Thus a 0.25 M solu-

Example 2 CALCULATION OF IONIC STRENGTHS

Question Calculate the ionic strength of (i) 0.1 M NaCl, (ii) 0.1 M NaCl + 0.05 M KNO_3 + 0.01 M $Na_2 SO_4$.

Answer Ionic strength can be calculated using the equation $\mu = \frac{1}{2}\Sigma cz^2$.

(i) Calculating cz^2 for each ion:

$$Na^+ = 0.1 \times (+1)^2 = 0.1\,M$$

$$Cl^- = 0.1 \times (-1)^2 = 0.1\,M$$

Hence

$$\frac{1}{2}\Sigma cz^2 = 0.2/2 = 0.1\,M$$

(ii)

Na^+	$= 0.1 \times (+1)^2 + 0.02 \times (+1)^2 = 0.12\,M$	
Cl^-	$= 0.1 \times (-1)^2$	$= 0.10\,M$
K^+	$= 0.05 \times (+1)^2$	$= 0.05\,M$
NO_3^-	$= 0.05 \times (-1)^2$	$= 0.05\,M$
SO_4^{2-}	$= 0.01 \times (-2)^2$	$= 0.04\,M$

Hence

$$\frac{1}{2}\Sigma cz^2 = \frac{1}{2}(0.36) = 0.18\,M$$

Note 1: the unit of ionic strength is M.

Note 2: that for Na_2SO_4 $c = 0.02$, since there are $2Na^+$ per mole.

Note 3: that for a 1 M 1:1 electrolyte such as NaCl, the ionic strength is 1 M; for a 1 M 2:1 electrolyte such as $MgCl_2$, the ionic strength is 3 M, for a 1 M 2:2 electrolyte such as $MgSO_4$, the ionic strength is 4 M and for a 3:1 electrolyte such as $FeCl_3$, the ionic strength is 6 M.

Note 4: As the concentration and ionic strength increase, this type of calculation becomes progressively inaccurate owing to the importance of activity coefficients.

tion of $MgSO_4$ is 65% ionised (i.e. 65% consists of individual magnesium and sulphate ions in solution), the remaining 35% existing as ion-pairs. As a consequence of ion-pairing it is more difficult to calculate the ionic strength of solutions of salts of this type.

In aqueous solution, anions and cations are surrounded by an ionic atmosphere or shell owing to the attraction by the ion of oppositely charged species, including water molecules in which the $O-H$ bond is polarised to give a δ^+ on each of the hydrogen atoms and δ^- on the oxygen atom. This ionic atmosphere has a net charge that is opposite to, but smaller than, that of the ion it surrounds. Its presence results in a reduction of the effective charge of the central ion and hence its attraction for oppositely charged ions. This effect is enhanced by an increase in the ionic strength of the solution. This is the basis of the salting out of proteins (Section 8.3.4).

Activities and activity coefficients

Ionic strength influences the effective concentration of a compound that can ionise in solution such that the effective concentration, referred to as the *activity* (*A*), is related to the nominal concentration by a factor known as *the activity coefficient* (*γ*) as shown in equation 1.2:

$$A_X = [X]\, \gamma_x \tag{1.2}$$

where A_X is the activity of species X, [X] is the concentration of X, and γ_x is the activity coefficient of X. An activity coefficient is a measure of the deviation of the behaviour of a species from the expected. As the ionic strength increases, the activity coefficient decreases, reducing the activity relative to the concentration. Thus the activity coefficient for Na^+ is 0.964 at 0.001 M and 0.79 at 0.1 M. The reverse of this, namely that, as the ionic strength decreases, the activity coefficient approaches unity, is important, since it means that under these circumstances the activity and concentration of the ion converge. The implications of this will be discussed later in the context of pH (Section 1.3.2). If the ionisable species gives rise to multiply charged ions, the activity coefficient decreases, irrespective of the sign, + or −, of the ions. Thus the activity coefficient for Mg^{2+} and Fe^{3+}, each at 0.001 M, is 0.872 and 0.738, respectively, at 25 °C.

Practical biochemical studies quite commonly include the use of reactants that are subject to discrepancies between concentration and activity. The design of such experiments has to include an assessment of the importance of this effect. Clearly, the impact will be greatest in those cases where the effect of a particular ion on a process or response is being studied. It is also important to realise that electrodes, such as the pH electrode and ion-selective electrodes commonly used in biochemical work, respond to the activities rather than concentration of the ion being measured. In the majority of other types of study it is generally acceptable to assume that activity and concentration are interchangeable, bearing in mind that in most biochemical studies the concentrations of reagents are generally low. When needed, the values of activity coefficients of organic and inorganic ions can be found in tables of physical constants.

1.3 WEAK ELECTROLYTES

1.3.1 The biochemical importance of weak electrolytes

Many molecules of biochemical importance are weak electrolytes in that they are acids or bases that are only partially ionised in aqueous solution. Examples include the amino acids, peptides, proteins, nucleosides, nucleotides and nucleic acids. The biochemical function of many of these molecules is dependent upon their precise state of ionisation at the prevailing cellular or extracellular pH. The catalytic sites of enzymes, for example, contain functional carboxyl and amino groups, from the side-chains of constituent amino acids in the protein chain, that need to be in a specific ionised state to enable the catalytic function of the enzyme to be realised. Before the ionisation of these compounds is discussed in detail, it is necessary to appreciate the importance of the ionisation of water.

1.3.2 Ionisation of weak acids and bases

Ionisation of water

One of the most important weak electrolytes is water, since it ionises to a small extent to give hydrogen ions and hydroxyl ions. In fact there is no such species as a free hydrogen ion in aqueous solution, as it reacts with water to give a hydronium ion (H_3O^+):

$$H_2O \rightleftharpoons H^+ + HO^-$$

$$H^+ + H_2O \rightleftharpoons H_3O^+$$

Even though free hydrogen ions do not exist, it is conventional to refer to them rather than hydronium ions. The equilibrium constant for the ionisation of water has a value of 1.8×10^{-16} at 24 °C. Since the ionic strength of water is very low, the activity coefficients for the hydrogen ions and hydroxyl ions will both effectively be unity so that the activity of each of these two ions is equal to their concentration. As calculated previously, the molarity of pure water is 55.6. This can be incorporated into a new constant, K_w. Thus, effectively, the activity of water is set at unity. It follows that:

$$1.8 \times 10^{-16} \times 55.6 = [H^+][HO^-] = 1.0 \times 10^{-14} = K_w \tag{1.3}$$

K_w is known as the autoprotolysis constant of water and does not include an expression for the concentration of water. Its numerical value of exactly 10^{-14} relates specifically to 24 °C. At 0 °C K_w has a value of 1.14×10^{-15} and at 100 °C a value of 5.45×10^{-13}. The stoichiometry in equation 1.3 shows that hydrogen ions and hydroxyl ions are produced in a 1 : 1 ratio; hence both of them must be present at a concentration of 1.0×10^{-7} M. Since the Sörensen definition of pH is that it is equal to the negative logarithm of the hydrogen ion activity, it follows that the pH of pure water is 7.0. This is the definition of neutrality.

This theoretical background to the pH of water is well known, but what is not so well appreciated is the influence on the pH of water of adding a salt such as NaCl.

Salt is a strong electrolyte and is virtually completely ionised in dilute aqueous solution, but it does not result in the production of either hydrogen ions or hydroxyl ions. It might therefore be expected that it would not affect the pH of water. This assumption, however, ignores the concomitant change in the ionic strength of the solution. For example, if NaCl is added to a concentration of 0.1 M, the activity coefficients of the hydrogen ions and hydroxyl ions are lowered to 0.83 and 0.76, respectively. Hence the following position now prevails:

$$K_w = 1.0 \times 10^{-14} = [H^+]0.83 \times [HO^-]0.76$$

As before, the hydrogen ions and hydroxyl ions are produced in equal amounts so that it can be calculated from the above that each is equal to 1.26×10^{-7} M. The activity of the hydrogen ions in solution is therefore equal to $1.26 \times 10^{-7} \times 0.83 = 1.05 \times 10^{-7}$ M. Hence the pH of the 0.1 M NaCl is 6.90. Whilst this may seem a very small change from that of the original pure water, this is misleading owing to the logarithmic nature of pH as it actually represents a 26% increase in the hydrogen ion concentration and 20% in hydrogen ion activity relative to that of pure water. Once again, this highlights the importance of considering activities rather than concentrations when the ionic strength of an experimental solution could influence the interpretation of experimental data.

Ionisation of carboxylic acids and amines

As previously stressed, many biochemically important compounds contain a carboxyl group (-COOH) or a primary (RNH_2), secondary (R_2NH) or tertiary (R_3N) amine that can donate or accept a hydrogen ion on ionisation. The tendency of a weak acid, generically represented as HA, to ionise is expressed by the equilibrium reaction:

$$\begin{array}{ccc} HA & \rightleftharpoons H^+ + & A^- \\ \text{weak acid} & & \text{conjugate} \\ & & \text{base (anion)} \end{array}$$

This reversible reaction can be represented by an equilibrium constant, K_a, known as the acid dissociation constant (equation 1.4). Numerically, it is very small.

$$K_a = \frac{[H^+][A^-]}{[HA]} \tag{1.4}$$

Note that the ionisation of a weak acid results in the release of a hydrogen ion and the conjugate base of the acid, both of which are ionic in nature.

Similarly, amino groups (primary, secondary and tertiary) as weak bases can exist in ionised and unionised forms and the concomitant ionisation process represented by an equilibrium constant, K_b (equation 1.5):

$$\begin{array}{cccc} RNH_2 & + H_2O \rightleftharpoons & RNH_3^+ & + HO^- \\ \text{weak base} & & \text{conjugate acid} & \\ \text{(primary amine)} & & \text{(substituted} & \\ & & \text{ammonium ion)} & \end{array}$$

$$K_b = \frac{[RNH_3^+][HO^-]}{[RNH_2][H_2O]} \qquad (1.5)$$

In this case, the non-ionised form of the base abstracts a hydrogen ion from water to produce the conjugate acid, which is ionised. If this equation is viewed from the reverse direction it is of a format similar to that of equation 1.4. Equally, equation 1.4 viewed in reverse is similar in format to equation 1.5.

From our previous consideration of concentration, activity and activity coefficients, it is evident that equations 1.2 and 1.3 are incorrect in that they lack an activity coefficient term for each of the reaction species. Thus the correct form of equation 1.4 is:

$$K_a = \frac{[H^+]_{\gamma_{H^+}}[A^-]_{\gamma_{A^-}}}{[HA]_{\gamma_{HA}}} \qquad (1.6)$$

where γ_H^+, γ_A^- and γ_{HA} are the activity coefficients for the three species.

The practical implications of including expressions for the activity coefficients will be discussed later but, in general, if the difference between concentration and activity of a species under investigation is such as to compromise the quantitative outcome to the study, then activity coefficients must be taken into account.

A specific and simple example of the ionisation of a weak acid is that of acetic (ethanoic) acid, CH_3COOH:

$$CH_3COOH \rightleftharpoons CH_3COO^- + H^+$$

acetic acid $\qquad$ acetate anion

Acetic acid and its conjugate base, the acetate anion, are known as a conjugate acid–base pair. The acid dissociation constant can be written as:

$$K_a = \frac{[CH_3COO^-]_{\gamma_{Ac}}[H^+]_{\gamma_{H^+}}}{[CH_3COOH]_{\gamma_{HAc}}} = \frac{[\text{conjugate base}]_{\gamma_{Ac}}[H^+]_{\gamma_{H^+}}}{[\text{weak acid}]_{\gamma_{HAc}}}$$

where γ_{HAc} and γ_{Ac} are the activity coefficients for acetic acid and the acetate anion respectively.

K_a has a value of 1.75×10^{-5}. Hence its negative logarithm, pK_a (i.e. $-\log K_a$), is equal to 4.75. It can be seen from equation 1.4 that pK_a is numerically equal to the pH at which 50% of the acid is protonated (unionised) and 50% is deprotonated (ionised).

It is possible to write an expression for the K_b of the acetate anion as a conjugate base:

$$CH_3COO_3^- + H_2O \rightleftharpoons CH_3COOH + HO^-$$

$$K_b = \frac{[CH_3COOH]_{\gamma_{HAc}}[HO^-]_{\gamma_{HO^-}}}{[CH_3COO^-]_{\gamma_{HAc}}}$$

K_b has a value of 1.77×10^{-10}, hence $pK_b = 9.25$.

Multiplying these two expressions together results in the important relationship:

$$K_a \times K_b = K_w = 1.0 \times 10^{-14} \text{ at } 24\,^{\circ}\text{C}$$

hence

$$pK_a + pK_b = pK_w = 14 \tag{1.7}$$

This relationship holds for all acid–base pairs and enables one pK_a value to be calculated from knowledge of the other.

Many biologically important molecules are amphoteric, i.e. they have both acidic and basic groups and therefore in aqueous solution can accept or donate protons. The amino acids are a case in point and this aspect of their properties is discussed in Section 8.1.

In the case of the ionisation of weak bases, the most common convention is to quote the K_a or the pK_a of the conjugate acid rather than the K_b or pK_b of the weak base itself. Examples of the pK_a values of some weak acids and bases are given in Table 1.6. Remember that the smaller the numerical value of pK_a the stronger the acid (more ionised) and the weaker its conjugate base. Weak acids will be predominantly unionised at low pH values and ionised at high values. In contrast, weak bases will be predominantly ionised at low pH values and unionised at high values. This sensitivity to pH of the state of ionisation of weak electrolytes is important both physiologically and in *in vitro* studies employing such analytical techniques as electrophoresis and ion-exchange chromatography.

Ionisation of polyprotic weak acids and bases

Polyprotic weak acids and bases are capable of donating or accepting more than one hydrogen ion. Each ionisation stage can be represented by a K_a value using the convention that K_a^1 refers to the acid with the most ionisable hydrogen atoms and K_a^n the acid with the least number of ionisable hydrogen atoms. One of the most important biochemical examples is phosphoric acid, H_3PO_4:

$$H_3PO_4 \rightleftharpoons H^+ + H_2PO_4^- \qquad pK_a^1 \qquad 1.96$$

$$H_2PO_4^- \rightleftharpoons H^+ + HPO_4^{2-} \qquad pK_a^2 \qquad 6.70$$

$$HPO_4^{2-} \rightleftharpoons H^+ + PO_4^{3-} \qquad pK_a^3 \qquad 12.30$$

Example 3 **CALCULATION OF pH AND THE EXTENT OF IONISATION OF A WEAK ELECTROLYTE**

Calculate the pH of a 0.01 M solution of acetic acid and its fractional ionisation given that its K_a is 1.75×10^{-5}.

To calculate the pH we can write:

$$K_a = \frac{[\text{acetate}^-][\text{H}^+]}{[\text{acetic acid}]} = 1.75 \times 10^{-5}$$

Since acetate and hydrogen ions are produced in equal quantities, if $x =$ the concentration of each then the concentration of unionised acetic acid remaining will be $0.01 - x$. Hence:

$$1.75 \times 10^{-5} = \frac{(x)(x)}{0.01 - x}$$

$$1.75 \times 10^{-7} - 1.75 \times 10^{-5}x = x^2$$

This can now be solved either by use of the quadratic formula or, more easily, by neglecting the x term since it is so small. Adopting the latter alternative gives:

$$x^2 = 1.75 \times 10^{-7}$$

hence

$$x = 4.18 \times 10^{-4}\,\text{M}$$

hence

$$\text{pH} = 3.38$$

Note that this solution has ignored the activity coefficients of the acetate and hydrogen ions. They are 0.90 and 0.91 respectively at 0.01 M and 25 °C. Inserting these values into the above expression and assuming that the activity coefficient of acetic acid is unity gives:

$$1.75 \times 10^{-5} = \frac{(x)0.90(x)0.91}{0.01 - x}$$

Solving this equation for x gives a value of $4.61 \times 10^{-4}\,\text{M}$, and hence a pH of 3.33. This illustrates the relatively small influence of activity coefficients in this case.

The fractional ionisation (α) of the acetic acid is defined as the fraction of the acetic acid that is in the form of acetate and is therefore given by the equation:

$$\alpha = \frac{[\text{acetate}]}{[\text{acetate}] + [\text{acetic acid}]}$$

$$= \frac{4.18 \times 10^{-4}}{4.18 \times 10^{-4} + 0.01 - 4.18 \times 10^{-4}}$$

$$= \frac{4.18 \times 10^{-4}}{0.01}$$

$$= 4.18 \times 10^{-2} \quad \text{or } 4.18\%$$

Thus the majority of the acetic acid is present as the unionised form. If the pH is increased above 3.33 the proportion of acetate present will increase in accordance with the Henderson–Hasselbalch equation.

1.4 BUFFER SOLUTIONS – THEIR NATURE AND PREPARATION

1.4.1 Titration curves

If a solution of a weak acid, such as acetic acid, is titrated with a strong base, such as sodium hydroxide, and the change in pH monitored continuously by use of a calibrated pH electrode and meter, it will be observed that the initial pH of around 3 (see Example 3) will gradually increase then begin to plateau as half-neutralisation is reached. As the titration continues, this plateau of small change in pH eventually ceases and the pH increases again more rapidly until the acid is fully neutralised. The same shape of titration curve will be observed irrespective of the weak acid chosen, the only differences being the initial pH and the prevailing pH in the region of half-neutralisation. If a diprotic acid, such as succinic acid, is titrated, two plateau regions will be observed and in the case of a triprotic acid, such as phosphoric acid, three plateau regions will be evident. In all cases the pH at the mid-point of the plateau region will be equal to the pK_a of the acid and the extent of the plateau approximately $pK_a \pm 1$ pH unit. This plateau region gives a clue as to the nature of a buffer solution; that is, one that resists a change in pH on the addition of acid or alkali. At half-neutralisation the titration solution contains equal amounts of the conjugate base of the acid and unionised acid. This is the characteristic of all buffer solutions. The conjugate base neutralises added acid whilst the unionised acid neutralises added base.

1.4.2 Henderson–Hasselbalch equation

The Henderson–Hasselbalch equation is of central importance in the preparation of buffer solutions. It can be expressed in a variety of forms. For a buffer based on a weak acid:

$$pH = pK_a + \log \frac{[\text{conjugate base}]}{[\text{weak acid}]} \tag{1.8a}$$

or

$$pH = pK_a + \log \frac{[\text{ionised form}]}{[\text{unionised form}]} \tag{1.8b}$$

For a buffer based on the conjugate acid of a weak base:

$$pH = pK_a + \log \frac{[\text{weak acid}]}{[\text{conjugate base}]} \tag{1.9a}$$

or

$$pH = pK_a + \log \frac{[\text{unionised form}]}{[\text{ionised form}]} \tag{1.8b}$$

For total correctness, all four forms should contain expressions for the activity coefficients of each species, but these have been omitted for clarity.

1.4.3 Buffer capacity

It can be seen from the Henderson–Hasselbalch equation that when the concentration (or more strictly the activity) of the weak acid and base is equal, their ratio is 1 and their logarithm zero so that $pH = pK_a$. This rationalises the shape of titration curves with their plateau at the mid-point of neutralisation. The ability of

| Table 1.6 | pKₐ values of some acids and bases that are commonly used as buffer solutions |

Table 1.6 pK_a values of some acids and bases that are commonly used as buffer solutions

Acid or base	pK_a
Acetic acid	4.75
Barbituric acid	3.98
Carbonic acid	6.10, 10.22
Citric acid	3.10, 4.76, 5.40
Glycylglycine	3.06, 8.13
Hepes[a]	7.50
Phosphoric acid	1.96, 6.70, 12.30
Phthalic acid	2.90, 5.51
Pipes[a]	6.80
Succinic acid	4.18, 5.56
Tartaric acid	2.96, 4.16
Tris[a]	8.14

[a] See list of abbreviations at the front of the book.

a buffer solution to resist a change in pH on the addition of strong acid or alkali is expressed by its buffer capacity (β). This is defined as the amount (moles) of acid or base required to change the pH by one unit, i.e.:

$$\beta = \frac{db}{dpH} = \frac{-da}{dpH} \tag{1.10}$$

where db and da are the amount of base and acid respectively, and dpH is the resulting change in pH. In practice, β is largest within the pH range p$K_a \pm 1$ confirming the earlier observation about the size of the plateau in the titration curve. Table 1.6 lists some weak acids and bases commonly used in the preparation of buffer solutions.

1.4.4 Preparation of buffer solutions

Buffer solutions may be prepared either by adding a strong base, such as 0.5 M NaOH, to the calculated quantity of the weak acid, based on a Henderson–Hasselbalch calculation, or by mixing the calculated quantities of the weak acid and its sodium salt. In both cases the resulting mixture is adjusted to a volume just short of the required volume, checked for the correct pH using a calibrated pH electrode and pH meter and finally adjusted to the correct total volume in a volumetric flask. Methods based on the addition of the calculated quantities of weak acid and its conjugate weak base should, in principle, automatically give rise to the required pH but in practice this may not be the case for a number of reasons including, first, that most commonly the calculations will have been based on molarities rather than activities and, secondly, because the temperature and hence the pK_a may not be correct. As previously emphasised, pH is sensitive to the ionic strength of the solution so appropriate precautions must be taken when adding other reagents to a stock buffer solution. However, simple dilution of a stock buffer solution should have little impact on its pH. It will, however, decrease the buffer capacity.

Selection of a buffer

When selecting a buffer for a particular experimental study, several factors should be taken into account:

- select the one with a pK_a as near as possible to the required experimental pH and within the range p$K_a \pm 1$, as outside this range there will be too little weak acid or weak base present to maintain an effective buffer capacity;
- select an appropriate concentration of buffer to have adequate buffer capacity for the particular experiment. Most commonly buffers are used in the range 0.05–0.5 M;
- ensure that the selected buffer does not form insoluble complexes with any anions or cations essential to the reaction being studied (phosphate buffers tend to precipitate polyvalent cations, for example, and may be a metabolite or inhibitor of the reaction);
- ensure that the proposed buffer has other desirable properties such as being non-toxic, able to penetrate membranes, and does not absorb in the visible or ultraviolet region.

Example 4 **PREPARATION OF A PHOSPHATE BUFFER**

Question

How would you prepare 1 dm^3 of 0.1 M phosphate buffer, pH 7.1, given that pK_a^2 for phosphoric acid is 6.8 and that the atomic masses for Na, P and O are 23, 31 and 16 daltons respectively?

Answer

The buffer will be based on the ionisation:

$$H_2PO_4^- \rightleftharpoons HPO_4^{2-} + H^+ \qquad pK_a^2 = 6.8$$

and will therefore involve the use of solid sodium dihydrogen phosphate (NaH_2PO_4) and disodium hydrogen phosphate (Na_2HPO_4).

Applying the appropriate Henderson–Hasselbalch equation (equation 1.8) gives:

$$7.1 = 6.8 + \log \frac{[HPO_4^{2-}]}{[H_2PO_4^-]}$$

$$0.3 = \log \frac{[HPO_4^{2-}]}{[H_2PO_4^-]^2}$$

$$2.0 = \frac{[HPO_4^{2-}]}{[H_2PO_4^-]^2}$$

Since the total concentration of the two species needs to be 0.1 M it follows that [$H_2PO_4^{2-}$] must be 0.067 M and [$H_2PO_4^-$] 0.033 M. Their molecular masses are 142 and 120 daltons, respectively; hence the weight of each required is $0.067 \times 142 = 9.51$ g (Na_2HPO_4) and $0.033 \times 120 = 3.96$ g (NaH_2PO_4). These weights would be dissolved in approximately 800 cm^3 of pure water, the pH measured and adjusted as necessary, and the volume finally made up to 1 dm^3.

1.5 pH AND OXYGEN ELECTRODES

1.5.1 Reference electrodes

Half-cells and galvanic cells

One of the most common needs in biochemical experiments is the requirement to measure and control the pH (i.e. the hydrogen ion activity) of a reaction mixture. A close second, in terms of routine need, is the measurement of the oxygen tension of a solution. These needs are best met by the use of special electrodes that respond specifically to the particular ion or molecule (the analyte). These electrodes work on the basis that the analyte in question can accept an electron from, or donate one to, an electrode, which is most commonly made of platinum. This transfer of electrons is the basis of oxidation and reduction reactions: acceptance of an electron by the analyte resulting in its reduction; the donation of an electron by the analyte resulting in its oxidation. In general terms an oxidation–reduction reaction such as this can be represented as follows, where X is a chemical species capable of being reduced, Y a species capable of being oxidised, e^- is an electron and a, n and b are small integers:

$$a\mathrm{X} + ne^- \rightleftharpoons b\mathrm{Y}$$

oxidised   reduced

analyte   analyte

The transfer of electrons to or from the electrode establishes a so-called indicator (or sensing) half-cell and a potential (E) at the electrode. This potential can be quantified by coupling the half-cell to a reference half-cell, which generates a constant and known potential so that the experimentally measured potential, which is the net sum of the potentials generated by the two half-cells, can be correlated to that produced by the indicator half-cell. The two half-cells must be linked via a salt bridge, which allows electrons to flow between the two, thus maintaining electrical neutrality. Two half-cells linked in this manner constitute a galvanic cell.

The experimental potential (E) generated by any half-cell is given by the Nernst equation:

$$E = E^0 - 2.303\,(RT/nF)\log\,(A_\mathrm{Y}/A_\mathrm{X})$$
$$= E^0\,(-0.0592/n)\log\,(A_\mathrm{Y}/A_\mathrm{X})\text{ volts at }25\,^\circ\mathrm{C} \tag{1.11}$$

where E^0 is the standard reduction potential (also called a standard potential or a standard redox potential), A_Y and A_X are the activities of the reduced and oxidised species respectively, F is the Faraday (electrical charge of one mole of electrons) ($9.648 \times 10\,\mathrm{J\,V^{-1}\,mol^{-1}}$), R is the molar gas constant ($8.314\,\mathrm{J\,mol^{-1}\,K^{-1}}$), n is the number of moles of electrons per mole of reactant transferred in the half-cell, T is the absolute temperature, $(2.303RT)/F$ is the Nernst factor that at $25\,^\circ\mathrm{C}$ is equal to $0.059159\,\mathrm{V}$.

When the activities of the oxidised and reduced species are equal, their ratio will be one and their logarithm zero so that $E = E^0$. It is important to note that it is the ratio of the two activities rather than their absolute values that determines the value of the experimental potential E. The Nernst equation therefore defines the potential of a half-cell whose reactive species are not present at unit activity.

The calomel electrode and the silver/silver chloride electrode are the two most commonly used reference electrodes to measure the potential of an indicator half-cell.

Saturated calomel electrode

This consists of two concentric tubes, the smaller central one containing a platinum electrode in contact with a paste of mercury, mercurous chloride and potassium chloride. At the base of this inner tube is a small opening to the outer tube, which contains a saturated solution of potassium chloride as the salt bridge to link the half-cell to the indicator half-cell via a porous plug (Fig. 1.1a). The half-cell can be represented as follows;

$Hg \mid Hg_2Cl_2 \mid KCl \mid \mid$ test solution

where the double line represents the salt bridge linking the half-cell to the indicator half-cell.

The calomel electrode generates a potential according to the following equation:

$$\frac{1}{2}Hg_2Cl_2 \quad + e^- \rightleftharpoons Hg + Cl^-$$

mercurous chloride   mercury
(calomel)

The standard reduction potential (E^0) of the half-cell is +0.241 V.

Silver/silver chloride electrode

This consists of a deposit of silver chloride on the surface of metallic silver inserted in a saturated solution of silver chloride and potassium chloride contained in a tube the end of which is open to the test solution via a porous plug covered with solid potassium chloride. The half-cell generates a potential according to the following reaction;

$AgCl + e^- \rightleftharpoons Ag + Cl^-$

The standard reduction potential (E^0) of the half-cell is +0.197 V.

The use of saturated potassium chloride in both these two reference electrodes ensures that the concentrations of their reactive species remain constant.

Standard hydrogen electrode

Although the calomel and silver/silver chloride reference electrodes are in common use, their standard reduction potentials have in turn to be measured against an international standard. This is the standard hydrogen electrode. It consists of a platinum electrode in a solution of hydrochloric acid, the activity of which is unity, through which hydrogen gas at one atmosphere pressure

Table 1.7	Standard redox potentials of biochemical interest (at 25 °C)

$E^{0'}(V)$	Half-reaction
−0.42	$2H^+ + 2e^- \rightleftharpoons H_2$
−0.32	$NAD^+ + H^+ + 2e^- \rightleftharpoons NADH$
−0.22	$FAD + 2H^+ + 2e^- \rightleftharpoons FADH_2$
−0.20	Acetaldehyde $+ 2H^+ + 2e^- \rightleftharpoons$ ethanol
−0.19	Pyruvate $+ 2H^+ + 2e^- \rightleftharpoons$ lactate
−0.17	Oxaloacetate $+ 2H^+ + 2e^- \rightleftharpoons$ malate
−0.03	Fumarate $+ 2H^+ + 2e^- \rightleftharpoons$ succinate
+0.08	Cytochrome $b (Fe^{3+}) + e^- \rightleftharpoons$ cytochrome $b (Fe^{2+})$
+0.25	Cytochrome $c (Fe^{3+}) + e^- \rightleftharpoons$ cytochrome $c (Fe^{2+})$
+0.29	Cytochrome $a (Fe^{3+}) + e^- \rightleftharpoons$ cytochrome $a (Fe^{2-})$
+0.30	$\frac{1}{2}O_2 + H_2O + 2e^- \rightleftharpoons H_2O_2$
+0.80	$O_2 + 2H^+ + 2e^- \rightleftharpoons H_2O$

(101 325 Pa) (so that its activity is also unity) is bubbled to enable the following equilibrium to be established:

$$H^+ + e^- \rightleftharpoons \frac{1}{2}H_2$$

When the activities of the hydrogen ions and hydrogen gas are unity, the electrode is arbitrarily assigned a standard reduction potential of 0.00V at 25 °C. The electrode is too cumbersome for routine laboratory use.

The use of standard reduction potentials (E^0), developed initially by chemists, presents biochemists with a difficulty, since they are based on unit activity of hydrogen ions (i.e. pH 0). The majority of biochemical reactions occurring in living cells take place around neutrality (i.e. pH 7). Biochemists have therefore introduced an alternative scale of standard reduction potentials based on pH 7. These are referred to as $E^{0'}$ (spoken as E nought dash). These values are less positive than their E^0 counterparts. Table 1.7 gives some examples of standard redox potentials of biochemical interest. Positive $E^{0'}$ values represent a more oxidising system and negative values a more reducing system than the standard hydrogen electrode. Half-cells of the type shown in Table 1.7 operate as coupled pairs such that one is oxidised and the other reduced. The driving force for such a coupled reaction is the free energy change ($\Delta G^{0'}$) resulting from the potential difference ($\Delta E^{0'}$) between the two half-cells:

$$\Delta G^{0'} = -nF\Delta E^{0'}$$

where

$$\Delta E^{0'} = (\Delta E^{0'}_{\text{oxidising half-cell}} - E^{0'}_{\text{reducing half-cell}})$$

Some artificial redox half-cells have the attraction that they have different colours in their oxidised and reduced states. These so-called redox dyes are particularly useful for the study of enzyme reactions. This is discussed further in Section 15.2.2. Examples of redox dyes are given in Table 1.8.

Table 1.8	Standard redox potentials of some redox dyes (at 25 °C)
$E^{0\prime}$ (V)	Redox dye
−0.45	Methyl viologen
−0.36	Benzyl viologen
−0.36	Potassium ferricyanide
−0.22	2,6-Dichlorophenol indophenol (DCPIP)
−0.08	2,3,5-Triphenyltetrazolium chloride (TTC)
−0.08	Phenazine methosulphate (PMS)
−0.01	Methylene blue

1.5.2 The pH electrode and other ion-selective electrodes

Principle of the pH electrode

The pH electrode is an example of an ion-selective electrode (ISE) that responds to one specific ion in solution. Unlike the calomel and silver/silver chloride electrodes, the underlying mechanism of action of ISEs is not based on an oxidation–reduction reaction but on ion gradients. However, they all rely on the technique of potentiometry, which involves the measurement of a potential of an electrode without a current flowing.

The pH electrode consists of a thin, glass, porous membrane sealed at the end of a hard glass tube containing 0.1 M hydrochloric acid into which is immersed a silver wire coated with silver chloride. This silver/silver chloride electrode acts as an internal reference that generates a constant potential. The porous membrane is typically 0.1 mm thick, the outer and inner 10 nm consisting of a hydrated gel layer containing exchange binding sites for hydrogen or sodium ions. On the inside of the membrane the exchange sites are predominantly occupied by hydrogen ions from the hydrochloric acid, whilst on the outside the exchange sites are occupied by sodium and hydrogen ions. The bulk of the membrane is a dry silicate layer in which all exchange sites are occupied by sodium ions. Most of the coordinated ions in both hydrated layers are free to diffuse into the surrounding solution, whilst hydrogen ions in the test solution can diffuse in the opposite direction, replacing bound sodium ions in a process called ion-exchange equilibrium. Any other types of cation present in the test solution are unable to bind to the exchange sites, thus ensuring the high specificity of the electrode. Note that hydrogen ions do not diffuse across the dry glass layer but sodium ions can. Thus, effectively, the membrane consists of two hydrated layers containing different hydrogen ion activities separated by a sodium ion transport system.

The principle of operation of the pH electrode is based upon the fact that if there is a gradient of hydrogen ion activity across the membrane this will generate a potential the size of which is given by the Nernst equation (equation 1.11). In this case, however, the potential is determined solely by the hydrogen ion gradient across the membrane rather than by the ratio of oxidised to reduced species. Moreover, since the hydrogen ion activity on the inside is constant (owing to the use of 0.1 M hydrochloric acid) the observed potential is directly dependent upon

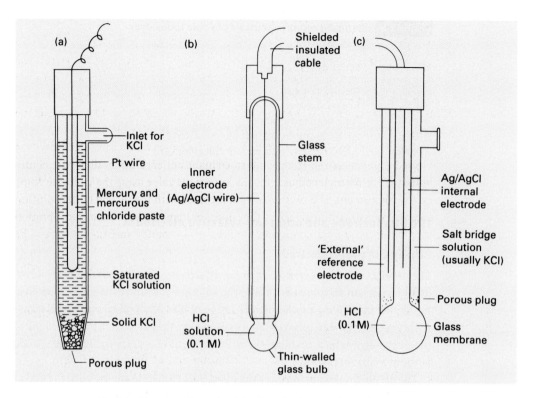

Fig. 1.1. Common electrodes: (a) calomel reference electrode; (b) glass electrode; (c) combination electrode.

the hydrogen ion activity of the test solution. It is evident from equation 1.11 that if the hydrogen ion activities on the two sides of the membrane were equal (i.e. the test solution consisted of 0.1 M hydrochloric acid), the resulting potential should be zero volts. In practice it is not, owing to a small junction or asymmetry potential (E^*) in part created by linking the glass electrode to the reference electrode. The observed potential across the membrane is therefore given by the equation:

$$E = E^* + 0.059\,\text{pH}$$

Since the precise composition of the porous membrane varies with time, so too does the asymmetry potential. This contributes to the need for the frequent recalibration of the electrode. For each 10-fold change in the hydrogen ion activity across the membrane (equivalent to a pH change of 1 in the test solution) there will be a potential difference change of 59.2 mV across the membrane. The presence of a term in the Nernst equation for the absolute temperature explains the sensitivity of pH measurements to the prevailing temperature.

The most common forms of pH electrode are the glass electrode (Fig. 1.1b) and the combination electrode (Fig. 1.1c), which contains an in-built calomel reference electrode.

Operation and calibration of a pH electrode

The glass membrane of a pH electrode is fragile and easily damaged. It is important that its surface remains hydrated and so it should be kept immersed in water when not in use. Electrodes that have been allowed to dry out should be soaked in 6 M hydrochloric acid followed by water prior to recalibration. Calibration should normally be carried out using two standard buffer solutions that span the pH range for which the electrode is to be used. Buffers of pH 4.008 (0.05 M potassium hydrogen phthalate) and 9.18 (0.01 M borax) are commonly used. The clean and blotted-dry electrode should be immersed in the buffer solution, allowed to equilibrate and the pH meter adjusted to the known pH value using the 'calibrate' knob on the instrument. The process is then repeated with the second buffer solution and any adjustment made using the 'slope' or 'temperature' knob. Recalibration may be necessary after 1–2 h of use. A well-calibrated instrument should be capable of reading to ± 0.2 pH units.

Errors in the measurement of pH

The measurement of pH is subject to several sources of error. These may be caused by a variety of factors including:

- the failure to provide adequate temperature control of the test solution;
- the failure to correctly maintain and calibrate the electrode;
- the failure to allow adequate equilibration time before the pH of the test solution is recorded;
- the presence of salts that ionise in the test solution, thereby altering the activity coefficients of the buffer components;
- the addition of organic solvents such as ethanol to the test solution, resulting in a change in the activity coefficients of the buffer components;
- the presence of proteins in the test solution that can coat the glass membrane and thereby affect the ion-exchange process at the hydrated membrane surface;
- the fact that, at pH values above 12, the low hydrogen ion concentration allows sodium ions in the test solution to replace hydrogen ions in the outer hydrated layer, in turn allowing the electrode to respond to sodium ions so that the recorded pH is lower than the actual pH. This is referred to as the sodium or alkaline error. Special glass electrodes, in which sodium ions are replaced by lithium, are available for measurements at high pH values.

Ion-selective electrodes

Electrodes exist for the measurement of many other ions including Li^+, K^+, Na^+, Ca^{2+}, Cl^- and NO_3^-. Their principle of operation is very similar to that of the pH electrode. In these cases, the permeable membrane may be made of special aluminosilicate glass or an inorganic crystal. The fluoride electrode, for example, uses a crystal of LaF_3 that responds selectively to the adsorption of fluoride ions onto its surface. A problem with most of these electrodes is their lack of absolute specificity for the test ion. Selectivity is expressed by a selectivity coefficient that expresses the ratio of the response to the competing ions relative to that for the desired ion. The specificity of the electrode is therefore inversely proportional to the selectivity coefficient. Most commercial ISEs have both a good linear response to the desired ion and a fast response time. ISEs are used routinely in clinical biochemistry laboratories for the measurement of sodium, potassium, calcium and chloride using autoanalyser techniques (Section 1.7.2).

Gas-sensing electrodes

Electrodes responding to gases such as CO_2 and NH_3 are commercially available and are based on principles similar to those of ISEs. In the case of a CO_2 electrode the outer glass membrane of a pH electrode is sealed inside a CO_2-permeable membrane bag made of polytetrafluoroethylene (PTFE) or polyethylene containing 0.1M KCl plus a weak bicarbonate buffer. CO_2 diffuses across the membrane from the test sample until its concentration is equal across both sides. Inside the membrane it forms carbonic acid that ionises to bicarbonate and hydrogen ions. Since the bicarbonate concentration in the bag is virtually constant owing to the presence of the bicarbonate buffer, the measurement of pH can be linked directly to the concentration of CO_2 in the test sample.

Biosensors and optical sensors

Biosensors are derived from ISEs or gas-sensing electrodes by incorporating an immobilised enzyme or cell onto the surface of the electrode that then responds, via a suitable transducer (a means of converting a chemical change into an electrical or optical signal), to either the test analyte or a metabolite of it. Important biochemical examples are the glucose, urea and cholesterol biosensors. The urea biosensor consists of urease immobilised onto the surface of an ammonia-sensing electrode. The urease converts the urea in the test sample to ammonia, which is detected by the electrode:

$$CO(NH_2)_2 + H_2O \rightleftharpoons 2NH_3 + CO_2$$

The glucose and cholesterol biosensors are based on the oxidation of the test analyte (by glucose oxidase and cholesterol oxidase, respectively) and either on the amperometric measurement of the generated hydrogen peroxide by its reduction at the anode or on the direct measurement, via an oxygen electrode, of the uptake of oxygen by the oxidase:

$$\beta\text{-D-glucose} + O_2 \rightleftharpoons \text{D-glucose-1,5-lactone} + H_2O_2$$

$$\text{cholesterol} + O_2 \rightleftharpoons \text{4-cholesten-3-one} + H_2O_2$$

Optical sensors, such as that for the measurement of ATP, detect light emitted by the action of luciferase (Section 15.2.2). A photomultiplier detects and enhances the light signal, creating a very sensitive method for the measurement of ATP.

1.5.3 **The oxygen electrode**

Principle of operation

The utilisation of oxygen during respiration and the evolution of oxygen during photosynthesis are two of the most fundamental life processes. Early studies of these processes used the technique of manometry, which involves the measurement of gross changes in gas volume. However, the advent of the oxygen electrode has revolutionised biochemical studies of the mechanistic detail underlying the processes of oxidative phosphorylation in mitochondria and of photosynthesis in chloroplasts. The oxygen electrode is an electrochemical cell containing a platinum cathode and a silver anode, both of which are separated from the test solution by an oxygen-permeable membrane. A polarising potential of 0.6 V is applied across the electrodes so that oxygen near the cathode surface is reduced by electrons, whilst at the anode electrons are released as a result of an oxidation process:

At the cathode $O_2 + 4H^+ + 4e^- \rightleftharpoons 2H_2O$ reduction

At the anode $4Ag + 4Cl^- \rightleftharpoons 4AgCl + 4e^-$ oxidation

The reductive removal of the oxygen at the cathode surface allows more oxygen in the test solution to diffuse across the permeable membrane and for the process of reduction at the cathode to continue. This generates a current, the size of which is directly proportional to the amount of oxygen (referred to as the oxygen tension) in the test solution. The oxygen electrode is therefore based on the process of amperometry (the measurement of a current flowing through an electrode at a constant potential).

It is important to ensure that the diffusion of oxygen from the bulk of the test solution to the membrane surface does not become a limiting factor for the generation of the current. To avoid this problem, the test solution must be stirred efficiently. The oxygen electrode gives a continuous record of the oxygen tension in the test solution, for example during oxidative phosphorylation (Fig. 1.2). Prior to each experiment the electrode has to be calibrated by the use of air-saturated water and oxygen-depleted water (usually achieved by the addition of a crystal of sodium dithionite to the water). The concentration of oxygen in air-saturated water at various temperatures is recorded in tables of physical constants.

Oxygen electrodes are available commercially in many forms. One of the most widely used is the Rank electrode shown diagrammatically in Fig. 1.3. The reaction vessel has a volume of about 3 cm³. The oxygen-permeable membrane may be made of Teflon™, Cellophane™ or silicone rubber. All membranes are sensitive to contamination particularly by proteins. The anode and cathode are connected to each other via a solution of potassium chloride.

Applications of the oxygen electrode

The use of an oxygen electrode is the method of choice for the study of any biochemical process in which there is the uptake or evolution of oxygen. The method has proved particularly successful in the study of respiratory control, the effect of

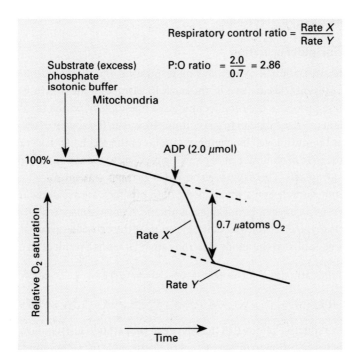

Fig. 1.2. A typical experimental trace of oxygen consumption for intact mitochondria obtained using an oxygen electrode.

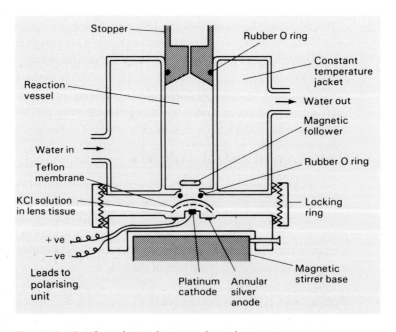

Fig. 1.3. Section through a Rank oxygen electrode.

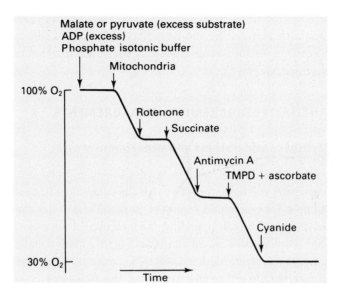

Fig. 1.4. Oxygen electrode trace showing the effect of inhibitors of electron transport and electron donors on mitochondrial respiration TMPD, tetramethylphenylenediamie.

inhibitors on mitochondrial respiration, and the measurement of P:O ratios in oxidative and photosynthetic phosphorylation. Fig. 1.2 records oxygen consumption in intact mitochondria. The trace shows slow oxygen consumption by the mitochondria until ADP is added. This stimulates oxygen uptake by the promotion of ATP production (rate X) until all the ADP has been consumed, at which point the rate declines to Y. The ratio of X to Y is a measure of the respiratory control ratio. From knowledge of the ADP added and the oxygen consumed the P:O ratio can be calculated. The sites of action of respiratory inhibitors on the two processes and the way the inhibition can be overcome by electron donors can also be studied, as shown in Fig. 1.4.

Variants of the Rank electrode are available that allow the study of oxygen exchange in the gas phase rather than in aqueous solution.

1.5.4 Electrochemical study of single cells

In recent years the miniaturisation of electrodes has stimulated studies of quantitative cellular analysis. Microelectrodes with a tip diameter in the range 1–5 μm, response time of a few microseconds and capability of measuring at the level of zeptomoles (zmol, i.e. 10^{-21} mol, representing approximately 600 molecules) have been developed that have enabled the dynamics of cellular processes to be investigated. The electrodes are most commonly made of carbon fibre and have been constructed in disc-shaped and cylindrical geometries. Microelectrodes of the ion-selective type have been used to monitor intracellular levels of H^+, Li^+, Ca^{2+} and Mg^{2+}, whilst platinum microelectrodes have been used to study compounds that readily undergo oxidation or reduction at the surface of the electrode. Such compounds include dopamine, enabling its release from single nerve cells to be studied. Microelectrodes have also been used to study the dynamics of exocytosis. Studies with cultured bovine medullary chromaffin cells, for example, have demonstrated that an average of 5–10 attomoles (i.e. 10^{-18} moles) of serotonin are released per exocytotic event.

1.6 QUANTITATIVE BIOCHEMICAL MEASUREMENTS

1.6.1 Analytical considerations and experimental error

Many biochemical investigations involve the quantitative determination of the concentration and/or amount of a particular component (the analyte) present in a test sample. For example, in studies of the mode of action of enzymes, transmembrane transport and cell signalling, the measurement of a particular reactant or product is investigated as a function of a range of experimental conditions and the data used to calculate kinetic or thermodynamic constants. These in turn are used to deduce details of the mechanism of the biological process taking place. Irrespective of the experimental rationale for undertaking such quantitative studies, all quantitative experimental data must first be questioned and validated in order to give credibility to the derived data and the conclusions that can be drawn from it. This requires that the experimental data be assessed and confirmed as an acceptable estimate of the 'true' values by the application of one or more standard statistical tests. Evidence of the validation of quantitative data by the application of such tests is a standard requirement by the editors of peer-refereed journals for the acceptance for publication of draft research papers. The following sections will address the theoretical and practical considerations behind these statistical tests.

The test sample

The test material for quantitative analysis may be of a widely diverse nature. Examples include a preparation of a purified protein or nucleic acid, an organelle preparation, a cell suspension or homogenate, a tissue homogenate, a sample of physiological fluid such as urine, serum, plasma or whole blood, or the eluant from a chromatographic column. The matrix (the nature of medium in which the analyte is present such as water, saline, serum, urine) will influence the process of sampling. Sampling is the process by which a representative portion is taken for analysis. Homogeneous, aqueous test solutions present no problem in this respect but if the sample is viscous the accurate sampling of a given volume is more difficult. If the test material is heterogeneous it is particularly difficult to ensure that the sample taken for analysis is representative of the whole. For example, it might be appropriate to grind plant material in a pestle and mortar to ensure the representation of the selected sample for the analysis. Alternatively, it may be necessary to undertake some form of preliminary extraction so that the selected sample is in a form suitable for analysis. Possible extraction techniques include liquid extraction, in which the test material is continuously extracted with an organic solvent such as dichloromethane or chloroform, and solid-phase extraction, which is a form of adsorption or ion-exchange chromatography. Some potential test samples may be too concentrated for direct analysis and in such cases the question of a suitable diluent arises. For example, if the concentration of an analyte in serum or plasma is too high, dilution of the sample with water would automatically alter the activity as well as the concentration of the analyte and dilution with a 'blank' serum or plasma sample would not be possible.

Selecting an analytical method

The nature of the quantitative analysis to be carried out will require a decision to be taken on the analytical technique to be employed. A variety of methods may be capable of achieving the desired analysis and the decision to select one may depend on a variety of issues. These include:

- the availability of specific pieces of apparatus;
- the precision, accuracy and detection limits of the competing methods;
- the precision, accuracy and detection limit acceptable for the particular analysis;
- the number of other compounds present in the sample that may interfere with the analysis;
- the potential cost of the method (particularly important for repetitive analysis);
- the possible hazards inherent in the method and the appropriate precautions needed to minimise risk;
- the published literature method of choice;
- personal preference.

The most common biochemical quantitative analytical methods are visible, ultra-violet and fluorimetric spectrophotometry, chromatographic techniques such as high performance liquid chromatography (HPLC) and gas–liquid chromatography (GLC) coupled to spectrophotometry or mass spectrometry, ion-selective electrodes and immunological methods such as the enzyme-linked immunosorbent assay (ELISA). Once a method has been selected it must be developed and/or validated using the approaches discussed in the following sections. If it is to be used over a prolonged period of time, measures will need to be put in place to ensure that there is no drift in response. This normally entails an internal quality control approach using reference test samples covering the analytical range that are measured each time the method is applied to test samples. Any deviation from the known values for these reference samples will require the whole batch of test samples to be reassayed.

The nature of experimental errors

Every quantitative measurement has some uncertainty associated with it. This uncertainty is referred to as the experimental error, which is a measure of the difference between the 'true' value and the experimental value. The 'true' value normally remains unknown except in cases where a standard sample (i.e. one of known composition) is being analysed. In other cases it has to be estimated from the analytical data by the methods that will be discussed later. The consequence of the existence of experimental errors is that the measurements recorded can be accepted with a high, medium or low degree of confidence depending upon the sophistication of the technique employed, but seldom, if ever, with absolute certainty.

Experimental error may be of two kinds: systematic error and random error.

Systematic error (also called determinate error)

Systematic errors are consistent errors that can be identified and either eliminated or reduced. They are most commonly caused by a fault or inherent limitation in the apparatus being used but may also be influenced by poor experimental design. Common causes include the misuse of manual or automatic pipettes, the incorrect preparation of stock solutions, and the incorrect calibration and use of pH meters. They may be constant (i.e. have a fixed value irrespective of the amount of test analyte present in the test sample under investigation) or proportional (i.e. the size of the error is dependent upon the amount of test analyte present). Thus the overall effect of the two types in a given experimental result will differ. Both of these types of systematic error have three common causes:

- *Analyst error:*   This is best minimised by good training and/or by the automation of the method.
- *Instrument error:*   This may not be eliminable and hence alternative methods should be considered. Instrument error may be electronic in origin or may be linked to the matrix of the sample.
- *Method error:*   This can be identified by comparison of the experimental data with that obtained by the use of alternative methods.

Identification of systematic errors

Systematic errors are always reproducible and may be positive or negative, i.e. they increase or decrease the experimental value relative to the 'true' value. The crucial characteristic, however, is that their cause can be identified and corrected. There are four common means of identifying this type of error:

- *Use of a blank sample:*   This is a sample that you know contains none of the analyte under test so that if the method gives a non-zero answer then it must be responding in some unintended way. The use of blank samples is difficult in cases where the matrix of the test sample is complex, for example serum.
- *Use of a standard reference sample:*   This is a sample of the test analyte of known composition so the method under evaluation must reproduce the known answer.
- *Use of an alternative method:*   If the test and alternative methods give different results for a given test sample then at least one of the methods must have an in-built flaw.
- *Use of an external quality assessment sample:*   This is a standard reference sample that is analysed by other investigators based in different laboratories employing the same or different methods. Their results are compared and any

differences in excess of random errors (see below) identify the systematic error for each analyst. The use of external quality assessment schemes is standard practice in clinical biochemistry laboratories (Section 1.7.3).

Random error (also called indeterminate error)

Random errors are caused by unpredictable and often uncontrollable inaccuracies in the various manipulations involved in the method. These errors may be variably positive or negative and are caused by factors such as difficulty in the process of sampling, random electrical 'noise' in an instrument, or by the analyst being inconsistent in the operation of the instrument or of recording readings from it.

Standard operating procedures

The minimisation of both systematic and random errors is essential in cases where the analytical data are used as the basis for a crucial diagnostic or prognostic decision as is common, for example, in routine clinical biochemical investigations and in the development of new drugs. In such cases it is normal for the analyses to be conducted in accordance with standard operating procedures (SOPs) that define in full detail the quality of the reagents, the preparation of standard solutions, the calibration of instruments and the methodology of the actual analytical procedure that must be followed.

1.6.2 Assessment of the performance of an analytical method

All analytical methods can be characterised by a number of performance indicators that define how the selected method performs under specified conditions. Knowledge of these performance indicators allows the analyst to decide whether or not the method is acceptable for the particular application. The major performance indicators are:

- *Precision (also called imprecision and variability):* This is a measure of the reproducibility of a particular set of analytical measurements on the same sample of test analyte. If the replicated values agree closely with each other, the measurements are said to be of high precision (or low imprecision). In contrast, if the values diverge, the measurements are said to be of poor or low precision (or high imprecision). In analytical biochemical work the normal aim is to develop a method that has as high a precision as possible within the general objectives of the investigation. However, precision commonly varies over the analytical range (see below) and over periods of time. As a consequence, precision may be expressed as either within batch or between batch. Within-batch precision is the variability when the same test sample is analysed repeatedly during the same batch of analyses on the same day. Between-batch precision is the variability when the same test sample is analysed repeatedly during different batches of analyses over a period of time. Since there is more opportunity for the analytical conditions to change for the assessment of between-batch precision, it is the higher of the two types of assessment. Results that are of high precision may nevertheless be a poor estimate of the 'true' value (i.e. of low accuracy or high bias) because of the presence of unidentified errors. Methods for the assessment of precision of a data set are discussed below. The term imprecision is preferred in particular by clinical biochemists, since they believe that it best describes the variability that occurs in replicated analyses.

- *Accuracy (also called bias and inaccuracy):*   This is the difference between the mean of a set of analytical measurements on the same sample of test analyte and the 'true' value for the test sample. As previously pointed out, the 'true' value is normally unknown except in the case of standard measurements. In other cases accuracy has to be assessed indirectly by use of an internationally agreed reference method and/or by the use of external quality assessment schemes (see above) and/or by the use of population statistics that are discussed below.

- *Detection limit (also called sensitivity):*   This is the smallest concentration of the test analyte that can be distinguished from zero with a defined degree of confidence. Concentrations below this limit should simply be reported as 'less than the detection limit'. All methods have their individual detection limits for a given analyte and this may be one of the factors that influence the choice of a specific analytical method for a given study. Thus the Bradford, Lowry and bicinchoninic acid methods for the measurements of proteins have detection limits of 20, 10 and 0. 5 μg protein cm^{-3}, respectively. In clinical biochemical measurements, sensitivity is often defined as the ability of the method to detect the analyte without giving false negatives (Section 1.7.1).

- *Analytical range:*   This is the range of concentrations of the test analyte that can be measured reproducibly, the lower end of the range being the detection limit. In most cases the analytical range is defined by an appropriate calibration curve (Section 1.6.6). As previously pointed out, the precision of the method may vary across the range.

- *Analytical specificity (also called selectivity):*   This is a measure of the extent to which other substances that may be present in the sample of test analyte may interfere with the analysis and therefore lead to a falsely high or low value. A simple example is the ability of a method to measure glucose in the presence of other hexoses such as mannose and galactose. In clinical biochemical measurements, selectivity is an index of the ability of the method to give a consistent negative result for known negatives (Section 1.7.1).

- *Analytical sensitivity:*   This is a measure of the change in response of the method to a defined change in the quantity of analyte present. In many cases analytical sensitivity is expressed as the slope of a linear calibration curve.

- *Robustness:*   This is a measure of the ability of the method to give a consistent result in spite of small changes in experimental parameters such as pH, temperature, or amount of reagents added. For routine analysis, the robustness of a method is an important practical consideration.

These performance indicators are established by the use of well-characterised test and reference analyte samples. The order in which they are evaluated will depend on the immediate analytical priorities, but initially the three most important may be specificity, detection limit and analytical range. Once a method is in routine use, the question of assuring the quality of analytical data by the implementation of quality assessment procedures comes into play (Section 1.7.3).

1.6.3 Assessment of precision

After a quantitative study has been completed and an experimental value for the amount and/or concentration of the test analyte in the test sample obtained, the experimenter must ask the question 'How confident can I be that my result is an acceptable estimate of the "true" value?' (i.e. is it accurate?). An additional question may be 'Is the quality of my analytical data comparable with that in the published scientific literature for the particular analytical method?' (i.e. is it precise?). Once the answers to such questions are known, a result that has a high probability of being correct can be accepted and used as a basis for the design of further studies, whilst a result that is subject to unacceptable error can be rejected. Unfortunately it is not possible to assess the precision of a single quantitative determination. Rather, it is necessary to carry out analyses in replicate (i.e. the experiment is repeated several times on the same sample of test analyte) and to subject the resulting data set to some basic statistical tests.

If a particular experimental determination is repeated numerous times and a graph constructed of the number of times a particular result occurs against its value, it is normally bell shaped, with the results clustering symmetrically about a mean value. This type of distribution is called a Gaussian or normal distribution. In such cases the precision of the data set is a reflection of random error. However, if the plot is skewed to one side of the mean value, then systematic errors have not been eliminated. Assuming that the data set is of the normal distribution type, there are three statistical parameters that can be used to quantify precision.

Standard deviation, coefficient of variation and variance – measures of precision

These three statistical terms are different ways of expressing the scatter of the values within a data set about the mean (calculated by summing their total value and dividing by the number of individual values). Each term has its individual merit. In all three cases the term is actually measuring the width of the normal distribution curve such that the narrower the curve the smaller the value of the term and the higher the precision of the analytical data set.

The standard deviation (s) of a data set is calculated by use of equation 1.12 or 1.13:

$$s = \sqrt{\frac{\sum (x_i - \bar{x})^2}{n - 1}} \tag{1.12}$$

$$s = \sqrt{\frac{\sum x_i^2 - \left[\left(\sum x_i\right)^2 / n\right]}{n-1}} \qquad (1.13)$$

$(x_i - \bar{x})$ is the difference between an individual experimental value (x_i) and the calculated mean $(\bar{x})$ of the individual values. Since these differences may be positive or negative, and since the distribution of experimental values about the mean is symmetrical, if they were simply added together they would cancel each other out. The differences are therefore squared to give consistent positive values. To compensate for this, the square root of the resulting calculation has to be taken to obtain the standard deviation.

Standard deviation (SD) has the same units as the actual measurements and this is one of its attractions. The mathematical nature of a normal distribution curve is such that 68.2% of the area under the curve (and hence 68.2% of the individual values within the data set) is within one standard deviation either side of the mean, 95.5% of the area under the curve is within two standard deviations and 99.7% within three standard deviations. Exactly 95% of the area under the curve falls between the mean and 1.96 standard deviations. The precision (or imprecision) of a data set is commonly expressed as ± 1 SD of the mean.

The term $(n-1)$ is called the degrees of freedom of the data set and is an important variable. The initial number of degrees of freedom possessed by a data set is equal to the number of results (n) in the set. However, when another quantity characterising the data set, such as the mean or standard deviation, is calculated, the number of degrees of freedom of the set is reduced by 1 and by 1 again for each new derivation made. Many modern calculators and computers include programs for the calculation of standard deviation. However, some use variants of equation 1.12 in that they use n as the denominator rather than $n-1$ as the basis for the calculation. If n is large, greater than 30 for example, then the difference between the two calculations is small, but if n is small, and certainly if it is less than 10, the use of n rather than $n-1$ will significantly underestimate the standard deviation. This may lead to false conclusions being drawn about the precision of the data set. Thus, for most analytical biochemical studies, it is imperative that the calculation of the standard deviation is based on the use of $n-1$.

The coefficient of variation (CV) (also known as relative standard deviation) of a data set is the standard deviation expressed as a percentage of the mean, as shown in equation 1.14.

$$CV = \frac{s\,100\%}{\bar{x}} \qquad (1.14)$$

Since the mean and standard deviation have the same units, the coefficient of variation is simply a percentage. This independence of the unit of measurement allows methods based on different units to be compared.

The variance of a data set is the mean of the squares of the differences between each value and the mean of the values. It is also the square of the standard deviation, hence the symbol s^2. It has units that are the square of the original units and this makes it appear rather cumbersome, which explains why standard deviation and coefficient of variation are the preferred ways of expressing the variability of data sets. The importance of variance will be evident in later discussions of the ways of making a statistical comparison of two data sets.

To appreciate the relative merits of the standard deviation and coefficient of variation as measures of precision, consider the following scenario. Suppose that two serum samples, A and B, were each analysed 20 times for serum glucose by the glucose oxidase method (Section 15.2.5) such that sample A gave a mean value of 2.00 mM with a standard deviation of ±0.10 mM and sample B a mean of 8.00 mM and a standard deviation of ± 0.41 mM. On the basis of the standard deviation values it might be concluded that the method had given a better precision for sample A than for sample B. However, this ignores the absolute values of the two samples. If this is taken into account by calculating the coefficient of variation, the two values are 5.0% and 5.1%, respectively, showing that the method had given the same precision for both samples. This illustrates the fact that the standard deviation is an acceptable assessment of precision for a given data set but, if it is necessary to compare the precision of two or more data sets, particularly ones with different mean values, then the coefficient of variation should be used. The majority of well-developed analytical methods have a coefficient of variation within the analytical range of less than 5% and many, especially automated methods, of less than 2%.

1.6.4 Assessment of accuracy

Population statistics

Whilst standard deviation and coefficient of variation give a measure of the precision of the data set they do not quantify how well the mean of the data set approaches the 'true' value. To address this issue it is necessary to introduce the concepts of population statistics and confidence level and confidence interval. If a data set is made up of a very large number of individual values so that n is a large number, then the mean of the set would equal the population mean mu (μ) and the standard deviation would equal the population standard deviation sigma (σ). Note that Greek letters represent the population parameters and the roman alphabet the sample parameters. These two population parameters are the best estimates of the 'true' values, since they are based on the largest number of individual measurements, so the influence of random errors is minimised. In practice the population parameters are seldom measured for obvious practicality reasons and the sample parameters have a larger uncertainty associated with them. The uncertainty of the sample mean deviating from the population mean decreases in proportion to the reciprocal of the square root of the number of values in the data set, i.e. $1/\sqrt{n}$. Thus, to decrease the uncertainty by a factor of 2, the number of experimental values would have to be increased 4-fold and for a factor of 10 the number of measurements would need to be increased 100-fold. The nature of this relationship again emphasises the importance of evaluating the acceptable degree

Example 5 ASSESSMENT OF THE PRECISION OF AN ANALYTICAL DATA SET

Question

Five measurements of the fasting serum glucose concentration were made on the same sample taken from a diabetic patient. The values obtained were 2.3, 2.5, 2.2, 2.6 and 2.5 mM. Calculate the precision of the data set.

Answer

Precision is normally expressed either as one standard deviation of the mean or as the coefficient of variation of the mean. These statistical parameters therefore need to be calculated.

Mean

$$\bar{x} = \frac{2.2 + 2.3 + 2.5 + 2.5 + 2.6}{5} = 2.42 \text{ mM}$$

Standard deviation
Using both equations 1.12 and 1.13 to calculate the value of s:

x_i	$x_i - \bar{x}$	$(x_i - \bar{x})^2$	x_i^2
2.2	−0.22	0.0484	4.84
2.3	−0.12	0.0144	5.29
2.5	+0.08	0.0064	6.25
2.5	+0.08	0.0064	6.25
2.6	+0.18	0.0324	6.75
Σx_i 12.1	Σ0.00	Σ0.1080	Σ29.39

Using equation 1.12

$$s = \sqrt{(0.108/4)} = 0.164 \text{ mM}$$

Using equation 1.13

$$s = \sqrt{\frac{29.39 - (12.1)^2/5}{4}} = \sqrt{\frac{29.39 - 29.28}{4}} = 0.166 \text{ mM}$$

Coefficient of variation
Using equation 1.9

$$CV = \frac{0.165 \times 100\%}{2.42}$$

$$= 6.82\%$$

Discussion

In this case it is easier to appreciate the precision of the data set by considering the coefficient of variation: 6.82% is moderately high for this type of analysis. Automation of the method would certainly reduce it by at least half. Note that it is legitimate to quote the answers to these calculations to one more digit than was present in the original data set. In practice, it is advisable to carry out the statistical analysis on a far larger data set than that presented in this example.

of uncertainty of the experimental result before the design of the experiment is completed and the practical analysis begun. Modern automated analytical instruments recognise the importance of multiple results by facilitating repeat analyses at maximum speed. It is good practice to report the number of measurements on which the mean and standard deviation are based, as this gives a clear indication of the quality of the calculated data.

Confidence intervals, confidence level and the Student's *t* factor

Accepting that the population mean is the best estimate of the 'true' value, the question arises 'How can I relate my experimental sample mean to the population mean?' The answer is by using the concept of confidence. Confidence level expresses the level of confidence, expressed as a percentage, that can be attached to the data. Its value has to be set by the experimenter to achieve the objectives of the study. Confidence interval is a mathematical statement relating the sample mean to the population mean. A confidence interval gives a range of values about the sample mean within which there is a given probability (determined by the confidence level) that the population mean lies. The relationship between the two means is expressed in terms of the standard deviation of the data set, the square root of the number of values in the data set and a factor known as Student's *t* (equation 1.15):

$$\mu = \bar{x} \pm \frac{ts}{\sqrt{n}} \tag{1.15}$$

where $\bar{x}$ is the measured mean, μ is the population mean, s is the measured standard deviation, n is the number of measurements, and t is the Student's t factor. The term $s/\sqrt{n}$ is known as the standard error of the mean and is a measure of the reliability of the sample mean as a good estimate of the population mean.

Confidence level can be set at any value up to 100%. For example, it may be that a confidence level of only 50% would be acceptable for a particular experiment. However, a 50% level means that that there is a 1 in 2 chance that the sample mean is not an acceptable estimate of the population mean. In contrast, the choice of a 95% or 99% confidence level would mean that there was only a 1 in 20 or a 1 in 100 chance, respectively, that the best estimate had not been achieved. In practice, most analytical biochemists choose a confidence level in the range 90–99% and most commonly 95%.

Student's t is a way of linking probability with the size of the data set and is used in a number of statistical tests. Student's t values for varying numbers in a data set (and hence with varying degrees of freedom) at selected confidence levels are available in statistical tables. Some values are shown in Table 1.9. The numerical value of t is equal to the number of standard errors of the mean that must be added and subtracted from the mean to give the confidence interval at a given confidence level. Note that, as the sample size (and hence the degrees of freedom) increases, the confidence levels converge. When n is large and if we wish to calculate the 95% confidence interval, the value of t approximates to 1.96 and

Table 1.9   Values of Student's *t*

Degrees of freedom	Confidence level (%)					
	50	90	95	98	99	99.9
2	0.816	2.920	4.303	6.965	9.925	31.598
3	0.765	2.353	3.182	4.541	5.841	12.924
4	0.741	2.132	2.776	3.747	4.604	8.610
5	0.727	2.015	2.571	3.365	4.032	6.869
6	0.718	1.943	2.447	3.143	3.707	5.959
7	0.711	1.895	2.365	2.998	3.500	5.408
8	0.706	1.860	2.306	2.896	3.355	5.041
9	0.703	1.833	2.262	2.821	3.250	4.798
10	0.700	1.812	2.228	2.764	3.169	4.587
15	0.691	1.753	2.131	2.602	2.947	4.073
20	0.687	1.725	2.086	2.528	2.845	3.850
30	0.683	1.697	2.042	2.457	2.750	3.646

some texts quote equation 1.15 in this form. The term Student's *t* factor may give the impression that it was devised specifically with students' needs in mind. In fact 'Student' was the pseudonym of a statistician, by the name of W. S. Gossett, who in 1908 first devised the term and who was not permitted by his employer to publish his work under his own name.

Criteria for the rejection of outlier experimental data – *Q*-test

A very common problem in quantitative biochemical analysis is the need to decide whether or not a particular result is an outlier and should therefore be rejected before the remainder of the data set is subjected to statistical analysis. It is important to identify such data as they have a disproportionate effect on the calculation of the mean and standard deviation of the data set. When faced with this problem, the first action should be to check that the suspected outlier is not due to a simple experimental or mathematical error. Once the suspect figure has been confirmed its validity is checked by application of Dixon's *Q*-test. Like other tests to be described later, the test is based on a null hypothesis, namely that there is no difference in the values being compared. If the hypothesis is proved to be correct then the suspect value cannot be rejected. The suspect value is used to calculate an experimental rejection quotient, Q_{exp}. Q_{exp} is then compared with tabulated critical rejection quotients, Q_{table}, for a given confidence level and the number of experimental results (Table 1.10). If Q_{exp} is less than Q_{table} the null hypothesis is confirmed and the suspect value should not be rejected, but if it is greater then the value can be rejected. The basis of the test is the fact that, in a normal distribution, 95.5% of the values are within the range of two standard deviations of the mean. In setting limits for the acceptability or rejection of data, a compromise has to be made on the confidence level chosen. If a high confidence level is chosen, the limits of acceptability are set wide and therefore there is a risk of accepting values

Example 6 **ASSESSMENT OF THE ACCURACY OF AN ANALYTICAL DATA SET**

Question

Calculate the confidence intervals at the 50%, 95% and 99% confidence levels of the fasting serum glucose concentrations given in Example 5.

Answer

Accuracy in this type of situation is expressed in terms of confidence intervals that express a range of values over which there is a given probability that the 'true' values lies.

As previously calculated, $\bar{x} = 2.42$ mM and s $= 0.16$ mM. Inspection of Table 1.9 reveals that, for 4 degrees of freedom (the number of experimental values minus 1) and a confidence level of 50%, $t = 0.741$ so that the confidence interval for the population mean is given by:

$$\text{Confidence interval} = 2.42 \pm \frac{(0.741)(0.16)}{\sqrt{5}}$$

$$= 2.42 \pm 0.05 \text{ mM}$$

For the 95% confidence level and the same number of degrees of freedom, $t = 2.776$, hence the confidence interval for the population mean is given by:

$$\text{Confidence interval} = 2.42 \pm \frac{(2.776)(0.16)}{\sqrt{5}}$$

$$= 2.42 \pm 0.20 \text{ mM}$$

For the 99% confidence level and the same number of degrees of freedom, $t = 4.604$; hence the confidence interval for the population mean is given by:

$$\text{Confidence interval} = 2.42 \pm \frac{(4.604)(0.16)}{\sqrt{5}}$$

$$= 2.42 \pm 0.33 \text{ mM}$$

Discussion

These calculations show that there is a 50% chance that the population mean lies in the range 2.37–2.47 mM, a 95% chance that the population mean lies within the range 2.22–2.62 mM and a 99% chance that it lies in the range 2.09–2.75 mM. Note that as the confidence level increases the range of potential values for the population mean also increases. You can calculate for yourself that if the mean and standard deviation had been based on 20 measurements (i.e. a 4-fold increase in the number of measurements) then the 50% and 95% confidence intervals would have been reduced to 2.42 ± 0.02 mM and 2.42 ± 0.07 mM, respectively. This re-emphasises the beneficial impact of multiple experimental determinations but at the same time highlights the need to balance the value of multiple determinations against the accuracy with which the experimental mean is required within the objectives of the individual study.

that are subject to error. If the confidence level is set too low, the acceptability limits will be too narrow and therefore there will be a risk of rejecting legitimate data. In practice a confidence level of 90% or 95% is most commonly applied. The Q_{table} values in Table 1.10 are based on a 95% confidence level.

Table 1.10 Values of Q for the rejection of outliers	
Number of observations	Q (95% confidence)
4	0.83
5	0.72
6	0.62
7	0.57
8	0.52

The calculation of Q_{exp} is based upon equation 1.16, which requires the calculation of the separation of the questionable value from the nearest acceptable value (gap) coupled with knowledge of the range covered by the data set:

$$Q_{exp} = \frac{x_n - x_{n-1}}{x_n - x_1} = \frac{gap}{range} \tag{1.16}$$

where x is the value under investigation in the series $x_1, x_2, x_3, \ldots, x_{n-1}, x_n$.

Example 7 IDENTIFICATION OF AN OUTLIER EXPERIMENTAL RESULT

Question   If the data set in Example 6 contained an addition value of 3.0 mM, could this value be regarded as an outlier point at the 95% confidence level?

Answer   From equation 1.16

$$Q_{exp} = \frac{3.0 - 2.6}{3.0 - 2.2} = \frac{0.4}{0.8} = 0.5$$

Using Table 1.11 for six data points, $Q_{table} = 0.62$.

Since Q_{exp} is smaller than Q_{table} the point should not be rejected as there is a more than 5% chance that it is part of the same data set as the other five values. It is easy to show that an additional data point of 3.3 rather than 3.0 mM would give a Q_{exp} of 0.64 and could be rejected.

1.6.5 Validation of an analytical method – the use of *t*-tests

A *t*-test in general is used to address the question of whether or not two data sets have the same mean. Both data sets need to have a normal distribution and equal variances. There are three types:

- *Unpaired t-test:* Used to test whether two data sets have the same mean.
- *Paired t-test:* Used to test whether two data sets have the same mean, where each value in one set is paired with a value in the other set.
- *One-sample t-test:* Used to test whether the mean of a data set is equal to a particular value.

Each test is based on a null hypothesis, which is that there is no difference between the means of the two data sets. The tests measures how likely the hypothesis is to be true. The attraction of such tests is that they are easy to carry out and interpret.

Analysis of a standard solution – one-sample *t*-test

Once the choice of the analytical method to be used for a particular biochemical assay has been made, the normal first step is to carry out an evaluation of the method in the laboratory. This evaluation entails the replicated analysis of a known standard solution of the test analyte and the calculation of the mean and standard deviation of the resulting data set. The question is then asked 'Does the mean of the analytical results agree with the known value of the standard solution within experimental error?' To answer this question a *t*-test is applied.

In the case of the analysis of a standard solution the calculated mean and standard deviation of the analytical results are used to calculate a value of the Student's t (t_{calc}) using equation 1.17. It is then compared with table values of t (t_{table}) for the particular degrees of freedom of the data set and at the required confidence level (Table 1.10).

$$t_{calc} = \frac{(\text{known value} - \bar{x})\sqrt{n}}{s} \tag{1.17}$$

These table values of t represent critical values that mark the border between different probability levels. If t_{calc} is greater than t_{table} the analytical results are deemed not to be from the same data set as the known standard solution at the selected confidence level. In such cases the conclusion is therefore drawn that the analytical results do not agree with the standard solution and hence that there are unidentified errors in them. There would be no point in applying the analytical method to unknown test analyte samples until the problem has been resolved.

Comparing two competitive analytical methods – unpaired *t*-test

In quantitative biochemical analysis it is frequently helpful to compare the performance of two alternative methods of analysis in order to establish whether or not they give the same quantitative result within experimental error. To address this need, each method is used to analyse the same test sample using replicated analysis. The mean and standard deviation for each set of analytical data is then calculated and a Student's *t*-test applied. In this case the *t*-test measures the overlap between the data sets such that the smaller the value of t_{calc} the greater the overlap between the two data sets. This is an example of an unpaired *t*-test.

In using the tables of critical *t*-values, the relevant degrees of freedom is the sum of the number of values in the two data sets (i.e. $n_1 + n_2$) minus 2. The larger the number of degrees of freedom the smaller the value of t_{calc} needs to be to exceed the critical value at a given confidence level. The formulae for calculating t_{calc} depend on whether or not the standard deviations of the two data sets are the same. This is often obvious by inspection, the two standard deviations being similar. However,

Example 8 VALIDATING AN ANALYTICAL METHOD

Question

A standard solution of glucose is known to be 5.05 mM. Samples of it were analysed by the glucose oxidase method (for details see Section 15.2.5) that was being used in the laboratory for the first time. A calibration curve obtained using least mean square linear regression was used to calculate the concentration of glucose in the test sample. The following experimental values were obtained: 5.12, 4.96, 5.21, 5.18, 5.26 mM. Does the experimental data set for the glucose solution agree with the known value within experimental error?

Answer

It is first necessary to calculate the mean and standard deviation for the set and then to use it to calculate a value for Student's t.

Applying equations 1.12 and 1.13 to the data set gives $\bar{x} = 5.15$ mM and $s = \pm 0.1$ mM.

Now applying equation 1.17 to give t_{calc}:

$$t_{calc} = \frac{(5.05 - 5.15)\sqrt{5}}{0.1} = 2.236$$

Note that the negative difference between the two mean values in this calculation is ignored. From Table 1.9 at the 95% confidence level with 4 degrees of freedom, $t_{table} = 2.776$. t_{calc} is therefore less than t_{table} and the conclusion can be drawn that measured mean value does agree with the known value. Using equation 1.14, the coefficient of variation for the measured values can be calculated to be 1.96%.

if in doubt, an F-test, named after Fisher who introduced it, can be applied. An F-test is based on the null hypothesis that there is no difference between the two variances. The test calculates a value for $F(F_{calc})$, which is the ratio of the larger of the two variances to the smaller variance. It is then compared with critical F-values (F_{table}) available in statistical tables or computer packages (Table 1.11). If the calculated value of F is less than the table value, the null hypothesis is proved and the two standard deviations are considered to be similar. If the two variances are of the same order, then equations 1.18 and 1.19 are used to calculate t_{calc} for the two data sets. If not, equations 1.20 and 1.21 are used.

$$t_{calc} = \frac{\bar{x}_1 - \bar{x}_2}{S_{pooled}} \sqrt{\frac{n_1 n_2}{n_1 + n_2}} \tag{1.18}$$

$$S_{pooled} = \sqrt{\frac{s_1^2(n_1 - 1) + s_2^2(n_2 - 1)}{n_1 + n_2 - 2}} \tag{1.19}$$

$$t_{calc} = \frac{\bar{x}_1 - \bar{x}_2}{\sqrt{(s_1^2/n_1) + (s_2^2/n_2)}} \tag{1.20}$$

$$\text{Degrees of freedom} = \left\{ \frac{(s_1^2/n_1 + s_2^2/n_2)^2}{[(s_1^2/n_1)^2/(n_1 + 1)] + [(s_2^2/n_2)^2/(n_2 + 1)]} \right\} - 2 \tag{1.21}$$

where $\bar{x}_1$ and $\bar{x}_2$ are the calculated means of the two methods, s_1^2 and s_2^2 are the calculated standard deviations of the two methods, and n_1 and n_2 are the number of measurements in the two methods.

At first sight these four equations may appear daunting, but closer inspection reveals that they are simply based on variance (s^2), mean ($\bar{x}$) and number of analytical measurements (n) and that the mathematical manipulation of the data is relatively easy.

Example 9 **COMPARISON OF TWO ANALYTICAL METHODS USING REPLICATED ANALYSIS OF A SINGLE TEST SAMPLE**

Question

A sample of fasting serum was used to evaluate the performance of the glucose oxidase and hexokinase methods for the quantification of serum glucose concentrations (for details, see Section 15.2.5). The following replicated values were obtained: for the glucose oxidase method 2.3, 2.5, 2.2, 2.6 and 2.5 mM and for the hexokinase method 2.1, 2.7, 2.4, 2.4 and 2.2 mM. Establish whether or not the two methods gave the same results at the 95% confidence level.

Answer

Using the standard formulae (equations 1.12 and 1.14) we can calculate the mean, standard deviation and variance for each data set.

Glucose oxidase method:

$\bar{x} = 2.42\,\text{mM}, \quad s = 0.16\,\text{mM}, \quad s^2 = 0.026\,(\text{mM})^2$

Hexokinase method:

$\bar{x} = 2.36\,\text{mM}, \quad s = 0.23\,\text{mM}, \quad s^2 = 0.053\,(\text{mM})^2$

We can then apply the *F*-test to the two variances to establish whether or not they are the same:

$$F_{\text{calc}} = \frac{0.053}{0.026} = 2.04$$

F_{table} for the two sets of data each with 4 degrees of freedom and for the 95% confidence level is 6.39 (Table 1.11).

Since F_{calc} is less than F_{table} we can conclude that the two variances are not significantly different. Therefore, using equations 1.18 and 1.19, we can calculate that:

$$S_{\text{pooled}} = \sqrt{\frac{0.16(4) + 0.23(4)}{8}} = \sqrt{\frac{0.64 + 0.92}{8}} = \sqrt{0.195} = 0.442$$

$$t_{\text{calc}} = \frac{2.42 - 2.36}{0.442}\sqrt{\frac{(5)(5)}{10}} = (0.06/0.442)(1.58) = 0.21$$

Using Table 1.9 at the 95% confidence level and for 8 degrees of freedom t_{table} is 2.306. Thus t_{calc} is far less than t_{table} and so the two sets of data are not significantly different, i.e. the two methods have given the same result at the 95% confidence level.

| Table 1.11 | Critical values of F at the 95% confidence level |

Degrees of freedom for S_2	Degrees of freedom for S_1							
	2	3	4	6	10	15	30	∞
2	19.0	19.2	19.2	19.3	19.4	19.4	19.5	19.5
3	9.55	9.28	9.12	8.94	8.79	8.70	8.62	8.53
4	6.94	6.59	6.39	6.16	5.96	5.86	5.75	5.63
5	5.79	5.41	5.19	4.95	4.74	4.62	4.50	4.36
6	5.14	4.76	4.53	4.28	4.06	3.94	3.81	3.67
7	4.74	4.35	4.12	3.87	3.64	3.51	3.38	3.23
8	4.46	4.07	3.84	3.58	3.35	3.22	3.08	2.93
9	4.26	3.86	3.63	3.37	3.14	3.01	2.86	2.71
10	4.10	3.71	3.48	3.22	2.98	2.84	2.70	2.54
15	3.68	3.29	3.06	2.79	2.54	2.40	2.25	2.07
20	3.49	2.10	2.87	2.60	2.35	2.20	2.04	1.84
30	3.32	2.92	2.69	2.42	2.16	2.01	1.84	1.62
∞	3.00	2.60	2.37	2.10	1.83	1.67	1.46	1.00

Comparison of two competitive analytical methods – paired t-test

A variant of the previous type of comparison of two analytical methods, based upon the analysis of a common standard sample, is the case in which a series of test samples is analysed once by the two different analytical methods. In this case there is no replication of analysis of any test sample by either method. The t-test is applied to the differences between the results of each method for each test sample. This is an example of a paired t-test. The formula for calculating t_{calc} in this case is given by equation 1.22:

$$t_{calc} = \frac{\bar{d}}{s_d}\sqrt{n} \qquad (1.22)$$

$$s_d = \sqrt{\frac{\Sigma(d_i - \bar{d})^2}{n-1}} \qquad (1.23)$$

where d_i is the difference between the paired results, $\bar{d}$ is the mean difference between the paired results, n is the number of paired results, and s_d is the standard deviation of the differences between the pairs.

Example 10 **COMPARISON OF TWO ANALYTICAL METHODS USING DIFFERENT TEST SAMPLES**

Question

Ten fasting serum samples were each analysed by the glucose oxidase and hexokinase methods. The following results, in mM, were obtained:

Glucose oxidase (mM)	Hexokinase (mM)	Difference, d_i	Difference minus mean of difference	(Difference minus mean of difference)^2
1.1	0.9	0.2	0.08	0.0064
2.0	2.1	−0.1	−0.22	0.0484
3.2	2.9	0.3	0.18	0.0324
3.7	3.5	0.2	0.08	0.0064
5.1	4.8	0.3	0.18	0.0324
8.6	8.7	−0.1	−0.22	0.0484
10.4	10.6	−0.2	−0.32	0.1024
15.2	14.9	0.3	0.18	0.0324
18.7	18.7	0.0	−0.12	0.0144
25.3	25.0	0.3	0.18	0.0324
		Mean ($\bar{d}$) 0.12		Σ 0.3560

Do the two methods give the same results at the 95% confidence level?

Answer

Before addressing the main question, note that the 10 samples analysed by the two methods were chosen to cover the whole analytical range for the methods. To assess whether or not the two methods have given the same result at the chosen confidence level, it is necessary to calculate a value for t_{calc} and to compare it with t_{table} for the 9 degrees of freedom in the study. To calculate t_{calc}, it is first necessary to calculate the value of s_d in equation 1.23. The appropriate calculations are shown in the table above.

$$s_d = \sqrt{[\Sigma(d_i - \bar{d})^2]/(n-1)}$$

$$= \sqrt{(0.356/9)}$$

$$= 0.199$$

From equation 1.22

$$t_{calc} = \frac{\bar{d}\sqrt{n}}{s_d}$$

$$= (0.12\sqrt{10})/0.199$$

$$= 1.907$$

Using Table 1.9, t_{table} at the 95% confidence level and for 9 degrees of freedom is 2.262. Since t_{calc} is smaller than t_{table} the two methods do give the same results at the 95% confidence level. Inspection of the two data sets shows that the glucose oxidase method gave a slightly high value for 7 of the 10 samples analysed.

An alternative approach to the comparison of the two methods is to plot the two data sets as an x/y plot and to carry out a regression analysis of the data. If this is done using the glucose oxidase data as the y variable, the following results are obtained:

Slope: 1.0016,   intercept: 0.1057,   correlation coefficient r: 0.9997

The slope of very nearly 1 confirms the similarity of the two data sets, whilst the small positive intercept on the y-axis confirms that the glucose oxidase method gives a slightly higher, but insignificantly different, value from that of the hexokinase method.

1.6.6 **Calibration methods**

Quantitative biochemical analyses often involve the use of a calibration curve produced by the use of known amounts of the analyte using the selected analytical procedure. A calibration curve is a record of the measurement (absorbance, peak area, etc.) produced by the analytical procedure in response to a range of known quantities of the standard analyte. It involves the preparation of a standard solution of the analyte and the use of a range of aliquots in the test analytical procedure. It is good practice to replicate each calibration point and to use the mean ± 1 SD for the construction of the calibration plot. Inspection of the compiled data usually reveals a scatter of the points about a linear relationship but such that there are several options for the 'best' fit. The technique of fitting the best fit 'by eye' is not recommended, as it is highly subjective and irreproducible. The method of least mean squares linear regression (LMSLR) is the most common mathematical way of fitting a straight line to data but, in applying the method, it is important to realise that the accuracy of the values for slope and intercept that it gives are determined by experimental error built into the x and y values.

The mathematical basis of LMSLR is complex and will not be considered here, but the principles upon which it is based are simple. If the relationship between the two variables, such as the concentration or amount of analyte and response, is linear, then the 'best' straight line will have the general form $y = mx + c$, where x and y are the two variables, m is the slope of the line and c is the intercept on the y-axis. It is assumed first, correctly in most cases, that the errors in the measurement of y are much greater than those for x (it does not assume that there are no errors in the x values) and, secondly, that uncertainties (standard deviations) in the y values are all of the same magnitude. The method uses two criteria. The first is that the line will pass through the point $(\bar{x},\bar{y})$ where $\bar{x}$ and $\bar{y}$ are the mean of the x and y values respectively. The second is that the slope (m) is based on the calculation of the optimum values of m and c that give minimum variation between individual experimental y values and their corresponding values as predicted by the 'best' straight line. Since these variations can be positive or negative (i.e. the experimental values can be greater or smaller than those predicted by the 'best' straight line), in the process of arriving at the best slope the method measures the deviations between the experimental and candidate straight line values, squares them (so they are all positive), sums them and then selects the values of m and c that give the minimum deviations. The end result of the regression analysis is the equation for the best-fit straight line for the experimental data set. This is then used to construct the calibration curve and subsequently to analyse the test analyte(s). Most modern calculators will carry out this type of analysis and will simultaneously report the 95% confidence limits for the m and c values and/or the standard deviation associated with the two values together with the 'goodness-of-fit' of the data as expressed by a correlation coefficient r or a coefficient of determination r^2. The stronger the correlation between the two variables, the closer the value of r approaches $+1$ or -1. Values of r are quoted to four decimal places and for good correlations commonly exceed 0.99. Values of 0.98 and less should be considered with care, since even slight curvature can give *r* values of this order.

In the routine construction of a calibration curve, a number of points have to be borne in mind:

- *Selection of standard values:* A range of standard analyte amounts/ concentrations should be selected to cover the expected values for the test analyte(s) in such a way that the values are equally distributed along the calibration curve. Test samples should not be estimated outside this selected range, as there is no evidence that the regression analysis relationship holds outside the range. It is good practice to establish the analytical range and the limit of detection for the method. It is also advisable to determine the precision (standard deviation) of the method at different points across the analytical range and to present the values on the calibration curve. Such a plot is referred to as a precision profile. It is common for the precision to decrease (standard deviation to increase) at the two ends of the curve and this may have implications for the routine use of the curve. For example, the determination of testosterone in male and female serum requires the use of different methods, since the two values (reference range 10–30 nM for males, <3 nM for females) cannot be accommodated with acceptable precision on one calibration curve.

- *Use of a 'blank' sample:* This is where no standard analyte is present. One should be included in the experimental design when possible (it will not be possible, for example, with analyses based on serum or plasma). Any experimental value, for example absorbance, obtained for it must be deducted from all other measurements. This may be achieved automatically in spectrophotometric measurements by the use of a double-beam spectrophotometer in which the blank sample is placed in the reference cell.

- *Shape of curve:* It should not be assumed that all calibration curves are linear. They may be curved, and best represented by a quadratic equation of the type $y = ax^2 + bx + c$ where *a*, *b* and *c* are constants, or they may be logarithmic.

- *Recalibration:* A new calibration curve should be constructed on a regular basis. It is not acceptable to rely on a calibration curve produced on a much earlier occasion.

1.6.7 Internal standards

An additional approach to the control of time-related minor changes in a calibration curve and the quantification of an analyte in a test sample is the use of an internal standard. An ideal internal standard is a compound that has a molecular structure and physical properties as similar as possible to those of the test analyte and which gives a response to the analytical method similar to that of the test analyte. This response, expressed on a unit quantity basis, may be different from that for the test analyte but, provided that the relative response of the two compounds is constant, the advantages of the use of the internal standard are not compromised. Quite commonly the internal standard is a structural or geometrical isomer of the test analyte.

A known fixed quantity of the standard is added to each test sample and analysed alongside the test analyte by the standard analytical procedure. The resulting response for the standard and the range of amounts or concentrations of the test analyte is used to calculate a relative response for the test analyte and used in the construction of the calibration curve. The curve therefore consists of a plot of the relative response to the test analyte against the range of quantities of the analyte.

Internal standards are commonly used in liquid and gas–liquid chromatography, since they help to compensate for small temporal variations in the flow of liquid or gas through the chromatographic column. In such applications it is, of course, essential that the internal standard runs near to, but distinct from, the test analyte on the chromatograph.

If the analytical procedure involves preliminary sampling procedures, such as solid-phase extraction, it is important that a known amount of the internal standard is introduced into the test sample at as early a stage as possible and is therefore taken through the preliminary procedures. This ensures that any loss of the test analyte during these preliminary stages will be compensated for by identical losses to the internal standard, so that the final relative response of the method to the two compounds is a true reflection of the quantity of the test analyte.

1.7 PRINCIPLES OF CLINICAL BIOCHEMICAL ANALYSIS

1.7.1 Basis of analysis of body fluids for diagnostic, prognostic and monitoring purposes

Many human diseases are either the result of abnormal metabolism or the cause of a perturbation of normal cellular activity. In both cases there is a characteristic and significant change in the biochemical profile of body fluids. The application of quantitative analytical biochemical tests to a large range of biological analytes in body fluids and tissues is a valuable aid to the diagnosis and management of the prevailing disease state. In this section the general biological and analytical principles underlying these tests will be discussed and related to the general principles of quantitative chemical analysis discussed in Section 1.6.

Body fluids such as blood, cerebrospinal fluid and urine in both healthy and diseased states contain a large number of inorganic ions and organic molecules. Whilst the normal biological function of some of these chemical species lies within that fluid, for the majority it does not. The presence of this latter group of chemical species within the fluid is due to the fact that normal cellular secretory mechanisms, and the temporal synthesis and turnover of individual cells and their organelles within the major organs of the body, all result in the release of cell components, particularly those located in the cytoplasm, into the surrounding extracellular fluid and eventually into the blood circulatory system. This in turn transports them to the main excretory organs, namely the liver, kidneys and lungs, so that these cell components and/or their degradation products are eventually excreted in faeces, urine and expired air. Examples of cell components in this category include enzymes, hormones, intermediary metabolites and small organic and inorganic ions.

The concentration, amount or activity of a given cell component that can be detected in these fluids of a healthy individual at any point in time depends on many factors that can be classified into one of three categories, namely chemical characteristics of the component, endogenous factors characteristic of the individual, and exogenous factors that are imposed on the individual.

- *Chemical characteristics:* Some molecules are inherently unstable outside their normal cellular environment. For example, some enzymes are reliant on the presence of their substrate and/or coenzyme for their stability and these may be absent or in too low concentrations in the extracellular fluid. Molecules that can act as substrates of catabolic enzymes found in extracellular fluids, in particular blood, will also be quickly metabolised. Cell components that fall into these two categories therefore have a short half-life outside the cell and are normally present in low concentrations in fluids such as blood.
- *Endogenous factors:* These include age, gender, body mass and pregnancy. For example:

  (a) serum cholesterol concentrations are higher in men than in pre-menopausal women, but the differences decreases post-menopause;
  (b) serum alkaline phosphatase activity is higher in children than in adults and is raised in women during pregnancy;
  (c) serum insulin and triglyceride concentrations are higher in obese individuals than in the lean;
  (d) serum creatinine, a metabolic product of creatine important in muscle metabolism, is higher in individuals with a large muscle mass;
  (e) serum sex hormone concentrations differ between males and females and change with age.

- *Exogenous factors:* These include time, exercise, food intake and stress. Several hormones are secreted in a time-related fashion. Thus cortisol and to a lesser extent thyroid-stimulating hormone (TSH) and prolactin all show a diurnal rhythm in their secretion. In the case of cortisol, its secretion peaks around 9:00 a.m. and declines during the day, reaching a trough between 11:00 p.m. and 5:00 a.m. The secretion of female sex hormones varies during the menstrual cycle, and that of 25-hydroxycholecalciferol (vitamin D_3) varies with the seasons, peaking during the late summer months. The concentrations of glucose, triglycerides and insulin in blood rise shortly after the intake of a meal. Stress, including that imposed by the process of taking a blood sample by puncturing a vein (venipuncture), can stimulate the secretion of a number of hormones and neurotransmitters including prolactin, cortisol, adrenocorticotrophic hormone (ACTH) and adrenaline.

The influence of these various factors on the extent of release of cell components into extracellular fluids inevitably means that, even in healthy individuals, there is a considerable intra-individual variation (i.e. variation from one occasion to another in one individual) in the value of any chosen test analyte of diagnostic importance and an even larger inter-individual variation (i.e. variation between individuals). More importantly, the superimposition of a disease state onto these causes of intra- and inter-individual variation will result in an even greater variability between test occasions.

Many clinical conditions compromise the integrity of cells located in the organs affected by the condition. This may result in the cells becoming more 'leaky' or, in more severe cases, actually dying (necrosis) and releasing their contents into the surrounding extracellular fluid. In the vast majority of cases the extent of release of specific cell components into the extracellular fluid, relative to the healthy reference range, will reflect the extent of organ damage and this relationship forms the basis of diagnostic clinical biochemistry. If the cause of the organ damage continues for a prolonged time and is essentially irreversible (i.e. the organ does not undergo self-repair), as is the case in cirrhosis of the liver for example, then the mass of cells remaining to undergo necrosis will progressively decline so that eventually the release of cell components into the surrounding extracellular fluid will decrease even though organ cells are continuing to be damaged. In such cases the measured amounts will not reflect the extent of organ damage.

Clinical biochemical tests have been developed to complement in four main ways a provisional clinical diagnosis based on the patient's medical history and clinical examination:

- *To support or reject a provisional diagnosis* by detecting and quantifying abnormal amounts of test analytes consistent with the diagnosis. For example, serum myoglobin, troponin I (part of the cardiac contractile muscle), creatine kinase (specifically the CK-MB isoform; Section 1.7.3) and aspartate transaminase all rise following a myocardial infarction (heart attack), which results in cell death in some heart tissue. Tests can also help a differential diagnosis, for example in distinguishing the various forms of jaundice (yellowing of the skin owing to the presence of the yellow pigment bilirubin, a metabolite of haem) by the measurement of alanine transaminase and aspartate transaminase activities and by determining whether or not the bilirubin is conjugated with β-glucuronic acid.
- *To monitor recovery following treatment* by repeating the tests on a regular basis and monitoring the return of the test values to those within the reference range. Following a myocardial infarction, for example, the raised serum enzyme activities referred to above usually return to reference range values within 10 days (Section 1.7.3, see Fig. 1.6). Similarly, the measurement of serum tumour markers such as CA125 can be used to follow recovery or recurrence after treatment for ovarian cancer.
- *To screen for latent disease* in apparently healthy individuals by testing for raised levels of key analytes; for example, measuring serum glucose for diabetes mellitus and immunoreactive trypsin for cystic fibrosis. It is now common for serum cholesterol levels to be used as a measure of the risk of an individual

developing heart disease. This is particularly important for individuals with a family history of the disease. An action limit of serum cholesterol <5.2 mM has been set by the British Hyperlipidaemia Association for an individual to be counselled on the importance of a healthy (low fat) diet and regular exercise and a higher action limit of serum cholesterol >6.6 mM for cholesterol-lowering 'statin' drugs to be prescribed and clinical advice given.

● *To detect toxic side-effects of treatment*, for example in patients receiving hepatotoxic drugs, by undertaking regular liver function tests. An extension of this is therapeutic drug monitoring, in which patients receiving drugs such as phenytoin and carbamezepine (both of which are used in the treatment of epilepsy) that have a low therapeutic index (ratio of the dose required to produce a toxic effect relative to the dose required to produce a therapeutic effect) are regularly monitored for drug levels and liver function to ensure that they are receiving effective and safe therapy.

Reference ranges

For a biochemical test for a specific analyte to be routinely used as an aid to clinical diagnosis, it is essential that the test has the required performance indicators (Section 1.6.2) especially specificity and sensitivity. Sensitivity expresses the proportion of patients with the disease who are correctly identified by the test. Specificity expresses the proportion of patients without the disease who are correctly identified by the test. These two parameters may be expressed mathematically as follows:

$$\text{sensitivity} = \frac{\text{true positive tests} \times 100\%}{\text{total patients with the disease}}$$

$$\text{specificity} = \frac{\text{true negative tests} \times 100\%}{\text{total patients without the disease}}$$

Ideally both of these indicators for a particular test should be 100% but this is not always the case. This problem is most likely to occur in cases where the change in the amount of the test analyte in the clinical sample is small as compared with the reference range values found in healthy individuals. Both of these indicators express the performance of the test but it is equally important to be able to quantify the probability that the patient with a positive test has the disease in question. This is best achieved by the predictive power of the test. This expresses the proportion of patients with a positive test who are correctly diagnosed as disease positive:

$$\text{positive predictive value} = \frac{\text{true positive patients}}{\text{total positive tests}}$$

$$\text{negative predictive value} = \frac{\text{true negative patients}}{\text{total negative tests}}$$

The concept of predictive power can be illustrated by reference to fetal screening for Down's syndrome and neural tube defects. Preliminary tests for these conditions in unborn children are based on the measurement of α-fetoprotein (AFP), human chorionic gonadotrophin (hCG) and unconjugated oestriol (uE_3) in the mother's blood. The presence of these conditions results in an increased hCG and decreased AFP and uE_3 relative to the average in healthy pregnancies. The results of the tests are used in conjunction with the gestational and maternal ages to calculate the risk of the baby suffering from these conditions. If the risk is high, further tests are undertaken, including the recovery of some fetal cells for genetic screening from the amniotic fluid surrounding the fetus in the womb by inserting a hollow needle into the womb (amniocentesis). The three tests detect two out of three cases (67%) of Down's syndrome and four out of five cases (80%) of neural tube defects. Thus the performance indicators of the tests are not 100% but they are sufficiently high to justify their routine use.

The correct interpretation of all biochemical test data is heavily dependent upon the use of the correct reference range against which the test data are to be judged. As pointed out above, the majority of biological analytes of diagnostic importance are subject to considerable inter- and intra-individual variation in healthy adults, and the analytical method chosen for a particular analyte assay will have its own precision, accuracy and selectivity that will influence the analytical results. In view of these biological and analytical factors, individual laboratories must establish their own reference range for each test analyte, using their chosen methodology and a large number (hundreds) of 'healthy' individuals. The recruitment of individuals to be included in reference range studies presents a considerable practical and ethical problem owing to the difficulty of defining 'normal' and of using invasive procedures, such as venipuncture, to obtain the necessary biological samples. The establishment of reference ranges for children, especially neonates, is a particular problem.

Reference ranges are most commonly expressed as the range that covers the mean ± 1.96 standard deviations of the mean of the experimental population. This range covers 95% of the population. The majority of reference ranges are based on a normal distribution of individual values but, in some cases, the experimental data is asymmetric, often being skewed to the upper limits. In such cases it is normal to use logarithmic data to establish the reference range but, even so, the range may overlap with values found in patients with the test disease state. Typical reference ranges are shown in Table 1.12.

1.7.2 The operation of clinical biochemistry laboratories

The clinical biochemistry laboratory in a typical general hospital in the UK serves a population of about 400 000, containing approximately 60 general practitioner (GP) groups, depending upon the location in the UK. This population will generate approximately 1200 requests from GPs and hospital doctors each weekday for clinical biochemical tests on their patients. Each patient request will require the laboratory to undertake an average of seven specific analyte tests. The result is that a typical general hospital laboratory will carry out between 2.5 and 3 million tests each year. The majority of clinical biochemistry laboratories offers the local

Table 1.12   Typical reference ranges for biochemical analytes

Analyte	Reference range	Comment
Sodium	133–145 mM	
Potassium	3.5–5.0 mM	Values increased by haemolysis or prolonged contact with cells
Urea	3.5–6.5 mM	Range varies with sex and age, e.g. values up to 12.1 will be found in males over the age of 70
Creatinine	75–115 mM (males) 58–93 mM (females)	Creatinine (a metabolite of creatine) production relates to muscle mass and is also a reflection of renal function. Values for both sexes increase by 5–20% in the elderly
Aspartate transaminase (AST)	$<40 \, IU \, dm^{-3}$	Perinatal levels are $<80 \, IU \, dm^{-3}$ and fall to adult values by the age of 18 years. Some slightly increased values up to $60 \, IU \, dm^{-3}$ may be found in females over the age of 50 years. Results are increased by haemolysis
Alanine transaminase (ALT)	$<40 \, IU \, dm^{-3}$	Higher values are found in males up to the age of 60 years
Alkaline phosphatase (AP)	$<122 \, IU \, dm^{-3}$ (adults) $<455 \, IU \, dm^{-3}$ (children <12 yr)	Significantly raised results of up to 2- or 3-fold would be experienced during growth spurts through teenage years. Slightly raised levels also seen in the elderly and in women during pregnancy
Cholesterol	No reference range but recommended value of <5.2 mM	The measurement of cholesterol in an adult 'well' population does not show a Gaussian distribution but a very tailed distribution with relatively few low results. The majority are <10 mM but there is a long tail up to over 20 mM. There is a tendency for males to have a higher cholesterol than females of the same age but, after the menopause, female values revert to those of males. Generally values increase with age

medical community as many as 200 different clinical biochemical tests that can be divided into eight categories as shown in Table 1.13.

Most of the requests for biochemical tests will arise on a routine daily basis but some will arise from emergency medical situations at any time of the day. The large number of daily test samples coupled with the need for a 24 hour, 7 days per week service dictates that the laboratory must rely heavily on automated analysis to carry out the tests and on information technology to process the data.

To achieve an effective service, a clinical biochemistry laboratory has three main functions:

● to advise the requesting GP or hospital doctor on the appropriate tests for a particular medical condition and on the collection, storage and transport of the patient samples for analysis;

Table 1.13 Examples of biochemical analytes used to support clinical diagnosis

Type of analyte	Examples
Food stuffs entering the body	Cholesterol, glucose, fatty acids, triglycerides
Waste products	Bilirubin, creatinine, urea
Tissue-specific messengers	Adrenocorticotrophic hormone (ACTH), follicle-stimulating hormone (FSH), lutenising hormone (LH), thyroid-stimulating hormone (TSH)
General messengers	Cortisol, insulin, thyroxine
Response to messengers	Glucose tolerance test assessing the appropriate secretion of insulin. Tests of pituitary function
Organ function	Adrenal function – cortisol, ACTH Renal function – K^+, Na^+, urea, creatinine Thyroid function – free thyroxine (FT_4), free tri-iodothyronine (FT_3), TSH
Organ disease markers	Heart – troponin I, creatine kinase (CK-MB), AST, lactate dehydrogenase (LD) Liver – ALT, AP, γ-glutamyl transferase (GGT), bilirubin, albumin
Disease specific markers	Specific proteins ('tumour markers') secreted from specific organs – prostate-specific antigen (PSA), CA-125 (ovary), calcitonin (thyroid), α_1-fetoprotein (liver)

- to provide a quality analytical service for the measurement of biological analytes in an appropriate and timely way;
- to provide the requesting doctor with a data interpretation and advice service on the outcome of the biochemical tests and possible further tests.

The advice given to the clinician is generally supported by a User Handbook, prepared by senior laboratory personnel, which includes a description of each test offered, instructions on sample collection and storage, normal laboratory working hours and the approximate time it will take the laboratory to undertake each test. This turnaround time will vary from less than 1 h to several weeks, depending upon the speciality of the test. The vast majority of biochemical tests are carried out on serum or plasma derived from a blood sample. Serum is the preferred matrix for biochemical tests but the concentrations of most test analytes are almost the same in the two fluids. Serum is obtained by allowing the blood to clot and removing the clot by centrifugation. To obtain plasma it is necessary to add an anticoagulant to the blood sample and removing red cells by centrifugation. The two most common anticoagulants are heparin and EDTA, the choice depending on the particular biochemical test required. For example, EDTA complexes calcium ions so that calcium in EDTA plasma would be undetectable. For the measurement of glucose, fluoride/oxalate is added to the sample not as an anticoagulant but to inhibit glycolysis during the transport and storage of the sample. Special vacuum collection tubes containing specific anticoagulants or other additives are available for the storage of blood samples. Collection tubes are also available containing clot enhancers to speed the clotting process for serum preparation. Many containers incorporate a gel with a specific gravity designed to float the gel between cells and serum providing a barrier between the two for up to 4 days. Biochemical tests may also be carried out on whole blood, urine, cerebrospinal fluid (the fluid surrounding the spinal cord and brain), faeces, sweat, saliva and amniotic fluid. It is essential that the samples are collected in the appropriate container at the correct time (particularly important if the test is for the measurement of hormones such as cortisol subject to diurnal release) and labelled with appropriate patient and biohazard details. Samples submitted to the laboratory for biochemical tests are accompanied by a request form, signed by the requesting clinician, that gives details of the tests required and brief details of the reasons for the request to aid data interpretation and to help identify other appropriate tests.

Laboratory reception

On receipt in the laboratory both the sample and the request form will be assigned an acquisition number, usually in an optically readable form but with a bar code. A check is made of the validity of the sample details on both the request form and sample container to ensure that the correct container for the tests required has been used. Samples may be rejected at this stage if details are not in accordance with the set protocol. Correct samples are then split from the request form and prepared for analysis typically by centrifugation to prepare serum or plasma. The request form is processed into the computer system that identifies the patient against the sample acquisition number, and the tests requested by the clinician typed into the database. It is vital at this reception phase that the sample and patient data match and that the correct details are placed in the database. These details must be adequate to uniquely identify the patient, bearing in mind the number of potential patients in the catchment area, and will include name, address, date of birth, hospital or Accident & Emergency number and acquisition number.

Analytical organisation

The analytical organisation of the majority of clinical biochemical laboratories is based on three work areas:

- autoanalyser section,
- immunoassay section,
- manual section.

Autoanalyser section

Autoanalysers dedicated to clinical biochemical analysis are available from many commercial manufacturers. A typical analyser layout is shown in Fig. 1.5. Analysers have carousels for holding the test samples in racks each carrying up to 15 samples, one or two carousels each for up to 50 different reagents, which are identified by a unique bar code, carousels for sample washing/preparation and a

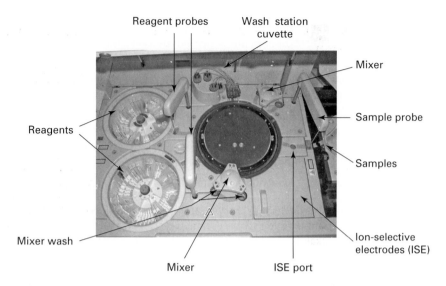

Fig. 1.5. The Olympus 640 autoanalyser (Reproduced by permission of Olympus Diagnostic Division, UK.)

reaction carousel containing up to 200 cuvettes for initiating and monitoring individual test reactions. The analysers have a high throughput capacity with a time cycle that allows additions or readings to be taken in a given cuvette every 4–20 s depending on the analyser model. Multiple analyte test reactions will be taking place and being monitored at any given time. The total reaction time for a given analyte sample will depend on the specific reaction being monitored, but a typical cycle is that for the analysis of serum glucose based on the hexokinase and glucose-6-phosphate dehydrogenase reactions and the monitoring of the increase in absorption at 340 nm due to NADH (Section 15.2.5):

- *Time* 0: Add reagent 1 (ATP, Mg^{2+} and hexokinase in Pipes buffer, pH 7.6) to reaction cuvette. Dilute with deionised water and mix.
- *Time* 30 s: Add serum test sample. Dilute with deionised water and mix. Monitor absorption at 340 nm for 3 min to obtain sample blank reading.
- *Time* 3 *min* 30 s: Add reagent 2 (glucose-6-phosphate dehydrogenase, NAD^+). Mix. Total reaction volume 250 mm^3. Monitor absorption at 340 nm every 20 s.
- *Time* 8 *min*: Record final absorption change due to NADH, allowing for sample blank. Calculate glucose concentration in test sample and record on database. Rinse cuvette. Cycle complete. If the absorption change is outside the calibration range, the analyser will automatically initiate a repeat analysis using a smaller test sample.

The analysers operate with a state-of-the-art spectrophotometer with fibre optics that has multiple read-centres around the reaction carousel that can take readings at several wavelengths simultaneously. Measurements can also be taken with an oxygen electrode and three or four different ion-selective electrodes. The reaction cuvettes may be disposable and automatically loaded and unloaded onto

Table 1.14 Examples of analytical techniques used to quantify analytes by autoanalysers

Analytical technique	Examples of analytes
Ion-selective electrodes	K^+, Na^+, Li^+, Cl^-
Visible and UV spectrophotometry	Urea, creatinine, calcium, urate
Turbidimetric	IgG, IgA, IgM, D-dimer (a metabolic product of fibrinogen)
Reaction rate	Enzymes – AST, ALT, GGT, AP, CK, LD
EMIT	Therapeutic drug monitoring – phenytoin, carbamezapine

UV, ultraviolet; EMIT, enzyme multiplier immunoassay test; AST, aspartate transaminase; ALT, alanine aminotransaminase; GGT, γ-glutamyl transferase; AP, alkaline phosphatase; CK, creatine kinase; LD, lactate dehydrogenase.

the carousel or may be reusable, in which case they are laundered by a sophisticated wash station that uses cycles of acid, alkali and alcohol in various combinations followed by a water wash and an air dry. Disposable cuvettes are collected in sealable containers for disposal and all liquid waste is pumped into containers containing powerful disinfectants. Internal computers as well as an external interface with the main laboratory computer and database control the operation of the analyser. Most analysers have about 25 pre-programmed methods of analysis for a range of analytes, based on five main analytical modes (Table 1.14), but also allow 'in-house' methods to be programmed by laboratory personnel.

Each laboratory will have at least two analysers each offering a similar analytical repertoire so that one can back up the other. The analyser reads the bar code acquisition number for each sample and, on the basis of the reading, interrogates the host computer database to identify the tests to be carried out on the sample. The identified tests are then automatically prioritised into the most efficient order and the analyser programmed to take the appropriate volume of sample by means of a sampler that may also be capable of detecting microclots in the sample, add the appropriate volume of reagents in a specified order and to monitor the progress of the reaction. Internal quality control samples are also analysed on an identical basis at regular intervals. The analyser automatically monitors the use of all reagents so that it can identify when each will need replenishing. When the test results are calculated, the operator can validate them either on the analyser or on the main computer database. When it is appropriate, the results can also be checked against previous results on the same patient.

Immunoassay section

Immunoassay procedures undertaken by modern autoanalysers are based mostly on fluorescence or polarised fluorescence techniques. The range of analytes varies from manufacturer to manufacturer but usually involves basic endocrinology (e.g. thyroid fuction tests), therapeutic drugs (theophylline, digoxin) and drugs of abuse (opiates, cannabis). The operation of autoanalysers in immunoassay mode is similar to that described above and the results are generally reported on the same day, and are compared with the previous set of results for the patient.

Manual assays section

This approach to biochemical tests is generally more labour intensive than the other two sections and covers a range of analytical techniques such as acetate or gel electrophoresis, immunoelectrophoresis and some more difficult basic spectrophotometric assays. Examples include the assays for catecholamines (for the diagnosis of phaeochromocytoma), 5-hydroxyindole acetic acid (for the diagnosis of carcinoid syndrome) or haemoglobinA$_{1c}$ (for the monitoring of diabetes).

Result reporting

The instrument operator or the section leader initially validates analytical results. This validation process will, in part, be based on the use of internal quality control procedures for individual analytes. Quality control samples are analysed at least twice daily or are included in each batch of test analytes. The analytical results are then subject to an automatic process that identifies results that are either significantly abnormal or require clinical comment or interpretation against rules set by senior laboratory staff.

1.7.3 Diagnostic enzymology

The measurement of the activities or masses of selected enzymes in serum is a long established aid to clinical diagnosis and prognosis. The enzymes found in serum can be divided into three categories based on the location of their normal physiological function:

- *Serum-specific enzymes:* The normal physiological function of these enzymes is based in serum. Examples include the enzymes associated with lipoprotein metabolism and with the coagulation of blood.
- *Secreted enzymes:* These are closely related to the serum-specific enzymes. Examples include pancreatic lipase, prostatic acid phosphatase and salivary amylase.
- *Non-serum-specific enzymes:* These enzymes have no physiological role in serum. They are released into the extracellular fluid and, as a consequence, appear in serum as result of normal cell turnover or, more abundantly, as a result of cell membrane damage, cell death or morphological changes to cells such as those in cases of malignancy. Their normal substrates and/or cofactors may be absent or in low concentrations in serum.

Serum enzymes in the third category are of the greatest diagnostic value. When a cell is damaged, the contents of the cell are released over a period of several hours, with enzymes of the cytoplasm appearing first, since their release is dependent only on the impairment of the integrity of the plasma membrane. The release of these enzymes following cell membrane damage is facilitated by their large concentration gradient, in excess of 1000-fold, across the membrane. The integrity of the cell membrane is particularly sensitive to events that impair energy production, for example by the restriction of oxygen supply. It is also sensitive to toxic chemicals including some drugs, microorganisms, certain immunological conditions and genetic defects. Enzymes released from cells by such events may not necessarily be found in serum in the same relative amounts as were originally present in the cell. Such variations reflect differences in the rate of their metabolism and excretion from the body and hence of differences in their serum half-lives. This may be as short as a few hours (intestinal alkaline phosphatase, glutathione S-transferase, creatine kinase) or as long as several days (liver alkaline phosphatase, alanine aminotransferase, lactate dehydrogenase).

The clinical exploitation of non-serum-specific enzyme activities is influenced by several factors:

- *Organ specificity:* Few enzymes are unique to one particular organ but fortunately some enzymes are present in much larger amounts in some tissues than in others. As a consequence, the relative proportions (pattern) of a number of enzymes found in serum are often characteristic of the organ of origin.
- *Isoenzymes:* Some clinically important enzymes exist in isoenzyme forms and in many cases the relative proportion of the isoenzymes varies considerably between tissues so that measurement of the serum isoenzymes allows their organ of origin to be deduced.
- *Reference ranges:* The activities of enzymes present in the serum of healthy individuals are invariably smaller than that in the serum of individuals with a diagnosed clinical condition such as liver disease. In many cases, the extent to which the activity of a particular enzyme is raised by the disease state is a direct indicator of the extent of cellular damage to the organ of origin.
- *Variable rate of increase in serum activity:* The rate of increase in the activity of released enzymes in serum following cell damage in a particular organ is a characteristic of each enzyme. Moreover, the rate at which the activity of each enzyme decreases towards the reference range following the event that caused cell damage and the subsequent treatment of the patient is a valuable indicator of the patient's recovery from the condition.

The practical implication of these various points to the applications of diagnostic enzymology is illustrated by its use in the management of heart disease and liver disease.

Ischaemic heart disease and myocardial infarction

The healthy functioning of the heart is dependent upon the availability of oxygen. This oxygen availability may be compromised by the slow deposition of cholesterol-rich atheromatous plaques in the coronary arteries. As these deposits increase, a point is reached at which the oxygen supply cannot be met at times of peak demand, for example at times of strenuous exercise. As a consequence, the heart becomes temporarily ischaemic ('lacking in oxygen') and the individual experiences severe chest pain, a condition known as angina pectoris ('angina of effort'). Although the pain may be severe during such events, the cardiac cells temporarily deprived of oxygen are not damaged and do not release their cellular contents. However, if the arteries become completely blocked either by the plaque or by a small thrombus (clot) that is prevented from flowing through the artery by the plaque, the patient experiences a myocardial infarction ('heart attack', MI) characterised by the same severe chest pain, but in this case the pain is accompanied by the irreversible damage to the cardiac cells and the release of their cellular contents. This release is not immediate, but occurs over a period of many hours. From the point of view of the clinical management of the patient, it is important for the clinician to establish whether or not the chest pain was accompanied by a MI. In about one-fifth of the cases of a MI event the patient does not experience the characteristic chest pain ('silent MI') but again it is important for the clinician to be aware that the event has occurred. Electrocardiogram (ECG) patterns are a primary indicator of these events but in atypical presentations ECG changes may be ambiguous and additional evidence is sought in the form of changes in serum enzyme activities. The activities of three enzymes are commonly measured:

- *Creatine kinase (CK):* This enzyme converts phosphocreatine (important in muscle metabolism) to creatine. CK is a dimeric protein composed of two monomers, one denoted as M (muscle) the other as B (brain), so that three isoforms exist, CK-MM, CK-MB and CK-BB. The tissue distribution of these isoenzymes is significantly different such that heart muscle consists of 80–85% MM and 15–20% MB, skeletal muscle 99% MM and 1% MB and brain, stomach, intestine and bladder predominantly BB. CK activity is raised in a number of clinical conditions but since the CK-MB form is almost unique to the heart, its raised activity in serum gives unambiguous support for a MI even in cases in which the total CK activity remains within the reference range. A rise in total serum CK activity is detectable within 6 h of the MI and the serum activity reaches a peak after 24–36 h. However, a rise in CK-MB is detectable within 3–4 h, has 100% sensitivity within 8–12 h and reaches a peak within 10–24 h. It remains raised for 2–4 days.
- *Aspartate aminotransferase (AST):* This is one of a number of transaminases involved in intermediary metabolism. It is found in most tissues but is abundant in heart and liver. Its activity in serum is raised following a MI and reaches a peak between 48 and 60 h. It has little clinical value in the early diagnosis of heart muscle damage but is of use in the case of delayed presentation with chest pain.
- *Lactate dehydrogenase (LD):* This is a tetrameric protein made of two monomers denoted as H (heart) and M (muscle) so that five isoforms exist: LD-1 (H4), LD-2 (H3M), LD-3 (H2M2), LD-4 (HM3) and LD-5 (M5). LD-1 predominates in heart, brain and kidney and LD-5 in skeletal muscle and liver. Total LD activity and LD-1 activity in serum increases following a MI and reaches a peak after 48–72 h. The subsequent decline in activity is much slower that that of CK or AST. The diagnostic value of LD activity measurement is mainly confined to monitoring the patient's recovery from the MI event.

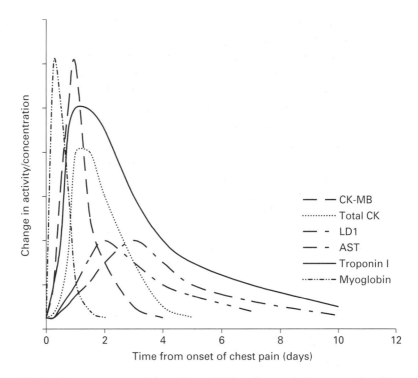

Fig. 1.6. Serum enzyme activity and myoglobin and troponin I concentration changes following a myocardial infarction. Changes are expressed as a multiple of the upper limit of the reference range. Values vary according to the severity of the event, but the time course of each profile is characteristic of all events. CK, creatine kinase; LD, lactate dehydrogenase; AST, aspartate transaminase.

Typical changes in the activities of these three enzymes following a MI are shown in Fig. 1.6. All three enzymes are assayed by an automated method based on the following reactions.

- *Total CK activity:* This is assessed by coupled reactions (Section 15.2.2) with hexokinase and glucose-6-phosphate dehydrogenase in the presence of *N*-acetylcysteine as activator, and the measurement of increase in absorbance at 340 nm or by fluorescence polarisation (primary wavelength 340 nm, reference wavelength 378 nm):

$$\text{creatine phosphate} + \text{ADP} \rightleftharpoons \text{creatine} + \text{ATP}$$
$$\text{ATP} + \text{D-glucose} \rightleftharpoons \text{ADP} + \text{D-glucose 6-phosphate}$$
$$\text{D-glucose 6-phosphate} + \text{NAD(P)}^+ \rightleftharpoons \text{D-6-phosphogluconate} + \text{NAD(P)H} + \text{H}^+$$

- *CK-MB activity:* This is assessed by the inhibition of the activity of the M monomer by the addition to the serum sample of an antibody to the M monomer. This inhibits CK-MM and the M unit of CK-MB. The activity of CK-BB is unaffected but is normally undetectable in serum, hence the remaining activity in serum is due to the B unit of CK-MB. It is assayed by the above coupled assay procedure and the activity doubled to give an estimate of the CK-MB activity. An alternative assay uses a double antibody technique: CK-MB is bound to anti-CK-MB coated on microparticles, the resulting complex washed to remove non-bound forms of CK and anti-CK-MM conjugated to added alkaline phosphatase. It binds to the antibody–antigen complex, is washed to remove unbound materials and assayed using 4-methyl-umbelliferone phosphate as substrate, the released 4-methylumbelliferone being measured by its fluorescence and expressed as a concentration (ng cm^{-3}) rather than as activity.

- *Aspartate aminotransferase activity:*   This is assessed by a coupled assay with malate dehydrogenase and the measurement of the decrease in absorbance at 340 nm:

$$\text{L-aspartate} + \text{2-oxoglutarate} \rightleftharpoons \text{oxaloacetate} + \text{L-glutamate}$$

$$\text{oxaloacetate} + \text{NADH} + \text{H}^+ \rightleftharpoons \text{malate} + \text{NAD}^+$$

- *Lactate dehydrogenase:*   The measurement of total activity is based on the measurement of the increase in absorbance at 340 nm using lactate as substrate. The measurement of LD-1 is based on the use of 2-hydroxybutyrate as substrate, since only LD-1 and LD-2 can use it:

$$\text{Total LD:}\quad \text{lactate} + \text{NAD}^+ \rightleftharpoons \text{pyruvate} + \text{NADH} + \text{H}^+$$

$$\text{LD-1:}\quad \text{2-hydroxybutyrate} + \text{NAD}^+ \rightleftharpoons \text{2-ketobutyrate} + \text{NADH} + \text{H}^+$$

The clinical importance of obtaining early unambiguous evidence of a myocardial infarction has encouraged the development of markers other than enzyme activities and currently two tests are commonly run alongside enzyme activities. These are based on myoglobin and troponin I:

Myoglobin: Concentrations of this protein in serum, assayed by HPLC or immunoassay, increase more rapidly than CK-MB after a MI. An increase is detectable within 1–2 h, has 100% sensitivity and reaches a peak within 4–8 h and returns to normal within 12–24 h. However, myoglobin changes are not specific for a MI, since similar changes also occur in other syndromes such as muscle damage or crush injury such as that following a road accident.

Troponin I: This is one of three proteins (the others being troponin T and troponin C) of a complex that regulate the contractility of the myocardial cells. Its activity in serum increases at the same rate as CK-MB after a myocardial infarction, has a similar time for 100% sensitivity and for peak time, but it remains raised for up to 4 days after the onset of symptoms. Its reference range is less than 1 ng cm^{-3} but its concentration in serum is raised to up to 30–50 ng cm^{-3} within 24 h of a MI event. It is assayed by a 'sandwich' immunological assay in which the antibody is labelled with alkaline phosphatase. Using 4-methylumbelliferone phosphate as substrate, the release of 4-methylumbelliferone is measured by fluorescence. The measurement of serum troponin I is widely used to exclude cardiac damage in patients with chest pain since it remains raised for several days following a MI, but the timing of the test sample is important as a sample taken too early may give a false negative result. A limitation of its use is that its release into serum is not specific to MI, an increase in serum mass may occur following a crush injury.

The measurement of enzyme activities and myoglobin and troponin I concentrations, together with plasma potassium, glucose and arterial blood gases, is routinely used to monitor the recovery of patients following a MI. A patient may experience a second MI within a few days of the first. In such cases the pattern of serum enzymes shown in Fig. 1.6 is repeated, the pattern being superimposed on the remnants of the first profile. CK-MB is the best initial indicator of a second infarction, since the levels of troponin I may not reflect a secondary event.

The sensitivity and specificity (Section 1.7.1) of ECG and diagnostic enzymology in the management of heart disease are complementary. Thus the specificity of ECG is 100% whilst that of enzyme measurements is 90%, and the sensitivity of ECG is 70% whilst that of enzyme measurements is 95%.

Liver disease

Diagnostic enzymology is routinely used to discriminate between several forms of liver disease including:

- *Hepatitis:* General inflammation of the liver most commonly caused by viral infection but which may also be a consequence of blood poisoning (septicaemia) or glandular fever. It results in only mild necrosis of the hepatic cells and hence of a modest release of cellular enzymes.
- *Cirrhosis:* A general destruction of the liver cells and their replacement by fibrous tissue. It is most commonly caused by excess alcohol intake but is also a result of prolonged hepatitis, various autoimmune diseases and genetic conditions. They all result in extensive cell damage and release of hepatic cell enzymes.
- *Malignancy:* Primary and secondary tumours.
- *Cholestasis:* The prevention of bile from reaching the gut due either to blockage of the bile duct by gallstones or tumours or to liver cell destruction as a result of cirrhosis or prolonged hepatitis. This gives rise to obstructive jaundice (presence of bilirubin, a yellow metabolite of haem, in the skin).

Patients with these various liver diseases often present to their doctor with similar symptoms and a differential diagnosis needs to be made on the basis of a range of investigations including imaging techniques especially ultrasonography (ultrasound), magnetic resonance imaging (MRI), computed tomography (CT) scanning, microscopic examination of biopsy samples and liver function tests. Five enzymes are routinely assayed to aid differential diagnosis:

- *Aspartate aminotransferase (AST) and alanine aminotransferase (ALT):* As previously stated, these enzymes are widely distributed but their ratios in serum are characteristic of the specific cause of liver cell damage. For example, an AST:ALT ratio of less than 1 is found in acute viral hepatitis and fresh obstructive jaundice, a ratio of about 1 in obstructive jaundice caused by viral hepatitis, and a ratio of greater than 1 in cases of cirrhosis.

- *γ-Glutamyl transferase (GGT):*   This enzyme transfers a γ-glutamyl group between substrates and may be assayed by the use of γ-glutamyl 4-nitroaniline as substrate and monitoring the release of 4-nitroaniline at 400 nm. GGT is widely distributed and is abundant in liver, especially bile canaliculi, kidney, pancreas and prostate but these do not present themselves by contributing to serum levels. Raised activities are found in cirrhosis, secondary hepatic tumours and cholestasis, and tend to parallel increases in the activity of alkaline phosphatase, especially in cholestasis. Its synthesis is induced by alcohol and some drugs also cause its serum activity to rise.

- *Alkaline phosphatase (AP):*   This enzyme is found in most tissues but is especially abundant in the bile canaliculi, kidney, bone and placenta. It may be assayed by using 4-nitrophenylphosphate as substrate and monitoring the release of 4-nitrophenol at 400 nm. Its activity is raised in obstructive jaundice and, when measured in conjunction with ALT, can be used to distinguish between obstructive jaundice and hepatitis, since its activity is raised more than that of ALT in obstructive jaundice. Decreasing serum activity of AP is valuable in confirming an end of cholestasis. Raised serum AP levels can also be present in various bone diseases and during growth and pregnancy.

1.7.4 Quality assessment procedures

In order to validate the analytical precision and accuracy of the biochemical tests conducted by a clinical biochemistry department, the department will participate in external quality assessment schemes in addition to routinely carrying out internal quality control procedures that involve the repeated analysis of reference samples covering the full analytical range for the test analyte. In the UK there are two main national clinical biochemistry external quality assessment schemes: the UK National External Quality Assessment Scheme (UK NEQAS: website <www.ukneqas.org.uk>) coordinated at the Queen Elizabeth Medical Centre, Birmingham and the Wales External Quality Assessment Scheme (WEQAS: website <www.weqas.com>) coordinated at the University Hospital of Wales, Cardiff. The majority of UK hospital clinical biochemistry departments subscribe to both schemes. UK NEQAS and WEQAS distribute test samples on a fortnightly basis, the samples being human serum based. In the case of UK NEQAS the samples contain multiple analytes each at an undeclared concentration within the analytical range. The concentration of each analyte is varied from one distribution to the next. In contrast, WEQAS distributes four or five test samples containing the test analytes at various concentrations within the analytical range. Both UK NEQAS and WEQAS offer a number of quality assessment schemes in which the distributed test samples contain groups of related analytes such as general chemistry analytes, peptide hormones, steroid hormones and therapeutic drug-monitoring analytes. Participating laboratories elect to subscribe to schemes relevant to their analytical services.

The participating laboratories are required to analyse the external quality assessment samples alongside routine clinical samples and to report the results to the organising centre. Each centre undertakes a full statistical analysis of all the submitted results and reports them back to the individual laboratories on a confidential basis. The statistical data record the individual laboratory's data in comparison with all the submitted data and with the compiled data broken down into individual methods (e.g. the glucose oxidase and hexokinase methods for glucose) and for specific manufacturers' systems. Results are presented in tabular, histogram and graphic form and are compared with the results from recent previously submitted samples. This comparison with previous performance data allows longer-term trends in analytical performance for each analyte to be monitored. Laboratory data that are regarded as unsatisfactory are identified and followed up. Selected data from typical UK NEQAS and WEQAS reports are presented in Table 1.15 and Fig. 1.7.

Clinical audit and accreditation

In addition to participating in external quality assessment schemes, clinical laboratories are also subject to clinical audit. This is a systematic and critical assessment of the general performance of the laboratory against its own declared standards and procedures and against nationally agreed standards. In the context of analytical procedures, the audit evaluates the laboratory performance in terms of: the appropriateness of the use of the tests offered by the laboratory; the clinical interpretation of the results; and the procedures that operate for the receipt, analysis and reporting of the test samples. Thus, whilst it includes the evaluation of analytical data, the audit is concerned primarily with processes leading to the test data with a view to implementing change and improvement. The ultimate objective of the audit is to ensure that the patient receives the best possible care and support in a cost-effective way. The audit is normally undertaken by junior doctors from the hospital, lasts for several days, and involves interaction with all laboratory personnel.

Closely allied to the process of clinical audit is that of accreditation. However, whereas clinical audit is carried out primarily for the local benefit of the laboratory and its staff and ultimately for the patient, accreditation is a public and national recognition of the professional quality and status of the laboratory and its personnel. The accreditation process and assessment is the responsibility of either a recognised public professional body or a government department or agency. Different models operate in different countries. In the UK, accreditation of clinical biochemistry laboratories is voluntary and is carried out by either Clinical Pathology Accreditation (UK) Ltd (CPA) or less commonly the United Kingdom Accreditation Service (UKAS). In the USA, accreditation is mandatory and may be carried out by one of a number of 'deemed authorities' such as the College of American Pathologists. Accreditation organisations also exist for non-clinical analytical laboratories. Examples in the UK include the National Measurement

Table 1.15 Selected UK NEQAS and WEQAS quality assessment data for serum glucose (mM)

(a) **UK NEQAS report** © The data are reproduced by permission of UK NEQAS, Wolfson EQA Laboratory, Birmingham

Analytical method	n	Mean	SD	CV (%)
All methods	635	18.68	0.60	3.2
Beckman Glucose Analyser	62	18.22	0.41	2.2
Beckman Synchron CX3/CX7	59	18.25	0.38	2.1
Glucose oxidase/dehydrogenase	148	18.78	0.63	3.4
Roche Hitachi/Modular	75	18.60	0.52	2.8
Other discrete analysers	47	18.89	0.82	4.4
Hexokinase + G6PDH	297	18.84	0.61	3.2
Discrete analyser	47	18.57	0.59	3.2
Olympus systems	132	19.05	0.51	2.7
Roche Integra	51	18.86	0.62	3.3
Ortho Vitros	112	18.46	0.37	2.0
700/750/950	47	18.39	0.40	2.2
250	59	18.52	0.35	1.9

SD, standard deviation; CV, coefficient of variation.

The Beckman Glucose Analyser uses the glucose oxidase method and measures oxygen consumption using an oxygen electrode. The Vitros method is a so-called 'dry chemistry' method that involves placing the sample on a slide, similar to a photographic slide, that has the reagents of the glucose oxidase method impregnated in the emulsion. A blue colour is produced and its intensity measured by reflected light.

These data are for a laboratory that used the hexokinase method and reported a result of 18.7 mM. UK NEQAS calculate a method laboratory trimmed mean (MLTM) as a target value. It is the mean value of all the results returned by all laboratories using the same method with results ±2 SD outside the mean omitted. Its value was 18.84. On the basis of the difference between the MLTM and the laboratory's result, UK NEQAS also calculates a score of the specimen accuracy and bias together with a measurement of the laboratory's consistency of bias. This involves aggregating the bias data from all specimens of that analyte submitted by the laboratory, within the previous 6 months, representing the 12 most recent distributions. This score is an assessment of the tendency of the laboratory to give an over-positive or under-negative estimate of the target MLTM values. The score indicated that the laboratory was consistently underestimating the MLTM but within an acceptable laboratory performance.

The results embodied in this table are shown in histogram form in Fig. 1.7.

Accreditation Service (NAMAS) and the British Standards Institution (BSI). The International Laboratory Accreditation Cooperation (ILAC), the European Co-operation for Accreditation (EA) and the Asia-Pacific Laboratory Accreditation Co-operation (APLAC) are three of many international fora for the harmonisation of national standards of accreditation for analytical laboratories.

Assessors appointed by the accreditation body assess the compliance by the laboratory with standards set by the accreditation body. The standards cover a wide range of issues such as those of accuracy and precision, timeliness of results,

Table 1.15 *(Cont.)*

(b) **WEQAS report** © The data are reproduced by permission of WEQAS, Directorate
of Laboratory Medicine, University Hospital of Wales, Cardiff

		Sample number			
Analytical method		1	2	3	4
Reported result		7.2	3.7	17.2	8.7
Hexokinase	Mean	6.9	3.6	17.0	8.4
	SD	0.2	0.1	0.5	0.3
	Number	220	221	219	219
Aeroset	Mean	7.2	3.8	17.3	8.5
	SD	0.15	0.08	0.045	0.2
	Number	8	8	9	8
Overall	Mean	7.0	3.7	17.2	8.6
	SD	0.28	0.20	0.54	0.33
	Number	388	392	388	389
WEQAS SD		0.26	0.16	0.6	0.3
SDI		1.15	0.63	0.33	1.0

SD, standard deviation; SDI, standard deviation index.

These data are for a laboratory that used the hexokinase method for glucose using an
Aeroset instrument. Accordingly, the WEQAS report includes the results submitted by
all laboratories using the hexokinase method and all results for the method using an
Aeroset. The overall results refer to all methods irrespective of instrument. All the data
are 'trimmed' in that results outside ±2 SD of the mean are rejected, which explains
why the total number for each test sample varies slightly. WEQAS SD is calculated from
the precision profiles for each analyte and the SDI is equal to (the laboratory result
minus method mean result)/WEQAS SD at that level. SDI is a measure of total error and
includes components of inaccuracy and imprecision. The four SDIs for the laboratory
are used to calculate an overall analyte SDI, in this case 0.78. A value of less than 1
indicates that all estimates were within ±1 SD and is regarded as a good performance.
A value greater than 2 would be indicative of an unacceptable performance.

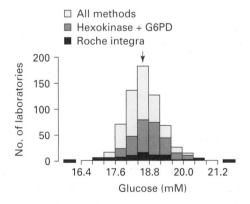

Fig. 1.7. Histogram of UK NEQAS quality assessment data for serum glucose based on data
in Table 1.15a. The arrow indicates the location of the value submitted by the participating
laboratory. (Reproduced by permission of UK NEQAS, Wolfson EQA Laboratory,
Birmingham.)

clinical relevance of the tests performed, competence to carry out the tests as judged by the training and qualifications of the laboratory staff, health and safety, the quality of administrative and technical support systems and the quality of the laboratory management systems and document control. The successful outcome of an assessment is the national recognition that the laboratory is in compliance with the standards and hence provides quality healthcare. The accreditation normally lasts for 3 years.

1.8 SAFETY IN THE LABORATORY

Virtually all experiments conducted in a biochemistry laboratory present a potential risk to the wellbeing of the investigator. In planning any experiment it is essential that careful thought be given to all aspects of safety before the experimental design is finalised. Health hazards come from a variety of sources:

- *Chemical hazards:* All chemicals are, to varying extents, capable of causing damage to the body. First, they may be irritants and cause a short-term effect on exposure. Secondly, they may be corrosive and cause severe and often irreversible damage to the skin. Examples include strong acids and alkalis. Thirdly, they may be toxic once they have gained access to the body by ingestion, inhalation or absorption across the skin. Once in the body their effect may range from slight to the extremes of being a poison (e.g. cyanide), a carcinogen (e.g. benzene and vinyl chloride) or a teratogen (e.g. thalidomide). Finally there is the special case of the use of radioactive compounds that are discussed in detail in Chapter 14.
- *Biological hazards:* Examples include human body fluids that may carry infections such as the human immunodeficiency virus (HIV), laboratory animals that may cause allergic reactions or transmit certain diseases, pathogenic animal and cell tissue cultures, and all microorganisms, including genetically engineered forms. In the UK, animal experiments must be conducted in accordance with Home Office regulations and guidelines. All experiments with tissue and cell cultures should be conducted in microbiological cabinets that are provided with a sterile airflow away from the operator.
- *Electrical and mechanical hazards:* All electrical apparatus should be used and maintained in accordance with the manufacturers' instructions. Electrophoresis equipment presents a particular potential for safety problems. Centrifuges, especially high speed varieties, also need careful use especially in the correct use and balance of the rotors.
- *General laboratory hazards:* Common examples include syringe needles, broken glassware and liquid nitrogen flasks.

Routine precautions that should be taken to minimise personal exposure to these hazards include the wearing of laboratory coats, which should be of the high-necked buttoned variety for work with microorganisms, safety spectacles and lightweight disposable gloves. It is also good practice not to work alone in a laboratory so that help is to hand if needed. In the UK, laboratory work is subject to legislation including the Health and Safety at Work Act, 1974, the Control of Substances Hazardous to Health (COSHH) Regulations 1994 and the Management of Health and Safety at Work Regulations 1999. This legislation requires a risk assessment to be carried out prior to laboratory work being undertaken. As the name implies, a risk assessment requires potential hazards to be identified and an assessment made of their potential severity and probability of occurrence. Action must be taken in cases where the potential severity and probability of an adverse event are medium to high. Such assessments require knowledge of the toxicity of all the chemicals used in the study. Toxicity data are widely available via computer packages and published handbooks and should be on reference in all laboratories. Once the toxicity data are known, consideration may be given to the use of alternative and less toxic compounds or, if it is decided to proceed with the use of toxic compounds, precautions taken to minimise their risk and plans laid for dealing with an accident should one occur. These include arranging access to first-aiders and other emergency services. It is normal for all laboratories to have a nominated Safety Officer whose responsibility it is to give advice on safety issues. To facilitate good practice, procedures for the disposal of organic solvents, radioactive residues, body fluids, tissue and cell cultures and microbiological cultures are posted in all laboratories. The outcome of the risk assessment is recorded on an approved form, signed by the investigator and countersigned by an approved senior person such as the Safety Officer. In all laboratory work it is essential to observe routine good practice including:

- always use an automatic pipette, such as the Gilson Pipetman^R, to pipette liquids: never be tempted to pipette by mouth, however, apparently innocuous the liquid;
- use a fume cupboard for potentially hazardous chemicals, ensuring that you conform to its correct operating procedure;
- use gas cylinders according to the suppliers specification;
- make sure you are aware of the location of safety equipment such as eyebaths and fire extinguishers;
- dispose of biological material, used glassware, pipette tips, broken glassware etc. according to laboratory procedures.

1.9 SUGGESTIONS FOR FURTHER READING

Analytical chemistry

BURNETT, D. (2002). *A Practical Guide to Accreditation in Laboratory Medicine*. ACB Ventures, London. (A comprehensive and highly user-friendly guide to this important aspect of quality assurance in clinical biochemistry.)

HARRIS, D. C. (2003). *Quantitative Chemical Analysis*, 6th edn. Freeman, New York. (An excellent undergraduate textbook covering all aspects of chemical analysis.)

KENKEL, J. (2000). *A Primer on Quality in the Analytical Laboratory*. Lewis, Boca Raton, FL. (A good introductory text on the general issues of quality control.)

SAUNDERS, G. C. and PARKES, H. C. (1999). *Analytical Molecular Biology*, LGC, Teddington, Middx. (Contains a very good chapter on quality in the molecular biology laboratory.)

Clinical biochemistry

BURTIS, C. A. and ASHWOOD, E. R. (2001). *Tietz Fundamentals of Clinical Chemistry*, 5th edn. Saunders, Philadelphia. (A comprehensive coverage of the principles and practice of clinical biochemistry.)

SMITH, A. F. and BECKETT, G. J. (1998). *Lecture Notes on Clinical Biochemistry*, 6th edn. Blackwell Science, Oxford. (An excellent reference text for all aspects of clinical biochemistry.)

Data analysis

JONES, R. and PAYNE, B. (1997). *Clinical Investigation and Statistics in Laboratory Medicine.* ACB Ventures, London. (Written specifically for analytical studies in clinical biochemistry.)

TOWNEND, J. (2002). *Practical Statistics for Environmental and Biological Scientists.* Wiley, Chichester. (A concise, user-friendly, non-technical introduction to statistics.)

Research methodology

BALNAVES, M. and CAPUTI, P. (2001). *Introduction to Quantitative Research Methods: An Investigative Approach.* Sage Publications, London. (A clear and accessible text with a practical emphasis based on case studies. Includes a CD-ROM for tutorial use.)

FESLING, M. F. W. (2003). Principles: The need for better experimental design. *Trends in Pharmacological Sciences*, **24**, 341–345. (Illustrates the importance of good experimental design by using a model experiment.)

Safety

Control of Substances Hazardous to Health Regulations 2002. Approved Code of Practice and Guidance. HSE Books, Kingston upon Thames. (A step-by-step approach to understanding the practical implications of COSHH.)

Chapter 2

Cell culture techniques

2.1 INTRODUCTION

Cell culture is a technique that involves the isolation and maintenance *in vitro* of cells isolated from tissues or whole organs derived from animals, microbes or plants. In general, animal cells have more complex nutritional requirements and usually need more stringent conditions for growth and maintenance. By comparison, microbes and plants require less rigorous conditions and grow effectively with the minimum of needs. Regardless of the source of material used, practical cell culture is governed by the same general principles, requiring a sterile pure culture of cells, the need to adopt appropriate aseptic techniques and the utilisation of suitable conditions for optimal viable growth of cells.

Once established, cells in culture can be exploited in many different ways. For instance, they are ideal for studying intracellular processes including protein synthesis, signal transduction mechanisms and drug metabolism. They have also been widely used to understand the mechanisms of drug actions, cell–cell interaction and genetics. Additionally, cell culture technology has been adopted in medicine, where genetic abnormalities can be determined by chromosomal analysis of cells derived, for example from expectant mothers. Similarly, viral infections can be assayed both qualitatively and quantitatively on isolated cells in culture. In industry, cultured cells are used routinely to test both the pharmacological and toxicological effects of pharmaceutical compounds. This technology thus provides a valuable tool to scientists, offering a user-friendly system that is relatively cheap to run and the exploitation of which avoids the legal, moral and ethical questions generally associated with animal experimentation.

In this chapter, fundamental information required for cell culture, together with a series of principles and outline protocols used routinely in growing animal, bacterial and plant cells are discussed. This should provide the basic knowledge for those new to the field of cell culture and act as a revision aid for those with limited experience in the field. Particular attention is paid to the importance of the work environment, outlining safety considerations together with adequate descriptions of the essential equipment required for tissue culture work.

2.2 THE CELL CULTURE LABORATORY AND EQUIPMENT

2.2.1 The cell culture laboratory

The design and maintenance of the cell culture laboratory is perhaps the most important aspect of cell culture, since a sterile surrounding is critical for handling of cells and culture media, which should be free from contaminating microorganisms. Such organisms, if left unchecked, would outgrow the cells being cultured, eventually resulting in culture-cell demise owing to the release of toxins and/or depletion of nutrient from the culture medium.

Where possible, a cell culture laboratory should be designed in such a way that it facilitates preparation of media and allows for the isolation, examination, evaluation and maintenance of cultures under controlled sterile conditions. In an ideal situation, there should be a room dedicated to each of the above tasks. However, many cell culture facilities, especially in academia, form part of an open plan laboratory and as such are limited in space. It is not unusual therefore to find an open plan area where places are designated for each of the above functions. This is not a serious problem as long as a few basic guidelines are adopted. For instance, good aseptic techniques (discussed below) should be used at all times. There should also be adequate facilities for media preparation, sterilisation and all cell culture materials should be maintained under sterile conditions until used. In addition, all surfaces within the culture area should be non-porous to prevent adsorption of media and other materials that may provide a good breeding ground for microorganisms, resulting in the infection of the cultures. Surfaces should also be easy to clean and all waste generated should be disposed of immediately. The disposal procedure may require prior autoclaving of the waste, which can be carried out using pressurized steam at 121 °C under 105 kPa for a defined period of time. These conditions are required to destroy microorganisms.

For smooth running of the facilities, daily checks should be made of the temperature in incubators, and of the gas supply to the incubators, by checking the CO_2 cylinder pressure. Water baths should be kept clean at all times and areas under the work surfaces of the flow cabinets cleaned of any spills.

2.2.2 Equipment for cell culture

Several pieces of equipment are essential. These include a tissue culture hood, incubator(s), autoclave and microscope. A brief description will be given of these and other essential equipments.

Cell culture hoods

The cell culture hood is the central piece of equipment where all the cell handling is carried out and is designed not only to protect the cultures from the operator but in some cases to protect the operator from the cultures. These hoods are generally referred to as laminar flow hoods as they generate a smooth uninterrupted stream-lined flow (laminar flow) of sterile air which has been filtered through a high efficiency particulate air (HEPA) filter. There are two types of laminar flow hood classified as either vertical or horizontal. The horizontal hoods allow air to flow directly at the operator and as a result are generally used for media preparation or when one is working with non-infectious materials including those derived from plants. The vertical hoods (also known as biology safety cabinets) are best for working with hazardous organisms, since air within the hood is filtered before it passes into the surrounding environment.

Currently, there are at least three different classes of hood used which all offer various levels of protection to the cultures, the operator or both and these are described below.

Class I hoods   These hoods, as with the class II type, have a screen at the front that provides a barrier between the operator and the cells but yet allows access into the hood through an opening at the bottom of the screen (Fig. 2.1). This barrier prevents too much turbulence to air flow from the outside and, more importantly, provides good protection for the operator. Cultures are also protected but to a lesser extent when compared to the class II hoods as the air drawn in from the outside is sucked through the inner cabinet to the top of the hood. These hoods are suitable for use with low risk organisms and when operator protection only is required.

Class II hoods   Class II hoods are the most common units found in tissue culture laboratories. These hoods offer good protection to both the operator and the cell culture. Unlike with class I hoods, air drawn from the outside is passed through the grill in the front of the work area and filtered through the HEPA filter at the top of the hood before streaming down over the tissue culture (Fig. 2.1). This mechanism protects the operator and ensures that the air over the cultures is largely sterile. These hoods are adequate for animal cell culture, which involves low to moderate toxic or infectious agents, but are not suitable for use with high-risk pathogens, which may require a higher level of containment.

Class III hoods   Class III safety cabinets are required when the highest levels of operator and product protection are required. These hoods are completely sealed, providing two glove pockets through which the operator can work with material inside the cabinet (Fig. 2.1). Thus the operator is completely shielded, making class III hoods suitable for work with highly pathogenic organisms including tissue samples carrying known human pathogens.

Practical hints and safety aspects of using cell culture hoods   All hoods must be maintained in a clutter free and clean state at all times as too much clutter may affect air flow and contamination will introduce infections. Thus, as a rule of thumb, put only items that are required inside the cabinet and clean all work surfaces before and after use with industrial methylated spirit (IMS). The latter is used at an effective concentration of 70% (prepared by adding 70% v/v IMS to 30% Milli-Q water),

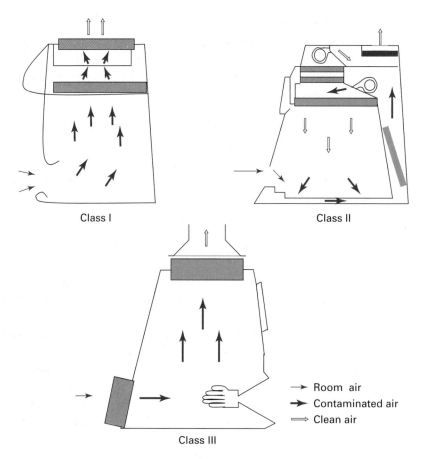

Fig. 2.1. Schematic representation of tissue culture cabinets.

which acts against bacteria and fungal spores by dehydrating and fixing cells, thus preventing contamination of cultures.

Some cabinets may be equipped with a short-wave ultraviolet light that can be used to irradiate the interior of the hood to kill microorganisms. When present, switch on the ultraviolet light for at least 15 min to sterilise the inside of the cabinet, including the work area. Note, however, that ultraviolet radiation can cause adverse damage to the skin and eyes and precaution should be taken at all times to ensure that the operator is not in direct contact with the ultraviolet light when using this option to sterilise the hood. Once finished, ensure that the front panel door (class I and II hoods) is replaced securely after use. In addition always turn the hood on for at least 10 min before starting work to allow the flow of air to stabilise. During this period, monitor the air flow and check all dials in the control panel at the front of the hood to ensure that they are within the safe margin.

CO_2 incubators

Water-jacketed incubators are required to facilitate optimal cell growth under strictly maintained and regulated conditions, normally requiring a constant temperature of 37 °C and an atmosphere of 5–10% CO_2 plus air. The purpose of the CO_2 is to ensure that the culture medium is maintained at the required physiological pH (usually pH 7.2–7.4). This is achieved by the supply of CO_2 from a gas cylinder into the incubator through a valve that is triggered to draw in CO_2 whenever the level fall below the set value of 5% or 10%. The CO_2 that enters the inner chamber of the incubator dissolves into the culture medium containing bicarbonate. The latter reacts with H^+ (generated from cellular metabolism), forming carbonic acid, which is in equilibrium with water and CO_2, thereby maintaining the pH in the medium at approximately pH 7.2.

$$HCO_3^- + H^+ \rightleftharpoons H_2CO_3 \rightleftharpoons CO_2 + H_2O$$

These incubators are generally humidified by the inclusion of a tray of sterile water to the bottom deck. The evaporation of water creates a highly humidified atmosphere, which helps to prevent evaporation of medium from the cultures.

An alternative to humidified incubators is the dry non-gassed unit that is not humidified and relies on the use of alternative buffering systems such as 4(2-hydroxyethyl)-1-piperazine-ethanesulphonic acid (Hepes) or morpholino-propane sulphonic acid (Mops) for maintaining a balanced pH within the culture medium. The advantage of this system is that it eliminates the risk from infections that can be posed by the tray of water in the humidified unit. The disadvantage, however, is that the culture medium will evaporate rapidly, thereby stressing the cells. One way round this problem is to place the cell culture plate in a sandwich box containing little pots of sterile water. With the sandwich box lid partially closed, evaporation of water from the pots will create a humidified atmosphere within the sandwich box, thus reducing the risk of evaporation of medium from the culture plate.

Practical hints and safety aspects of using cell culture incubators   The incubator should be maintained at 37 °C and supplied with 5% CO_2 at all times. A constant temperature can be maintained by keeping a thermometer in the incubator, preferably on the inside of the inner glass door. This can then be checked on a regular basis and adjustments made as required. CO_2 levels inside the unit can be monitored and adjusted by using a gas analyser such as the Fryrite Reader. Regular checks should also be made on the levels of CO_2 in the gas cylinders that supply CO_2 to the incubators and when necessary replaced when levels are very low. Most incubators are designed with an in-built alarm that sounds when the CO_2 level inside the chamber drops. At this point the gas cylinder must be replaced immediately to avoid stressing or killing the cultures. It is now possible to connect two gas cylinders to a cylinder change-over unit that switches automatically to the second source of gas supply when the first is empty. It is advisable therefore to use this device where possible.

When one is using a humidified incubator, it is essential that the water tray is maintained and kept free from microorganisms. This can be achieved by adding various agents to the water such as the antimicrobial agent Roccal at a concentration of 1%(w/v). Other products such as Thimerosal or SigmaClean from Sigma-Aldrich can also be used. Proper care and maintenance of the incubator should, however, include regular cleaning of the interior of the unit using any of the above reagents then swabbed with 70% IMS. More recently, copper-coated incubators have been introduced which, due to the antimicrobial properties of copper, are reported to reduce microbial contamination.

Microscopes

Inverted phase contrast microscopes (see Chapter 4) are routinely used for visualising cells in culture. These are expensive but easy to operate, with a light source located above and the objective lenses below the stage on which the cells are placed. Visualisation of cells by microscopy can provide useful information about the morphology and state of the cells. Early signs of cells stress may be easily identified and appropriate action taken to prevent loss of cultures.

Other general equipment

Several other pieces of equipment are required in cell culture. These include a centrifuge to spin down cells, a water bath for thawing frozen samples of cells and warming media to 37 °C before use, and a fridge and freezer for storage of media and other materials required for cell culture. Some cells need to attach onto a surface in order to grow and are therefore referred to as adherent. These cells are cultured in non-toxic polystyrene plastics that contain a biologically inert surface on which the cells attach and grow. Various types of plastics are available for this purpose and include Petri dishes, multi-well plates (with either 96, 24, 12 or 6 wells per plate) and screwcap flasks classified according to their surface areas: T-25, T-75, T-225 (cm² of surface area). A selection of these plastics is shown in Fig. 2.2.

2.3 SAFETY CONSIDERATIONS IN CELL CULTURE

Because of the nature of the work, safety in the cell culture laboratory must be of a major concern to the operator. This is particularly the case when one is working with pathogenic microbes or with fresh primate or human tissues or cells that may contain agents that use humans as hosts. One very good example of this would be working with fresh human lymphocytes, which may contain infectious agents such as the human immunodeficiency virus (HIV) and/or hepatitis B virus. Thus, when one is working with fresh human tissue, it is essential that the infection status of the donor is determined in advance of use and all necessary precautions taken to eliminate or limit the risks to which the operator is exposed. A recirculation class II cabinet would be a minimum requirement for this type of cell culture work and the operator should be provided with protective

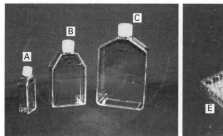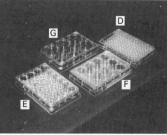

Fig. 2.2. Tissue culture plastics used generally for cell culture. (A–C) T-flasks; (D–G) representative of multi-well plates. (A) T–25 (25 cm²), (B) T-75 (75 cm²), (C) T–225 (225 cm²), (D) 96-well plate, (E) 24-well plate, (F) 12-well plate, and (G) 6-well plate.

clothing including latex gloves and a face mask if required. Such work should also be carried out under the guidelines laid down by the UK Advisory Committee on Dangerous Pathogens (ACDP).

Apart from the risks posed by the biological material being used, the operator should also be aware of his or her work environment and be fairly conversant with the equipment being used, as these may also pose a serious hazard. The culture cabinet should be serviced routinely and checked (approximately every 6 months) to ensure its safety to the operator. Additionally the operator could ensure his or her own safety by adopting some common precautionary measures such as refraining from eating or drinking whilst working in the cabinet and using a pipette aid as opposed to mouth pipetting to prevent ingestion of unwanted substances. Gloves and adequate protective clothing such as a clean laboratory coat should be worn at all times and gloves must be discarded after handling of non-sterile or contaminated material.

2.4 ASEPTIC TECHNIQUES AND GOOD CELL CULTURE PRACTICE

2.4.1 Good practice

In order to maintain a clean and safe culture environment, adequate aseptic or sterile technique should be adopted at all times. This simply involves working under conditions that prevent contaminating microorganisms from the environment from entering the cultures. Part of the precaution taken involves washing hands with antiseptic soap and ensuring that all work surfaces are kept clean and sterile by swabbing with 70% IMS before starting work. Moreover, all procedures, including media preparation and cell handling, should be carried out in a cell culture cabinet that is maintained in a clean and sterile condition.

Other essential precautions should include avoiding talking, sneezing or coughing into the cabinet or over the cultures. A clean pipette should be used for each different procedure and under no circumstance should the same pipette be used between different bottles of media, as this will significantly increase the risk of cross-contamination. All spillages must be cleaned quickly to avoid contamination from microorganisms that may be present in the air. Failing to do so may result in infections to the cultures, which may be reduced by using antibiotics. However, this is not always guaranteed and good aseptic techniques should eliminate the need for antibiotics. In the event of cultures becoming contaminated, these should be removed immediately from the laboratory, disinfected and autoclaved to prevent the contamination spreading. Under no circumstance can an infected culture be opened inside the cell culture cabinet or incubator. Moreover, all waste generated must be decontaminated and disposed of immediately after completing the work. This should be carried out in accordance with the national legislative requirements, which state that cell culture waste including media be inactivated using a disinfectant before disposal and that all contaminated materials and waste be autoclaved before being discarded or incinerated.

The risk from infections is the most common cause for concern in cell culture. Various factors can contribute to this, including poor work environment, poor aseptic techniques and indeed poor hygiene of the operator. The last of these is important, since most of the common sources of infections such as bacteria, yeast and fungus originate from the worker. Maintaining a clean environment and adopting good laboratory practice and aseptic techniques should, therefore, help to reduce the risks of infection. However, should infections occur, it is advisable to address this immediately and eradicate the problem. To do this, it helps to know the types of infection to expect and what to look for.

In animal cell cultures, bacterial and fungal infections are relatively easy to identify and isolate. The other most common contamination originates from mycoplasma. These are the smallest (approximately 0.3 μm in diameter) self-replicating prokaryotes in existence. They lack a rigid cell wall and generally infect the cytoplasm of mammalian cells. There are at least five species known to contaminate cells in culture: *Mycoplasma hyorhinis*, *Mycoplasma arginini*, *Mycoplasma orale*, *Mycoplasma fermentans* and *Acholeplasma laidlawii*. Infections caused by these organisms are more problematic and not easily identified or eliminated. Moreover, if left unchecked, mycoplasma contamination will cause subtle but adverse effects on cultures, including changes in metabolism, DNA, RNA and protein synthesis, morphology and growth. This can lead to non-reproducible, unreliable experimental results and unsafe biological products.

2.4.2 Identification and eradication of bacterial and fungal infections

Both bacterial and fungal contaminations are easily identified as the infective agents are readily visible to the naked eye even in the early stages. This is usually made noticeable by the increase in turbidity and the change in colour of the culture medium owing to the change in pH caused by the infection. In addition, bacteria can be easily identified under microscopic examination as motile round bodies. Fungi on the other hand are distinctive by their long hyphal growth and by the fuzzy colonies they form in the medium. In most cases the simplest solution to these infections is to remove and dispose of the contaminated cultures. In the early stages of an infection, attempts can be made to eliminate the infecting microorganism using repeated washes and incubations with antibiotics or anti-fungal agents but this is not advisable as handling infected cultures in the sterile work environment increases the chances of the infection spreading.

As part of the good laboratory practice, sterile testing of cultures should be carried out regularly to ensure that cultures are free from microbial organisms. This is particularly important when preparing cell culture products or generating cells for storage. Generally, the presence of these organisms can be detected much earlier and necessary precautions taken to avoid a full-blown contamination crisis in the laboratory. The testing procedure usually involves culturing a suspension of cells or products in an appropriate medium such as tryptone soya broth (TSB) for bacterial or thioglycollate medium (TGM) for fungal detection. The mixture is incubated for up to 14 days but examined daily for turbidity, which is used as an indication of microbial growth. It is essential that both positive and negative controls are set up in parallel with the sample to be tested. For this purpose a suspension of bacteria such as *Bacillus subtilis* or fungus such as *Clostridium sporogenes* is used instead of the cells or product to be tested. Uninoculated flasks containing only the growth medium are used as negative controls. Any contamination in the cell cultures will result in the broth appearing turbid, as would the positive controls. The negative controls should remain clear. Infected cultures should be discarded, whilst clear cultures would be safe to use or keep.

2.4.3 Identification of mycoplasma infections

Mycoplasma contaminations are more prevalent in cell culture than many workers realise. The reason for this is that mycoplasma contaminations are not evident under light microscopy nor do they result in a turbid growth in culture. Instead the changes induced are more subtle and manifest themselves mainly as a slow-down in growth and in changes in cellular metabolism and functions. However, cells generally return to their native morphology and normal proliferation rates relatively rapidly after eradication of mycoplasma.

The presence of mycoplasma contamination in cultures has, until recently, been difficult to determine and samples had to be analysed by specialist laboratories. There are, however, improved techniques now available for detection of mycoplasma in cell culture laboratories. These involve either microbiological cultures of infected cells or an indirect DNA staining technique using the fluorochrome dye Hoechst 33258. With the former technique, cells in suspension are inoculated into liquid broth and then incubated under aerobic conditions at 37 °C for 14 days. A non-inoculated flask of broth is used as a negative control. Aliquots of broth are taken every 3 days and inoculated onto an agar plate, which is incubated anaerobically as above. All plates are then examined under an inverted microscope at a magnification of 300× after 14 days of incubation. Positive cultures will show the typical mycoplasma colony formation, which has an opaque granular central zone surrounded by a translucent border, giving a 'fried egg' appearance (Fig. 2.3). It may be necessary to set up positive controls in parallel,

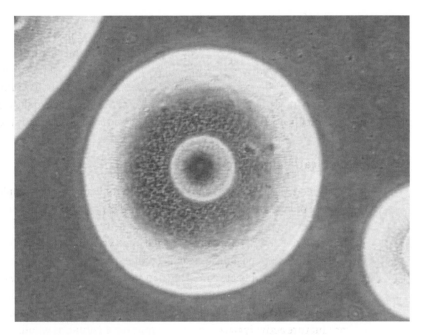

Fig. 2.3. Photograph of mycoplasma, showing the characteristic opaque granular central zone surrounded by a translucent border, giving a 'fried egg' appearance.

in which case plates and broth should be inoculated with a known strain of mycoplasma such as *Mycoplasma orale* or *Mycoplasma pneumoniae*.

The DNA binding method offers a rapid alternative for detecting mycoplasma and works on the principle that Hoechst 33258 fluoresces under ultraviolet light once bound to DNA. Thus, in contaminated cells, the fluorescence will be fairly dispersed in the cytoplasm of the cells owing to the presence of mycoplasma. In contrast, uncontaminated cells will show localised fluorescence in their nucleus only.

The Hoechst 33258 assay, although rapid, is relatively less sensitive when compared with the culture technique described above. For this assay, an aliquot of the culture to be tested is placed on a sterile coverslip in a 35 mm culture dish and incubated at 37 °C in a cell culture incubator to allow cells to adhere. The coverslip is then fixed by adding a fixative consisting of 1 part glacial acetic acid and 3 parts methanol, prepared fresh on the day. A freshly prepared solution of Hoechst 33258 stain is added to the fixed coverslip, incubated in the dark at room temperature to allow the dye to bind to the DNA and then viewed under ultraviolet fluorescence at 1000×. All positive cultures will show fluorescence of mycoplasma DNA, which will appear as small cocci or filaments in the cytoplasm of the contaminated cells (Fig. 2.4b, see colour section). Negative cultures will show only fluorescing nuclei of uncontaminated cells against a dark cytoplasmic background (Fig. 2.4a, see colour section). However, this technique is prone to errors, including false-negative results. To avoid the latter, cells should be cultured in antibiotic-free medium for two to three passages before being used. A positive control using a strain of mycoplasma seeded onto a cover slip is essential. Such controls should be handled away from the cell culture laboratory to avoid contaminating clean cultures of cells. It is also important to ensure that the fluorescence detected is not due to the presence of bacterial contamination or debris embedded into the plastics during manufacture. The former normally appear larger than the fluorescing cocci or filaments of mycoplasma. Debris, on the other hand, would show a non-uniform fluorescence owing to the variation in size of the particles usually found in plastics.

2.4.4 Eradication of mycoplasma

Until recently, the most common approach for eradicating mycoplasma has been the use of antibiotics such as gentamycin. This approach is, however, not always effective, as not all strains of mycoplasma are susceptible to this antibiotic. Moreover antibiotic therapy does not always result in long-lasting successful elimination and most drugs can be cytotoxic to the cell culture. More recently, a new generation of bactericidal antibiotic preparation referred to as Plasmocin™ was introduced and has been shown to be effective against mycoplasma even at relatively low, non-cytotoxic concentrations. The antibiotics contained in this product are actively transported into cells, thus facilitating killing of intracellular mycoplasma but without any adverse effects on actual cellular metabolism.

Apart from antibiotics, various products have also been introduced into the cell culture market that the manufacturers claim eradicate mycoplasma efficiently and quickly without causing any adverse effects to the cells. One such product is Mynox®, a biological agent that integrates into the membrane of mycoplasma, compromising its integrity and eventually initiating its disintegration. This process apparently occurs within an hour of applying Mynox® and may have the added advantage that it is not an antibiotic and as a result will not lead to the development of resistant strains. It is safe to cultures and eliminated once the medium has been replaced. Moreover, this reagent is highly sensitive, detecting as little as 1–5 fg of mycoplasma DNA, which corresponds to two to five mycoplasma per sample and is effective against many of the common mycoplasma contaminations encountered in cell culture.

2.5 TYPES OF ANIMAL CELL AND THEIR CHARACTERISTICS IN CULTURE

The cell types used in cell culture fall into two categories generally referred to as either a primary culture or a cell line.

2.5.1 Primary cell cultures

Primary cultures are cells derived directly from tissues following enzymatic dissociation or from tissue fragments referred to as explants. These are usually the cells of preference, since it is argued that primary cultures retain their characteristics and reflect the true activity of the cell type *in vivo*. The disadvantage in using primary cultures, however, is that their isolation can be labour intensive and may produce a heterogeneous population of cells. Moreover primary cultures have a relatively limited life span and can be used over only a limited period of time in culture.

Primary cultures can be obtained from many different tissues and the source of tissue used generally defines the cell type isolated. For instance, cells isolated from the endothelium of blood vessels are referred to as endothelial cells whilst those isolated from the medial layer of the blood vessels and other similar tissues are smooth muscle cells. Although both can be obtained from the same vessels, endothelial cells are different in morphology and function, generally growing as a single monolayer characterised by a cobble-stoned morphology. Smooth muscle cells on the other hand are elongated, with spindle-like projections at either end and grow in layers even when maintained in culture. In addition to these cell types there are several other widely used primary cultures derived from a diverse range of tissues, including fibroblasts from connective tissue, lymphocytes from blood, neurones from nervous tissues and hepatocytes from liver tissue.

2.5.2 Continuous cell lines

Cell lines consist of a single cell type that has gained the ability for infinite growth. This usually occurs after transformation of cells by one of several means that include treatment with carcinogens or exposure to viruses such as the monkey Simian virus 40 (SV40), Epstein–Barr virus (EBV) or Abelson murine leukaema virus (A-MuLV) amongst others. These treatments cause the cells to lose their ability to regulate growth. As a result, transformed cells grow continuously and, unlike primary culture, have an infinite life span (become 'immortalised'). The drawback to this is that transformed cells generally lose some of their original *in vivo* characteristics. For instance, certain established cell lines do not express particular tissue-specific genes. One good example of this is the inability of liver cell lines to produce clotting factors. Continuous cell lines, however, have several advantages over primary cultures, not least because they are immortalised. In addition, they require less serum for growth, have a shorter doubling time and can grow without necessarily needing to attach or adhere to the surface of the flask.

Many different cell lines are currently available from various cell banks, which makes it easier to obtain these cells without having to generate them. One of the largest organisations that supplies cell lines is the European Collection of Animal Cell Cultures (ECACC) based in Salisbury, UK. A selection of the different cell lines supplied by this organisation is listed in Table 2.1.

2.5.3 Cell culture media and growth requirements for animal cells

The cell culture medium used for animal cell growth is a complex mixture of nutrients (amino acids, a carbohydrate such as glucose, and vitamins), inorganic salts (e.g. containing magnesium, sodium, potassium, calcium, phosphate, chloride, sulphate, and bicarbonate ions) and broad-spectrum antibiotics. In

Table 2.1	Some commonly used cell lines supplied by cell banks		
Cell line	Morphology	Species	Tissue origin
BAE-1	Endothelial	Bovine	Aorta
BHK-21	Fibroblast	Syrian hamster	Kidney
CHO	Fibroblast	Chinese hamster	Ovary
COS-1/7	Fibroblast	African green monkey	Kidney
HeLa	Epithelial	Human	Cervix
HEK-293	Epithelial	Human	Kidney
HT-29	Epithelial	Human	Colon
MRC-5	Fibroblast	Human	Lung
NCI-H660	Epithelial	Human	Lung
NIH/3T3	Fibroblast	Mouse	Embryo
THP-1	Monocytic	Human	Blood
V-79	Fibroblasts	Chinese hamster	Lung
HEP1	Hepatocytes	Human	Liver

certain situations it may be essential to include a fungicide such as amphotericin B, although this may not always be necessary. For convenience and ease of monitoring the status of the medium, the pH indicator phenol red may also be included. This will change from red at pH 7.2–7.4 to yellow or fuchsia as the pH becomes either acidic or alkaline, respectively.

The other key basic ingredient in the cell culture medium is serum, usually bovine or fetal calf. This is used to provide a buffer for the culture medium, but, more importantly, enhances cell attachment and provides additional nutrients and hormone-like growth factors that promote healthy growth of cells. An attempt to culture cells in the absence of serum does not usually result in successful or healthy cultures, even though cells can produce growth factors of their own. However, despite these benefits, the use of serum is increasingly being questioned not least because of many of the other unknowns that can be introduced, including infectious agents such as viruses and mycoplasma. The more recent resurgence of 'mad cow disease' (bovine spongioform encephalitis) has introduced an additional drawback, posing a particular risk for the cell culturist and has increased the need for alternative products. In this regard, several cell culture reagent manufacturers have now developed serum-free medium supplemented with various components including albumin, transferrin, insulin, growth factors and other essential elements required for optimal cell growth. This is proving very useful, particularly for the pharmaceutical and biotechnology companies involved in the manufacture of drugs or biological products for human and animal consumption.

2.5.4 Preparation of animal cell culture medium

Preparation of the culture medium is perhaps taken for granted as a simple straightforward procedure that is often not given due care and attention. As a result, most infections in cell culture laboratories originate from infected media. Following the simple yet effective procedures outlined in Section 2.4.1 should prevent or minimise the risk of infecting the media when they are being prepared.

Preparation of the medium itself should also be carried out inside the culture cabinet and usually involves adding a required amount of serum together with antibiotics to a fixed volume of medium. The amount of serum used will depend on the cell type but usually varies between 10% and 20%. The most common antibiotics used are penicillin and streptomycin, which inhibit a wide spectrum of Gram-positive and Gram-negative bacteria. Penicillin acts by inhibiting the last step in bacterial cell wall synthesis whilst streptomycin blocks protein synthesis.

Once prepared, the mixture, which is referred to as complete growth medium, should be kept at 4 °C until used. To minimise wastage and risk of contamination it is advisable to make just the required volume of medium and use this within a short period of time. As an added precaution it is also advisable always to check the clarity of the medium before use. Any infected medium, which will appear cloudy or turbid, should be discarded immediately. In addition to checking the clarity, a close eye should also be kept on the colour of the medium, which should be red at physiological pH owing to the presence of phenol red. Media that looks acidic (yellow) or alkaline (fuchsia) should be discarded, as these extremes will affect the viability and thus growth of the cells.

2.5.5 Subculture of cells

Subculturing is the process by which cells are harvested, diluted in fresh growth medium and replaced in a new culture flask to promote further growth. This process, also known as passaging, is essential if the cells are to be maintained in a healthy and viable state, otherwise they may die after a certain period in continuous culture. The reason for this is that adherent cells grow in a continuous layer that eventually occupies the whole surface of the culture dish and at this point they are said to be confluent. Once confluent, the cells stop dividing and go into a resting state where they stop growing (senesce) and eventually die. Thus, to keep cells viable and facilitate efficient transformation, they must be subcultured before they reach full contact inhibition. Ideally, cells should be harvested just before they reach a confluent state.

Cells can be harvested and subcultured using one of several techniques. The precise method used is dependent to a large extent on whether the cells are adherent or in suspension.

Subculture of adherent cells   Adherent cells can be harvested either mechanically, using a rubber spatula (also referred to as a rubber policeman) or enzymatically using proteolytic enzymes. Cells in suspension are simply diluted in fresh medium by taking a given volume of cell suspension and adding an equal volume of medium.

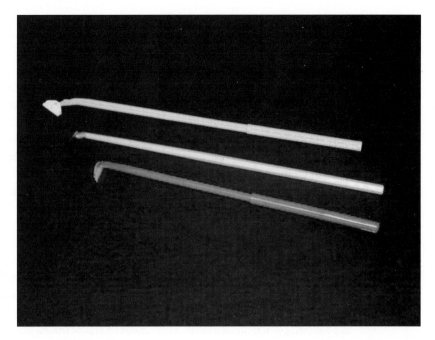

Fig. 2.5. Cell scrapers.

Harvesting of cells mechanically   This method is simple and easy. It involves gently scraping cells from the growth surface into the culture medium using a rubber spatula that has a rigid polystyrene handle with a soft polyethylene scraping blade (Fig. 2.5). This method is not suitable for all cell types as the scraping may result in membrane damage and significant cell death. Before adopting this approach it is important to carry out some test runs where cell viability and growth are monitored in a small sample of cells following harvesting.

Harvesting of cells using proteolytic enzymes   Several different proteolytic enzymes can be exploited including trypsin, a proteolytic enzyme that destroys proteinaceous connections between cells and between cells and the surface of the flask in which they grow. As a result, harvesting of cells using this enzyme results in the release of single cells, which is ideal for subculturing as each cell will then divide and grow, thus enhancing the propagation of the cultures.

Trypsin is commonly used in combination with EDTA, which enhances the action of the enzyme. EDTA alone can also be effective in detaching adherent cells as it chelates the Ca^{2+} required by some adhesion molecules that facilitate cell–cell or cell–matrix interactions. Although EDTA alone is much gentler on the cells than trypsin, some cell types may adhere strongly to the plastic, requiring trypsin to detach.

The standard procedure for detaching adherent cells using trypsin and EDTA involves making a working solution of 0.1% trypsin plus 0.02% EDTA in Ca^{2+}/Mg^{2+}-free phosphate-buffered saline. The growth medium is aspirated from confluent cultures and washed at least twice with a serum-free medium such as Ca^{2+} or Mg^{2+}-free PBS to remove traces of serum that may inactivate the trypsin. The trypsin-EDTA solution (approximately $1\,cm^3$ per $25\,cm^2$ of surface area) is then added to the cell monolayer and swirled around for a few seconds. Excess trypsin-EDTA is aspirated, leaving just enough to form a thin film over the monolayer. The flask is then incubated at $37\,°C$ in a cell culture incubator for 2–5 min but monitored under an inverted light microscope at intervals to detect when the cells are beginning to round up and detach. This is to ensure that the cells are not overexposed to trypsin, as this may result in extensive damage to the cell surface, eventually resulting in cell death. It is important therefore that the proteolysis reaction is quickly terminated by the addition of complete medium containing serum that will inactivate the trypsin. The suspension of cells is collected into a sterile centrifuge tube and spun at 1000 r.p.m. for 10 min to pellet the cells, which are then resuspended in a known volume of fresh complete culture medium to give a required density of cells per cubic centimetre volume.

As with all tissue culture procedures, aseptic techniques should be adopted at all times. This means that all the above procedures should be carried out in a tissue culture cabinet under sterile conditions. Other precautions worth noting include the handling of the trypsin stock. This should be stored frozen at $-20\,°C$ and, when needed, placed in a waterbath just to the point where it thaws. Any additional time in the $37\,°C$ waterbath will inactivate the enzymatic activity of the trypsin. The working solution should be kept at $4\,°C$ once made and can be stored for up to 3 months.

Subculture of cells in suspension   For cells in suspension it is important initially to examine an aliquot of cells under a microscope to establish whether cultures are growing as single cells or clumps. If cultures are growing as single cells, an aliquot is counted as described in Section 2.5.6 below and then reseeded at the desired seeding density in a new flask by simply diluting the cell suspension with fresh medium, provided the original medium in which the cells were growing is not spent. However, if the medium is spent and appears acidic, then the cells must be centrifuged at 1000 r.p.m. for 10 min, resuspended in fresh medium and transferred into a new flask. Cells that grow in clumps should first be centrifuged and resuspended in fresh medium as single cells using a glass Pasteur or fine-bore pipette.

2.5.6 Cell quantification

It is essential that when cells are subcultured they are seeded at the appropriate seeding density that will facilitate optimum growth. If cells are seeded at a lower seeding density they may take longer to reach confluency and some may expire before getting to this point. On the other hand, if seeded at a high density, cells will reach confluency too quickly, resulting in irreproducible experimental results. This is because trypsin can digest surface proteins, including receptors for drugs, and these will need time (sometimes several days) to renew. Failure to allow these

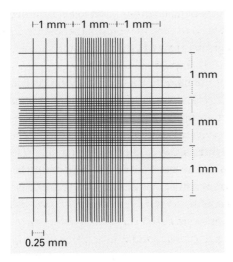

Fig. 2.6. Haemocytometer.

proteins to be regenerated on the cell surface may therefore result in variable responses to drugs specific for such receptors.

Several techniques are now available for quantification of cells and of these the most common method involves the use of a haemocytometer. This has the added advantage of being simple and cheap to use. The haemocytometer itself is a thickened glass slide that has a small chamber of grids cut into the glass. The chamber has a fixed volume and is etched into nine large squares, of which the large corner squares contain 16 small squares each; each large square measures 1 mm × 1 mm and is 0.1 mm deep (see Fig. 2.6).

Thus, with a coverslip in place, each square represents a volume of 0.1 mm^3 (1.0 mm^2 area × 0.1 mm depth) or 10^{-4} cm^3. Knowing this, the cell concentration (and the total number of cells) can therefore be determined and expressed per cubic centimetre. The general procedure involves loading approximately 10 µl of a cell suspension into a clean haemocytometer chamber and counting the cells within the four corner squares with the aid of a microscope set at 20× magnification. The count is mathematically converted to the number of cells/cm^3 of suspension.

To ensure accuracy, the coverslip must be firmly in place and this can be achieved by moistening a coverslip with exhaled breath and gently sliding it over the haemocytometer chamber, pressing firmly until Newton's refraction rings (usually rainbow-like) appear under the coverslip. The total number of cells in each of the four 1 mm^3 corner squares should be counted, with the proviso that only cells touching the top or left borders but not those touching the bottom and right borders are counted. Moreover, cells outside the large squares, even if they are within the field of view, should not be counted. When present, clumps should be counted as one cell. Ideally >100 cells should be counted to ensure a high degree of accuracy in counting. If the total cell count is less than 100 or if more than 10% of the cells counted appear to be clustered, then the original cell suspension should be thoroughly mixed and the counting procedure repeated. Similarly, if the total cell count is greater than 400, the suspension should be diluted further to get counts of between 100 and 400 cells.

Since some cells may not survive the trypsinisation procedure it is usually advisable to add an equal volume of the dye trypan blue to a small aliquot of the cell suspension before counting. This dye is excluded by viable cells but taken up by dead cells. Thus, when viewed under the microscope, viable cells will appear as bright translucent structures while dead cells will stain blue (see Section 2.5.12). The number of dead cells can therefore be excluded from the total cell count, ensuring that the seeding density accurately reflects viable cells.

Calculating cell number

Cell number is usually expressed per cubic centimetre and is determined by multiplying the average of the number of cells counted by a conversion factor that is constant for each haemocytometer. The conversion factor is estimated at 1000, based on the fact that each large square counted represents a total volume of $10^{-4} cm^3$.
Thus:

$$\text{cells cm}^{-3} = \frac{\text{number of cells counted}}{\text{number of squares counted}} \times \text{conversion factor}$$

If the cells were diluted before counting then the dilution factor should also be taken into account. Therefore:

$$\text{cells cm}^{-3} = \frac{\text{number of cells counted}}{\text{number of squares counted}} \times \text{conversion factor} \times \text{dilution factor}$$

To find the total number of cells harvested, the number of cells determined per cubic centimetre should be multiplied by the original volume of fluid from which the cell sample was removed, i.e.:

$$\text{total cells} = \text{cells cm}^{-3} \times \text{total volume of cells}$$

Alternative methods for determination of cell number

Several other methods are available for quantifying cells in culture, including direct measurement using an electronic Coulter counter. This is an automated method of counting and measuring the size of microscopic particles. The instrument itself consists of a glass probe with an electrode that is connected to an oscilloscope (Fig. 2.7). The probe has a small aperture of fixed diameter near its bottom end. When immersed in a solution of cell suspension, cells are flushed through the aperture causing a brief increase in resistance owing to a partial interruption of current flow. This will result in spikes being recorded on the oscilloscope and each spike is counted as a cell. One disadvantage of this method, however, is that it does not distinguish between viable and dead cells.

Example 1 CALCULATION OF CELL NUMBER

Question

Calculate the total number of cells suspended in a final volume of 5 cm³, taking into account that the cells were diluted 1:2 before counting and the number of cells counted with the haemocytometer was 400.

Answer

$$\text{cells cm}^{-3} = \frac{\text{number of cells counted}}{\text{large squares counted}} \times \text{conversion factor}$$

$$= \frac{400}{4} \times 1000$$

$$= 100\,000 \text{ cells cm}^{-3}$$

Because there is a dilution factor of 2, the correct number of cells cm⁻³ is given as:

100 000 × 2 = 200 000 cells cm⁻³

Thus, in a final volume of 5 cm³, the total number of cells present is:

200 000 × 5 = 1 000 000 cells

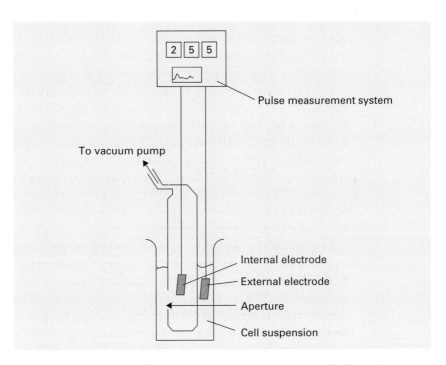

Fig. 2.7. Coulter counter. Cells entering the aperture create a pulse of resistance between the internal and external electrodes that is recorded on the oscilloscope.

Indirectly, cells can be counted by determining total cell protein and using a protein versus cell number standard curve to determine cell number in test samples. However, protein content per cell can vary during culture and may not give a true reflection of cell number. Alternatively, the DNA content of cells may be used as an indicator of cell number, since the DNA content of diploid cells is usually constant. However, the DNA content of cells may change during the cell cycle and therefore not give an accurate estimate of cell number.

2.5.7 Seeding cells onto culture plates

Once counted, cells should then be seeded at a density that promotes optimal cell growth. It is essential therefore that when cells are subcultured they are seeded at the appropriate seeding density. If cells are seeded at a lower density they may take longer to reach confluency and some may die before getting to this point. On the other hand, if seeded at too high a density cells will reach confluency too quickly, resulting in irreproducible experimental results as already discussed above (see Section 2.5.6). The seeding density will vary depending on the cell type and on the surface area of the culture flask into which the cells will be placed. These factors should therefore be taken into account when deciding on the seeding density of any given cell type and the purpose of the experiments carried out.

2.5.8 Maintenance of cells in culture

It is important that after seeding, flasks are clearly labelled with the date, cell type and the number of times the cells have been subcultured or passaged. Moreover, a strict regime of feeding and subculturing should be established that permits cells to be fed at regular intervals without allowing the medium to be depleted of nutrients or the cells to overgrow or become super confluent. This can be achieved by following a standard but routine procedure for maintaining cells in a viable state under optimum growth conditions. In addition, cultures should be examined daily under a inverted microscope, looking particularly for changes in morphology and cell density. Cell shape can be an important guide when determining the status of growing cultures. Round or floating cells in subconfluent cultures are not usually a good sign and may indicate distressed or dying cells. The presence of abnormally large cells can also be useful in determining the well-being of the cells, since the number of such cells increases as a culture ages or becomes less viable. Extremes in pH should be avoided by regularly replacing spent medium with fresh medium. This may be carried out on alternate days until the cultures are approximately 90% confluent, at which point the cells are either used for experimentation or trypsinised and subcultured following the procedures outlined in Section 2.5.5.

The volume of medium added to the cultures will depend on the confluency of the cells and the surface area of the flasks in which the cells are grown. As a guide, cells which are under 25% confluent may be cultured in approximately 1 cm^3 of medium per 5 cm^2 and those between 25% and 40% or $\geq$45% confluency should be supplemented with 1. 5 cm^3 or 2 cm^3 culture medium per 5 cm^2, respectively. When changing the medium it is advisable to pipette the latter on either to the sides or the opposite surface of the flask from where the cells are attached. This is to avoid making direct contact with the monolayers as this will damage or dislodge the cells.

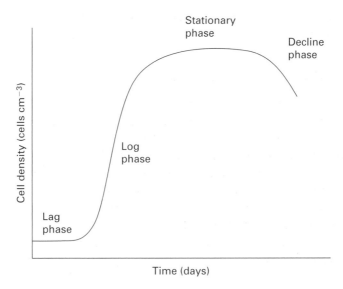

Fig. 2.8. Growth curve showing the phases of cell growth in culture.

2.5.9 **Growth kinetics of animal cells in culture**

When maintained under optimum culture conditions, cells follow a characteristic growth pattern (Fig. 2.8), exhibiting an initial lag phase in which there is enhanced cellular activity but no apparent increase in cell growth. The duration of this phase is dependent on several factors including the viability of the cells, the density at which the cells are plated and the media component.

The lag phase is followed by a log phase in which there is an exponential increase in cell number with high metabolic activity. These cells eventually reach a stationary phase where is there no further increase in growth due to depletion of nutrients in the medium, accumulation of toxic metabolic waste or a limitation in available growth space. If left unattended, cells in the stationary phase will eventually begin to die, resulting in the decline phase on the growth curve.

2.5.10 **Cryopreservation of cells**

Cells can be preserved for later use by freezing stocks in liquid nitrogen. This process is referred to as cryopreservation and is an efficient way of sustaining stocks. Indeed, it is advisable that, when good cultures are available, aliquots of cells should be stored in the frozen state. This provides a renewable source of cells that could be used in future without one necessarily having to culture new batches from tissues. Freezing can, however, result in several lethal changes within the cells, including formation of ice crystals and changes in the concentration of electrolytes and in pH. To minimise these risks a cryoprotective agent such as DMSO is usually added to the cells prior to freezing in order to lower the freezing point and prevent ice crystals from forming inside the cells. In addition, the freezing process is carried out in stages, allowing the cells initially to cool down slowly from room temperature to $-80\,°C$ at a rate of 1–3 deg.C min^{-1}. This initial stage can be carried out using a freezing chamber or alternatively a cryo freezing container ('Mr Frosty') filled with isopropanol, which provides the critical, repeatable -1 deg.C min^{-1} cooling rate required for successful cell cryopreservation. When this process is complete, the cryogenic vials, which are polypropylene tubes that can withstand temperatures as low as $-190\,°C$, are removed and immediately placed in a liquid nitrogen storage tank where they can remain for an indefinite period or until required.

The actual cryogenic procedure is itself relatively straightforward and involves harvesting cells as described in Section 2.5.5 and resuspending them in 1 cm^3 of freezing medium, which is basically culture medium containing 40% serum. The cell suspension is counted and appropriately diluted to give a final cell count of between 10^6 and 10^7 cells cm^{-3}. A 0.9 cm^3 aliquot is transferred into a cryogenic vial labelled with the cell type, passage number and date harvested. This is then made up to 1 cm^3 by adding 100 mm^3 of DMSO to give a final concentration of 10%. The cells should then be mixed gently by rotating or inverting the vial and placed in a 'Mr. Frosty' cryo freezing container. The container and cells should then be placed in a $-80\,°C$ freezer and allowed to freeze overnight. The frozen vials may then be transferred into a liquid nitrogen storage container. At this stage cells can be stored frozen until required for use.

All procedures should be carried out under sterile conditions to avoid contaminating cultures as this will appear once the frozen stocks are recultured. As an added precaution it is advisable to replace the growth medium in the 24 h period prior to harvesting cells for freezing. Moreover, cells used for freezing should be in the log phase of growth and not too confluent in case they may already be in growth arrest.

2.5.11 Resuscitation of frozen cells

When required, frozen stocks of cells may be revived by removing the cryogenic vial from storage in liquid nitrogen and placed in a waterbath at 37 °C for 1–2 min or until the ice crystals melt. It is important that the vials are not allowed to warm up to 37 °C as this may cause the cells to rapidly die. The thawed cell suspension may then be transferred into a centrifuge tube, to which fresh medium is added and centrifuged at 1000 r.p.m. for 10 min. The supernatant should be discarded to remove the DMSO used in the freezing process and the cell pellet resuspended in 1 cm^3 of fresh medium, ensuring that clumps are dispersed into single cells or much smaller clusters using a glass Pasteur pipette. The required amount of fresh pre-warmed growth medium is placed in a culture flask and the cells pipetted into the flask, which is then placed in a cell culture incubator and the cells allowed to adhere and grow.

2.5.12 Determination of cell viability

Determination of cell viability is extremely important, since the survival and growth of the cells may depend on the density at which they are seeded. The degree of viability is most commonly determined by differentiating living from dead cells using the dye exclusion method. Basically, living cells exclude certain dyes that are readily taken up by dead cells. As a result, dead cells stain the colour of the dye used whilst living cells remain refractile owing to the inability of the dye to penetrate into the cytoplasm. One of the most commonly used dyes in such assays is trypan blue. This is incubated at a concentration of 0.4% with cells in suspension and applied to a haemocytometer. The haemocytometer is then viewed under an inverted microscope set at $100\times$ magnification and the cells counted as described in Section 2.5.6, keeping separate counts for viable and non-viable cells.

The total number of cells is calculated using the following equation, as described previously:

$$\text{cells cm}^{-3} = \frac{\text{number of cells counted}}{\text{number of squares counted}} \times \text{conversion factor} \times \text{dilution factor}$$

and the percentage of viable cells determined using the following formula:

$$\% \text{ viability} = \frac{\text{number of unstained cells counted}}{\text{total number of cells counted}} \times 100$$

To avoid underestimating cell viability it is important that the cells are not exposed to the dye for more than 5 min before counting. This is because uptake of trypan blue is time sensitive and the dye may be taken up by viable cells during prolonged incubation periods. Additionally, trypan blue has a high affinity for serum proteins and as such may produce a high background staining. The cells should therefore be free from serum, which can be achieved by washing the cells with PBS before counting.

2.6 BACTERIAL CELL CULTURE

As with animal cells, pure bacterial cultures (cultures that contain only one species of organism) are cultivated routinely and maintained indefinitely using standard sterile techniques that are now well defined. However, since bacterial cells exhibit a much wider degree of diversity in terms of both their nutritional and environmental requirements, conditions for their cultivation are diverse and the precise requirements highly dependent on the species being cultivated. Outlined below are general procedures and precautions adopted in bacterial cell culture.

2.6.1 Safety considerations for bacterial cells culture

Culture of microbial cells, like that involving cells of animal origin, requires care and sterile techniques, not least of all to prevent accidental contamination of pure cultures with other organisms. More importantly, utmost care should be given towards protecting the operator, especially from potentially harmful organisms. Aseptic techniques and safety conditions described for animal cell culture should be adopted at all times. Additionally, instruments used during the culturing procedures should be sterilised before and after use by heating in a Bunsen burner flame. Moreover, to avoid spread of bacteria, areas of work must be decontaminated after use using germicidal sprays and/or ultraviolet radiation. This is to prevent airborne bacteria from spreading rapidly. In line with these precautions, all materials used in microbial cell culture work must be disposed of appropriately; for instance, autoclaving of all plastics and tissue culture waste before disposal is usually essential.

2.6.2 Nutritional requirements of bacteria

The growth of bacteria requires much simpler conditions than those described for animal cells. However, due to their diversity, the composition of the medium used may be variable and largely determined by the nutritional classification of the organisms to be cultured. These generally fall into two main categories classified as either autotrophs (self-feeding organisms that synthesise food in the form of sugars using light energy from the sun) or heterotrophs (non-self-feeding organisms that derive chemical energy by breaking down organic molecules consumed). These in turn are subgrouped into chemo or photo autotrophs or heterotrophs. Both chemo- and photoautotrophs rely on carbon dioxide as a source of carbon but derive energy from completely different sources, with the chemoautotrophs utilising inorganic substances whilst the photoautotrophs use light. Chemoheterotrophs and photoheterotrophs both use organic compounds as the main source of carbon with the photoheterotrophs using light for energy and the chemo subgroup getting their energy from the metabolism of organic substances.

2.6.3 Culture media for bacterial cell culture

Several different types of medium are used to culture bacteria and these can be categorised as either complex or defined. The former usually consist of natural substances, including meat and yeast extract, and as a result are less well defined, since their precise composition is largely unknown. Such media are, however, rich in nutrients and therefore generally suitable for culturing fastidious organisms that require a mixture of nutrients for growth. Defined media, by contrast, are relatively simple. These are usually designed to the specific needs of the bacterial species to be cultivated and as a result are made up of known components put together in the required amounts. This flexibility is usually exploited to select or eliminate certain species by taking advantage of their distinguishing nutritional requirements. For instance, bile salts may be included in media when selective cultivation of enteric bacteria (rod-shaped Gram-negative bacteria such as *Salmonella* or *Shigella*) is required, since growth of most other Gram-positive and Gram-negative bacteria will be inhibited.

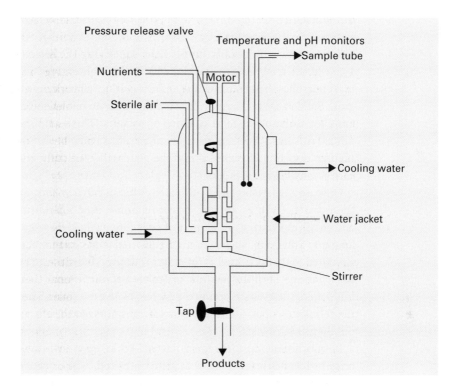

Fig. 2.9. Schematic representation of a fermenter.

2.6.4 **Culture procedures for bacterial cells**

Bacteria can be cultured in the laboratory using either liquid or solid media. Liquid media are normally dispensed into flasks and inoculated with an aliquot of the organism to be grown. This is then agitated continuously on a shaker that rotates in an orbital manner, mixing and ensuring that cultures are kept in suspension. For such cultures, sufficient space should be allowed above the medium to facilitate adequate diffusion of oxygen into the solution. Thus, as a rule of thumb, the volume of medium added to the flasks should not exceed more than 20% of the total volume of the flask. This is particularly important for aerobic bacteria and less so for anaerobic microorganisms.

In large-scale culture, fermenters or bioreactors equipped with stirring devices for improved mixing and gas exchange may be used. The device (Fig. 2.9) is usually fitted with probes that monitor changes in pH, oxygen concentration and temperature. In addition most systems are surrounded by a water jacket with fast flowing cold water to reduce the heat generated during fermentation. Outlets are also included to release CO_2 and other gases produced by cell metabolism.

When fermenters are used, precautions should be taken to reduce potential contamination with airborne microorganisms when air is bubbled through the cultures. Sterilisation of the air may therefore be necessary and can be achieved by introducing a filter (pore size of approximately 0.2 μm) at the point of entry of the air flow into the chamber.

Solid medium is usually prepared by solidifying the selected medium with 1–2% of the seaweed extract agar, which, although organic, is not degraded by most microbes thereby providing an inert gelling medium on which bacteria can grow. Solid agar media are widely used to separate mixed cultures and form the basis for isolation of pure cultures of bacteria. This is achieved by streaking diluted cultures of bacteria onto the surface of an agar plate by using a sterile inoculating loop. Cells streaked across the plate will eventually grow into a colony, each colony being the product of a single cell and thus of a single species.

Once isolated, cells can be cultivated either in batch or continuous cultures. Of these, batch cultures are the most commonly used for routine liquid growth and entail inoculating an aliquot of cells into a sterile flask containing a finite amount of medium. Such systems are referred to as closed, since nutrient supply is limited to that provided at the start of culture. Under these conditions, growth will continue until the medium is depleted of nutrients or there is an excessive build-up of toxic waste products generate by the microbes. Thus, in this system, the cellular composition and physiological status of the cells will vary throughout the growth cycle.

In continuous cultures (also referred to as open systems) the medium is refreshed regularly to replace that spent by the cells. The objective of this system is to maintain the cells in the exponential growth phase by enabling nutrients, biomass and waste products to be controlled through varying the dilution rate of the cultures. Continuous cultures, although more complex to set up, offer certain advantages over batch cultures in that they facilitate growth under steady-state conditions in which there is tight coupling between cell division and biosynthesis. As a result, the physiological status of the cultures is more clearly defined, with very little variation in the cellular composition of the cells during the growth cycle. The main concern with the open system is the high risk of contamination associated with the dilution of the cultures. However, applying strict aseptic techniques during feeding or harvesting cells may help to reduce the risk of such contaminations. In addition, the whole system can be automated by connecting the culture vessels to their reservoirs through solenoid valves that can be triggered to open when required. This minimises direct contact with the operator or outside environment and thus reduces the risk of contamination.

2.6.5 Determination of growth of bacterial cultures

Several methods are available for determining the growth of bacterial cells in culture, including directly counting cells using a haemocytometer as described (Section 2.5.6). This is, however, suitable only for cells in suspension. When cells are grown on solid agar plates, colony counting can be used instead to estimate growth. This method assumes that each colony is derived from a single cell, which may not always be the case, since errors in dilution and/or streaking may result in clumps rather than single cells producing colonies. In addition, suboptimal culture conditions may cause poor growth, thus leading to an underestimation of the true cell count. When cells are grown in suspension, changes in the turbidity of the growth medium could be determined using a spectrophotometer and the absorbance value converted to cell number using a standard curve of absorbance versus cell number. This should be constructed for each cell type by taking the readings of a series of known numbers of cells in suspension (see also Section 12.4.1).

2.7 PLANT CELL CULTURE

Plant cells, by being totipotent (i.e. capable of developing by regeneration into a whole new adult) are exploited in the laboratory for tissue culture purposes. Various techniques are used routinely to facilitate the regeneration of new plants from fully differentiated cells. This is achieved by inducing cells with various agents, including hormones (auxins, cytokinins), to undergo a new developmental programme and regenerate an entire new individual plant. As with all other tissue culture procedures, plant tissue culture requires a sterile environment, aseptic manipulation of specimens and defined growth conditions. The general laboratory requirements are similar to those outlined previously for animal cells but with certain modifications specific to plant tissue culture. For instance, a plant growth chamber or a controlled-environment room may be used instead of the standard CO_2 incubators required for animal cells. Other environmental conditions required for optimum growth will vary depending on the species but, in general, consideration should be given to the diurnal temperature variations, light quality and intensity and the relative length of light–dark cycles required by the plants.

2.7.1 Health and safety considerations for plant cell culture

The safety concerns in this case are relatively trivial when compared to the precautions that need to be taken when one is working with animal or bacterial cells. However, some plant tissues may pose a risk if contaminated with microorganisms and certain precautions should therefore be taken to prevent transfer or spread of the contaminant and, more importantly, protect the operator from inhaling spores. These should include surface sterilisation of the specimen using appropriate agents such as hypochlorite solution (1–10%, w/v). These agents pose an additional risk, as they can be harmful to the operator. Hypochlorite, for instance, can cause severe bronchial irritation if inhaled.

2.7.2 Plant culture media

Models for plant cell culture used *in vitro* involve incubating parts of a plant in a suitable medium under defined conditions. For this purpose, a wide range of different types of media that are chemically defined is now available from various commercial suppliers. Some of the most commonly used media include Murashige and Skoog, Gamborg B5, Nitsche, Shenck and Hildebrandt and McCown's Woody Plant Medium.

In addition to the balanced mixture, the medium may be supplemented with macro- (nitrogen, phosphorus, potassium, calcium, magnesium and sulphur) and micronutrients (iron, manganese, zinc, boron, copper, molybdenum and chlorine), vitamins (B vitamins) and a carbon source, which is usually sucrose or D-glucose. Growth regulators including cytokinins such as zeatin (naturally occurring) or its synthetic analogue 6-furfurylaminopurine (kinetin) may also be included to stimulate cell division. Some cultures may require auxin-like regulators that promote cell expansion and this may include the naturally occurring indol-3-yl acetic acid (IAA) or synthetic compounds such as 2,4-dichlorophenoxyacetic acid. Growth may be further enhanced by including oxygen-saturated perfluorochemicals (PFCs) such as perfluorodecalin (Flutec PP5), which improves oxygen supply to cells and thus stimulates growth. Non-ionic surfactants such as the polyoxyethylene–polypropylene copolymer Pluronic F68 are sometimes included in the media to increase plasma membrane permeability. Some media may contain activated charcoal (0–3%) or polyvinylpyrrolidone (PVP) and antioxidants to prevent browning due to phenol release, oxidation and polymerisation. Although antibiotics are not normally included, they may be employed when essential to clean up highly contaminated explants. Growth-retarding chemicals such as Paclobutrazol may also be added to the medium to ameliorate anatomical and physiological abnormalities associated with tissue incubation for long periods. Such verification is reduced when the medium is solidified with agar to approximately 1% (w/v) final concentration.

2.7.3 Plant cell culture systems

Setting up a plant cell or tissue culture begins with the excision and surface sterilisation of explants, which may be chosen from any part of the plant, depending on the objective of the study. Leaves are frequently preferred for protoplast isolation (cells without walls), anthers for production of haploids, shoot meristems for proliferating shoot cultures, and root tips for root cultures.

Explants

Explants may be excised either in the field or from glasshouse-grown plants or seedlings incubated under aseptic conditions. Surface sterilisation most frequently employs several minutes exposure to a 1–10% (w/v) sodium hypochlorite solution in which chlorine gas acts as a biocide. After the set time (of the order of 5 min) excess hypochlorite must be removed immediately by copious washing in sterile distilled water.

Explants are most likely to survive *in vitro* when the tissue chosen is physiologically active (i.e. not dormant). Many types of explant contain meristematic tissue capable of cell division. Undifferentiated callus is formed soon after excision and comprises cells with a small amount of cytoplasm but large vacuoles. Such tissue may develop localised growth centres called meristemoids from which caulogenesis (shoot indication), rhizogenesis (root initiation), or both may ensue. The ability of callus to undergo such organogenesis is genetically controlled but may be encouraged *in vitro* by manipulating the cytokinin to auxin ratio in the medium. A high cytokinin to auxin ratio usually favours shoot proliferation, whereas a low cytokinin to auxin ratio usually promotes rooting. In practical terms, whole plantlets can be produced *in vitro* from organogenic callus by first encouraging shoot proliferation on a cytokinin-rich medium and then transferring leafy shoots to auxin-rich medium for root induction.

Roots may also be developed *in vivo*, provided plants are protected from desiccation. Organogenesis from callus is not generally recommended for plantlet multiplication *in vitro* (micropropagation) because there is considerable evidence that it results in genetically aberrant plants being recovered. A greater degree of chromosomal stability can be achieved by using shoot meristems as initial explants for reasons that are as yet ill defined. Meristem cultures are consequently a convenient starting material for micropropagation. Meristem culture can also be used sometimes to cure plants infected with viruses, following the use of high temperature treatment (thermotherapy) and/or chemicals (chemotherapy).

Calluses

Callus (an undifferentiated tissue formed at a wound in a plant) is often used as the starting material for suspension culture in which a mixture of both single cells and cell aggregates are incubated in a liquid medium that has to be artificially aerated to prevent the cells from becoming waterlogged. The ease of suspension formation is largely genetically controlled but friability can be improved empirically in certain cases by reducing calcium levels in the medium, altering the gas mix, changing the plant growth regulator regime or adding anti-oxidants or combinations of such variables.

Cell suspension

Cell suspension may grow as batch, fed-batch or continuous culture on a small, medium or large scale. For example, single individual cells may be grown in incubated microscope slide chambers where knowledge of the clonal origin of the plant is a prerequisite for the study. The wide-necked Erlenmeyer flask, shaken on a horizontal platform orbital shaker is a favourite container for small-scale batch culture. Fermenters with capacities of 1 to 50 000 dm^3 have been designed for large-scale cultures.

Cell suspensions provide excellent model systems for studies on cell division, cell expansion, cell differentiation and intermediary metabolism, because of the ease of adding test compounds and of harvesting cells and medium for analysis. The physiological properties of plant suspensions, however, render them more difficult to exploit than microbial cells. Moreover, the higher cost of plant culture medium, longer fermentation time (usually of the order of weeks), higher downstream processing costs and potential changes in the number of sets of chromosomes (i.e. ploidy instability) expressed in cells on prolonged subculture, significantly detracts from their usefulness for commercial exploitation (i.e. as important drugs, food additives, perfumes, biocides etc.). Despite these difficulties, research is being conducted into using cell fermenters for plant secondary product synthesis because such compounds are either not possible or economically impractical to synthesise chemically. Since many desirable compounds are derived from plants found only in environmentally sensitive areas, there is added pressure on chemical manufacturers to turn to alternative sources of supply.

Plant cell culture suspensions are useful in experiments in which mutants are selected by growing colonies in the presence of the selecting agent. Ideally, suspensions comprising only single haploid cells should be used for mutant selection. Single-cell suspensions may be obtained by sequential filtration through a graded series of filters down to 50 μm pore size. Single-cell colonies selected for superior yields are usually transferred to a production medium, possibly involving mild stress, which suppresses cell division whilst promoting some degree of differentiation.

Protoplast

A protoplast is a spherical, osmotically sensitive cell with an intact cell membrane but lacking a cell wall. This can be prepared from whole cells following the removal of the cell wall either enzymatically using pectinase in conjunction with cellulases, or mechanically by dispersing plasmolysed tissues in which the protoplasts have shrunk away from the cell wall following incubations in a concentrated osmoticum such as mannitol (at approximately 500 mM). Of the two protocols, enzymatic isolations give much higher yields of uniform protoplast. However, incubation conditions must be carefully defined and monitored to avoid overexposure to the wall-degrading enzymes that may alter metabolism with deleterious consequences.

Protoplasts may be isolated from healthy leaves that have initially been sterilised in a solution of hypochlorite for approximately 10 min. The lower epidermis is peeled off and the leaf cut into small sections and incubated with the digesting enzyme mixture in the dark at 25 °C overnight. Protoplasts released into the suspension can then be separated from cell debris and purified by a combination of filtration using a fine nylon mesh, centrifugation at low speed and washing. The quality of the yield may be verified by checking their viability using dyes such as fluorescein diacetate or Evans Blue. The former is accumulated by viable protoplasts and subsequently converted by endogenous esterases to fluorescein, which can be visualised using ultraviolet microscopy. In contrast, Evans Blue is excluded by viable protoplasts and thus can be used to distinguish these from dead isolates.

Protoplasts will start to undergo division and form new calluses within 24 h of culture, following the regeneration of a new cell wall. To facilitate this, freshly isolated protoplasts should be counted to find an effective inoculum density for growth (10^4 cells cm^{-3}) prior to plating. As with previous counting procedures, this can be performed using a haemocytometer. For certain experimental purposes, protoplast fusion may be required. This may be particularly valuable in plant breeding experiments where sexual incompatibility between genera may be a limiting factor. Protoplast fusion can be induced by either chemical or physical means (electrofusion). Chemically, fusogens such as polyethyleneglycol (PEG, approximately 30%) or a high pH calcium solution (1.1% (w/v) $CaCl_2.6H_2O$ in 10% (w/v) mannitol, pH 10.4) may be used to initiate this process, which can be achieved in less than 30 min.

Electrofusion is carried out in two steps. In the first, protoplasts are placed in a medium of low conductivity between two electrodes (platinum wires arranged in parallel on a microscope slide). A high frequency alternating field (0.5–1.5 MHz) is applied between the electrodes, which causes the protoplasts to align in a process known as di-electrophoresis. In the second step, one or more short (10–200 μs) direct current pulses (of 1–3 kVcm^{-1}) are applied, which causes pores to form in the membranes of protoplasts and allows fusion to take place where there is close membrane contact. This technique allows a higher degree of control over the fusion process than do chemical methods.

2.8 POTENTIAL USE OF CELL CULTURES

Cell cultures of various sorts from animals, plants and microbes are becoming increasingly exploited not only by scientists for studying the activity of cells in isolation but also by various biotechnology and pharmaceutical companies for the production of valuable biological products including viral vaccines (e.g. polio vaccine), antibodies (e.g. OKT3 used in suppressing immunological organ rejection in transplant surgery) and various recombinant proteins. The application of recombinant DNA techniques has led to an ever-expanding list of improved products, from both mammalian and bacterial cells, for therapeutic use in humans. These products include the commercial production of factor VIII for haemophilia, insulin for diabetes, interferon-β and α for anticancer chemotherapy and erthyropoietin for anaemia. Bacterial cultures have also been widely used for other industrial purposes, including the large-scale production of cell proteins, growth regulators, organic acids, alcohols, solvents, sterols, surfactants, vitamins, amino acids and many more products. In addition, degradation of waste products, particularly those from the agricultural and food industries, are another important industrial application of microbial cells. They are also exploited in the bioconversion of waste to useful end-products, and in toxicological studies where some of these organisms are rapidly replacing animals in preliminary toxicological testing of xenobiotics. More recently, both mammalian and bacterial cell systems are being developed to replace and supplement the use of animals in toxicological studies. Mammalian and bacterial cells are by no means the only systems being exploited. Plant cell cultures are used in genetic transformation and somatic hybridization, and protoplast fusion is proving especially valuable in plant breeding experiments, where it is used to overcome sexual incompatibility mechanisms between genera that prevent the formation of viable zygotes.

2.9 SUGGESTIONS FOR FURTHER READING

BALL, A. S. (1997). *Bacterial Cell Culture: Essential Data*. John Wiley & Sons, Inc., New York.
(Gives an adequate background into bacterial cell culture and techniques.)

DAVIS, J. M. (2002). *Basic Cell Culture: A Practical Approach*, 2nd edn. Oxford University Press, Oxford. (A comprehensive coverage of basic cell culture techniques.)

DIXON, R. A and GONZALES, R. A. (1994). *Plant Cell Culture: A Practical Approach.* Oxford University Press, Oxford. (Provides a good background on plant tissue culture techniques and application.)

FRESHNEY, R.I. (2000). *Culture of Animal Cells: A Manual of Basic Technique*, 4th edn. John Wiley & Sons, Inc., New York. (A comprehensive coverage of animal cell culture techniques and applications.)

FURR, A. K. (ed.) (1995). *CRC Handbook of Laboratory Safety*, 4th edn. CRC Press, Boca Raton, FL. (A complete guide to laboratory safety.)

HSC ADVISORY COMMITTEE ON DANGEROUS PATHOGENS (2001). *The Management Design and Operation of Microbiological Containment Laboratories.* HSE books, Sudbury. (Provides guidance, legal requirements and detailed technical information on the design, management and operation of containment laboratories.)

PAREKH, S. R. and VINCI, V. A. (2003). *Handbook of Industrial Cell Culture: Mammalian, Microbial, and Plant Cells.* Humana Press, Totowa, NJ. (Provides a good coverage of state-of-the-art techniques for industrial screening, cultivation and scale-up of mammalian, microbial, and plant cells.)

Chapter 3

Centrifugation

3.1 **INTRODUCTION**

The biochemical analysis of subcellular structures, supramolecular complexes and isolated macromolecules is of central importance for our understanding of the molecular biology of the cell. An important prerequisite for studying the biochemical and physiological properties of organelles and biomolecules is the preservation of their biological functions and properties during the separation of cellular components. A key technique for separating and analysing the various elements of a cellular homogenate is represented by centrifugation. The development of the first analytical ultracentrifuge by Svedberg in the late 1920s and the technical refinement of the preparative centrifugation technique by Albert Claude and colleagues in the 1940s positioned centrifugation technology at the centre of biological and biomedical research for many decades. Today, centrifugation techniques are an indispensable tool of modern biochemistry and employed in almost all invasive subcellular studies. While analytical centrifugation is concerned mainly with the study of purified macromolecules or isolated supramolecular assemblies, preparative centrifugation methodology is devoted to the actual separation of cells, subcellular structures, membrane vesicles and other particles of biochemical interest.

Most undergraduate students will be exposed to preparative centrifugation protocols during practical classes and might also experience a demonstration of analytical centrifugation techniques. This chapter is accordingly divided into a short introduction to the theoretical background of sedimentation, an overview of practical aspects of using centrifuges in the biochemical laboratory, an outline of preparative centrifugation and a description of the usefulness of ultracentrifugation techniques in the biochemical characterisation of macromolecules. To aid in the understanding of the basic principles of centrifugation, the general design of various rotors and separation processes is diagrammatically represented. Often the learning process of undergraduate students is hampered by a lack of a proper linkage between theoretical knowledge and practical applications. To overcome this problem, the description of preparative centrifugation techniques is accompanied by an explanatory flow chart and the detailed discussion of the subcellular fractionation protocol of a specific tissue preparation. Taking the isolation of fractions from skeletal muscle homogenates as an example, the rationale behind individual preparative steps is explained. Since affinity isolation methods not only represent an extremely powerful tool in purifying biomolecules (see Section 11.8) but can also be utilised to separate intact organelles and membrane vesicles by centrifugation, lectin affinity agglutination of highly purified plasmalemma vesicles from skeletal muscle is described. Traditionally, marker enzyme activities are used to determine the overall yield and enrichment of particular structures within subcellular fractions following centrifugation. As an example, the distribution of key enzyme activities in mitochondrial subfractions from liver is given. However, most modern fractionation procedures are evaluated by more convenient methods, such as protein gel analysis in conjunction with immunoblot analysis. Miniature gel and blotting equipment can produce highly reliable results within a few hours, making it an ideal analytical tool for high throughput testing. Since electrophoretic techniques are introduced in Chapter 10 and are routine methods used in biochemical laboratories, the protein gel analysis of the distribution of typical marker proteins in affinity isolated plasmalemma fractions is graphically represented and discussed here.

Although monomeric peptides and proteins are capable of performing complex biochemical reactions, many physiologically important elements do not exist in isolation under native conditions. Therefore, if one considers individual proteins as the basic units of the proteome (see Section 8.5), protein complexes actually form the functional units of cell biology. This gives investigations into the supramolecular structure of protein complexes a central place in biochemical research. To illustrate this point, the sedimentation analysis of a high molecular mass membrane assembly, the dystrophin–glycoprotein complex of skeletal muscle, is shown and the use of sucrose gradient centrifugation explained.

3.2 **BASIC PRINCIPLES OF SEDIMENTATION**

From every-day experience, the effect of sedimentation due to the influence of the earth's gravitational field ($g = 981$ cm s^{-2}) versus the increased rate of sedimentation in a centrifugal field ($g > 981$ cm s^{-2}) is apparent. To give a simple, but illustrative example, sand particles added to a bucket of water travel slowly to the bottom of the bucket by gravitation, but sediment much faster when the bucket is swung around in a circle. Similarly, biological structures exhibit a drastic increase in sedimentation when they undergo acceleration in a centrifugal field. The relative centrifugal field is usually expressed as a multiple of the acceleration due to gravity. For a detailed description of the forces acting on biological particles suspended in a liquid medium the reader is referred to textbooks on centrifugation listed in Section 3.6. Below is a short description of equations used in practical centrifugation classes.

When designing a centrifugation protocol, it is important to keep in mind that:

- the more dense a biological structure is, the faster it sediments in a centrifugal field,
- the more massive a biological particle is, the faster it moves in a centrifugal field,

- the denser the biological buffer system is, the slower the particle will move in a centrifugal field,
- the greater the frictional coefficient is, the slower a particle will move,
- the greater the centrifugal force is, the faster the particle sediments,
- the sedimentation rate of a given particle will be zero when the density of the particle and the medium are equal.

Biological particles moving through a viscous medium experience a frictional drag, whereby the frictional force acts in the opposite direction to sedimentation and equals the velocity of the particle multiplied by the frictional coefficient. The frictional coefficient depends on the size and shape of the biological particle. As the sample moves towards the bottom of a centrifuge tube, its velocity will increase owing to the increase in radial distance. At the same time the particles also encounter a frictional drag that is proportional to their velocity. The frictional force of a particle moving through a viscous fluid is the product of its velocity and its frictional coefficient, and acts in the direction opposite to sedimentation.

From equation 3.1 for the calculation of the relative centrifugal field it becomes apparent that when the conditions for the centrifugal separation of a biological particle are described, a detailed listing of rotor speed, radial dimensions and duration of centrifugation has to be provided. Basically, the rate of sedimentation is dependent upon the applied centrifugal field (cm s^{-2}), G, that is determined by the radial distance, r, of the particle from the axis of rotation (in cm) and the square of the angular velocity, ω, of the rotor (in radians per second):

$$G = \omega^2 r \tag{3.1}$$

Example 1 **CALCULATION OF CENTRIFUGAL FIELD**

Question

What is the applied centrifugal field at a point equivalent to 5 cm from the centre of rotation and an angular velocity of 3000 rad s^{-1}?

Answer

The centrifugal field, G, at a point 5 cm from the centre of rotation may be calculated using the equation $G = \omega^2 r$

$$G = (3000)^2 \times 5 \text{ cm s}^{-2} = 4.5 \times 10^7 \text{ cm s}^{-2}$$

The average angular velocity of a rigid body that rotates about a fixed axis is defined as the ratio of the angular displacement in a given time interval. One radian, usually abbreviated as 1 rad, represents the angle subtended at the centre of a circle by an arc with a length equal to the radius of the circle. Since 360° equals 2π radians, one revolution of the rotor can be expressed as 2π rad. Accordingly, the angular velocity of the rotor can be expressed in terms of rotor speed in revolutions (rev) per minute:

$$\omega = \frac{2\pi \text{ rev min}^{-1}}{60} \tag{3.2}$$

and therefore the centrifugal field can be expressed as:

$$G = \frac{4\pi^2 (\text{rev min}^{-1})^2 r}{3600} \tag{3.3}$$

Example 2 CALCULATION OF ANGULAR VELOCITY

Question

For the pelleting of the microsomal fraction from a liver homogenate, an ultra-centrifuge is operated at a speed of 40 000 r.p.m. What is the angular velocity, ω, in radians per second?

Answer   The angular velocity, ω, may be calculated using the equation:

$$\omega = \frac{2\pi \,\text{rev min}^{-1}}{60}$$

$$\omega = 2 \times 3.1416 \times 40\,000/60 \,\text{rad s}^{-1} = 4188.8 \,\text{rad s}^{-1}$$

The centrifugal field is generally expressed in multiples of the gravitational field, g (981cm s^{-2}). The relative centrifugal field, RCF, which is the ratio of the centrifugal acceleration at a specified radius and the speed to the standard acceleration of gravity, can be calculated from the following equation:

$$\text{RCF} = \frac{4\pi^2 (\text{rev min}^{-1})^2 r}{3600 \times 981} \tag{3.4}$$

RCF units are therefore expressed in '$\times g$' and revolutions per minute are usually abbreviated as 'r.p.m.' More simply RCF = 1.12×10^{-5} r.p.m.^{2} r.

Although the relative centrifugal force can be calculated easily, centrifugation manuals usually contain a nomograph for convenient conversion between relative centrifugal force and speed of the centrifuge at different radii of the centrifugation spindle to a point along the centrifuge tube. A nomograph consists of three columns representing the radial distance (in millimeters), the relative centrifugal force ($\times g$) and the rotor speed (in r.p.m.). For the conversion between relative centrifugal force and speed of the centrifuge spindle in r.p.m. at different radii, a straight line is drawn through known values in two columns, then the desired figure is read where the straight line intersects with the third column. See Fig. 3.1 for an illustration of the usage of a nomograph.

In a suspension of biological particles, the rate of sedimentation is dependent not only upon the applied centrifugal field but also on the nature of the particle, i.e. its density and radius, and also the viscosity of the surrounding medium. Stokes law describes these relationships for the sedimentation of a rigid spherical particle:

$$v = \frac{2}{9} \frac{r^2 (\rho_p - \rho_m)}{\eta} \times g \tag{3.5}$$

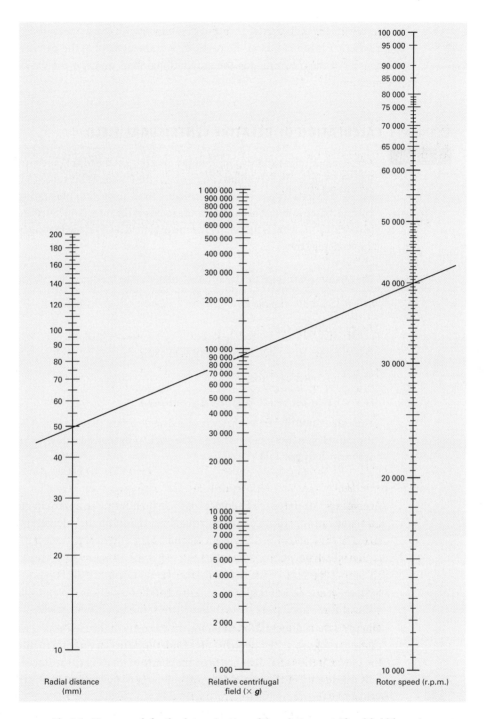

Fig. 3.1. Nomograph for the determination of the relative centrifugal field for a given rotor speed and radius. The three columns represent the radial distance (in mm), the relative centrifugal force ($\times$ *g*) and the rotor speed (in r.p.m.). For the conversion between relative centrifugal force and speed of the centrifuge spindle in r.p.m. at different radii, draw a straight line through known values in two columns. The desired figure can then be read where the straight line intersects the third column. (Courtesy of Beckman–Coulter.)

where v is the sedimentation rate of the sphere, 2/9 is the shape factor constant for a sphere, r is the radius of the particle, ρ_p is the density of the particle, ρ_m is the density of the medium, g is the gravitational field, and η is the viscosity of the medium.

Example 3 CALCULATION OF RELATIVE CENTRIFUGAL FIELD

Question

A fixed-angle rotor exhibits a minimum radius, r_{min}, at the top of the centrifuge tube of 3.5 cm, and a maximum radius, r_{max}, at the bottom of the tube of 7.0 cm. See Fig. 3.2a for a cross-sectional diagram of a fixed-angle rotor illustrating the position of the minimum and maximum radius. If the rotor is operated at a speed of 20 000 r.p.m., what is the relative centrifugal field (RCF) at the top and bottom of the centrifuge tube?

Answer

The relative centrifugal field may be calculated using the equation:

$$RCF = 1.12 \times 10^{-5} \, \text{r.p.m.}^2 \, r$$

Top of centrifuge tube:

$$RCF = 1.12 \times 10^{-5} \times (20\,000)^2 \times 3.5 \, g = 15\,680 \, g$$

Bottom of centrifuge tube:

$$RCF = 1.12 \times 10^{-5} \times (20\,000)^2 \times 7.0 \, g = 31\,360 \, g$$

This calculation illustrates that, with fixed-angle rotors, the centrifugal field at the top and bottom of the centrifuge tube might differ considerably, in this case approximately two-fold.

Accordingly, a mixture of biological particles exhibiting an approximately spherical shape can be separated in a centrifugal field based on their density and/or their size. The time of sedimentation (in seconds) for a spherical particle is:

$$t = \frac{9}{2} \frac{\eta}{\omega^2 r_p^2 (\rho_p - \rho_m)} \times \ln \frac{r_b}{r_t} \tag{3.6}$$

where t is the sedimentation time, η is the viscosity of the medium, r_p is the radius of the particle, r_b is the radial distance from the centre of rotation to the bottom of the tube, r_t is the radial distance from the centre of rotation to the liquid meniscus, ρ_p is the density of the particle, ρ_m is the density of medium, and ω is the angular velocity of the rotor.

The sedimentation rate or velocity of a biological particle can also be expressed as its sedimentation coefficient (s), whereby:

$$s = \frac{v}{\omega^2 r} \tag{3.7}$$

Since the sedimentation rate per unit centrifugal field can be determined at different temperatures and with various media, experimental values of the sedimentation coefficient are corrected to a sedimentation constant theoretically obtainable in water at 20°C, yielding the $S_{20,W}$ value. The sedimentation coefficients of biological macromolecules are relatively small, and are usually expressed (Section 3.5) as Svedberg units, S. One Svedberg unit equals 10^{-13} s.

3.3 TYPES, CARE AND SAFETY ASPECTS OF CENTRIFUGES

3.3.1 Types of centrifuge

Centrifugation techniques take a central position in modern biochemical, cellular and molecular biological studies. Depending on the particular application, centrifuges differ in their overall design and size. However, a common feature in all centrifuges is the central motor that spins a rotor containing the samples to be separated. Particles of biochemical interest are usually suspended in a liquid buffer system contained in specific tubes or separation chambers that are located in specialised rotors. The biological medium is chosen for the specific centrifugal application and may differ considerably between preparative and analytical approaches. As outlined below, the optimum pH value, salt concentration, stabilising cofactors and protective ingredients such as protease inhibitors have to be carefully evaluated in order to preserve biological function. The most obvious difference between centrifuges are:

- the maximum speed at which biological specimens are subjected to increased sedimentation,
- the presence or absence of a vacuum,
- the potential for refrigeration or general manipulation of the temperature during a centrifugation run,
- the maximum volume of samples and capacity for individual centrifugation tubes.

Many different types of centrifuge are commercially available, including:

- large-capacity low speed preparative centrifuges,
- refrigerated high speed preparative centrifuges,
- analytical ultracentrifuges,
- preparative ultracentrifuges,
- large-scale clinical centrifuges,
- small-scale laboratory microfuges.

Some large-volume centrifuge models are quite demanding on space and also generate considerable amounts of heat and noise, and are therefore often centrally positioned in special instrument rooms in biochemistry departments. However, the development of small-capacity bench-top centrifuges for biochemical applications, even in the case of ultracentrifuges, has led to the introduction of these models in many individual research laboratories.

The main types of centrifuge encountered by undergraduate students during introductory practicals may be divided into microfuges (so called because they centrifuge small volume samples in Eppendorf tubes), large-capacity preparative centrifuges, high speed refrigerated centrifuges and ultracentrifuges. Simple bench-top centrifuges vary in design and are used mainly to collect small amounts of biological material such as blood cells. To prevent denaturation of protein samples, non-refrigerated microfuges are often used in cold rooms. Modern refrigerated microfuges are equipped with adapters to accommodate standardised plastic tubes for the sedimentation of 0.5–1.5 cm^3 volumes. They can provide centrifugal fields of approximately 10 000 g and sediment biological samples in minutes, making microfuges an indispensable separation tool for many biochemical methods. Microfuges can also be used to concentrate protein samples. For example, the dilution of protein samples eluted by column chromatography can often represent a challenge for subsequent analyses. Accelerated ultrafiltration with the help of plastic tube-associated filter units, spun at low g forces in a microfuge, can overcome this problem. Depending on the proteins of interest, the biological buffers used and the molecular mass cut-off point of the particular filters, a 10- to 20-fold concentration of samples can be achieved within minutes. Larger preparative bench-top centrifuges develop maximum centrifugal fields of 3000–7000 g and can be used for the spinning of various types of container. Depending on the range of available adapters, considerable quantities of 5–250 cm^3 plastic tubes or 96-well enzyme-linked immunosorbent assay (ELISA) plates can be accommodated. This gives simple and relatively inexpensive bench centrifuges a central place in many high throughput biochemical assays where the quick and efficient separation of coarse precipitates or whole cells is of importance.

High speed and supra-speed refrigerated centrifuges are absolutely essential for the sedimentation of protein precipitates, large intact organelles, cellular debris derived from tissue homogenisation and microorganisms. As outlined in Section 3.4, the initial bulk separation of cellular elements prior to preparative ultracentrifugation is performed by these kinds of centrifuge. They operate at maximum centrifugal fields of approximately 100 000 g. Such centrifugal force is not sufficient to sediment smaller microsomal vesicles or ribosomes, but can be employed to differentially separate nuclei, mitochondria or chloroplasts. In addition, bulky protein aggregates can be sedimented using high speed refrigerated centrifuges. An example is the contractile apparatus released from muscle fibres by homogenisation, mostly consisting of myosin and actin macromolecules aggregated in filaments. In order to harvest yeast cells or bacteria from large volumes of culture media, high speed centrifugation may also be used in a continuous flow mode with zonal rotors. This approach does therefore not use centrifuge tubes but a continuous flow of medium. As the medium enters the moving rotor, biological particles are sedimented against the rotor periphery and excess liquid removed through a special outlet port.

Ultracentrifugation has decisively advanced the detailed biochemical analysis of subcellular structures and isolated biomolecules. Preparative ultracentrifugation can be operated at relative centrifugal fields of up to 600 000 g. In order to minimise excessive rotor temperatures generated by frictional resistance between the spinning rotor and air, the rotor chamber is sealed, evacuated and refrigerated. Depending on the type, age and condition of a particular ultracentrifuge, cooling to the required running temperature and the generation of a stable vacuum might take a considerable amount of time. To avoid delays during biochemical procedures involving ultracentrifugation, the cooling and evacuation system of older centrifuge models should be switched on at least an hour prior to the centrifugation run. On the other hand, modern ultracentrifuges can be started even without a fully established vacuum and will proceed in the evacuation of the rotor chamber during the initial acceleration process. For safety reasons, heavy armour plating encapsulates the ultracentrifuge to prevent injury to the user in case of uncontrolled rotor movements or dangerous vibrations. A centrifugation run cannot be initiated without proper closing of the chamber system. To prevent unfavourable fluctuations in chamber temperature, excessive vibrations or operation of rotors above their maximum rated speed, newer models of ultracentrifuges contain sophisticated temperature regulation systems, flexible drive shafts and an over-speed control device. Although slight rotor imbalances can be absorbed by modern ultracentrifuges, a more severe misbalance of tubes will cause the centrifuge to switch off automatically. This is especially true for swinging-bucket rotors. The many safety features incorporated into modern ultracentrifuges make them a robust piece of equipment that tolerates a certain degree of misuse by an inexperienced operator. See Sections 3.3.3 and 3.3.4 for a more detailed discussion of safety and centrifugation. In contrast to preparative ultracentrifuges, analytical ultracentrifuges contain a solid rotor that, in its simplest form, incorporates one analytical cell and one counterbalancing cell. An optical system enables the sedimenting material to be observed throughout the duration of centrifugation. Using a light absorption system, a Schlieren system or a Raleigh interferometric system, concentration distributions in the biological sample are determined at any time during ultracentrifugation. The Raleigh and Schlieren optical systems detect changes in the refractive index of the solution caused by concentration changes and can thus be used for sedimentation equilibrium analysis. This makes analytical ultracentrifugation a relatively accurate tool for the determination of the molecular mass of an isolated macromolecule. It can also provide crucial information about the thermodynamic properties of a protein or other large biomolecules.

3.3.2 **Types of rotor**

To illustrate the difference in design of fixed-angle rotors, vertical tube rotors and swinging-bucket rotors, Fig. 3.2 outlines cross-sectional diagrams of these three main types of rotor. Companies usually name rotors according to their type of design, the maximum allowable speed and sometimes the material composition. Depending on the use in a simple low speed centrifuge, a high speed centrifuge or an ultracentrifuge, different centrifugal forces are encountered by a spinning rotor. Accordingly, different types of rotor are made from different materials. Low speed rotors are made from steel or brass, while high speed rotors consist of

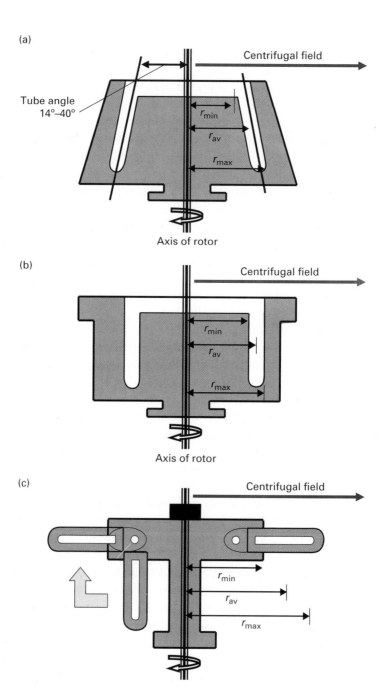

Fig. 3.2. Design of the three main types of rotor used in routine biochemical centrifugation techniques. Shown are cross-sectional diagrams of (a) a fixed-angle rotor, (b) a vertical tube rotor, and (c) a swinging-bucket rotor. A fourth type of rotor is represented by the class of near-vertical rotors.

aluminium, titanium or fibre-reinforced composites. The exterior of specific rotors might be finished with protective paints. For example, rotors for ultracentrifugation made out of titanium alloy are covered with a polyurethane layer. Aluminium rotors are protected from corrosion by an electrochemically formed tough layer of aluminium oxide. In order to avoid damage to these protective layers, care should be taken during rotor handling.

Fixed-angle rotors are an ideal tool for pelleting during the differential separation of biological particles whose sedimentation rates are significantly different; for example, when separating nuclei, mitochondria and microsomes. In addition, isopycnic banding may also be routinely performed with fixed-angle rotors. For isopycnic separation, centrifugation is continued until the biological particles of interest have reached their isopycnic position in a gradient. This means that the particle has reached a position where the sedimentation rate is zero because the densities of the biological particle and the surrounding medium are equal. Centrifugation tubes are held at a fixed angle of between 14° and 40° to the vertical in this class of rotor (Fig. 3.2a). Particles move radially outwards and, since the centrifugal field is exerted at an angle, they have only to travel a short distance until they reach their isopycnic position in a gradient using an isodensity technique or before colliding with the outer wall of the centrifuge tube using a differential centrifugation method. Vertical rotors (Fig. 3.2b) may be divided into true vertical rotors and near-vertical rotors. Sealed centrifuge tubes are held parallel to the axis of rotation in vertical rotors and are restrained in the rotor cavities by screws, special washers and plugs. Since samples are not separated down the length of the centrifuge tube, but across the diameter of the tube, isopycnic separation time is significantly shorter as compared with swinging-bucket rotors. In contrast to fixed-angle rotors, near-vertical rotors exhibit a reduced tube angle of 7°–10° and also employ quick-seal tubes. The reduced angle results in much shorter run times as compared with fixed-angle rotors. Near-vertical rotors are useful for gradient centrifugation of biological elements that do not properly participate in conventional gradients. Hinge pins or a crossbar is used to attach rotor buckets in swinging-bucket rotors (Fig. 3.2c). They are loaded in a vertical position and during the initial acceleration phase, rotor buckets swing out horizontally and then position themselves at the rotor body for support.

To illustrate the separation of particles in the three main types of rotor, Fig. 3.3 outlines the movement of biological samples during the initial acceleration stage, the main centrifugal separation phase, de-acceleration and the final harvesting of separated particles in the rotor at rest. In the case of isopycnic centrifugation in a fixed-angle rotor, the centrifuge tubes are gradually filled with a suitable gradient, the sample carefully loaded on top of this solution and then the tubes placed at a specific fixed-angle into the rotor cavities. During rotor acceleration, the sample solution and the gradient undergo reorientation in the centrifugal field, followed by the separation of particles with different sedimentation properties (Fig. 3.3a). The gradient returns to its original position during the deacceleration phase and separated particle bands can be taken from the tubes once the rotor is at rest. By analogy, similar reorientation of gradients and banding of particles occurs in a ver-

(a)

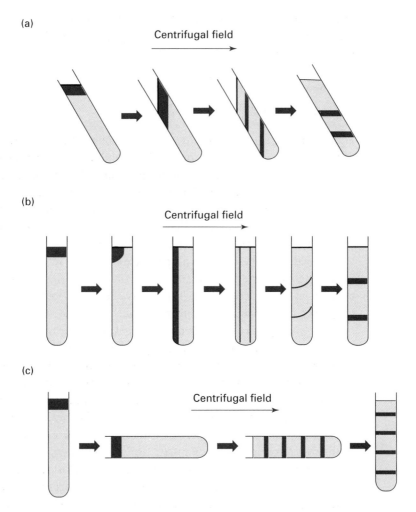

(b)

(c)

Fig. 3.3. Operation of the three main types of rotor used in routine biochemical centrifugation techniques. Shown are cross-sectional diagrams of a centrifuge tube positioned in (a) a fixed-angle rotor, (b) a vertical tube rotor, and (c) a swinging-bucket rotor (c). The diagrams illustrate the movement of biological samples during the initial acceleration stage, the main centrifugal separation phase, de-acceleration and the final harvesting of separated particles in the rotor at rest. Using a fixed-angle rotor, the tubes are filled with a gradient, the sample loaded on top of this solution and then the tubes placed at a specific fixed-angle into the rotor cavities. The sample and the gradient undergo reorientation in the centrifugal field during rotor acceleration, resulting in the separation of particles with different sedimentation properties. Similar reorientation of gradients and banding of particles occurs in a vertical tube rotor system. A great variety of gradients can be used with swinging-bucket rotors, making them the method of choice when maximum resolution of banding zones is required.

tical rotor system (Fig. 3.3b). Although run times are reduced and these kinds of rotor can usually hold a large number of tubes, resolution of separated bands during isopycnic centrifugation is less when compared with swinging-bucket applications. Since a greater variety of gradients exhibiting different steepness can be used with swinging-bucket rotors, they are the method of choice when maximum resolution of banding zones is required (Fig. 3.3c), such as in rate zonal studies based on the separation of biological particles as a function of sedimentation coefficient.

3.3.3 Care and maintenance of centrifuges

Corrosion and degradation due to biological buffer systems used within rotors or contamination of the interior or exterior of the centrifuge via spillage may seriously affect the lifetime of this equipment. Another important point is the proper balancing of centrifuge tubes. This is not only important with respect to safety, as outlined below, but might also cause vibration-induced damage to the rotor itself and the drive shaft of the centrifuge. Thus proper handling and care, as well as regular maintenance of both centrifuges and rotors, is an important part of keeping this biochemical method available in the laboratory. In order to avoid damage to the protective layers of rotors, such as polyurethane paint or aluminium oxide, care should be taken in the cleaning of the rotor exterior. Coarse brushes that may scratch the finish should not be used and only non-corrosive detergents employed. Corrosion may be triggered by long-term exposure of rotors to alkaline solutions, acidic buffers, aggressive detergents or salt. Thus rotors should be thoroughly washed with distilled or deionised water after every run. For overnight storage, rotors should be first left upside down to drain excess liquid and then be positioned in a safe and dry place. To avoid damage to the hinge pins of swinging-bucket rotors, the rotor assembly should be dried with tissue paper following removal of biological buffers and washing with water. Centrifuge rotors are often not properly stored in a clean environment; this can quickly lead to the destruction of the protective rotor coating and should thus be avoided. It is advisable to keep rotors in a special clean room, physically separated from the actual centrifugation facility, with dedicated places for individual types of rotor. Some researchers might prefer to pre-cool their rotors prior to a centrifugation run by transferring them to a cold room. Although this is an acceptable practice and might, for example, keep proteolytic degradation to a minimum, rotors should not undergo long-term storage in a wet and cold environment. Regular maintenance of rotors and centrifuges by engineers is important for ensuring the safe operation of a centralised centrifugation facility. In order to properly judge the need for replacement of a rotor or parts of a centrifuge, it is essential that all users of core centrifuge equipment participate in proper book-keeping. Accurate record-keeping of run times and centrifugal speeds is important, since cyclic acceleration and deacceleration of rotors may lead to metal fatigue.

3.3.4 Safety and centrifugation

Modern centrifuges are not only highly sophisticated but also relatively sturdy pieces of biochemical equipment that incorporate many safety features. Rotor chambers of high speed centrifuges and ultracentrifuges are always enclosed in heavy armour plating. Most centrifuges are designed to buffer a certain degree of imbalance and are usually equipped with an automatic switch-off mode. However, even in a well-balanced rotor, tube cracking during a centrifugation run might cause severe imbalance resulting in dangerous vibrations. Rotors must never be loaded with an odd number of tubes. When the rotor can only be partially loaded, the tubes must be located diametrically opposite each other in order that the load is distributed evenly around the rotor axis. This is not only important for ultracentrifugation with enormous centrifugal fields, but also for both small and large capacity bench centrifuges where the rotors are usually mounted on a more rigid suspension. When using swinging-bucket rotors, it is important always to load all buckets with their caps properly screwed on. Even if only two tubes are loaded with solutions, the empty swinging buckets have also to be assembled, since they form an integral part of the overall balance of the rotor system. In some swinging-bucket rotors, individual rotor buckets are numbered and should not be interchanged between their designated positions on similarly numbered hinge pins. To avoid the disturbance of delicate gradients, centrifugation runs with swinging-bucket rotors are usually initiated under fully established vacuum, and started and terminated at low acceleration and de-acceleration speeds, respectively. This practice also avoids the occurrence of sudden imbalances due to tube deformation or cracking and thus eliminates potentially dangerous vibrations.

Generally, safety and good laboratory practice are important aspects of all research projects and the awareness of the exposure to potentially harmful substances should be a concern for every biochemist. If you use dangerous chemicals, potentially infectious material or radioactive substances during centrifugation protocols, refer to up-to-date safety manuals and the safety statement of your individual department. Perform mock runs of important experiments in order to avoid the loss of precious specimens or expensive chemicals. As with all other biochemical procedures, experiments should never be rushed and protective clothing worn at all times. Centrifuge tubes should be handled slowly and carefully so as not to disturb pellets, bands of separated particles or unstable gradients. With respect to choosing the right kind of centrifuge tube for a particular application, the manufacturers of rotors usually give detailed recommendation of suitable materials. For safety reasons and to guarantee experimental success, it is important to make sure that individual centrifuge tubes are chemically resistant to the solvents used, have the right capacity for sample loading, can be used in the designated type of rotor and are able to withstand the maximum centrifugal forces and temperature range of a particular centrifuge. In fixed-angle rotors, large centrifugal forces tend to cause a collapse of centrifuge tubes making thick-walled tubes the choice for these rotors. In contrast, swinging-bucket rotor tubes are better protected from deformation and usually thin-walled polyallomer tubes are used. An important safety aspect is the proper handling of separated biological particles following centrifugation. In order to perform postcentrifugation analysis of individual fractions, centrifugation tubes often have to be punctured or sliced. For example, separated vesicle bands can be harvested from the pierced bottom of the centrifuge tube or are collected by slicing of the tube following quick freezing. If samples have been pre-incubated with radioactive markers or toxic ligands, the contamination of the centrifugation chamber and rotor cavities or buckets should be avoided. If centrifugal separation processes have to be performed routinely with a potentially harmful substance, it makes sense to dedicate a particular centrifuge and accompanying rotors for this work and thereby eliminate the potential for cross-contamination.

3.4 PREPARATIVE CENTRIFUGATION

3.4.1 Differential centrifugation

Cellular and subcellular fractionation techniques are indispensable methods used in biochemical research. Although the proper separation of many subcellular structures is absolutely dependent on preparative ultracentrifugation, the isolation of large cellular structures, the nuclear fraction, mitochondria, chloroplasts or large protein precipitates can be achieved by conventional high speed refrigerated centrifugation. Differential centrifugation is based upon the differences in the sedimentation rate of biological particles of different size and density. Crude tissue homogenates containing organelles, membrane vesicles and other structural fragments are divided into different fractions by the stepwise increase of the applied centrifugal field. Following the initial sedimentation of the largest particles of a homogenate (such as cellular debris) by centrifugation, various biological structures or aggregates are separated into pellet and supernatant fractions, depending upon the speed and time of individual centrifugation steps and the density and relative size of the particles. To increase the yield of membrane structures and protein aggregates released, cellular debris pellets are often re-homogenised several times and then re-centrifuged. This is especially important in the case of rigid biological structures such as muscular or connective tissue, or in the case of small tissue samples as occurs with human biopsy material or primary cell cultures.

The differential sedimentation of a particulate suspension in a centrifugal field is shown diagrammatically in Fig. 3.4a. Initially all particles of a homogenate are evenly distributed throughout the centrifuge tube and then move down the tube at their respective sedimentation rates during centrifugation. The largest class of particles forms a pellet on the bottom of the centrifuge tube, leaving smaller-sized structures within the supernatant. However, during the initial centrifugation step smaller particles also become entrapped in the pellet, causing a certain degree of contamination. At the end of each differential centrifugation step, the pellet and supernatant fractions are carefully separated from each other. To minimise cross-contamination, pellets are usually washed several times by re-suspension in buffer and re-centrifugation under the same conditions. However, repeated washing steps may considerably reduce the yield of the final pellet fraction and are therefore omitted in preparations with limiting starting material. Resulting supernatant fractions are centrifuged at a higher speed and for a longer time to separate medium-sized and small-sized particles. With respect to the separation of

(a)

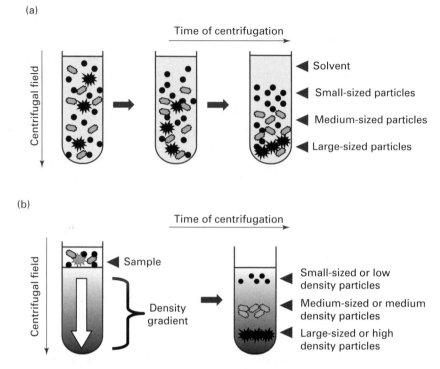

(b)

Fig. 3.4. Diagram of particle behaviour during differential and isopycnic separation. During differential sedimentation of a particulate suspension in a centrifugal field (a), the movement of particles is dependent upon their density, shape and size. For separation of biological particles using a density gradient (b), samples are carefully layered on top of a pre-formed density gradient prior to centrifugation. For isopycnic separation, centrifugation is continued until the desired particles have reached their isopycnic position in the liquid density gradient. In contrast, during rate separation, the required fraction does not reach its isopycnic position during the centrifugation run.

organelles and membrane vesicles, crude differential centrifugation techniques can be conveniently employed to isolate intact mitochondria and microsomes.

3.4.2 Density gradient centrifugation

To further separate biological particles of similar size but differing density, ultracentrifugation with pre-formed or self-establishing density gradients is the method of choice. Both rate separation or equilibrium methods can be used. In Fig. 3.4b, the preparative ultracentrifugation of low to high density particles is shown. A mixture of particles, such as is present in a heterogeneous microsomal membrane preparation, is layered on top of a pre-formed liquid density gradient. Depending on the particular biological application, a great variety of gradient materials are available. Caesium chloride is widely used for the banding of DNA and the isolation of plasmids, nucleoproteins and viruses. Sodium bromide and sodium iodide are employed for the fractionation of lipoproteins and the banding of DNA or RNA molecules, respectively. Various companies offer a range of gradient material for the separation of whole cells and subcellular particles, for example Percoll, Ficoll, Dextran, Metrizamide and Nycodenz. For the separation of membrane vesicles derived from tissue homogenates, ultrapure DNase-, RNase- and protease-free sucrose represents a suitable and widely employed medium for the preparation of stabile gradients. If one wants to separate all membrane species spanning the whole range of particle densities, the maximum density of the gradient must exceed the density of the most dense vesicle species. Both step gradient and continuous gradient systems are employed to achieve this. If automated gradient makers are not available, which is probably the case in most undergraduate practical classes, the manual pouring of a stepwise gradient with the help of a pipette is not that time-consuming or difficult. In contrast, the formation of a stable continuous gradient is much more challenging and requires a commercially available gradient maker. Following pouring, gradients are usually kept in a cold room for temperature equilibration and are moved extremely slowly in special holders so as to avoid mixing of different gradient layers. For rate separation of subcellular particles, the required fraction does not reach its isopycnic position within the gradient. For isopycnic separation, density centrifugation is continued until the buoyant density of the particle of interest and the density of the gradient are equal.

3.4.3 Practical applications of preparative centrifugation

To illustrate practical applications of differential centrifugation, density gradient ultracentrifugation and affinity methodology, the isolation of the microsomal fraction from muscle homogenates and subsequent separation of membrane vesicles with a differing density is described (Fig. 3.5), the isolation of highly purified sarcolemma vesicles outlined (Fig. 3.6), and the subfractionation of liver mitochondrial membrane systems shown (Fig. 3.7). Skeletal muscle fibres are highly specialised structures involved in contraction and the membrane systems that maintain the regulation of excitation–contraction coupling, energy metabolism and the stabilisation of the cell periphery are shown diagrammatically in Fig. 3.5a. The surface membrane consists of the sarcolemma and its invaginations, the transverse tubular membrane system. The transverse tubules may be subdivided into the non-junctional region and the triad part that forms contact zones with the terminal cisternae of the sarcoplasmic reticulum. Motorneurone-induced depolarisation of the sarcolemma travels into the transverse tubules and activates a voltage-sensing receptor complex that directly initiates the transient opening of a junctional calcium release channel. The membrane system that provides the luminal ion reservoir for the regulatory calcium cycling process is represented by the specialised endoplasmic reticulum. It forms membranous sheaths around the contractile apparatus whereby the longitudinal tubules are mainly involved in the uptake of calcium ions during muscle relaxation and the terminal cisternae provide the rapid calcium release mechanism that initiates muscle contraction. Mitochondria are the site of oxidative phosphorylation and exhibit a complex system of inner and outer membranes involved in energy metabolism.

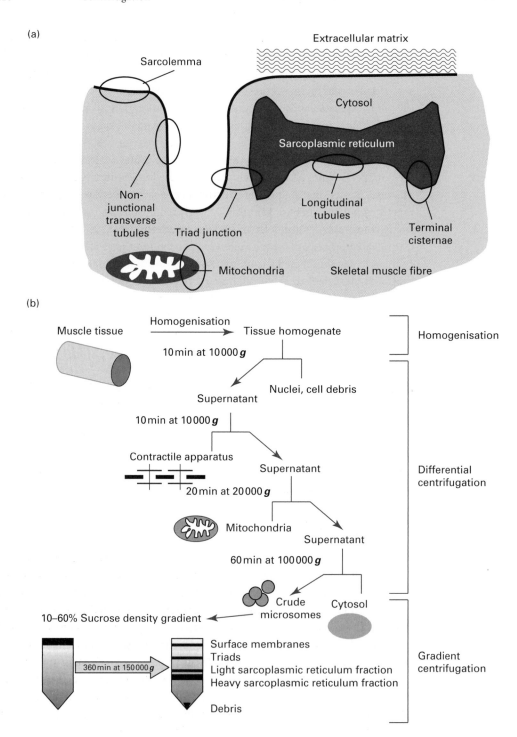

Fig. 3.5. Scheme of the fractionation of skeletal muscle homogenate into various subcellular fractions. Shown are (a) a diagrammatic presentation of the subcellular membrane system from skeletal muscle fibres and (b) a flow chart of the fractionation protocol of these membranes from tissue homogenates using differential centrifugation and density gradient methodology.

For the optimum homogenisation of tissue specimens, mincing of tissue has to be performed in the presence of a biological buffer system that provides the right pH value, salt concentration, stabilising cofactors and chelating agents. The optimum ratio between the wet weight of tissue and buffer volume, as well as the temperature (usually 4 °C) and presence of a protease inhibitor cocktail is also essential to minimise proteolytic degradation. Prior to the 1970s, neither protease inhibitors nor chelating agents were widely used in homogenisation buffers. This resulted in the degradation of many high molecular mass proteins. Since protective measures against endogenous enzymes have been routinely introduced into subcellular fractionation protocols, extremely large proteins have been isolated in their intact form, such as 427 kDa dystrophin, the 565 kDa ryanodine receptor, 800 kDa nebulin and the longest known polypeptide of 2200 kDa mass named titin. Commercially available protease inhibitor cocktails usually exhibit a broad specificity for the inhibition of cysteine proteases, serine proteases, aspartate proteases, metalloproteases and aminopeptidases. They are used in the micro-molar concentration range and are best added to buffer systems just prior to the tissue homogenisation process. Depending on the half-life of specific protease inhibitors, the length of a subcellular fractionation protocol and the amount of endogenous enzymes present in individual fractions, tissue suspensions might have to be replenished with a fresh aliquot of a protease inhibitor cocktail. Protease inhibitor kits for the creation of individualised cocktails are also available and consist of substances such as trypsin inhibitor, E-64, aminoethylbenzene-sulphonylfluoride, antipain, aprotinin, benzamidine, bestatin, chymostatin, ε-aminocaproic acid, N-ethylmaleimide, leupeptin, phosphoramidon and pepstatin. The most commonly used chelators of divalent cations for the inhibition of degrading enzymes such as of metalloproteases are EDTA and EGTA (ethylene glycol bis(aminoethylether)tetra-acetic acid).

3.4.4 Subcellular fractionation

A typical flow chart outlining a subcellular fractionation protocol is shown in Fig. 3.5b. Depending on the amount of starting material, which would usually range between 1 and 500 g in the case of skeletal muscle preparations, a particular type of rotor and size of centrifuge tube is chosen for individual stages of the isolation procedure. The repeated centrifugation at progressively higher speeds and longer centrifugation periods will fractionate the muscle homogenate into distinct fractions. Typical values for centrifugation steps are 10 min at 1000 g to pellet nuclei and cellular debris, 10 min at 10 000 g to pellet the contractile apparatus, 20 min at 20 000 g to pellet a fraction enriched in mitochondria, and 1 h at 100 000 g to separate the microsomal and cytosolic fractions. Mild salt washes can be carried out to remove myosin contamination of membrane preparations. Sucrose gradient centrifugation is then used to further separate microsomal subfractions derived from different muscle membranes. Using a vertical rotor or swinging-bucket rotor system at a sufficiently high g force, the crude surface membrane fraction, triad junctions, longitudinal tubules and terminal cisternae membrane vesicles can be separated. To collect bands of fractions, the careful removal of fractions from the top can be achieved manually with a pipette. Alternatively, in the case of relatively unstable gradients or tight banding patterns, membrane vesicles can be harvested from the bottom by an automated fraction collector. In this case, the centrifuge tube is pierced and fractions collected by gravity or slowly forced out of the tube by a replacing liquid of higher density. Another method for collecting fractions from unstable gradients is the slicing of the centrifuge tube after freezing. Both latter methods destroy the centrifuge tubes and are used routinely in research laboratories.

Cross-contamination of vesicular membrane populations is an inevitable problem during subcellular fractionation procedures. The technical reason for this is the lack of adequate control in the formation of various types of membrane during tissue homogenisation. Membrane domains originally derived from a similar subcellular location might form a variety of structures including inside-out vesicles, right-side-out vesicles, sealed structures, leaky vesicles and/or membrane sheets. In addition, smaller vesicles might become entrapped in larger vesicles. Different membrane systems might aggregate non-specifically or bind to or entrap abundant solubilised proteins. Hence, if highly purified membrane preparations are needed for sophisticated cell biological or biochemical studies, affinity separation methodology has to be employed. The flow chart and immunoblotting diagram in Fig. 3.6 illustrates both the preparative and analytical principles underlying such a biochemical approach. Modern preparative affinity techniques using centrifugation steps can be performed with various biological or chemical ligands. In the case of immunoaffinity purification, antibodies are used to specifically bind to their respective antigen.

3.4.5 Affinity purification of membrane vesicles

In Fig. 3.6a is shown a widely employed lectin agglutination method. Lectins are plant proteins that bind tightly to specific carbohydrate structures. The rationale behind using purified wheat germ agglutinin (WGA) lectin for the affinity purification of sarcolemma vesicles is that the muscle plasmalemma forms mostly right-side-out vesicles following homogenisation. By contrast, vesicles derived from the transverse tubules are mostly inside-out and thus do not expose their carbohydrates. Glycoproteins from the abundant sarcoplasmic reticulum do not exhibit carbohydrate moities that are recognised by this particular lectin species. Therefore only sarcolemma vesicles are agglutinated by the wheat germ lectin and the aggregate can be separated from the transverse tubular fraction by centrifugation for 2 min at 15 000 g. The electron microscopical characterisation of agglutinated surface membranes reveals large smooth sarcolemma vesicles that have electron-dense entrapments. To remove these vesicular contaminants, originally derived from the sarcoplasmic reticulum, immobilised surface vesicles are treated with low concentrations of the non-ionic detergent Triton X-100. This procedure does not solubilise integral membrane proteins, but introduces openings in the sarcolemma vesicles for the release of the much smaller sarcoplasmic reticulum

(a)

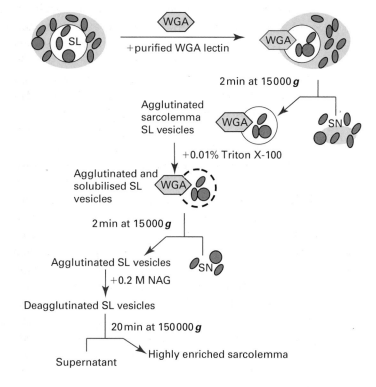

Crude surface membrane
Mixture of sarcolemma, transverse tubules and sarcoplasmic reticulum

(b)

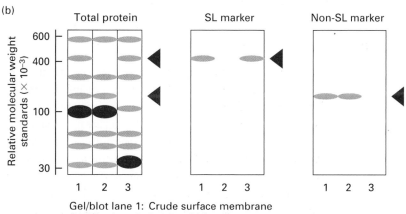

Gel/blot lane 1: Crude surface membrane
Gel/blot lane 2: Lectinvoid fraction
Gel/blot lane 3: Highly purified sarcolemma

Fig. 3.6. Affinity separation method using centrifugation of lectin agglutinated surface membrane vesicles from skeletal muscle. Shown are (a) a flow chart of the various preparative steps in the isolation of highly purified sarcolemma (SL) vesicles and (b) a diagram of the immunoblot analysis of this subcellular fractionation procedure. The SL and non-SL markers are surface-associated dystrophin of 427 kDa and the transverse-tubular α_{1S}-subunit of the dihydropyridine receptor of 170 kDa, respectively. NAG, N-acetylglycosamine; WGA, wheat germ agglutinin; SN, supernatant.

vesicles. Low g force centrifugation is then used to separate the agglutinated sarcolemma vesicles and the contaminants. To remove the lectin from the purified vesicles, the fraction is incubated with the competitive sugar N-acetylglucosamine, which eliminates the bonds between the surface glycoproteins and the lectin. A final centrifugation step for 20 min at 150 000 g results in a pellet of highly purified sarcolemma vesicles. A quick and convenient analytical method to confirm whether this subcellular fractionation procedure has resulted in the isolation of the muscle plasmalemma is immunoblotting with a mini electrophoresis unit. Fig. 3.6b shows a diagram of the protein and antigen banding pattern of crude surface membranes, the lectin void fraction and the highly purified sarcolemma fraction. Using antibodies to markers of the transverse tubules and the sarcolemma, such as the α_{1S}-subunit of the dihydropyridine receptor of 170 kDa and dystrophin of 427 kDa, respectively, the separation of both membrane species can be monitored. This analytical method is especially useful for the characterisation of membrane vesicles, when no simple and fast assay systems for testing marker enzyme activities are available.

In the case of the separation of mitochondrial membranes, the distribution of enzyme activities rather than immunoblotting is used routinely for determining the distribution of the inner membrane, contact zones and the outer membrane in density gradients. Binding assays or enzyme testing represents the more traditional way to characterise subcellular fractions following centrifugation. Fig. 3.7a outlines diagrammatically the microcompartments of liver mitochondria and the associated marker enzymes. While monoamino oxidase (MAO) is enriched in the outer membrane, the enzyme succinate dehydrogenase (SDH) is associated with the inner membrane system and a representative marker of contact sites between both membranes is glutathione transferase (GT). Membrane vesicles from intact mitochondria can be generated by consecutive swelling, shrinking and sonication of the suspended organelles. The vesicular mixture is then separated by sucrose density centrifugation into the three main types of mitochondrial membrane (Fig. 3.7b). The distribution of marker enzyme activities in the various fractions demonstrates that the outer membrane has a lower density compared to the inner membrane. The GT-containing contact zones are positioned in a band between the inner and outer mitochondrial membrane and contain enzyme activities characteristic for both systems (Fig. 3.7c). Routinely used enzymes as subcellular markers would be the Na^+/K^+-ATPase for the plasmalemma, glucose 6-phosphatase for the endoplasmic reticulum, galactosyl transferase for the Golgi apparatus, SDH for mitochondria, acid phosphatase for lysosomes, catalase for peroxisomes and lactate dehydrogenase for the cytosol.

3.5 ANALYTICAL CENTRIFUGATION

3.5.1 Applications of analytical ultracentrifugation

As biological macromolecules exhibit random thermal motion, the earth's gravitational field does not significantly affect their relatively uniform distribution in

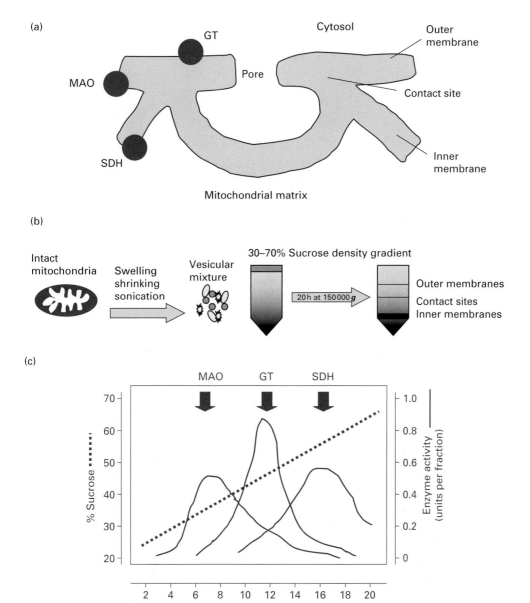

Fig. 3.7. Scheme of the fractionation of membranes derived from liver mitochondria. Shown are: (a) the distribution of marker enzymes in the microcompartments of liver mitochondria (MAO, monoamino oxidase; SDH, succinate dehydrogenase; GT, glutathione transferase); (b) the separation method to isolate fractions highly enriched in the inner cristae membrane, contact zones and the outer mitochondrial membrane and (c) the distribution of mitochondrial membranes after density gradient centrifugation.

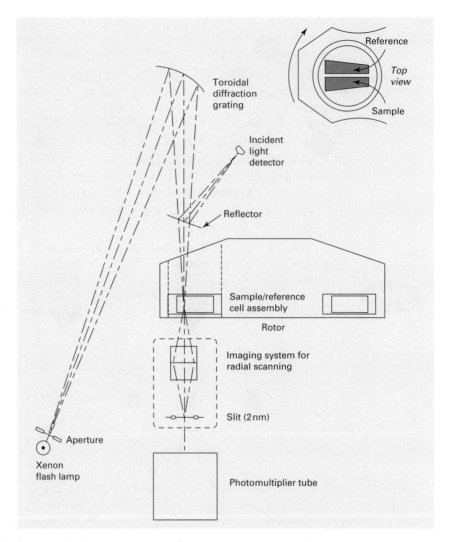

Fig. 3.8. Schematic diagram of the optical system of an analytical ultracentrifuge. The high intensity xenon flash lamp of the Beckman Optima XL-A analytical ultracentrifuge shown here allows the use of wavelengths between 190 nm and 800 nm. The high sensitivity of the absorbance optics allows the measurement of highly dilute protein samples below 230 nm. (Courtesy of Beckman–Coulter).

an aqueous environment. Isolated biomolecules in solution exhibit distinguishable sedimentation only when they undergo immense accelerations, for example in an ultracentrifugal field. A typical analytical ultracentrifuge can generate a centrifugal field of 250 000 g in its analytical cell. Within these extremely high gravitational fields, the ultracentrifuge cell has to allow light passage through the biological particles for proper measurement of the concentration distribution. The schematic diagram shown in Fig. 3.8 outlines the optical system of a modern analytical ultracentrifuge. The availability of high intensity xenon flash lamps and the advance in instrumental sensitivity and wavelength range has made the accurate measurement of highly dilute protein samples possible below 230 nm. Analytical ultracentrifuges such as the Beckman Optima XL-A allow the use of wavelengths between 190 and 800 nm. Sedimentation of isolated proteins or nucleic acids can be useful in the determination of the relative molecular mass, purity and shape of these biomolecules. Analytical ultracentrifugation for the determination of the relative molecular mass of a macromolecule can be performed by a sedimentation velocity approach or sedimentation equilibrium methodology. The hydrodynamic properties of macromolecules are described by their sedimentation coefficients and can be determined from the rate that a concentration boundary of the particular biomolecules moves in the gravitational field. Such studies on the solution behaviour of macromolecules can give detailed insight into the properties of large aggregates and thereby confirm results from biochemical analyses on complex formation. The sedimentation coefficient can be used to characterise changes in the size and shape of macromolecules with changing experimental conditions. This allows for the detailed biophysical analysis of the effect of variations in the pH value, temperature or cofactors on molecular shape.

Analytical ultracentrifugation is most often employed in:

- the determination of the purity of macromolecules,
- the determination of the relative molecular mass of solutes in their native state,
- the examination of changes in the relative molecular mass of supramolecular complexes,
- the detection of conformational changes,
- ligand-binding studies (Section 16.4.1).

The sedimentation velocity method can be employed to estimate sample purity. Sedimentation patterns can be obtained using the Schlieren optical system. This method measures the refractive index gradient at each point in the ultracentrifugation cell at varying time intervals. During the sedimentation velocity analysis, a homogeneous preparation forms a single, sharp, symmetrical, sedimenting boundary. This demonstrates that the biological macromolecules analysed exhibit the same relative molecular mass, shape and size. However, one cannot assume that the analysed particles exhibit an identical electrical charge or biological activity. Only additional biochemical studies using electrophoretic techniques and enzyme/bio-assays can differentiate between these minor subtypes of macromolecules with similar molecular mass. The great advantage of the sedimentation velocity method is that smaller or larger contaminants can be recognised clearly as shoulders on the main peak, asymmetry of the main peak and/or additional peaks. For a list of references please consult the review articles listed in Section 3.6. In addition, manufacturers of analytical ultracentrifuges have made available a large range of excellent brochures on the theoretical background of this method and its specific applications. These introductory texts are usually written by research biochemists and are well worth reading to become familiar with this field.

3.5.2 **Relative molecular mass determination**

For the accurate determination of the relative molecular mass of solutes in their native state, analytical ultracentrifugation presents an unrivalled technique. The method requires only small sample sizes (20–120 mm³) and low particle concentrations (0.01–1 g dm⁻³) and biological molecules with a wide range of relative molecular masses can be characterised. In conjunction with electrophoretic, chromatographic, crystallographic and sequencing data, the biochemical properties of a biological particle of interest can be determined in great detail. As long as the absorbance of the biomolecules to be investigated (such as proteins, carbohydrates or nucleic acids) is different from that of the surrounding solvent, analytical ultracentrifugation can be applied. At the start of an experiment using the boundary sedimentation method, the biological particles are uniformly distributed throughout the solution in the analytical cell. The application of a centrifugal field then causes a migration of the randomly distributed biomolecules through the solvent radially outwards from the centre of rotation. The solvent that has been cleared of particles and the solvent still containing the sedimenting material form a sharp boundary. The movement of the boundary with time is a measure of the rate of sedimentaion of the biomolecules. The sedimentation coefficient depends directly on the mass of the biological particle. The concentration distribution is dependent on the buoyant relative molecular mass. The movement of biomolecules in a centrifugal field can be determined and a plot of the natural logarithm of the solute concentration versus the squared radial distance from the centre of rotation (ln c versus r^2) yields a straight line with a slope proportional to the monomer molecular mass. Alternatively, the relative molecular mass of a biological macromolecule can be determined by the band sedimentation technique. In this case, the sample is layered on top of a denser solvent. During centrifugation, the solvent forms its own density gradient and the migration of the particle band is followed in the analytical cell. Relative molecular mass determination by analytical ultracentrifugation is applicable to values from a few hundred to several millions. It is therefore used for the analysis of small carbohydrates, proteins, nucleic acid macromolecules, viruses and subcellular particles such as mitochondria.

3.5.3 **Sedimentation coeffcient**

Biochemical studies over the last few decades have demonstrated clearly that biological macromolecules do not perform their biochemical and physiological functions in isolation. Many proteins were shown to be multifunctional and their activity is regulated by complex interactions within homogeneous and heterogeneous complexes. Cooperative kinetics and the influence of microdomains have been recognised to play a major role in the regulation of biochemical processes. Since conformational changes in biological macromolecules may cause differences in their sedimentation rates, analytical ultracentrifugation is an ideal experimental tool for the determination of such structural modifications. For example, a macromolecule that changes its conformation into a more compact structure decreases its frictional resistance in the solvent. In contrast, the frictional resistance increases

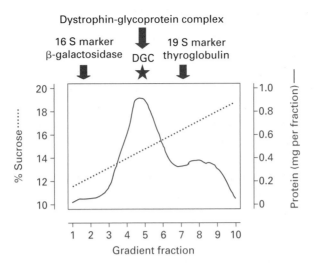

Fig. 3.9. Sedimentation analysis of a supramolecular protein complex. Shown is the sedimentation of the dystrophin–glycoprotein complex (DGC). Its size was estimated to be approximately 18 S by comparing its migration to that of the standards β-galactosidase (16 S) and thyroglobulin (19 S). Since the sedimentation coefficients of biological macromolecules are relatively small, they are expressed as Svedberg units (S), where 1 Svedberg unit equals 10^{-13} s.

when a molecular assembly becomes more disorganised. The binding of ligands (such as inhibitors, activators or substrates) or a change in temperature or buffering conditions may induce conformational changes in subunits of biomolecules that in turn can result in major changes in the supramolecular structure of complexes. Such modifications can be determined by distinct differences in the sedimentation velocity of the molecular species. Sedimentation equilibrium experiments can be used to determine the relative size of individual subunits participating in complex formation, the stoichiometry and size of a complex assembly under different physiological conditions and the strength of interactions between subunits.

When a new protein species is identified that appears to exist under native conditions in a large complex, several biochemical techniques are available to evaluate the oligomeric status of such a macromolecule. Gel filtration analysis, blot overlay assays, affinity chromatography, differential immunoprecipitation and chemical cross-linking are typical examples of such techniques. With respect to centrifugation, sedimentation analysis using a density gradient is an ideal method to support such biochemical data. For the initial determination of the size of a complex, the sedimentation of known marker proteins is compared with the novel protein complex. Biological particles with a different molecular mass, shape or size migrate with different velocities in a centrifugal field (Section 3.1). As can be seen in equation 3.7, the sedimentation coefficient has dimensions of seconds. The value of Svedberg units (S = 10^{-13} s) lies, for many macromolecules of biochemical interest, typically between 1 and 20, and for larger biological particles such as ribosomes, microsomes and mitochondria between 80 and several thousand. The prototype of a soluble protein, serum albumin of apparent relative molecular mass 66 000, has a sedimentation coefficient of 4.5 S. Fig. 3.9 illustrates the sedimentation analysis of the newly discovered dystrophin–glycoprotein complex (DGC). The size of this complex was estimated to be approximately 18 S by comparing its migration with that of the standards β-galactosidase (16 S) and thyroglobulin (19 S). When the membrane cytoskeletal element dystrophin was first identified, it was shown to bind to a lectin column, although it does not exhibit any carbohydrate chains. This suggested that dystrophin might exist in a complex with surface glycoproteins. Sedimentation analysis confirmed the existence of such a DGC and centrifugation, following various biochemical modifications of the protein assembly, led to a detailed understanding of its composition. Alkaline extraction, acid treatment or incubation with different types of detergent causes the differential disintegration of the DGC. It is now known that dystrophin is tightly associated with at least 10 different surface proteins that are involved in membrane stabilisation, receptor anchoring and signal transduction processes. The successful characterisation of the DGC by sedimentation analysis is an excellent example of how centrifugation methodology can be exploited quickly to gain biochemical knowledge of a newly discovered protein.

3.6 SUGGESTIONS FOR FURTHER READING

FINDLAY, J. B. C. and EVANS, W. H. (1987). *Biological Membranes*. Published in the Practical Approaches in Biochemistry Series, IRL Press, Oxford/Washington, DC. (Contains two extensive chapters on differential centrifugation procedures used in the subcellular fractionation of animal and plant cells.)

FISHER, D., FRANCIS, G. E. AND RICKWOOD, D. (eds.) (1998). *Cell Separation*. Published in the Practical Approaches in Biochemistry Series, IRL Press, Oxford/Washington, DC. (Outlines fractionation of cells by sedimentation methodology.)

GRAHAM, J. M. AND RICKWOOD, D. (eds.) (1997). *Subcellular Fractionation*. Published in the Practical Approaches in Biochemistry Series, IRL Press, Oxford/Washington, DC. (Provides a description of essential subcellular fractionation techniques.)

LAUE, T. M. (2001). Biophysical studies by ultracentrifugation. *Current Opinion in Structural Biology* **11**, 579–583. (Provides an excellent synopsis of the applicability of ultracentrifugation to the characterisation of macromolecular behaviour in complex solution.)

LAUE, T. M. and STAFFORD, W. F. III (1999). Modern applications of analytical ultracentrifugation. *Annual Reviews in Biophysics and Biomolecular Structures* **28**, 75–100. (Provides an overview of available information on analytical ultracentrifugation and how this analytical technique can be used in contemporary applications.)

MURRAY, B. E. and OHLENDIECK, K. (2000). Chemical cross-linking analysis of Ca^{2+}-ATPase from rabbit skeletal muscle. *Biochemical Education* **28**, 41–46. (Description of an undergraduate student experiment dealing with the subcellular fractionation of skeletal muscle homogenate.)

RALSTON, G. (1993). *Introduction to Analytical Ultracentrifugation*. Beckman Instruments, Fullerton, CA. (Describes the different types of experiment that can be performed with an analytical ultracentrifuge.)

Chapter 4

Microscopy

4.1 INTRODUCTION

Biochemical analysis is frequently accompanied by microscopic examination of tissue, cell or organelle preparations. Such examinations are used in many different applications; for example, to evaluate the integrity of samples during an experiment, to map the fine details of the spatial distribution of macromolecules within cells, or to directly measure biochemical events within living tissues.

There are two fundamentally different types of microscope: the light microscope and the electron microscope (Fig. 4.1). Light microscopes use a series of glass lenses to focus light in order to form an image whereas electron microscopes use electromagnetic lenses to focus a beam of electrons. Light microscopes are able to magnify to a maximum of approximately 1500 times whereas electron microscopes are capable of magnifying to a maximum of approximately 200 000 times.

Magnification is not, however, the best measure of a microscope. Rather, resolution, the ability to distinguish between two closely spaced points in a specimen, is a much more reliable estimate of a microscope's utility. Light microscopes have a resolution limit of about 0.5 micrometres (μm) for routine analysis. In contrast, electron microscopes have a resolution of up to 1 nanometre (nm). Both living and dead specimens are viewed with a light microscope, and often in real colour, whereas only dead ones are viewed with an electron microscope, and never in real colour. Recent advancements have improved upon the 0.2 μm resolution limit of the light microscope for some special applications (Section 4.8).

Applications of the microscope in biochemistry may be relatively simple and routine; for example, a quick check of the status of a cell preparation or of cells growing in tissue culture. Here, a simple bench-top light microscope is perfectly adequate. On the other hand, the application may be more involved, for example measuring the concentration of calcium in a living embryo over a millisecond time scale. Here a more advanced light microscope (often called an imaging system) is required. Alternatively, the application may require the location of macromolecules in membrane-bound compartments inside the cell. Here the electron microscope will be chosen for imaging, since it is the only instrument that is capable of the nanometre resolution required for such images.

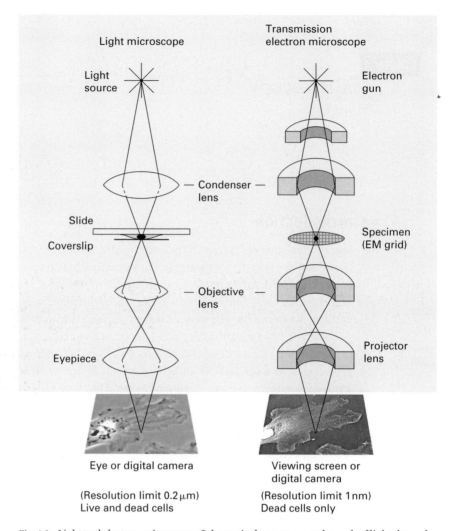

Fig. 4.1. Light and electron microscopy. Schematic that compares the path of light through a compound light microscope (LM) with the path of electrons through a transmission electron microscope (TEM). Light from a lamp (LM) or a beam of electrons from an electron gun (TEM) is focused at the specimen by a glass condenser lens (LM) or electromagnetic lenses (TEM). For the LM the specimen is mounted on a glass slide with a coverslip placed on top, and for the TEM the specimen is placed on a copper electron microscope grid. The image is magnified with an objective lens, glass in the LM and electromagnetic lens in the TEM, and projected onto a detector with the eyepiece lens in the LM or the projector lens in the TEM. The detector can be the eye or a digital camera in the LM or phosphorescent viewing screen or a digital camera in the TEM. (Light and EM images courtesy of Tatyana Svitkina.)

Some microscopes are more suited to specific applications than others. Images may be required from specimens of vastly different sizes and magnifications (Fig. 4.2); for example, for imaging whole animals (metres), through tissues and embryos (micrometres), and down to cells, proteins and DNA (nanometres). The study of living cells may require time resolution from days, for example when

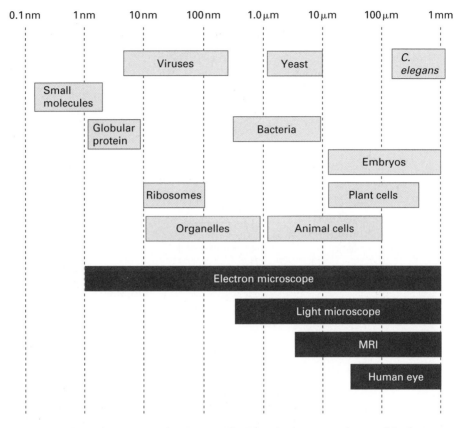

Fig. 4.2. The relative sizes of a selection of biological specimens and some of the devices used to image them. The range of resolution for each instrument is included in the dark purple bars at the base of the figure.

imaging neuronal development or disease processes, to milliseconds, for example when imaging cell signalling events.

The field of microscopy has undergone a renaissance over the past 20 years, with the addition of various technological advancements to the instruments. Most images produced by microscopes are now recorded electronically using digital imaging techniques – digital cameras, digital image acquisition software, digital printing and digital display methods. These advancements have allowed many more applications of the microscope in biochemistry, ranging from routine observations of cells and cell extracts to specialised techniques for directly measuring biochemical events in cells.

4.2 **THE LIGHT MICROSCOPE**

4.2.1 **Basic components of the light microscope**

The simplest form of light microscope consists of a single glass lens mounted in a metal frame – a magnifying glass (Fig. 4.3). Here the specimen requires very little

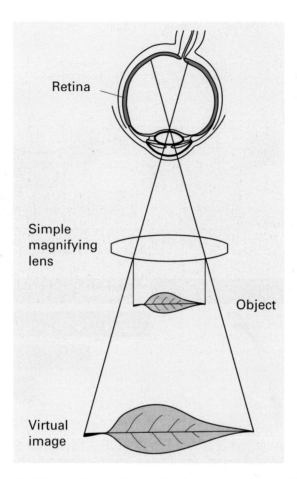

Fig. 4.3. Magnification in a simple microscope – a glass magnifying lens. The lens of the eye focuses light onto the retina – a collection of light-sensitive cells located at the back of the eye. The specimen is found by placing the convex lens between it and the eye. Magnification of the image of the specimen is achieved by the lens spreading the visual angle on the retina. Here the image appears as if it is on the same side of the lens as the specimen – this is called a virtual image.

preparation, and is usually held close to the eye in the hand. Focusing of the region of interest is achieved by moving the lens and the specimen relative to one another. The source of light is usually the sun or ambient indoor light. The detector is the human eye. The recording device is a hand drawing or an anecdote.

Compound microscopes

All modern light microscopes are made up of more than one glass lens in combination. The major components are the condenser lens, the objective lens and the eyepiece lens, and, such instruments are therefore called compound microscopes (Fig. 4.1). Each of these components is in turn made up of combinations of lenses, which are necessary to produce magnified images with reduced artefacts and aberrations. For example, chromatic aberration occurs when different

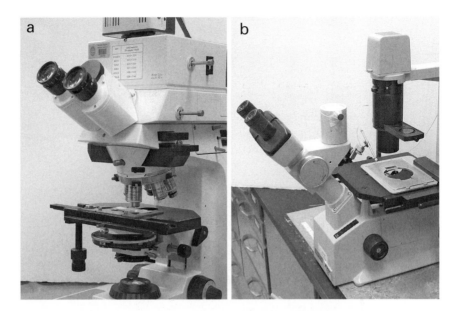

Fig. 4.4. Two basic types of compound light microscope. (a) An upright light microscope and (b) an inverted light microscope. Note how there is more room available on the stage of the inverted microscope (b). This instrument is set up for microinjection with a needle holder to the left of the stage.

wavelengths of light are separated and pass through a lens at different angles. This results in rainbow colours around the edges of objects in the image. This problem was encountered in the early microscopes of Antonie Van Leeuwenhoek and Robert Hooke, for example. All modern lenses are corrected to some degree in order to avoid this problem.

The main components of the compound light microscope include a light source that is focused at the specimen by a condenser lens. Light that either passes through the specimen (transmitted light) or is reflected back from the specimen (reflected light) is focused by the objective lens into the eyepiece lens. The image is either viewed directly by eye in the eyepiece or is most often projected onto a detector, for example photographic film or, more likely, a digital camera. The images are displayed on the screen of a computer imaging system, stored in a digital format and reproduced using digital methods.

The part of the microscope that holds all of the components firmly in position is called the stand. There are two basic types of compound light microscope stand – upright and inverted microscopes (Fig. 4.4). The light source is below the condenser lens in the upright microscope and the objectives are above the specimen stage. This is the most commonly used format for viewing specimens. The inverted microscope is engineered so that the light source and the condenser lens are above the specimen stage, and the objective lenses are beneath it. This allows additional room for manipulating the specimen directly on the stage, for example for the microinjection of macromolecules into tissue culture cells, for *in vitro* fertilisation of eggs, or for viewing developing embryos over time.

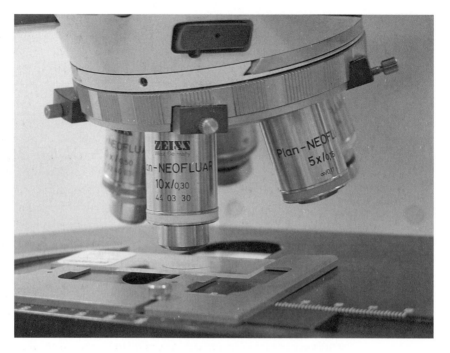

Fig. 4.5. The objective lens. A selection of objective lenses mounted on an upright research grade compound light microscope. From the inscription on the two lenses in focus they are relatively low magnification $10\times$ and $5\times$ of numerical aperture 0.3 and 0.16, respectively. Both lenses are Plan Neofluar, which means they are relatively well corrected. The $10\times$ lens is directly above a specimen mounted on a slide and coverslip, and held in place on the specimen stage.

The correct illumination of the specimen is critical for achieving high quality images and photomicrographs. This is achieved using a light source. Typically light sources are mercury lamps, xenon lamps or lasers. Light from the light source passes into the condenser lens, which is mounted beneath the microscope stage in an upright microscope (and above the stage in an inverted microscope) in a bracket that can be raised and lowered for focusing (Fig. 4.4). The condenser focuses light from the light source and illuminates the specimen with parallel beams of light. A correctly positioned condenser lens produces illumination that is uniformly bright and free from glare across the viewing area of the specimen (Köhler illumination). Condenser misalignment and an improperly adjusted condenser aperture diaphragm are major sources of poor images in the light microscope.

The specimen stage is a mechanical device that is finely engineered to hold the specimen firmly in place (Fig. 4.5). Any movement or vibration will be detrimental to the final image. The stage enables the specimen to be moved and positioned in fine and smooth increments, both horizontally and transversely, in the X and the Y directions, for locating a region of interest. The stage is moved vertically in the Z direction for focusing the specimen or for inverted microscopes, the objectives themselves are moved and the stage remains fixed. There are usually coarse and fine focusing controls for low magnification and high magnification viewing, respectively. The fine focus control can be moved in increments of 1 μm or better in the best research microscopes. The specimen stage can either be moved by hand or be controlled more accurately by a computer via stepper motors attached to the fine focus control of the microscope.

The objective lens is responsible for producing the magnified image, and can be the most expensive component of the light microscope (Fig. 4.5). Objectives are available in many different varieties, and there is a wealth of information inscribed on each one. This may include the manufacturer, magnification (4×, 10×, 20×, 40×, 60×, 100×), immersion requirements (air, oil or water), coverslip thickness (usually 0.17 mm) and often with more-specialised optical properties of the lens (Section 4.2.3). In addition, lens corrections for optical artefacts such as chromatic aberration and flatness of field may also be included in the lens description. For example, words such as fluorite, the least corrected (often shortened to 'fluo'), or plan apochromat, the most highly corrected (often shortened to 'plan' or 'plan apo'), may appear somewhere on the lens.

Lenses can either be dry or immersion lenses, and as a rule of thumb, most objectives below 40× are air (dry) objectives and those of 40× and above are immersion objective (oil, glycerol or water). Should the objective be designed to operate in oil it will be labelled 'OIL' or 'OEL'. Other immersion media include glycerol and water, and the lens will be marked to indicate this. Many lenses are colour coded to a manufacturer's specifications.

The numerical aperture (NA) is always marked on the lens. This is a number usually between 0.04 and 1.4. The NA is a measure of the ability of a lens to collect light from the specimen. Lenses with a low NA collect less light than those with a high NA. Resolution varies inversely with NA, which infers that higher NA objectives yield the best resolution. Generally speaking, the higher power objectives have a higher NA and better resolution than the lower power lenses with lower NAs. For example, 0.2 μm resolution can only be achieved using a 60× or a 100× plan-apochromat oil immersion lens with a NA of 1.4. Should there be a choice between two lenses of the same magnification, then it is usually best to choose the one of higher NA.

The objective lens is also the part of the microscope that can most easily be damaged by mishandling. Many lenses are coated with a protective coating but, even so, one scratch on the front of the lens can result in serious image degradation. Therefore great care should be taken when handling objective lenses. Objective lenses must be cleaned using a protocol recommended by the manufacturer, and only by a qualified person. A dirty objective lens is a major source of poor images.

The resolution of the lens measures the ability to distinguish between two objects in the specimen. The shorter the wavelengths of illuminating light, the higher is the resolving power of the microscope (Fig. 4.6). The limit of resolution for a microscope that uses visible light is about 300 nm with a dry lens (in air) and 200 nm with an oil immersion lens. By using ultraviolet light as a light source the resolution can be improved to 100 nm because of the shorter

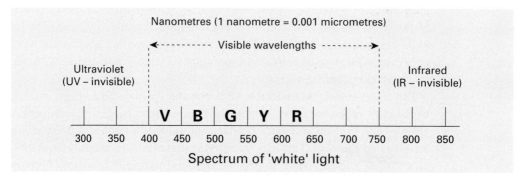

Fig. 4.6. The visible spectrum – the spectrum of white light visible to the human eye. Our eyes are able to detect colour in the visible wavelengths of the spectrum; usually in the region between 400 nm (violet) and 750 nm (red). Most modern electronic detectors are sensitive beyond the visible spectrum of the human eye. UV, ultraviolet; IR, infrared; V, violet; B, blue; G, green; Y, yellow; R, red.

wavelength of the light (200–300 nm). These limits of resolution are often difficult to achieve practically because of aberrations in the lenses and the poor optical properties of many biological specimens. More specialised research microscopes can now attain a resolution of around 20 nm in non-routine applications (Section 4.8).

The eyepiece (sometimes referred to as the ocular) works in combination with the objective lens to further magnify the image, and allows it to be detected by eye or more usually to project the image into a digital camera for recording purposes. Eyepieces usually magnify by 10×, since an eyepiece of higher magnification merely enlarges the image, with no improvement in resolution. There is an upper boundary to the useful magnification of the collection of lenses in a microscope. For each objective lens the magnification can be increased above a point where it is impossible to resolve any more detail in the specimen. Any magnification above this point is often called empty magnification. The best way to improve magnification is to use a higher magnification and higher NA objective lens. Should sufficient resolution not be achieved using the light microscope, then it will be necessary to use the electron microscope (Section 4.6).

In addition to the human eye and photographic film there are two types of electronic detector employed on modern light microscopes. These are area detectors that form an image directly, for example video cameras and charge-coupled devices (CCDs). Alternatively, point detectors can be used to measure intensities in the image; for example photomultiplier tubes (PMTs) and photodiodes. Point detectors are capable of producing images in scanning microscopy (Section 4.3).

4.2.2 **The specimen**

The specimen (sometimes called the sample) can be the entire organism or a dissected organ (whole mount), an aliquot collected during a biochemical protocol

Table 4.1 Generalised indirect immunofluorescence protocol

1. Fix in 1% formaldehyde for 30 min
2. Rinse in cold buffer
3. Block buffer
4. Incubate in primary antibody, e.g. mouse anti-tubulin[a]
5. Wash 4 times in buffer
6. Incubate in secondary antibody, e.g. fluorescein-labelled rabbit anti-mouse[a]
7. Wash 4 times in buffer
8. Incubate in anti-fade reagent, e.g. Vectashield[a]
9. Mount on slide with a coverslip
10. View using epifluorescence microscopy

[a] The incubation times vary with the tissue type, from 30 min for tissue culture cells (thin samples) to overnight for whole embryos (thick samples).

for a quick check of the preparation, or a small part of an organism (biopsy) or smear of blood or spermatozoa. In order to collect images from it, the specimen must be in a form that is compatible with the microscope. This is achieved using a published protocol. The end-product of a protocol is a relatively thin and somewhat transparent piece of tissue mounted on a piece of glass (slide) in a mounting medium (water, tissue culture medium or glycerol) with a thin square of glass mounted on top (coverslip).

Coverslips are graded by their thickness. The thinnest ones are labelled no. 1, which corresponds to a thickness of approximately 0.17 mm. The coverslip side of the specimen is always placed closest to the objective lens. It is essential to use a coverslip that is matched to the objective lens in order to achieve optimal resolution. This is critical for high-magnification imaging because if the coverslip is too thick it will be impossible to achieve an image using a high magnification objective lens.

Specimen preparation protocols can be relatively simple or they may involve many steps that take several days to complete (Table 4.1). A simple protocol would be to take an aliquot of a biological preparation, for example living spermatozoa, place a drop on a slide and put a coverslip onto the drop. The coverslip is sealed to the glass slide in some way, for example using nail polish or beeswax, so that it does not move. Shear forces from the movement of the coverslip over the glass slide can cause damage to the specimen or the objective lens.

Many specimens are too thick to be mounted directly onto a slide, and these are cut into thin sections using a device called a microtome. The tissue is usually mounted in a block of wax and cut with the knife of the microtome into thin sections (between 100 μm and 500 μm in thickness). The sections are then placed onto a glass slide, stained and sealed with mounting medium with a coverslip. Some samples are frozen and cut on a cryostat, which is basically a microtome that can keep a specimen in the frozen state, and produce frozen sections more suitable for immunolabelling (Section 4.2.3).

Prior to sectioning, the tissue is usually treated with a chemical agent called a fixative to preserve it. Popular fixatives include formaldehyde and glutaraldehyde, which act by cross-linking proteins, and alcohols, which act by precipitation. All of these fixatives are designed to maintain the structural integrity of the cell. After fixation the specimen is usually permeabilised in order to allow a stain to infuse the entire tissue. The amount of permeabilisation (time and severity) depends upon several factors; for example, the size of the stain or the density of the tissue. These parameters are found by trial and error for a new specimen, but are usually available in published protocols. The goal is to infiltrate the entire tissue with a uniform staining.

4.2.3 Contrast in the light microscope

Most cells and tissues are colourless and almost transparent, and lack contrast when viewed in a light microscope. Therefore to visualise any details of cellular components it is necessary to introduce contrast into the specimen. This is achieved either by optical means using a specific configuration of microscope components, or by staining the specimen with a dye or, more usually, using a combination of optical and staining methods. Different regions of the cell can be stained selectively with different stains.

Optical contrast

Contrast is achieved optically by introducing various elements into the light path of the microscope and using lenses and filters that change the pattern of light passing through the specimen and the optical system. This can be as simple as adding a piece of coloured glass or a neutral density filter into the illuminating light path, by changing the light intensity, or by adjusting the diameter of a condenser aperture. Usually all of these operations are adjusted until an acceptable level of contrast is achieved for imaging.

The most basic mode of the light microscope is called brightfield (bright background), which can be achieved with the minimum of optical elements. Contrast in brightfield images is usually produced by the colour of the specimen itself. Brightfield is therefore used most often to collect images from pigmented tissues or histological sections or tissue culture cells that have been stained with colourful dyes (Figs. 4.7a and 4.8b).

Several configurations of the light microscope have been introduced over the years specifically to add contrast to the final image. Darkfield illumination produces images of brightly illuminated objects on a black background (Figs. 4.7b and 4.8a). This technique has traditionally been used for viewing the outlines of objects in liquid media such as living spermatozoa, microorganisms, cells growing in tissue culture or for a quick check of the status of a biochemical preparation. For lower magnifications, a simple darkfield setting on the condenser will be sufficient. For more critical darkfield imaging at a higher magnification, a darkfield condenser with a darkfield objective lens will be required.

Phase contrast is used for viewing unstained cells growing in tissue culture and for testing cell and organelle preparations for lysis (Fig. 4.7c,d). The method

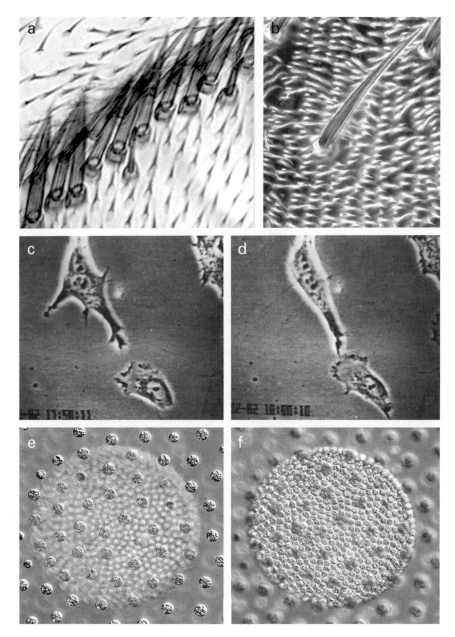

Fig. 4.7. Contrast methods in the light microscope. (a and b) A comparison of (a) brightfield and (b) darkfield images. Here the sensory bristles on the surface of a fly appear dark on a white background in the brightfield image (a) and white on a black background in a darkfield image (b). The dark colour in the larger bristles in (a) is produced by pigment. (c and d) Phase contrast view of cells growing in tissue culture. Two images extracted from a time-lapse video sequence (time between each frame is 5 min). The sequence shows the movement of a mouse 3T3 fibrosarcoma cell and a chick heart fibroblast. Note the bright 'phase halo' around the cells. (e and f) Differential interference contrast image of two focal planes of the multicellular alga *Volvox*. (Images (e) and (f) courtesy of Michael Davidson.)

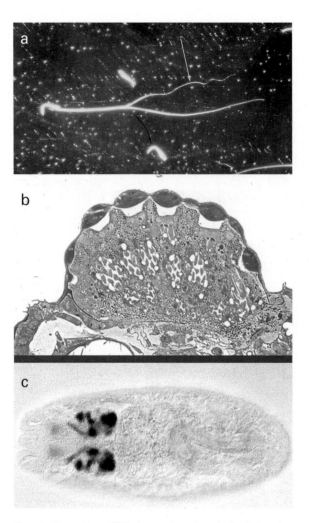

Fig. 4.8. Examples of different preparations in the light microscope. (a) Darkfield image of rat sperm preparation. An aliquot was collected from an experimental protocol in order to assess the amount of damage incurred during sonication of a population of spermatozoa. Many sperm heads can be seen in the preparation, and the fibres of the tail are starting to fray (arrowed). (b) A brightfield image of total protein staining on a section of a fly eye cut on a microtome, and stained with Coomassie Brilliant Blue. (c) DIC image of a stained *Drosophila* embryo – the DIC image shows the outline of the embryo with darker regions of neuronal staining. The DIC image of the whole embryo provides structural landmarks for placing the specific neuronal staining in the context of the anatomy.

images differences in the refractive index of cellular structures. Light that passes through thicker parts of the cell is held up relative to the light that passes through thinner parts of the cytoplasm. It requires a specialised phase condenser and phase objective lenses (both labelled 'ph'). Each phase setting of the condenser lens is matched with the phase setting of the objective lens. These are usually numbered as phase 1, phase 2 and phase 3, and are found on both the condenser and the objective lens.

(a)

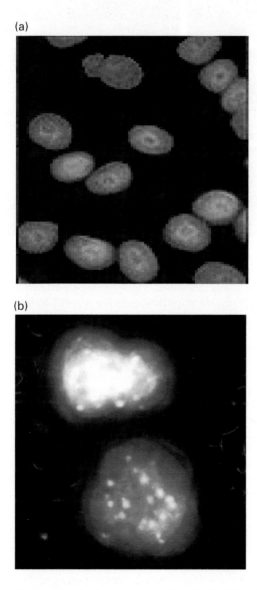

(b)

Fig. 2.4. Staining for mycoplasma in cells. (a) A Hoechst negative stain, with the dye staining cellular DNA in the nucleus and thus showing nuclear fluorescence. (b) A Hoechst positive stain, showing staining of mycoplasma DNA in the cytoplam of the cells.

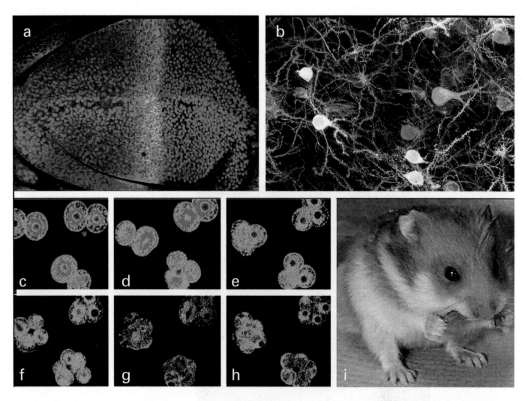

Fig. 4.13. Optical sectioning. Optical sections produced using LSCM (a and b) and multiple photon imaging (c). (a) Triple labelled *Drosophila* third instar wing imaginal disc. The images were produced using an air-cooled 25 mW krypton argon laser, which has three major lines at 488 nm (blue), 568 nm (yellow) and 647 nm (red). The three fluorochromes used were fluorescein (excitation 496 nm; emission 518 nm), lissamine rhodamine (excitation 572 nm; emission 590 nm) and cyanine 5 (excitation 649 nm; emission 666 nm). The images were collected simultaneously as single optical sections into the red, the green and the blue channels, respectively, and merged as a three-colour (red/green/blue) image (see Fig. 4.11). The image shows the expression of three wing-patterning genes; *vestigial* (in red), *apterous* (in blue) and *CiD* (in green). Regions of overlap of gene expression appear as an additive colour in the image. (b) Multicolour neurones labelled with combinations of lipophilic dyes. (c) Two photon images of three living hamster embryos labelled with the mitochondrial dye Mitotracker X rhodamine. The three embryos were imaged over a 24 h period. Images (c) to (h) are representative images collected from the time-lapse series. One of the three embryos was transferred to an adult female, who later produced 'Laser' – a living testament to the viability of multiple photon imaging. (Images kindly provided by (a) Jim Williams and Sean Carroll, (b) Wenbio Gan and Jeff Lichtman, and (c) Jayne Squirrell and Barry Bavister.)

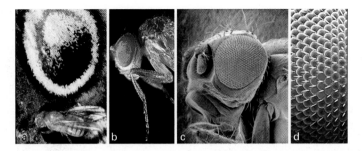

Fig. 4.17. Image surfaces using the light microscope (stereomicroscope) and in the electron microscope (scanning electron microscope). Images produced using the stereomicroscope (a) and (b) and the scanning electron microscope (c) and (d). A stereomicroscope view of a fly (*Drosophila melanogaster*) on a butterfly wing (*Precis coenia*). (a) Zoomed in to view the head region of the red-eyed fly (b). SEM image of a similar region of the fly's head (c) and zoomed more to view the individual ommatidia of the eye (d). Note that the stereomicroscope images can be viewed in real colour whereas those produced using the SEM are in greyscale. Colour can be added to EM images only digitally (d). (Images (b), (c) and (d) kindly provided by Georg Halder.)

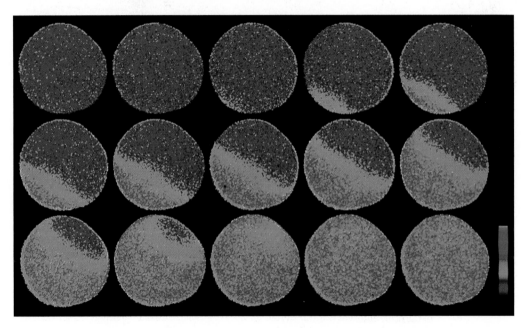

Fig. 4.21. Calcium imaging in living cells. A fertilisation-induced calcium wave in the egg of the starfish. The egg was microinjected with the calcium-sensitive fluorescent dye fluo-3 and subsequently fertilised by the addition of sperm during observation using time-lapse confocal microscopy with a 40× water immersion lens. An optical section located near the egg equator was collected every 4 s using the normal scan mode accumulated for two frames, and afterwards the images were corrected for offset and ratioed by linearly dividing the initial pre-fertilisation image into each successive frame of the time-lapse run. The ratioed images were then prepared as a montage and outputted with a pseudocolour look-up table: blue regions represent low ratios, and free calcium levels; green regions depict intermediary levels; and red areas depict high ratios and free calcium levels. Note that the wave sweeps through the entire ooplasm. (Image kindly provided by Steve Stricker).

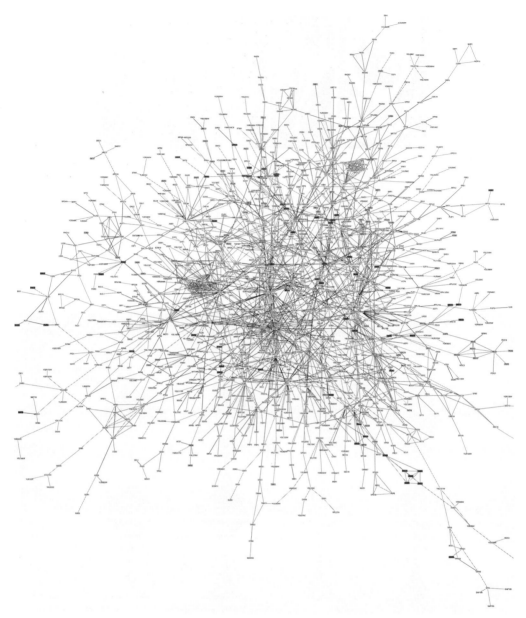

Fig. 8.11. An interaction map of the yeast proteome, assembled from published interactions (see text for details). (Courtesy of Benno Schwikowski, Peter Uetz and Stanley Fields. Reprinted with the permission of Nature Publishing Group.)

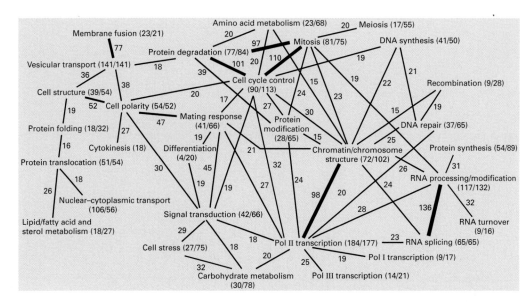

Fig. 8.12. A simplification of Fig. 8.11 identifying interactions between functional groups of proteins (see text for details). (Courtesy of Benno Schwikowski, Peter Uetz and Stanley Fields. Reprinted with the permission of Nature Publishing Group.)

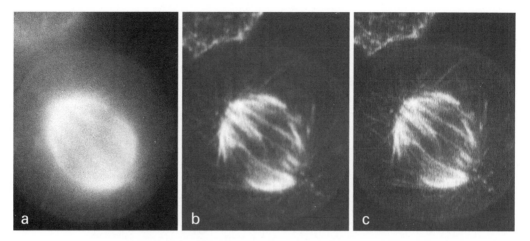

Fig. 4.9. Fluorescence microscopy. Comparison of epifluorescence and confocal fluorescence imaging of a mitotic spindle labelled using indirect immunofluorescence labelling with anti-tubulin (primary antibody) and a fluorescently labelled secondary antibody. The specimen was imaged using (a) conventional epifluorescence light microscopy or (b and c) using laser scanning confocal microscopy. Note the improved resolution of microtubules in the two confocal images (b) and (c) as compared with the conventional image (a). (b) and (c) represent two different resolution settings of the confocal microscope. Image (b) was collected with the pinhole set to a wider aperture than (c). (Image kindly provided by Brad Amos.)

Differential interference contrast (DIC) is a form of interference microscopy that produces images with a shadow relief (Fig. 4.7e,f). It is used for viewing unstained cells in tissue culture, eggs and embryos, and in combination with some stains. Here the overall shape and relief of the structure is viewed using DIC and a subset of the structure is stained with a coloured dye (Fig. 4.8c).

Fluorescence microscopy is currently the most widely used contrast technique (Fig. 4.9). The most commonly used fluorescence technique is called epifluorescence light microscopy, where 'epi' simply means 'from above'. Here, the light source comes from above the sample, and the objective lens acts as both condenser and objective lens (Fig. 4.10).

Fluorescence is popular because of the ability to achieve highly specific labelling of cellular compartments. The images usually consist of distinct regions of fluorescence (white) over large regions of no fluorescence (black), which gives excellent signal-to-noise ratios.

The light source is usually a high pressure mercury or xenon vapour lamp, which emits from the ultraviolet into the red wavelengths (Fig. 4.6). A specific wavelength of light is used to excite a fluorescent molecule or fluorophore in the specimen (Fig. 4.10). Light of longer wavelength from the excitation of the fluorophore is then imaged. This is achieved in the fluorescence microscope using combinations of filters that are specific for the excitation and emission characteristics of the fluorophore of interest. There are usually three main filters: an excitation filter, a dichromatic mirror (often called a dichroic) and a barrier filter, mounted in a single

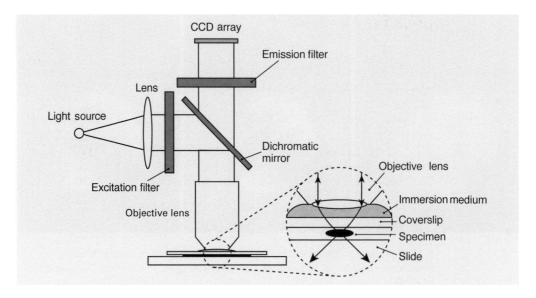

Fig. 4.10. Epifluorescence microscopy. Light from a xenon or mercury arc lamp (Light source) passes through a lens and the excitation filter and reflects off the dichromatic mirror into the objective lens. The objective lens focuses the light at the specimen via the immersion medium (usually immersion oil) and the glass coverslip (see exploded section). Any light resulting from the fluorescence excitation in the specimen passes back through the objective lens and, since it is of longer wavelength than the excitation light, it passes through the dichromatic mirror. The emission filter allows only light of the specific emission wavelength of the fluorochrome of interest to pass through to the detector, in this case a CCD array, where an image is formed.

housing above the objective lens. For example, the commonly used fluorophore fluorescein is optimally excited at a wavelength of 488 nm, and emits maximally at 518 nm (Table 4.2).

A set of glass filters for viewing fluorescein requires that all wavelengths of light from the lamp be blocked except for the 488 nm light. A filter is available that allows a maximum amount of 488 nm light to pass through it (the excitation filter). The 488 nm light is then directed to the specimen via the dichromatic mirror. Any fluorescein label in the specimen is excited by the 488 nm light, and the resulting 518 nm light that returns from the specimen passes through both the dichromatic mirror and the barrier filter to the detector. The emission filters only allow light of 518 nm to pass through to the detector, and ensure that only the signal emitted from the fluorochrome of interest reaches it. (For further details of fluorescence, see Sections 12.5 and 16.3.2.)

Chromatic mirrors and filters can be designed to filter two or three specific wavelengths for imaging specimens labelled with two or more fluorochromes (multiple labelling). The fluorescence emitted from the specimen is often too low to be detected by the human eye or it may be out of the wavelength range of detection of the eye, for example in the far-red wavelengths (Fig. 4.6). A sensitive digital camera easily detects such signals, for example a CCD or a PMT.

Table 4.2	Table of flurophores	
Dye	Excitation maximum (nm)	Emission maximum (nm)
Commonly used fluorophores		
Fluorescein (FITC)	496	518
Bodipy	503	511
CY3	554	568
Tetramethylrhodamine	554	576
Lissamine rhodamine	572	590
Texas Red	592	610
CY5	652	672
Nuclear dyes		
Hoechst 33342	346	460
DAPI	359	461
Acridine Orange	502	526
Propidium iodide	536	617
TOTO3	642	661
Ethidium bromide	510	595
Ethidium homodimer	528	617
Feulgen	570	625
Calcium indicators		
Fluo-3	506	526
Calcium Green	506	533
Reporter molecules		
Green fluorescent protein (GFP)	395/489	509
DsRed	558	583
Mitochondria		
JC-1	514	529
Rhodamine 123	507	529

DAPI, 4′,6′-diamidino-2-phenylindole.

Specimen stains

Contrast can be introduced into the specimen using one or more coloured dyes or stains. These can be non-specific stains, for example a general protein stain such as Coomassie Brilliant Blue (Fig. 4.8), or a stain that specifically labels an organelle, for example the nucleus, mitochondria, etc. Combinations of such dyes may be used to stain different organelles in contrasting colours. Many of these histological stains are usually observed using brightfield imaging. Other light microscopy techniques may also be employed in order to view the entire tissue along with the stained tissue. For example, using DIC to view the entire morphology of an embryo and a coloured stain to image the spatial distribution of the protein of interest within the embryo (Fig. 4.8).

More specific dyes are usually used in conjunction with fluorescence microscopy. Immunofluorescence microscopy is used to map the spatial distribution of macromolecules in cells and tissues. The method takes advantage of the highly specific binding of antibodies to proteins. Antibodies are raised to the protein of interest and labelled with a fluorescent probe. This probe is then used to label the protein of interest in the cell and can be imaged using fluorescence microscopy. In practice, cells are usually labelled using indirect immunofluorescence. Here the antibody to the protein of interest (primary antibody) is further labelled with a second antibody carrying the fluorescent tag (secondary antibody). Such a protocol gives a higher fluorescent signal than using a single fluorescently labelled antibody (Table 4.1).

A related technique, fluorescence *in situ* hybridisation (FISH) employs the specificity of fluorescently labelled DNA or RNA sequences. The nucleic acid probes are hybridised to chromosomes, nuclei or cellular preparations. Regions that bind the probe are imaged using fluorescence microscopy. Many different probes can be labelled with different fluorochromes in the same preparation. Multiple colour FISH is used extensively for clinical diagnoses of inherited genetic diseases. This technique has been applied to rapid screening of chromosomal and nuclear abnormalities in inherited diseases, for example Down's syndrome.

There are many different types of fluorescent molecules that can be attached to antibodies, DNA or RNA probes for fluorescence analysis (Table 4.2). All of these reagents, including primary antibodies, are available commercially or often from the laboratories that produced them. An active area of development is the production of the brightest fluorescent probes that are excited by the narrowest wavelength band and that are not damaged by light excitation (photobleaching). Traditional examples of such fluorescent probes include fluorescein and rhodamine. More modern examples include the Alexa range of dyes and the cyanine dyes. A recent addition to the list of fluorescent probes for imaging is the quantum dot. Quantum dots do not fluoresce but are nanocrystals that glow in different colours in laser light. The colours depend on the size of the dots, and they have the advantage that they are not photobleached.

4.3 OPTICAL SECTIONING

Many images collected from relatively thick specimens produced using epifluorescence microscopy are not very clear. This is because the image is made up of the optical plane of interest together with contributions from fluorescence above and below the focal plane of interest. Since the conventional epifluorescence microscope collects all of the information from the specimen, it is often referred to as a wide-field microscope. The 'out-of-focus fluorescence' can be removed using a variety of optical electronic techniques to produce optical sections (Fig. 4.9).

The term 'optical section' refers to a microscope's ability to produce sharper images of specimens than those produced using a standard wide-field epifluorescence microscope by removing the contribution from out-of-focus light to the image and, in most cases, without resorting to physical sectioning of the tissue. Such methods have revolutionised the ability to collect images from thick and fluorescently labelled specimens such as eggs, embryos and tissues. Optical sections can also be produced using high resolution DIC optics (Fig. 4.7e,f).

4.3.1 Laser scanning confocal microscopes

Optical sections are produced in the laser scanning confocal microscope (LSCM) by scanning the specimen point by point with a laser beam focused in the specimen and using a spatial filter, usually a pinhole (or a slit), to remove unwanted fluorescence from above and below the focal plane of interest (Fig. 4.11). The power of the confocal approach lies in the ability to image structures at discrete levels within an intact biological specimen.

There are two major advantages of using the LSCM in preference to conventional epifluorescence light microscopy. Glare from out-of-focus structures in the specimen is reduced and resolution is increased both laterally in the X and the Y directions (0.14 μm) and axially in the Z direction (0.23 μm). Image quality of some relatively thin specimens, for example chromosome spreads and the leading lamellipodium of cells growing in tissue culture (<0.2 μm thick), is not dramatically improved by the LSCM whereas thicker specimens such as fluorescently labelled multicellular embryos can only be imaged using the LSCM. For successful confocal imaging, a minimum number of photons should be used to efficiently excite each fluorescent probe labelling the specimen, and as many of the emitted photons from the fluorochromes as possible should make it through the light path of the instrument to the detector.

The LSCM has found many different applications in biomedical imaging. Some of these applications have been made possible by the ability of the instrument to produce a series of optical sections at discrete steps through the specimen (Fig. 4.12). This Z series of optical sections collected with a confocal microscope are all in register with each other, and can be merged together to form a single projection of the image (Z projection) or a three-dimensional (3D) representation of the image (3D reconstruction).

Multiple label images can be collected from a specimen labelled with more than one fluorescent probe, using multiple laser light sources for excitation (Fig. 4.13, see colour section). Since all of the images collected at different excitation wavelengths are in register, it is relatively easy to combine them into a single multicoloured image. Here, any overlap of staining is viewed as an additive colour change. Most confocal microscopes are able to image three or four different wavelengths simultaneously, and some more modern instruments are able to detect and separate up to 32 different wavelengths.

4.3.2 Spinning disc confocal microscopes

The spinning disc confocal microscope employs a scanning system different from that of the LSCM. Rather than scanning the specimen with a single beam, multiple beams scan the specimen simultaneously and optical sections are viewed in real time. Modern spinning disc microscopes have been improved

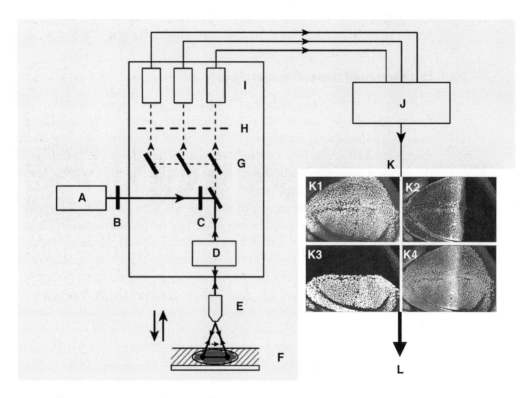

Fig. 4.11. Information flow in a generic laser scanning confocal microscope. Light from the laser (A) passes through a neutral density filter (B) and an excitation filter (C) on its way to the scanning unit (D). The scanning unit produces a scanned beam at the back focal plane of the objective lens (E) which focuses the light at the specimen (F). The specimen is scanned in the X and the Y directions in a raster pattern and in the Z direction by fine focusing (arrows indicate the movement of objective lens E). Any fluorescence from the specimen passes back through the objective lens and the scanning unit and is directed via dichromatic mirrors (G) to three pinholes (H). The pinholes act as spatial filters to block any light from above or below the plane of focus in the specimen. The point of light in the specimen is confocal with the pinhole aperture. This means that only distinct regions of the specimen are sampled. Light that passes through the pinholes strikes the PMT detectors (I) and the signal from the PMT is built into an image in the computer (J). The image is displayed on the computer screen (K) often as three greyscale images (K1, K2 and K3) together with a merged colour image of the three greyscale images (K4) and (Fig. 4.13a, see colour section). The computer synchronises the scanning mirrors with the build-up of the image in the computer framestore. The computer also controls a variety of peripheral devices. For example, the computer controls and correlates movement of a stepper motor connected to the fine focus of the microscope with image aquisition in order to produce a Z series. Furthermore the computer controls the area of the specimen to be scanned by the scanning unit so that zooming is easily achieved by scanning a smaller region of the specimen. In this way, a range of magnifications is imparted to a single objective lens so that the specimen does not have to be moved when the magnification is changed. Images are written to the hard disc of the computer or exported to various devices for viewing, hard copy production or archiving (L).

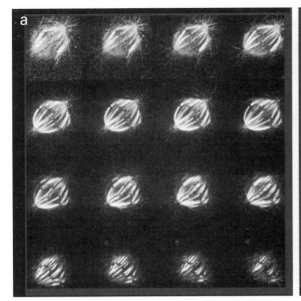 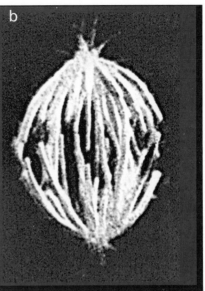

Fig. 4.12. Computer 3D reconstruction of confocal images. (a) Sixteen serial optical sections collected at 0.3 μm intervals through a mitotic spindle of a PtK1 cell stained with anti-tubulin and a second rhodamine-labelled antibody. Using the Z series macro program, a pre-set number of frames can be summed and the images transferred into a file on the hard disk. The stepper motor moves the fine focus control of the microscope by a pre-set increment. (b) Three-dimensional reconstruction of the data set produced using computer 3D reconstruction software. Such software can be used to view the data set from any specified angle or to produce videos of the structure rotating in 3D.

significantly by the addition of laser light sources and high quality CCD detectors to the instrument. Spinning disc systems are generally used in experiments where high resolution images are collected at a fast rate (high spatial and temporal resolution), and are used to follow the dynamics of fluorescently labelled proteins in living cells.

4.3.3 Multiple photon imaging

The multiple photon microscope has evolved from the confocal microscope. In fact, many of the instruments use the same scanning system as the LSCM or the spinning disk systems. The difference is that the light source is a high energy pulsed laser with tunable wavelengths, and the fluorochromes are excited by multiple rather than single photons. Optical sections are produced simply by focusing the laser beam in the specimen, since multiple photon excitation of a fluorophore occurs only where energy levels are high enough – statistically confined to the point of focus of the objective lens (Fig. 4.14).

Since red light is used in multiple photon microscopes, optical sections can be collected from deeper within the specimen than can those collected with the

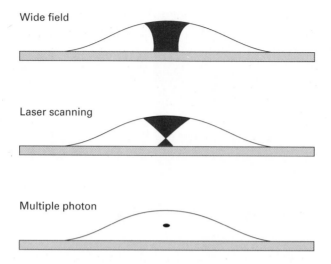

Fig. 4.14. Illumination in wide-field, confocal and multiple photon microscopes. The diagram shows a schematic of a side view of a fluorescently labelled cell on a microscope slide. The dark purple areas in each cell represent the volume of fluorescent excitation produced by each of the different microscopes in the cell. Conventional epifluorescence microscopy illuminates throughout the cell. In the LSCM, fluorescence illumination is throughout the cell but the pinhole in front of the detector excludes the out-of-focus light from the image. In the multiple photon microscope, excitation occurs only at the point of focus where the light flux is high enough.

LSCM. Multiple photon imaging is generally chosen for imaging fluorescently labelled living cells because red light is less damaging to living cells than are the shorter wavelengths usually employed in confocal microscopes. In addition, since the excitation of the fluorophore is restricted to the point of focus in the specimen, there is less chance of overexciting (photobleaching) the fluorescent probe and causing photodamage to the specimen itself.

4.3.4 **Deconvolution**

Optical sections can be produced using an image-processing method called deconvolution to remove the out-of-focus information from the digital image. Such images are computed from conventional wide-field microscope images. There are two basic types of deconvolution algorithm: deblurring and restoration. The approach relies upon knowledge of the point spread function of the imaging system. This is usually measured by imaging a point source, for example a small subresolution fluorescent bead (0.1 μm), and imaging how the point is spread out in the microscope. Since it is assumed that the real image of the bead should be a point, it is possible to calculate the amount of distortion in the image of the bead imposed by the imaging system. The actual image of the point can then be restored using a mathematical function, which can be applied to any subsequent images collected under identical settings of the microscope.

Early versions of the deconvolution method were relatively slow; for example, it could take some algorithms in the order of hours to compute a single optical section. Deconvolution is now much faster using today's fast computers and improved software, and the method compares favourably with the confocal approach for producing optical sections. Deconvolution is practical for multiple label imaging of both fixed and living cells, and excels over the scanning methods for imaging relatively dim and thin specimens, for example yeast cells. The method can also be used to remove additional background from images that were collected with the LSCM, the spinning disk microscope or a multiple photon microscope.

4.4 IMAGING LIVING CELLS AND TISSUES

There are two basically different approaches to imaging biochemical events over time. One strategy is to collect images from a series of fixed and stained tissues at different developmental ages. Each animal represents a single time point in the experiment. Alternatively, the same tissue can be imaged in the living state during its development. Here, the events of interest are captured directly. The second approach, imaging living cells and tissues, is technically more challenging than the first approach.

4.4.1 Avoidance of artefacts

The only way to eliminate artefacts from specimen preparation is to view the specimen in the living state. Many living specimens are sensitive to light, and especially those labelled with fluorescent dyes. This is because the excitation of fluorophores can release cytotoxic free radicals into the cell. Moreover, some wavelengths are more deleterious than others. Generally, the shorter wavelengths are more harmful than the longer ones and near-infrared light rather than ultraviolet light is preferred for imaging (Fig. 4.6). The levels of light used for imaging must not compromise the cells. This is achieved using extremely low levels of light, relatively bright fluorescent dyes and extremely sensitive photodetectors. Moreover, the viability of cells may also depend upon which cellular compartment has been labelled with the fluorochrome. For example, imaging the nucleus with a dye that is excited with a short wavelength will cause more cellular damage than imaging in the cytoplasm with a dye that is excited in the far red.

Great care has to be observed in order to maintain the tissue in the living state on the microscope stage. A live cell chamber is usually required for mounting the specimen on the microscope stage. This is basically a modified slide and coverslip arrangement that allows access to the specimen by the objective and condenser lenses. It also supports the cells in a constant environment and, depending on the cell type of interest, the chamber may have to provide a constant temperature, humidity, pH, carbon dioxide and/or oxygen levels. Many chambers have the facility for introducing fluids or perfusing the preparation with drugs for experimental treatments.

4.4.2 **Time-lapse imaging**

Time-lapse imaging continues to be used for the study of cellular dynamics. Here images are collected at predetermined time intervals (Fig. 4.13c–h, see colour section). Usually a shutter arrangement is placed in the light path so that the shutter is open only when an image is collected in order to reduce the amount of light energy impacting on the cells. When the images are played back in real time, a video of the process of interest is produced, albeit speeded up from real-time. Time-lapse is used to study cell behaviour in tissues and embryos and the dynamics of macromolecules within single cells. The event of interest and also the amount of light energy absorbed and tolerated by the cells govern the time interval used. For example, a cell in tissue culture moves relatively slowly and a time interval of 30 s between images might be used. Stability of the specimen and of the microscope is extremely important for successful time-lapse imaging. For example, the focus should not drift during the experiment.

All forms of light microscopy can be used for time-lapse imaging (Section 4.2.3 and Section 4.3). Phase contrast was the traditional choice for imaging cell movement and behaviour of cells growing in tissue culture. DIC or fluorescence microscopy is generally chosen for imaging the development of eggs and embryos. Computer imaging methods can be used in conjunction with DIC to improve resolution. Here, a background image is subtracted from each time-lapse frame and the contrast of the images is enhanced electronically. In this way microtubules assembled *in vitro* from tubulin in the presence of microtubule-associated proteins can be visualised on glass. These images are below the resolution of the light microscope. Such preparations have formed the basis of motility assays for motor proteins, for example kinesin and dynein.

4.4.3 **Fluorescent stains of living cells**

Relatively few cells possess any inherent fluorescence (autofluorescence) although some endogenous molecules are fluorescent and can be used for imaging, for example NAD(P)H. Relatively small fluorescent molecules are loaded into living cells using many different methods, including diffusion, microinjection, bead loading or electroporation. Relatively larger fluorescently labelled proteins are usually injected into cells, and after some time they are incorporated into the general protein pool of the cell for imaging.

Many reporter molecules are now available for recording the expression of specific genes in living cells using fluorescence microscopy (Table 4.2). The green fluorescent protein (GFP) is a very convenient reporter of gene expression because it is directly visible in the living cell using epifluorescence light microscopy with standard filter sets. The GFP gene can be linked to another gene of interest so that its expression is accompanied by GFP fluorescence in the living cell. No fixation, substrates or coenzymes are required. The fluorescence of GFP is extremely bright and is not susceptible to photobleaching. Spectral variants of GFP and additional reporters such as DsRed are now available for multiple labelling of living cells.

(a)   (b)   (c)

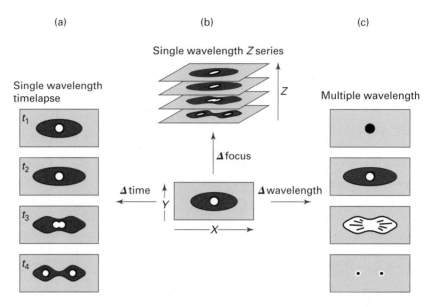

Fig. 4.15. Multidimensional imaging. (a) Single wavelength excitation over time or time-lapse X, Y imaging; (b) Z series or X, Y, Z imaging. The combination of (a) and (b) is 4D imaging. (c) Multiple wavelength imaging. The combination of (a) and (b) and (c) is 5D imaging.

These probes have revolutionised the ability to image living cells and tissues using light microscopy.

4.4.4 Multidimensional imaging

The collection of Z series over time is called four-dimensional (4D) imaging where individual optical sections (X and Y dimensions) are collected at different depths in the specimen (Z dimension) at different times (the fourth dimension), i.e. one time and three space dimensions (Fig. 4.15). Moreover multiple wavelength images can also be collected over time. This approach has been called 5D imaging. Software is now available for the analysis and display of such 4D and 5D data sets. For example, the movement of a structure through the consecutive stacks of images can be traced, changes in volume of a structure can be measured, and the 4D data sets can be displayed as series of Z projections or stereo videos. Multidimensional experiments can present problems for handling large amounts of data since gigabytes of information can be collected from a single 4D imaging experiment.

4.5 THE STEREOMICROSCOPE

A second type of light microscope, the stereomicroscope is used for the observation of the surfaces of large specimens (Fig. 4.16). The microscope is used when 3D information is required, for example for the observation of whole organisms (Fig. 4.17, see colour section). Stereomicroscopes are useful for micromanipulation and

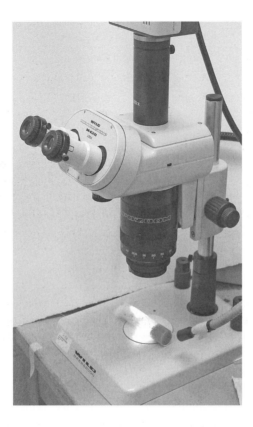

Fig. 4.16. A research grade stereomicroscope. Note the light source is from the side, which can give a shadow effect to the specimen – in this example a vial of flies. The large objective lens above the specimen can be rotated to zoom the image.

dissection where the wide field of view and the ability to zoom in and out in magnification is invaluable. A wide range of objectives and eyepieces are available for different applications. The light sources can be from above, from below the specimen, encircling the specimen using a ring light or from the side, giving a darkfield effect. These different light angles serve to add contrast or shadow relief to the images. Fluorescent stereomicroscopes are also available and are used for screening transgenic animals labelled with GFP and its variants.

4.6 THE ELECTRON MICROSCOPE

4.6.1 Principles

Electron microscopy is used when the greatest resolution is required. The images produced in an electron microscope (EM) reveal the ultrastructure of cells. There are two different types of electron microscope: the transmission electron microscope (TEM) and the scanning electron microscope (SEM). In the TEM, electrons that pass through the specimen are imaged. In the SEM, electrons that are reflected back from the specimen (secondary electrons) are collected, and the surfaces of specimens are imaged.

The equivalent of the light source in an electron microscope is the electron gun. When a high voltage of between 40 000 and 100 000 V (the accelerating voltage) is passed between the cathode and the anode, a tungsten filament emits electrons (Fig. 4.1). The negatively charged electrons pass through a hole in the anode forming an electron beam. The beam of electrons passes through a stack of electromagnetic lenses (the column). Focusing of the electron beam is achieved by changing the voltage across the electromagnetic lenses. When the electron beam passes through the specimen some of them are scattered whilst others are focused by the projector lens onto a phosphorescent screen or recorded using photographic film or a digital camera. The electrons have limited penetration power, which means that specimens must be thin (50–100 nm) to allow them to pass through.

Thicker specimens can be viewed by using a higher accelerating voltage, for example in the high voltage electron microscope (HVEM), which uses 1 000 000 V accelerating voltage or in the intermediate voltage electron microscope (IVEM), which uses an accelerating voltage of around 400 000 V. Here, stereo images are collected by collected two images at 8° to 10° tilt angles. Such images are useful in assessing the 3D relationships of organelles within cells when viewed in a stereoscope or with a digital stereoprojection system.

4.6.2 Preparation of specimens

Contrast in the EM depends on atomic number: the higher the atomic number the greater the scattering and the contrast. Thus heavy metals are used to add contrast in the EM, for example uranium, lead and osmium. Labelled structures appear black or electron dense in the image (Fig. 4.18).

All of the water has to be removed from any biological specimen before it can be imaged in the EM. This is because the electron beam can be produced and focused only in a vacuum. The major drawback of EM observation of biological specimens therefore is the non-physiological conditions necessary for their observation. Nevertheless, the improved resolution afforded by the EM has provided much information about biological structures and biochemical events within cells that could otherwise not have been collected using any other microscopical technique.

Extensive specimen preparation is required for EM analysis, and for this reason there can be issues of interpreting the images because of artefacts from specimen preparation. For example, specimens have been traditionally prepared for the TEM by fixation in glutaraldehyde to cross-link proteins, followed by osmium tetroxide to fix and stain lipid membranes. This is followed by dehydration in a series of alcohols to remove the water, and then embedding in a plastic such as Epon for thin sectioning (Fig. 4.18).

Small pieces of the embedded tissue are mounted and sectioned on an ultramicrotome using either a glass or a diamond knife. Ultrathin sections are cut to a thickness of approximately 60 nm. The ribbons of sections are floated onto the surface of

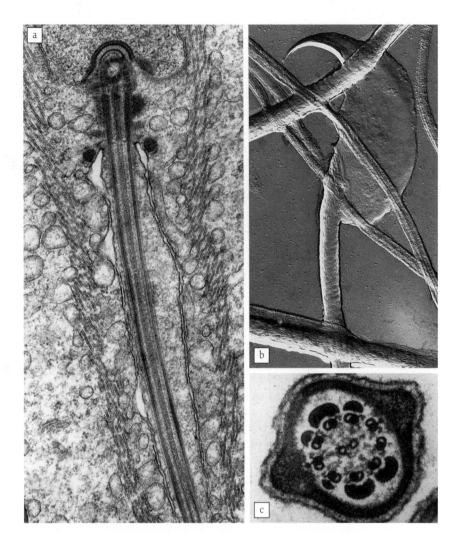

Fig. 4.18. Transmission electron microscopy. (a and c) Ultrathin Epon sections (60 nm thick) of developing sperm cells stained with uranyl acetate and lead citrate. (b) Carbon surface replica of a mouse sperm.

water and their interference colours are used to assess their thickness. The desired 60 nm section thickness has a silver/gold interference colour on the water surface. The sections are then mounted onto copper or gold EM grids, and are subsequently stained with heavy metals, for example uranyl acetate and lead citrate.

For the SEM, samples are fixed in glutaraldehyde, dehydrated through a series of solvents and dried completely either in air or by critical point drying. This method removes all of the water from the specimen instantly and avoids surface tension in the drying process, thereby avoiding artefacts of drying. The specimens are then mounted onto a special metal holder or stub and coated with a thin layer of gold before being viewed in the SEM (Fig. 4.17, see colour section). Surfaces can also be viewed in the TEM using either negative stains or carbon replicas of air-dried specimens (Fig. 4.18).

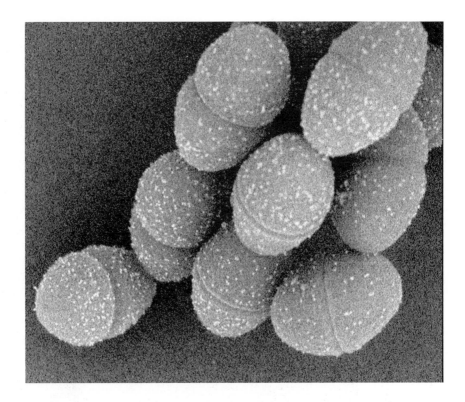

Fig. 4.19. Immunoelectron microscopy. Scanning electron microscope (SEM) imaging of microbes *Enterococcus faecalis* labelled with 10 nm colloidal gold for the surface adhesion protein 'aggregation substance'. This protein facilitates exchange of DNA during conjugation. The gold labels appear as white dots on the surface of the bacteria. (Image kindly provided by Stan Erlandsen.)

Immuno-EM methods allow the localisation of molecules within the cellular microenvironment for TEM and on the cell surface for SEM (Fig. 4.19). Cells are prepared in a similar way to indirect immunofluorescence, with the exception that, rather than a fluorescent probe bound to the secondary antibody, electron-dense colloidal gold particles are used. Multiple labelling can be achieved using different sizes of gold particles (10 nm) attached to antibodies to the proteins of interest. The method depends upon the binding of protein A to the gold particles, since protein A binds in turn to antibody fragments. Certain resins, for example Lowicryl and LR White, have been formulated to allow antibodies and gold particles to be attached to ultrathin sections for immunolabelling.

4.6.3 Recent developments in EM methods

New methods of fixation continue to be developed in an attempt to avoid the artefacts of specimen preparation and to observe the specimen more closely to its living state. Specimens are rapidly frozen in milliseconds by high pressure freezing. Under these conditions the biochemical state of the cell is more likely to be

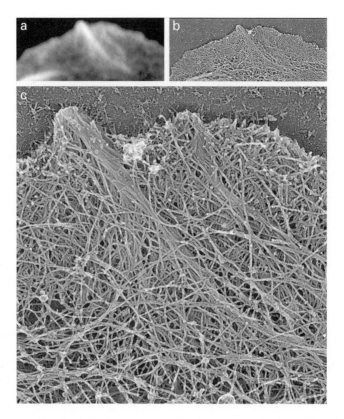

Fig. 4.20. Integrated microscopy. (a) Epifluorescence image and (b and c) whole mount TEM at different magnifications of the same cell. The fluorescence image is labelled with rhodamine phalloidin, which stains polymerised actin. A stress fibre at the periphery of the cell appears as a white line in the fluorescence image (a), and when viewed in the TEM the stress fibres appear as aligned densities of actin filaments. The TEM whole mount was prepared using detergent extraction, chemical fixation, critical point drying and platinum/carbon coating. (Image kindly provided by Tatyana Svitkina.)

preserved. Many of these frozen hydrated samples can be observed directly in the EM or they can be chemically fixed using freeze substitution methods. Here, fixatives are infused into the preparation at low temperature, after which the specimen is slowly warmed to room temperature.

Using cryo-electron tomography (Cryo-ET) the 3D structure of cells and macromolecules can be visualised at 5–8 nm resolution. Cells are frozen and mounted in an apparatus that moves the specimen through a range of tilt angles. A 2D digital EM image is collected at each one of these tilt angles, and, using computer software, a 3D representation of the specimen can be constructed.

4.6.4 **Integrated microscopy**

The same specimen can be viewed in the light microscope and subsequently in the EM. This approach is called integrated microscopy. The correlation of images of the same cell collected using the high temporal resolution of the light microscope and the high spatial resolution of the EM gives additional information to imaging using the two techniques separately (Fig. 4.20). The integrated approach also addresses the problem of artefacts. Probes are now available that are fluorescent in the light microscope and electron dense in the EM.

4.7 **IMAGING AND BIOCHEMISTRY**

Understanding the function of proteins within the context of the intact living cell is one of the main aims of contemporary biological research. The visualisation of specific cellular events has been greatly enhanced by modern microscopy. In addition to qualitative viewing of the images collected with a microscope, quantitative information can be gleaned from the images. The collection of meaningful measurements has been greatly facilitated by the advent of digital image processing. Subtle changes in intensity of probes of biochemical events can be detected with sensitive digital detectors. These technological advancements have allowed insight into the spatial aspects of molecular mechanisms.

Relatively simple measurements include counting features within a 2D image or measuring areas and lengths. Measurements of depth and volume can be made in 3D, 4D and 5D data sets. Images can be calibrated by collecting an image of a calibration grid at the same settings of the microscope as was used for collecting the images during the experiment. Many image-processing systems allow for a calibration factor to be added into the program, and all subsequent measurements will then be comparable.

The rapid development of fluorescence microscopy together with digital imaging and, above all, the development of new fluorescent probes of biological activity, have added a new level of sophistication to quantitative imaging. Most of the measurements are based on the ability to accurately measure the brightness of a fluorescent probe within a sample using a digital imaging system. This is also the basis of flow cytometry (Section 16.3.2), which measures the individual brightness of a population of cells as they pass through a laser beam. Cells can be sorted into different populations using a related technique, fluorescence-activated cell sorting (FACS).

The brightness of the fluorescence from the probe can be calibrated to the amount of probe present at any given location in the cell at high resolution. For example, the concentration of calcium is measured in different regions of living embryos using calcium indicator dyes (e.g. fluo-3) whose fluorescence increases in proportion to the amount of free calcium in the cell (Fig. 4.21, see colour section). Many probes have been developed for making such measurements in living tissues. Controls are a necessary part of such measurements, since photobleaching and various dye artefacts during the experiment can obscure the true measurements. This can be achieved by staining the sample with two ion-sensitive dyes and comparing their measured brightness during the experiment. These measurements are usually expressed as ratios (ratio imaging) and control for dye loading problems, photobleaching and instrument variation.

Fluorescently labelled proteins can be injected into cells where they are incorporated into macromolecular structures over time. This makes the structures accessible to time-lapse imaging using fluorescence microscopy. Such methods can lead to high background dye levels and can be difficult to interpret. In addition to optical sectioning methods (Section 4.3), several methods have been developed for avoiding high backgrounds for fluorescence measurements of biochemical events in cells.

Fluorescence recovery after photobleaching (FRAP) uses the high light flux from a laser to locally destroy fluorophores labelling the macromolecules to create a bleached zone (photobleaching). The subsequent movement of undamaged fluorophores into the bleached zone gives a measure of molecular mobility. This enables biochemical analysis within the living cell (Section 16.3.2). A second technique related to FRAP, photoactivation, uses a probe whose fluorescence can be induced by a pulse of short wavelength light. The activated probe is imaged using a longer wavelength of light. Here the signal-to-noise ratio of the images can be better than that for photobleaching experiments.

A third method, fluorescence speckle microscopy, was discovered as a chance observation but is now popular for imaging macromolecular dynamics inside living cells. Basically, a lower concentration of fluorescently labelled protein is injected into cells so that the protein of interest is not fully labelled inside the cell. When viewed in the microscope, structures inside cells that have been labelled in this way have a speckled appearance. The dark regions act as fiduciary marks for the observation of dynamics.

Fluorescence resonance energy transfer (FRET) is a fluorescence-based method that can take fluorescence microscopy past the theoretical resolution limit of the light microscope allowing the observation of protein–protein interactions *in vivo* (Fig. 4.22). FRET occurs between two fluorophores when the emission of the first one (the donor) serves as the excitation source for the second one (the acceptor). This will occur only when two fluorophore molecules are very close to one another, at a distance of 60 Å (6 nm) or less. An example of a FRET experiment would be to use spectral variants of GFP. Here the excitation of a cyan fluorescent protein (CFP)-tagged protein is used to monitor the emission of a yellow fluorescent protein (YFP)-tagged protein. YFP fluorescence will be observed under the excitation conditions of CFP only if the proteins are close together. Since this can be monitored over time, FRET can be used to measure direct binding of proteins or protein complexes (Section 16.3.2).

A more complex technique, fluorescence lifetime imaging (FLIM), measures the amount of time a fluorophore is fluorescent after excitation with a 10 ns pulse of laser light. FLIM is used for detecting multiple fluorophores with different fluorescent lifetimes and overlapping emission spectra.

4.8 SPECIALISED IMAGING TECHNIQUES

Technical advancements continue to impact on the field of microscopy and imaging, and enable yet more experimental approaches. Instruments continue to

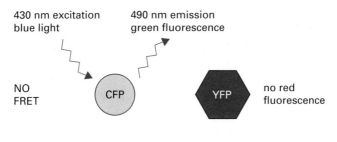

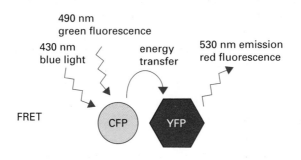

Fig. 4.22. Fluorescence resonance energy transfer (FRET). In the upper example (NO FRET) the cyan fluorescent protein (CFP) and the yellow fluorescent protein (YFP) are not close enough for FRET to occur (more than 60 Å (6 nm) separation). Here excitation with the 430 nm blue light results in the green 490 nm emission of the CFP only. Whereas, in the lower example (FRET), the CFP and YFP are close enough for 'energy transfer' or FRET to occur (closer than 60 nm). Here, excitation with the 430 nm blue light results in fluorescence of the CFP (green) and of the YFP (red).

Example 1 LOCATING AN UNKNOWN PROTEIN TO A SPECIFIC CELLULAR COMPARTMENT

Question

You have isolated and purified a novel protein from a biochemical preparation. How might you determine its subcellular distribution and possible function in the cell?

Answer

Many fluorescent probes are available that label specific cellular compartments. For example, TOTO3 labels the nucleus and fluorescent phalloidins label cell outlines. An antibody to your protein could be raised and used to immunofluorescently label cells. Using a multiple labelling approach and perhaps an optical sectioning technique such as laser scanning confocal microscopy the distribution of the protein in the cell relative to known distributions can be ascertained. For higher resolution immuno-EM or FRET studies could be performed.

be developed for specialised, non-routine applications in biochemistry. Most developments are designed to image more efficiently living cells and tissues at improved resolution.

Magnetic resonance imaging (MRI), whilst well developed for collecting 3D information from large structures such as whole body anatomy, has recently been adapted for the collection of relatively high resolution ($10\,\mu$m) images from deep into otherwise opaque microscopic tissues; for example, for the observation of the 3D anatomy of living embryos as they develop. Contrast agents are becoming available that can be used for both fluorescence microscopy and MRI of the same tissue. The MRI technique is able to penetrate the entire volume of the tissue whereas the fluorescence images can be collected from only a few micrometres within the embryo (see also Section 13.4.3).

Another area of active research is in the development of single molecule detection techniques. For example total internal reflection microscopy (TIRF) uses the properties of an evanescent wave close to the interface of two media (Fig. 4.23), for example the region between the specimen and the glass coverslip. The technique relies on the fact that the intensity of the evanescent field falls off rapidly so that the excitation of any fluorophore is confined to a region of just 100 nm above the glass interface. This is thinner than the optical section thickness achieved using confocal methods and allows the imaging of single molecules at the interface.

The atomic force microscope, rather than using a lens, probes the surface of a specimen with a sharp tip that is several micrometres in length and less than 10 nm in diameter at the point (near field imaging). The tip is at the end of a lever some 100–200 μm in length. As the tip moves across the specimen, forces between the two cause the lever to bend. The movement of the lever is detected using a computer, and an image is built up of the surface of the specimen from the minute deflections of the tip. The method produces images of surfaces at very high resolution (Table 4.3).

4.9 IMAGE ARCHIVING, PRESENTATION AND FURTHER INFORMATION

Most images produced by any kind of modern microscope are collected in a digital form. In addition to greatly speeding up the collection of the images (and experiment times), the use of digital imaging has allowed the use of digital image databases and the rapid transfer of information between laboratories across the World Wide Web. Moreover there is no loss in resolution or colour balance from the images collected at the microscope as they pass between laboratories and journal web pages.

International image databases are under development for the storage and access of microscope image data from many different locations. There is a trend for modern microscopes to produce more and more data, especially when multidimensional data sets are generated. This trend is continuing with the need to develop automated methods of image analysis of gene expression data from genomic screens.

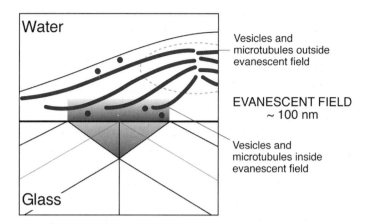

Fig. 4.23. Total internal reflection microscopy (TIRF). A 100 nm thick region of excitation is produced at the glass–water interface when illumination conditions are right for internal reflection. In this example, only those vesicles and microtubules within the evanescent field will contribute to the fluorescence image at 100 nm Z resolution.

Table 4.3 Resolution in optical imaging

	XY	Z
Standard microscope	0.5 μm	1.6 μm
Confocal/multiple photon	0.25 μm	0.7 μm
TIRF – evanescent wave	0.5 μm	0.3 μm
Atomic force – near field	0.05 μm	0.01 μm

TIRF, total internal reflection microscopy.

More detailed information on any of the microscopes and their applications in biochemistry can be accessed on the World Wide Web. Several websites have been included as starting points for further study (see Section 4.10). Should any of these listed websites become out of date, more information on any topic can be accessed using a Web search engine. The field of microscopy is moving very fast but the basic principles of light and electron microscopy remain unchanged.

4.10 SUGGESTIONS FOR FURTHER READING

ABRAMOWITZ, M. (2003). *Microscope Basics and Beyond.* Olympus of America Inc., Melville, NY. (Good, well-illustrated primer on all aspects of basic light microscopy – also available online as a pdf file.)

ALBERTS, B., JOHNSON, A., LEWIS, J., RAFF, M., ROBERTS, K. and WALTER, P. (2002). *Molecular Biology of the Cell*, 4th edn. Garland Science, New York. (Good introduction to all forms of microscopy and live cell imaging for the cell biologist.)

ANDREWS, P. D., HARPER, I. S. and SWEDLOW, J. R. (2002). To 5D and beyond: quantitative fluorescence microscopy in the postgenomic era. *Traffic*, **3**, 29–36. (Review of multidimensional imaging, methods of coping with large data sets and international image databases.)

BARUCH, A., JEFFERY, D. A. and BOFYO, M. (2004). Enzyme activity – it's all about image. *Trends in Cell Biology*, **14**, 29–35. (Recent review of biochemical experiments using fluorescence.)

BRAGA, P. C. and RICCI, D. (2003). *Atomic Force Microscopy – Biomedical Methods and Applications*. Methods in Molecular Biology, vol. 242. (Protocols-based methods and applications of atomic force microscopy.)

FRANKEL, F. (2002). *Envisioning Science: The Design and Craft of the Science Image*. MIT Press, Cambridge, MA. (Popular work on imaging with some great tips and trips for the stereomicroscope.)

HAUGLAND, R. (2003). *Handbook of Fluorescent Probes and Research Products*, 9th edn. Molecular Probes Inc., Eugene, OR. (A compendium of all modern fluorescent probes together with protocols and references – constant updates on the web.)

HURTLEY, S. M. and HELMUTH, L. (2003). Biological imaging. *Science*, **300**, 75–145. (Very good collection of papers on contemporary imaging topics.)

INOUE, S. and SPRING, K. (1997). *Video Microscopy, The Fundamentals*, 2nd edn. Plenum Publishing Corp., New York. (Excellent primer on live cell imaging, video microscopy and general microscopy.)

ISHIJIMA, A. and YANAGIDA, T. (2001). Single molecule nanobioscience. *Trends in Biochemical Sciences*, **26**, 438–444. (Review of single molecule imaging.)

LEWIS, A., TAHA, H., STRINKOVSKI, A., MANEVITCH, A., KHATCHATOURIANTS, A., DEKHTER, R. and AMMANN, E. (2003). Near-field optics: from subwavelength illumination to nanometric shadowing. *Nature Biotechnology*, **21**, 1378–1386. (Review of near-field optics and contemporary developments.)

MCINTOSH, J. R. (2001). Electron microscopy of cells: a new beginning for a new century. *Journal of Cell Biology*, **153**, F25–F32. (A good and brief start on modern EM techniques.)

PERIASAMY, A. (2001). *Methods in Cellular Imaging*. Oxford University Press, Oxford. (An excellent collection of advanced light microscopy including confocal, multiple photon and FRET.)

SCHULDT, A. and SMALLRIDGE, R. (2003). *Imaging in cell biology*. Supplement to Nature Cell Biology, **6**. (Recent overview of modern imaging techniques.)

SEDGEWICK, J. (2002). *Quick PhotoShop for Research: A Guide to Digital Imaging for PhotoShop*. Kluwer Academic/Plenum Publishing, New York. (Hands-on recipe based protocols for presentation of digital images from microscopes.)

SHAPIRO, H. M. (2003). *Practical Flow Cytometry*, 4th edn. John Wiley and Sons, New York. (Wonderfully written book on basic fluorescence and flow cytometry.)

SPECTOR, D. L. and GOLDMAN, R. D. (2004). *Live Cell Imaging: A Laboratory Manual*. Cold Spring Harbor Laboratory Press, Cold Spring Harbor, NY. (A good introduction to contemporary methods of imaging living cells.)

VAN ROESSEL, P. and BRAND, A. H. (2002). Imaging into the future: visualizing gene expression and protein interaction with fluorescent proteins. *Nature Cell Biology*, **4**, E15–E20. (Good primer on GFP and FRET.)

WALLACE, W., SCHAEFER, L. H. and SWEDLOW, J. R. (2001). Working person's guide to deconvolution in light microscopy. *BioTechniques*, **31**, 1076–1097. (Review of the deconvolution technique.)

ZHANG, J., CAMPBELL, R. E., TING, A. Y. and TSIEN, R.Y. (2002). Creating new fluorescent probes for cell biology. *Nature Reviews in Molecular Cell Biology*, **3**, 906–918. (Review of the development of fluorescent probes of biological activity especially reporter molecules.)

Websites of interest

General microscopy

<http://www.microscopyu.com/>
<http://www.microscopy.fsu.edu/>

<http://www.microscopy-analysis.com/>
<http://www.msa.microscopy.com/>
<http://www.rms.org.uk/>
<http://www.ou.edu/research/electron/mirror/web-subj.html>
<http://www.ou.edu/research/electron/www-vl/>

Fluorescent probes

<http://www.bdbiosciences.com/clontech/>
<http://www.qdots.com/>
<http://www.probes.com>
<http://www.jacksonimmuno.com/>

Image processing

<http://www.apple.com/quicktime/qtvr/>
<http://rsb.info.nih.gov/nih-image/>
<http://rsb.info.nih.gov/ij/>
<http://www.uiowa.edu/~dshbwww/>
<http://www.lemkesoft.de/en/index.htm>

Database

<http://www.openmicroscopy.org>

Chapter 5

Molecular biology, bioinformatics and basic techniques

5.1 INTRODUCTION

The completion of the Human Genome Project has been heralded as one of the major landmark events in science. The human genome contains the blueprint for human development and maintenance and may ultimately provide the means to understand human cellular and molecular processes in both health and disease. The genome is the full complement of DNA from an organism and carries all the information needed to specify the structure of every protein the cell can produce. The realisation that DNA lies behind all of the cell's activities led to the development of what is termed molecular biology. Rather than a discrete area of biosciences, molecular biology is now accepted as a very important means of understanding and describing complex biological processes. The development of methods and techniques for studying processes at the molecular level has led to new and powerful ways of isolating, analysing, manipulating and exploiting nucleic acids. Moreover, to keep pace with the explosion in biological information a new area termed bioinformatics has evolved and provides a vital role in current biosciences. The completion of the Human Genome Project and numerous other genome projects has allowed the continued development of new exciting areas of biological sciences such as biotechnology, genome mapping, molecular medicine and gene therapy.

In considering the potential utility of molecular biological techniques it is important to understand the basic structure of nucleic acids and gain an appreciation of how this dictates the function *in vivo* and *in vitro*. Indeed many techniques used in molecular biology mimic in some way the natural functions of nucleic acids such as replication and transcription. This chapter is therefore intended to provide an overview of the general features of nucleic acid structure and function and describe some of the basic methods used in its isolation and analysis.

5.2 **STRUCTURE OF NUCLEIC ACIDS**

5.2.1 **Primary structure of nucleic acids**

DNA and RNA are macromolecular structures composed of regular repeating polymers formed from nucleotides. These are the basic building blocks of nucleic acids and are derived from nucleosides that are composed of two elements: a five-membered pentose carbon sugar (2-deoxyribose in DNA and ribose in RNA) and a nitrogenous base. The carbon atoms of the sugar are designated 'prime' (1', 2', 3', etc.) to distinguish them from the carbon atoms of nitrogenous bases, of which there are two types – purines and pyrimidines. A nucleotide, or nucleoside phosphate, is formed by the attachment of a phosphate to the 5' position of a nucleoside by an ester linkage (Fig. 5.1). Such nucleotides can be joined together by the formation of a second ester bond by reaction between the terminal phosphate group of one nucleotide and the 3' hydroxyl of another, thus generating a 5' to 3' phosphodiester bond between adjacent sugars; this process can be repeated indefinitely to give long polynucleotide molecules (Fig. 5.2). DNA has two such polynucleotide strands; however, since each strand has both a free 5' hydroxyl group at one end and a free 3' hydroxyl at the other, each strand has a polarity or directionality. The polarities of the two strands of the molecule are in opposite directions, and thus DNA is described as an 'antiparallel' structure (Fig. 5.3).

The purine bases (composed of fused five- and six-membered rings), adenine (A) and guanine (G) are found in both RNA and DNA, as is the pyrimidine (a single six-membered ring) cytosine (C). The other pyrimidines are each restricted to one type of nucleic acid: uracil (U) occurs exclusively in RNA, whilst thymine (T) is limited to DNA. Thus it is possible to distinguish between RNA and DNA on the basis of the presence of ribose and uracil in RNA, and deoxyribose and thymine in DNA. However, it is the sequence of bases, which distinguishes one DNA (or RNA) molecule from another. It is conventional to write a nucleic acid sequence starting at the 5' end of the molecule, using single capital letters to represent each of the bases, for example CGGATCT. Note that there is usually no point in including the sugar or phosphate groups, since these are identical throughout the length of the molecule. Terminal phosphate groups can, when necessary, be indicated by use of a 'p'; thus 5' pCGGATCT 3' indicates the presence of a phosphate on the 5' end of the molecule.

5.2.2 **Secondary structure of nucleic acids**

The two polynucleotide chains in DNA are usually found in the shape of a right-handed double helix, in which the bases of the two strands lie in the centre of the molecule, with the sugar-phosphate backbones on the outside. A crucial feature of this double-stranded structure is that it depends on the sequence of bases in one strand being complementary to that in the other. A purine base attached to a sugar residue on one strand is always hydrogen bonded to a pyrimidine base attached to a sugar residue on the other strand. Moreover, adenine (A) always pairs with

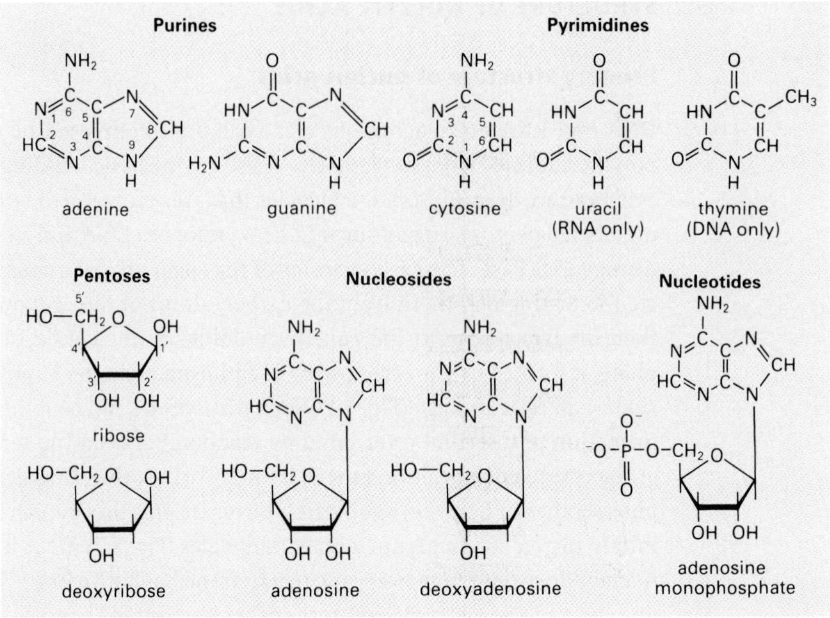

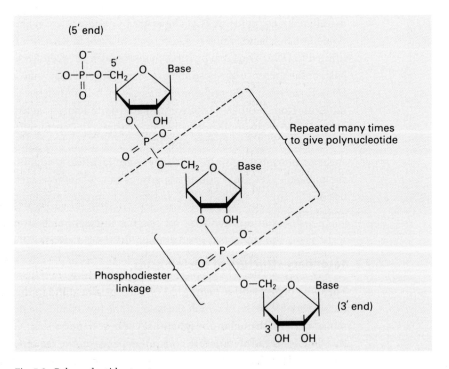

Fig. 5.1. Structure of bases, nucleosides and nucleotides.

Fig. 5.2. Polynucleotide structure.

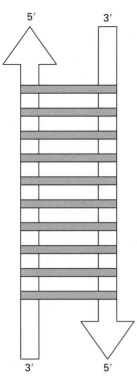

Fig. 5.3. The antiparallel nature of DNA. One strand in a double helix runs 5′ to 3′, whilst the other strand runs in the opposite direction 3′ to 5′. The strands are held together by hydrogen bonds between the bases.

thymine (T) or uracil (U) in RNA, via two hydrogen bonds, and guanine (G) always pairs with cytosine (C) by three hydrogen bonds (Fig. 5.4). When these conditions are met a stable double-helical structure results in which the backbones of the two strands are, on average, a constant distance apart. Thus, if the sequence of one strand is known, that of the other strand can be deduced. The strands are designated as plus (+) and minus (−) and an RNA molecule complementary to the minus (−) strand is synthesised during transcription (Section 5.5.3). The base sequence may cause significant local variations in the shape of the DNA molecule and these variations are vital for specific interactions between the DNA and various proteins to take place. Although the three-dimensional structure of DNA may vary it generally adopts a double helical structure termed the B form or B-DNA *in vivo*. There are also other forms of right-handed DNA, such as A and C, that are formed when DNA fibres are subjected to different relative humidities (Table 5.1).

The major distinguishing feature of B-DNA is that it has approximately 10 bases for one turn of the double helix; furthermore distinctive major and minor grooves may be identified (Fig. 5.5). In certain circumstances, where repeated DNA sequences or motifs are found, the DNA may adopt a left-handed helical structure termed Z-DNA. This form of DNA was first synthesised in the laboratory and is

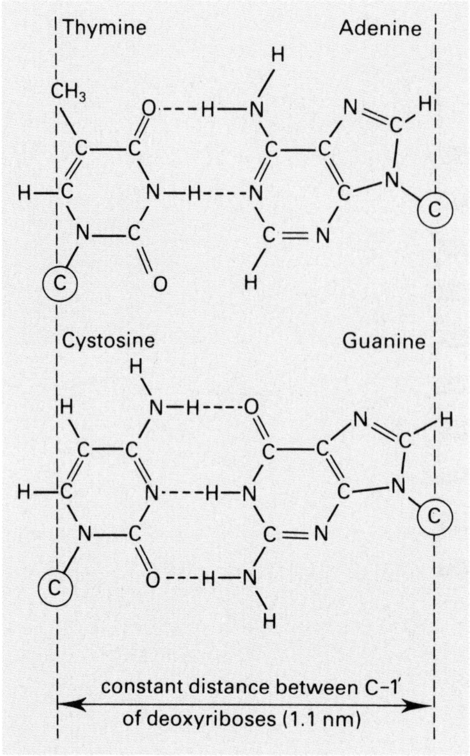

Fig. 5.4. Base-pairing in DNA. C in a circle represents carbon at the 1′ position of deoxyribose.

Table 5.1 **The various forms of DNA**

DNA form	% humidity	Helix direction	Base/turn helix	Helix diameter (A)
B	92%	RH	10	19
A	75%	RH	11	23
C	66%	RH	9.3	19
Z	$(Pu\text{-}Py)_n$	LH	12	18

RH, right-handed helix; LH, left-handed helix; Pu, Purine; Py, Pyrimidine.
Different forms of DNA may be obtained by subjecting DNA fibres to different relative humidities. The B form is the most common form of DNA whilst the A and C forms have been derived under laboratory conditions. The Z form may be produced with a DNA sequence made up from alternating purine and pyrimidine nucleotides.

thought is not to exist *in vivo*. The various forms of DNA serve to show that it is not a static molecule but dynamic and constantly in flux, and may be coiled, bent or distorted at certain times. Although RNA almost always exists as a single strand, it often contains sequences within the same strand which are self-complementary, and which can therefore base-pair if brought together by suitable folding of the

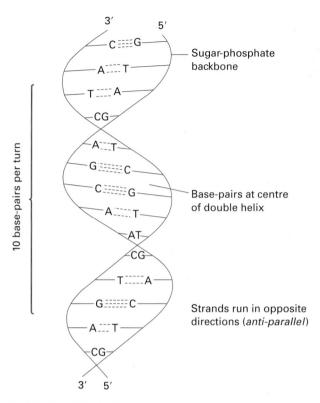

Fig. 5.5. The DNA double helix.

molecule. A notable example is transfer RNA (tRNA), which folds up to give a clover leaf secondary structure (Fig. 5.6).

5.2.3 **Separation of double-stranded DNA**

The two antiparallel strands of DNA are held together only by the weak forces of hydrogen bonding between complementary bases, and partly by hydrophobic interactions between adjacent, stacked base-pairs, termed base-stacking. Little energy is needed to separate a few base-pairs, and so, at any instant, a few short stretches of DNA will be opened up to the single-stranded conformation. However, such stretches immediately pair up again at room temperature, so the molecule as a whole remains predominantly double stranded.

If, however, a DNA solution is heated to approximately 90 °C or above there will be enough kinetic energy to denature the DNA completely, causing it to separate into single strands. This denaturation can be followed spectrophotometrically by monitoring the absorbance of light at 260 nm. The stacked bases of double-stranded DNA are less able to absorb light than the less constrained bases of single-stranded molecules, and so the absorbance of DNA at 260 nm increases as the DNA becomes denatured, a phenomenon known as the hyperchromic effect.

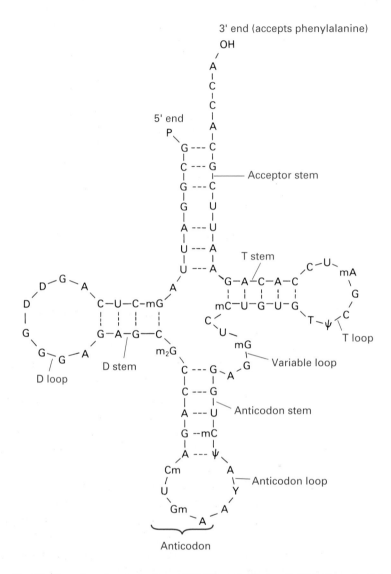

Fig. 5.6. Secondary structure of yeast tRNA^Phe. A single strand of 76 ribonucleotides forms four double-stranded 'stem' regions by base-pairing between complementary sequences. The anticodon will base-pair with UUU or UUC (both are codons for phenylalanine), phenylalanine is attached to the 3'-end by a specific aminoacyl tRNA synthetase. Several 'unusual' bases are present: D, dihydrouridine; T, ribothymidine; ψ, pseudouridine; Y, very highly modified, unlike any 'normal' base. mX indicates methylation of base X (m$_2$X shows dimethylation); Xm indicates methylation of ribose on the 2' position.

The absorbance at 260 nm may be plotted against the temperature of a DNA solution, which will indicate that little denaturation occurs below approximately 70 °C, but further increases in temperature result in a marked increase in the extent of denaturation. Eventually a temperature is reached at which the sample is totally denatured, or melted. The temperature at which 50% of the DNA is melted is termed the melting temperature or T_m, and this depends on the nature of the

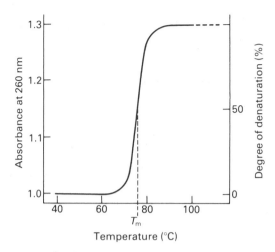

Fig. 5.7. Melting curve of DNA.

DNA (Fig. 5.7). If several different samples of DNA are melted, it is found that the T_m is highest for those DNA molecules that contain the highest proportion of cytosine and guanine, and T_m can actually be used to estimate the percentage (C + G) in a DNA sample. This relationship between T_m and (C + G) content arises because cytosine and guanine form three hydrogen bonds when base-paired, whereas thymine and adenine form only two. Because of the differential numbers of hydrogen bonds between A-T and C-G pairs those sequences with a predominance of C-G pairs will require greater energy to separate or denature them. The conditions required to separate a particular nucleotide sequence are also dependent on environmental conditions such as salt concentration.

If melted DNA is cooled it is possible for the separated strands to reassociate, a process known as renaturation. However, a stable double-stranded molecule will be formed only if the complementary strands collide in such a way that their bases are paired precisely, and this is an unlikely event if the DNA is very long and complex (i.e. if it contains a large number of different genes). Measurements of the rate of renaturation can give information about the complexity of a DNA preparation (Section 5.3).

Strands of RNA and DNA will associate with each other, if their sequences are complementary, to give double-stranded hybrid molecules. Similarly, strands of radioactively labelled RNA or DNA, when added to a denatured DNA preparation, will act as probes for DNA molecules to which they are complementary (Section 5.7). This hybridisation of complementary strands of nucleic acids is very useful for isolating a specific fragment of DNA from a complex mixture (Section 5.10). It is also possible for small single-stranded fragments of DNA (up to 40 bases in length) termed oligonucleotides to hybridise to a denatured sample of DNA. This type of hybridisation is termed annealing and again is dependent on the base sequence of the oligonucleotide and the salt concentration of the sample.

5.3 GENES AND GENOME COMPLEXITY

5.3.1 Gene complexity

Each region of DNA that codes for a single RNA or protein molecule is called a gene, and the entire set of genes in a cell, organelle or virus forms its genome. Cells and organelles may contain more than one copy of their genome. Genomic DNA from nearly all prokaryotic and eukaryotic organisms is also complexed with protein and termed chromosomal DNA. Each gene is located at a particular position along the chromosome, termed the locus, whilst the particular form of the gene is termed the allele. In mammalian DNA each gene is present in two allelic forms, which may be identical (homozygous) or may vary (heterozygous). Current estimates derived from the Human Genome Project indicate that there are approximately 35 000 genes present. However, various processing events may well increase the number of actual proteins found in the cell in relation to the number of genes. The occurrence of different alleles at the same site in the genome is termed polymorphism. In general the more complex an organism the larger its genome, although this is not always the case, since many higher organisms have non-coding sequences some of which are repeated numerous times and termed repetitive DNA. In mammalian DNA, repetitive sequences may be divided into low copy number and high copy number DNA. The latter is composed of repeat sequences that are dispersed throughout the genome and those that are clustered together. The repeat cluster DNA may be defined as so-called classical satellite DNA, minisatellite and microsatellite DNA, the last of these being composed mainly of dinucleotide repeats (Table 5.2). These sequences are termed polymorphic, collectively termed polymorphisms and vary between individuals; they also form the basis of genetic fingerprinting (Section 6.8.7).

Table 5.2 **Repetitive satellite sequences found in DNA, and their characteristics**

Types of repetitive DNA	Repeat unit size (bp)	Characteristics/motifs
Satellite DNA	5–200	Large repeat unit range (Mb) usually found at centromeres
Minisatellite DNA		
Telomere sequence	6	Found at the ends of chromosomes. Repeat unit may span up to 20 kb G-rich sequence
Hypervariable sequence	10–60	Repeat unit may span up to 20 kb
Microsatellite DNA	1–4	Mononucleotide repeat of adenine dinucleotide repeats common (CA). Usually known as VNTR (variable number tandem repeat)

bp, base-pairs; kb, kilobase-pairs.

5.3.2 **Single nucleotide polymorphisms**

In genomes, there is an additional source of polymorphic diversity termed single nucleotide polymorphisms (SNPs pronounced snips). SNPs are substitutions of one base at a precise location within the genome. Those that occur in coding regions are termed cSNPs. Estimates indicate that an SNP occurs once in every 300 bases and there are thought to be approximately 10 million in the human genome. Interest in SNPs lies in the fact that these differences may account for the differences in disease susceptibility, drug metabolism and response to environmental factors between individuals. There are now a number of initiatives to identify SNPs and produce a genome SNP map. A number of maps have been partially completed and a number of bioinformatics resources have been developed such as the SNP consortium.

5.3.3 **Chromosomes and karyotypes**

Higher organisms may be identified by using the size and shape of their genetic material at a particular point in the cell division cycle termed metaphase. At this point, DNA condenses to form a number of very distinct chromosome structures. Various morphological characteristics of chromosomes may be identified at this stage, including the centromere and the telomere. The array of chromosomes from a given organism may also be stained with dyes such as Giemsa stain and subsequently analysed by light microscopy. The complete array of chromosomes in an organism is termed the karyotype. In certain genetic disorders, aberrations in the size, shape and number of chromosomes may occur and thus the karyotype may be used as an indicator of the disorder (Section 6.8.2). Perhaps the best-known example of this is the correlation of Down's syndrome, where three copies of chromosome 21 (trisomy 21) exist rather than two as in the normal state.

5.3.4 **Renaturation kinetics and genome complexity**

When preparations of double-stranded DNA are denatured and allowed to renature, measurement of the rate of renaturation can give valuable information about the complexity of the DNA, i.e. how much information it contains (measured in base-pairs). The complexity of a molecule may be much less than its total length if some sequences are repetitive, but complexity will equal total length if all sequences are unique, appearing only once in the genome. In practice, the DNA is first cut randomly into fragments about 1 kb in length (Section 5.8), and is then completely denatured by heating above its T_m (Section 5.2.3). Renaturation at a temperature about 10 °C below the T_m is monitored either by decrease in absorbance at 260 nm (the hypochromic effect), or by passing samples at intervals through a column of hydroxylapatite, which will adsorb only double-stranded DNA, and measuring how much of the sample is bound. The degree of renaturation after a given time will

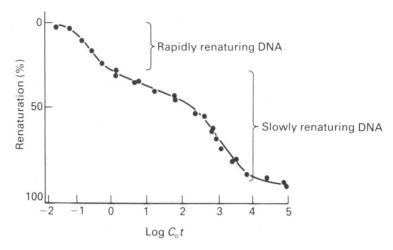

Fig. 5.8. Cot curve of human DNA. DNA was allowed to renature at 60 °C after being completely dissociated by heat. Samples were taken at intervals and passed through a hydroxylapatite column to determine the percentage of double-stranded DNA present. This percentage was plotted against log $C_0 t$ (original concentration of DNA × time of sampling).

depend on C_0, the concentration (in nucleotides per unit volume) of double-stranded DNA prior to denaturation, and t, the duration of the renaturation in seconds.

For a given C_0, it should be evident that a preparation of bacteriophage λ DNA (genome size 49 kb) will contain many more copies of the same sequence per unit volume than a preparation of human DNA (haploid genome size 3×10^6 kb), and will therefore renature far more rapidly, since there will be more molecules complementary to each other per unit volume in the case of λ DNA, and therefore more chance of two complementary strands colliding with each other. In order to compare the rates of renaturation of different DNA samples it is usual to measure C_0 and the time taken for renaturation to proceed half way to completion, $t_{1/2}$, and to multiply these values together to give a $C_0 t_{1/2}$ value. The larger the $C_0 t_{1/2}$, the greater the complexity of the DNA; hence λ DNA has a far lower $C_0 t_{1/2}$ than does human DNA.

In fact, the human genome does not renature in a uniform fashion. If the extent of renaturation is plotted against log $C_0 t$ (this is known as a Cot curve), it is seen that part of the DNA renatures quite rapidly, whilst the remainder is very slow to renature (Fig. 5.8). This indicates that some sequences have a higher concentration than others; in other words, part of the genome consists of repetitive sequences. These repetitive sequences can be separated from the single-copy DNA by passing the renaturing sample through a hydroxylapatite column early in the renaturation process, at a time that gives a low value of $C_0 t$. At this stage only the rapidly renaturing sequences will be double-stranded and they will therefore be the only ones able to bind to the column.

First position (5' end)	Second position				Third position (3' end)
	T	C	A	G	
T	Phe	Ser	Tyr	Cys	T
	Phe	Ser	Tyr	Cys	C
	Leu	Ser	**Stop**	**Stop**	A
	Leu	Ser	**Stop**	Trp	G
C	Leu	Pro	His	Arg	T
	Leu	Pro	His	Arg	C
	Leu	Pro	Gln	Arg	A
	Leu	Pro	Gln	Arg	G
A	Ile	Thr	Asn	Ser	T
	Ile	Thr	Asn	Ser	C
	Ile	Thr	Lys	Arg	A
	Met	Thr	Lys	Arg	G
G	Val	Ala	Asp	Gly	T
	Val	Ala	Asp	Gly	C
	Val	Ala	Glu	Gly	A
	Val	Ala	Glu	Gly	G

Fig. 5.9. The genetic code. Note that the codons in blue represent the start codon (ATG) and the three stop codons.

5.3.5 The nature of the genetic code

DNA encodes the primary sequence of a protein by utilising sets of three nucleotides, termed a codon or triplet, to encode a particular amino acid. The four bases (A, C, G and T) present in DNA allow a possible 64 triplet combinations; however, since there are only about 20 naturally occurring amino acids more than one codon may encode an amino acid. This phenomenon is termed the degeneracy of the genetic code. With the exception of a limited number of differences found in mitochondrial DNA and one or two other species, the genetic code appears to be universal. In addition to coding for amino acids, particular triplet sequences also indicate the beginning (Start) and the end (Stop) of a particular gene. Only one start codon exists (ATG) which also codes for the amino acid methionine, whereas three dedicated stop codons are available (TAT, TAG and TGA) (Fig. 5.9). A sequence flanked by a start and a stop codon containing a number of codons that may be read in-frame to represent a continuous protein sequence is termed an open reading frame (ORF).

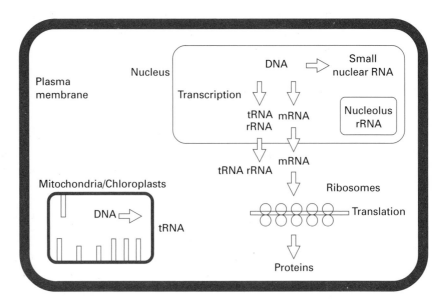

Fig. 5.10. Location of DNA and RNA molecules in eukaryotic cells and the flow of genetic information.

5.4 **LOCATION AND PACKAGING OF NUCLEIC ACIDS**

5.4.1 **Cellular compartments**

In general, DNA in eukaryotic cells is confined to the nucleus and organelles such as mitochondria or chloroplasts, which contain their own genome. The predominant RNA species are, however, normally located within the cytoplasm. The genetic information of cells and most viruses is stored in the form of DNA. This information is used to direct the synthesis of RNA molecules, which fall into three classes. Fig. 5.10 indicates the locations of nucleic acids in prokaryotic and eukaryotic cells.

- *Messenger RNA (mRNA):*   This contains sequences of ribonucleotides that code for the amino acid sequences of proteins. A single mRNA molecule codes for a single polypeptide chain in eukaryotes, but may code for several polypeptides in prokaryotes.
- *Ribosomal RNA (rRNA):*   This forms part of the structure of ribosomes, which are the sites of protein synthesis. Each ribosome contains only three or four different rRNA molecules, complexed with a total of between 55 and 75 proteins.
- *Transfer RNA (tRNA):*   These molecules carry amino acids to the ribosomes, and interact with the mRNA in such a way that their amino acids are joined together in the order specified by the mRNA. There is at least one type of tRNA for each amino acid.

In eukaryotic cells alone a further group of RNA molecules termed small nuclear RNA (snRNA) is present that function within the nucleus and promote the maturation of mRNA molecules. All RNA molecules are associated with their respective binding proteins and are essential for their cellular functions. Nucleic acids from prokaryotic cells are less well compartmentalised, although they serve similar functions.

5.4.2 The packaging of DNA

The DNA in prokaryotic cells resides in the cytoplasm, although is associated with nucleoid proteins, where it is tightly coiled and supercoiled by topoisomerase enzymes to enable it to physically fit into the cell. By contrast, eukaryotic cells have many levels of packaging of the DNA within the nucleus, involving a variety of DNA-binding proteins.

First-order packaging involves the winding of the DNA around a core complex of four small proteins repeated twice and termed histones (H2A, H2B, H3 and H4). These are rich in the basic amino acids lysine and arginine and form a barrel-shaped core octomer structure. Approximately 180 bp of DNA is wound twice around the structure, which is termed a nucleosome. A further histone protein, H1, is found to associate with the outer surface of the nucleosome. The compacting effect of the nucleosome reduces the length of the DNA by a factor of 6.

Nucleosomes also associate to form a second order of packaging termed the 30 nm chromatin fibre, thus further reducing the length of the DNA by a factor of 7 (Fig. 5.11). These structure may be further folded and looped through the interaction with other non-histone proteins and ultimately form chromosome structures.

DNA is found closely associated with the nuclear lamina matrix, which forms a protein scaffold within the nucleus. The DNA is attached at certain positions within the scaffold, usually coinciding with origins of replication. Many other DNA-binding proteins are also present, such as high mobility group (HMG) proteins, which assist in promoting certain DNA conformations during processes such as replication or active gene expression.

5.5 FUNCTIONS OF NUCLEIC ACIDS

5.5.1 DNA replication

The double-stranded nature of DNA provides a means of replication during cell division, since the separation of two DNA strands allows complementary strands to be synthesised upon them. Many enzymes and accessory proteins are required for *in vivo* replication, which in prokaryotes begins at a region of the DNA termed the origin of replication.

DNA has to be unwound before any of the proteins and enzymes needed for replication can act, and this involves separating the double-helical DNA into single strands. This process is carried out by the enzyme DNA helicase. Furthermore, in order to prevent the single strands from re-annealing, small proteins termed single-stranded DNA-binding proteins (SSBs) attach to the single DNA strands (Fig. 5.12).

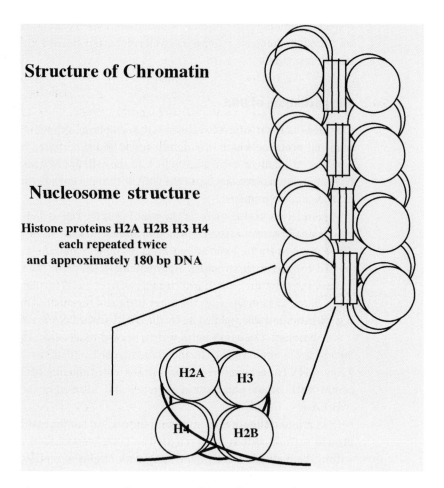

Fig. 5.11. Structure and composition of the nucleosome and chromatin.

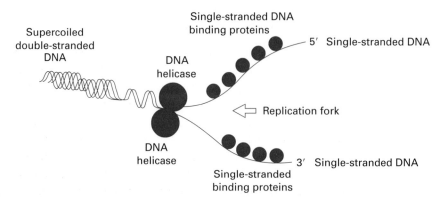

Fig. 5.12. Initial events at the replication fork involving DNA unwinding.

On each exposed single strand a short, complementary RNA chain termed a primer is first produced, using the DNA as a template. The primer is synthesised by an RNA polymerase enzyme known as a primase, which uses ribonucleoside triphosphates and itself requires no primer to function. Then DNA polymerase III (DNA pol III) also uses the original DNA as a template for synthesis of a DNA strand, using the RNA primer as a starting point. The primer is vital, since it leaves an exposed 3′ hydroxyl group. This is necessary, since DNA polymerase III can add new nucleotides only to the 3′ end and not the 5′ end of a nucleic acid. Synthesis of the DNA strand therefore occurs only in a 5′ to 3′ direction from the RNA primer. This DNA strand is usually termed the leading strand and provides the means for continuous DNA synthesis.

Since the two strands of double helical DNA are antiparallel, only one can be synthesised in a continuous fashion. Synthesis of the other strand must take place in a more complex way. The precise mechanism was worked out by Reiji Okazaki in the 1960s. Here, the strand, usually termed the lagging strand, is produced in relatively short stretches of 1–2 kb termed Okazaki fragments. This is still in a 5′ to 3′ direction, using many RNA primers for each individual stretch. Thus discontinuous synthesis of DNA takes place and allows DNA polymerase III to work in the 5′ to 3′ direction. The RNA primers are then removed by DNA polymerase I, which has a 5′ to 3′ exonuclease and the gaps are filled by the same enzyme acting as a polymerase. The separate fragments are joined together by DNA ligase to give a newly formed strand of DNA on the lagging strand (Fig. 5.13).

The replication of eukaryotic DNA is less well characterised, involves multiple origins of replication and is certainly more complex than that of prokaryotes; however, in both cases the process involves 5′ to 3′ synthesis of new DNA strands. The net result of the replication is that the original DNA is replaced by two molecules, each containing one 'old' and one 'new' strand; the process is therefore known as semi-conservative replication. The ideas behind DNA synthesis, replication and the enzymes involved in them have been adopted in many molecular biological techniques and form the basis of many manipulations in genetic engineering.

5.5.2 DNA protection and repair systems

Cellular growth and division require the correct and coordinated replication of DNA. Mechanisms that proofread replicated DNA sequences and maintain the integrity of those sequences are, however, complex and are only beginning to be elucidated for prokaryotic systems. Bacterial protection is afforded by the use of a restriction modification system based on differential methylation of host DNA, so as to distinguish it from foreign DNA such as viruses. The most common is type II and consists of a host DNA methylase and restriction endonuclease that recognises short (4–6 bp) palindromic sequences and cleaves foreign unmethylated DNA at a particular target sequence. The enzymes involved in this process have been of enormous benefit for the manipulation and analysis of DNA, as indicated in Section 5.8.

Repair systems allow the recognition of altered, mispaired or missing bases in double-stranded DNA and invoke an excision repair process. Bacterial repair

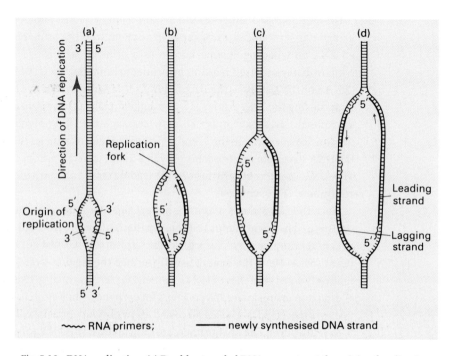

Fig. 5.13. DNA replication. (a) Double-stranded DNA separates at the origin of replication. RNA polymerase synthesises short DNA primer strands complementary to both DNA strands. (b) DNA polymerase III synthesises new DNA strands in a 5′ to 3′ direction, complementary to the exposed, old DNA strands, and continuing from the 3′ end of each RNA primer. Consequently DNA synthesis is in the same direction as DNA replication for one strand (the leading strand) and in the opposite direction for the other (the lagging strand). RNA primer synthesis occurs repeatedly to allow the synthesis of fragments of the lagging strand. (c) As the replication fork moves away from the origin of replication, DNA polymerase III continues the synthesis of the leading strand, and synthesises DNA between RNA primers of the lagging strand. (d) DNA polymerase I removes RNA primers from the lagging strand and fills the resulting gaps with DNA. DNA ligase then joins the resulting fragments, producing a continuous DNA strand.

systems are based on the length of repairable DNA either during replication (dam system) or in general repair (urr system). In some cases damage to DNA activates a protein termed RecA to produce an SOS response that includes the activation of many enzymes and proteins; however, this has yet to be fully characterised. The recombination–repair systems in eukaryotic cells may share some common features with prokaryotes, although the precise mechanism has yet to be established. Defects in DNA repair may result in the stable incorporation of errors into genomic sequences that may underscore several genetic-based diseases.

5.5.3 Transcription of DNA

Expression of genes is carried out initially by the process of transcription, whereby a complementary RNA strand is synthesised by an enzyme termed

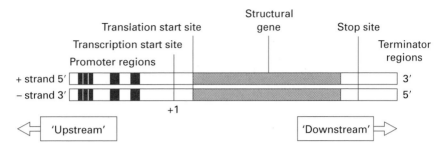

Fig. 5.14. Structure and nomenclature of a typical gene.

RNA polymerase from a DNA template encoding the gene. Most prokaryotic genes are made up of three regions. At the centre is the sequence that will be copied in the form of RNA, called the structural gene. To the 5′ side (upstream) from the strand that will be copied (the plus (+) strand) lies a region called the promoter, and downstream from the transcription unit is the terminator region. Transcription begins when DNA-dependent RNA polymerase binds to the promoter region and moves along the DNA to the transcription unit. At the start of the transcription unit the polymerase begins to synthesise an RNA molecule complementary to the minus (−) strand of the DNA, moving along this strand in a 3′ to 5′ direction, and synthesising RNA in a 5′ to 3′ direction, using ribonucleoside triphosphates. The RNA will therefore have the same sequence as the plus strand of the DNA, apart from the substitution of uracil for thymine. On reaching the stop site in the terminator region, transcription is stopped, and the RNA molecule is released. The numbering of bases in genes is a useful way of identifying key elements. Point or base +1 is the residue located at the transcription start site, positive numbers denote 3′ regions, whilst negative numbers denote 5′ regions (Fig. 5.14).

In eukaryotes, three different RNA polymerases exist, designated I, II and III. Messenger RNA is synthesised by RNA polymerase II, while RNA polymerases I and III catalyse the synthesis of rRNA (I), tRNA and snRNA (III). Many non-expressed genes tend to have residues that are methylated, usually the C of a GC dinucleotide, and, in general, active genes tend to be hypomethylated. This is especially prevalent at the 5′ flanking regions and is a useful means of discovering and identifying new genes.

5.5.4 Promoter and terminator sequences in DNA

Promoters are usually to the 5′ end or upstream from the structural gene and have been best characterised in prokaryotes such as *Escherichia coli*. They comprise two highly conserved sequence elements: the TATA box (consensus sequence 'TATATT'), which is centred approximately 10 bp upstream from the transcription initiation site (−10 in the gene numbering system), and a 'G + C-rich' sequence which is centred about −25 bp upstream from the TATA box. The G + C element is thought to be important in the initial recognition and binding of RNA polymerase

(a)

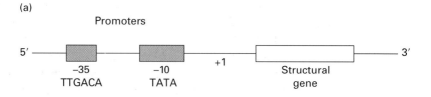

(b)

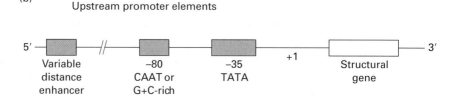

(c)

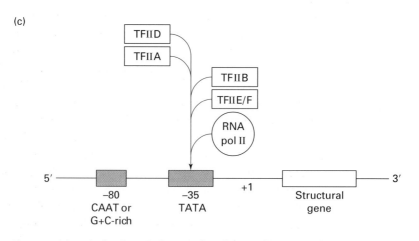

Fig. 5.15. (a) Typical promoter elements found in a prokaryotic cell (e.g. *E. coli*). (b) Typical promoter elements found in eukaryotic cells. (c) Generalised scheme of binding of transcription factors to the promoter regions of eukaryotic cells. Following the binding of the transcription factors IID, IIA, IIB, IIE and IIF a pre-initiation complex is formed. RNA polymerase II then binds to this complex and begins transcription from the start point +1.

to the DNA, while the −10 sequence is involved in the formation of a transcription initiation complex (Fig. 5.15a).

The promoter elements serve as recognition sites for DNA-binding proteins that control gene expression and these proteins are termed transcription factors or *trans*-acting factors. These proteins have a DNA-binding domain for interaction with promoters and an activation domain to allow interaction with other transcription factors. A well-studied example of a transcription factor (TF) is TFIID, which binds to the −35 promoter sequence in eukaryotic cells. Gene regulation occurs in most cases at the level of transcription, and primarily by the rate of transcription initiation, although control may also be by modulation of mRNA stability, or at other levels such as translation. Terminator sequences are less well characterised, but are thought to involve nucleotide sequences near the end of mRNA with the capacity to form a hairpin loop, followed by a run of U residues, which may constitute a termination signal for RNA polymerase.

In the case of eukaryotic genes, numerous short sequences spanning several hundred bases may be important for transcription, as compared with normally fewer than 100 bp for prokaryotic promoters. Particularly critical is the TATA box sequence, located approximately −35 bp upstream from the transcription initiation point in the majority of genes (Fig. 5.15b). This is analogous to the −10 sequence in prokaryotes. A number of other transcription factors also bind sequentially to form an initiation complex that includes RNA polymerase, subsequent to which transcription is initiated. In addition to the TATA box, a (CAT box (consensus GGCCAATCT) is often located at about −80 bp, which is an important determinant of promoter efficiency. Many upstream promoter elements (UPEs) have been described that are either general in their action or tissue (or gene) specific. GC elements that contain the sequence GGGCG may be present at multiple sites and in either orientation and are often associated with housekeeping genes such as those encoding enzymes involved in general metabolism. Some promoter sequence elements, such as the TATA box, are common to most genes, whilst others may be specific to particular genes or classes of genes.

Of particular interest is a class of promoter first investigated in simian virus 40 (SV40) and termed an enhancer. These sequences are distinguished from other promoter sequences by their unique ability to function over several kilobases either upstream or downstream from a particular gene in an orientation-independent manner. Even at such great distances from the transcription start point they may increase transcription by several hundred-fold. The precise interactions between transcription factors, RNA polymerase or other DNA-binding proteins and the DNA sequences to which they bind may be identified and characterised by the technique of DNA footprinting (Section 6.8.3). For transcription in eukaryotic cells to proceed, a number of transcription factors need to interact with the promoters and with each other. This cascade mechanism is indicated in Fig. 5.15c and is termed a pre-initiation complex. Once this has been formed around the −35 TATA sequence RNA polymerase II is able to transcribe the structural gene and form a complementary RNA copy (Section 5.5.6).

5.5.5 Transcription in prokaryotes

Prokaryotic gene organisation differs from that found in prokaryotes in a number of ways. Prokarotic genes are generally found as continuous coding sequences. Moreover they are frequently found clustered into operons, which contain genes that relate to a particular function such as the metabolism of a substrate or synthesis of a product. This is particularly evident in the best-known operon

(a)

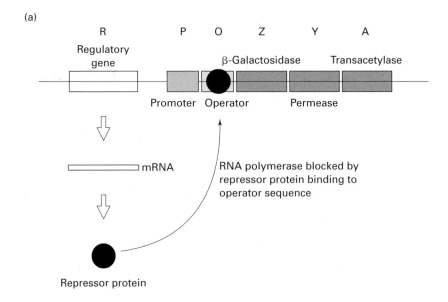

(b)

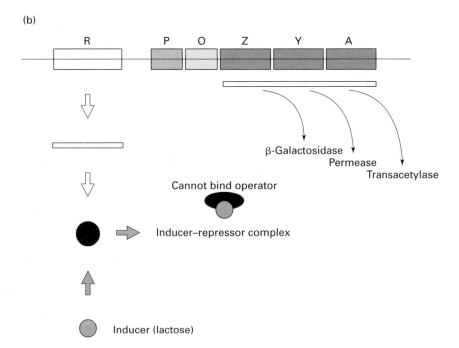

Fig. 5.16. Lactose operon (a) in a state of repression (no lactose present) and (b) following induction by lactose.

identified in *E. coli* termed the lactose operon, where three genes *lacZ*, *lacY* and *lacA* share the same promoter and are therefore switched on and off at the same time. In this model the absence of lactose results in a repressor protein binding to an operator region upstream of the *Z*, *Y* and *A* genes and prevents RNA polymerase from transcribing the genes (Fig. 5.16a). However, the presence of lactose

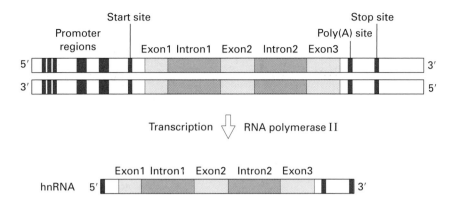

Fig. 5.17. Transcription of a typical eukaryotic gene to form heterogeneous nuclear RNA.

requires the genes to be transcribed to allow its metabolism. Lactose binds to the repressor protein and causes a conformational change in its structure. This prevents it binding to the operator and allows RNA polymerase to bind and transcribe the three genes (Fig. 5.16b). Transcription and translation in prokaryotes is also closely linked or coupled whereas in eukaryotic cells the two processes are distinct and take place in different cell compartments.

5.5.6 Post-transcriptional processing

Transcription of a eukaryotic gene results in the production of a heterogeneous nuclear RNA transcript (hnRNA) that faithfully represents the entire structural gene (Fig. 5.17). Three processing events then take place. The first processing step involves the addition of a methylated guanosine residue (m7Gppp) termed a cap to the 5′ end of the hnRNA. This may be a signalling structure or aid in the stability of the molecule (Fig. 5.18). In addition, 150 to 300 adenosine residues termed a poly (A) tail are attached at the 3′ end of the hnRNA by the enzyme poly (A) polymerase. The poly (A) tail allows the specific isolation of eukaryotic mRNA from total RNA by affinity chromatography (Section 5.7.2), its presence is thought to confer stability on the transcript.

Unlike prokaryotic transcripts, those from eukaryotes have their coding sequence (expressed regions or exons) interrupted by non-coding sequence (intervening regions or introns). Intron–exon boundaries are generally determined by the sequence GUAG and need to be removed or spliced before the mature mRNA is formed (Fig. 5.18). The process of intron splicing is mediated by small nuclear RNAs (snRNAs), which exist in the nucleus as ribonuclear protein particles. These are often found in a large nuclear structure complex termed the spliceosome, where splicing takes place. Introns are usually removed in a sequential manner from the 5′ to the 3′ end and their number varies between different genes. Some eukaryotic genes contain no introns, for example histone genes, whereas the gene for dystrophin, the gene responsible for muscular dystrophy, contains over 250 introns. In some cases, however, the same hnRNA transcript may be processed in

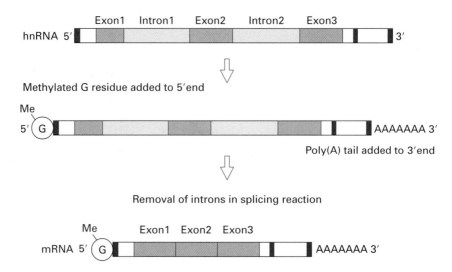

Fig. 5.18. Post-transcriptional modifications of heterogeneous nuclear RNA.

different ways to produce different mRNAs coding for different proteins in a process known as alternative splicing. Thus a sequence that constitutes an exon for one RNA species may be part of an excised intron in another. The particular type or amount of mRNA synthesised from a cell or cell type may be analysed by a variety of molecular biological techniques (Section 6.8.1).

5.5.7 Translation of mRNA

Messenger RNA molecules are read and translated into protein by complex RNA–protein particles termed ribosomes. The ribosomes are termed 70 S or 80 S depending on their sedimentation coefficient. Prokaryotic cells have 70 S ribosomes whilst those of the eukaryotic cytoplasm are 80 S. Ribosomes are composed of two subunits that are held apart by ribosomal binding proteins until translation proceeds. There are sites on the ribosome for the binding of one mRNA and two tRNA molecules and the translation process is in three stages.

- *Initiation:*   This involves the assembly of the ribosome subunits and the binding of the mRNA.
- *Elongation:*   This is where specific amino acids are used to form polypeptides, this being directed by the codon sequence in the mRNA.
- *Termination:*   This involves the disassembly of the components of translation following the production of a polypeptide.

Transfer RNA molecules is also essential for translation. Each of these is covalently linked to a specific amino acid, forming an aminoacyl tRNA, and each has a triplet of bases exposed that is complementary to the codon for that amino acid. This exposed triplet is known as the anticodon, and allows the tRNA to act as an 'adaptor' molecule, bringing together a codon and its corresponding amino acid.

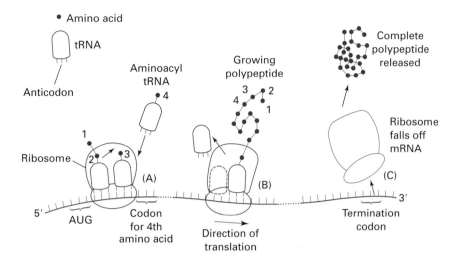

Fig. 5.19. Translation. Ribosome A has moved only a short way from the 5′ end of the mRNA, and has built up a dipeptide (on one tRNA) that is about to be transferred onto the third amino acid (still attached to tRNA). Ribosome B has moved much further along the mRNA and has built up an oligopeptide that has just been transferred onto the most recent aminoacyl tRNA. The resulting free tRNA leaves the ribosome and will receive another amino acid. The ribosome moves towards the 3′ end of the mRNA by a distance of three nucleotides, so that the next codon can be aligned with its corresponding aminoacyl tRNA on the ribosome. Ribosome C has reached a termination codon, has released the completed polypeptide, and has fallen off the mRNA.

The process of linking an amino acid to its specific tRNA is termed charging and is carried out by the enzyme aminoacyl tRNA synthetase.

In prokaryotic cells the ribosome binds to the 5′ end of the mRNA at a sequence known as the ribosome binding site or sometimes termed the Shine–Dalgarno sequence, after the discoverers of the sequence. In eukaryotes the situation is similar but involves a Kozak sequence located around the initiation codon. Following translation initiation the ribosome moves towards the 3′ end of the mRNA, allowing an aminoacyl tRNA molecule to base-pair with each successive codon, thereby carrying in amino acids in the correct order for protein synthesis. There are two sites for tRNA molecules in the ribosome: the A site and the P site. When these sites are occupied, directed by the sequence of codons in the mRNA, the ribosome allows the formation of a peptide bond between the amino acids. The process is also under the control of an enzyme, peptidyl transferase. When the ribosome encounters a termination codon (UAA, UGA or UAG) a release factor binds to the complex and translation stops, the polypeptide and its corresponding mRNA are released and the ribosome divides into its two subunits (Fig. 5.19). A myriad of accessory initiation and elongation protein factors are involved in this process. In eukaryotic cells the polypeptide may then be subjected to post-translational modifications such as glycosylation, and by virtue of specific amino acid signal sequences may be directed to specific cellular compartments or exported from the cell.

Since the mRNA base sequence is read in triplets, an error of one or two nucleotides in positioning of the ribosome will result in the synthesis of an incorrect polypeptide. Thus it is essential for the correct reading frame to be used during translation. This is ensured in prokaryotes by base-pairing between the Shine–Dalgarno sequence (Kozak sequence in eukaryotes) and a complementary sequence of one of the ribosome's rRNA molecules, thus establishing the correct starting point for movement of the ribosome along the mRNA. However, if a mutation such as a deletion/insertion takes place within the coding sequence, it will also cause a shift of the reading frame and result in an aberrant polypeptide. Genetic mutations and polymorphisms are considered in more detail in Section 6.8.5.

5.5.8 Control of protein production: RNA interference

There are a number of mechanisms by which protein production is controlled; however, the control may be at either the gene or the protein level. Typically this could include controlling levels of expression of mRNA, an increase or decrease in mRNA turnover, or controlling mRNA availability for translation. One recently discovered control mechanism that has also been adapted as a molecular biological technique to aid in the modulation of mRNA is termed RNA interference (RNAi). This involves the synthesis of short double-stranded RNA molecules that are cleaved into 21–23 nucleotide-long fragments to form an RNA-induced silencing complex (RISC). This complex potentially uses the short RNA molecules complementary to mRNA transcripts that, following hybridisation, allow an RNase to destroy the bound mRNA. The technique has important implications for medical conditions where, for example, increased levels of specific mRNA molecules in certain cancers and viral infections may be reduced using RNAi.

5.6 THE MANIPULATION OF NUCLEIC ACIDS: BASIC TOOLS AND TECHNIQUES

5.6.1 Enzymes used in molecular biology

The discovery and characterisation of a number of key enzymes has enabled the development of various techniques for the analysis and manipulation of DNA. In particular, the enzymes termed type II restriction endonucleases have come to play a key role in all aspects of molecular biology. These enzymes recognise certain DNA sequences, usually 4–6 bp in length, and cleave them in a defined manner. The sequences recognised are palindromic or of an inverted repeat nature; that is, they read the same in both directions on each strand. When cleaved they leave a flush-ended or staggered (also termed a cohesive-ended) fragment depending on the particular enzyme used (Fig. 5.20). An important property of staggered ends is that those produced from different molecules by the same enzyme are complementary (or 'sticky') and so will anneal to each other. The annealed strands are held together only by hydrogen bonding between complementary bases on opposite strands. Covalent joining of ends on each of the two

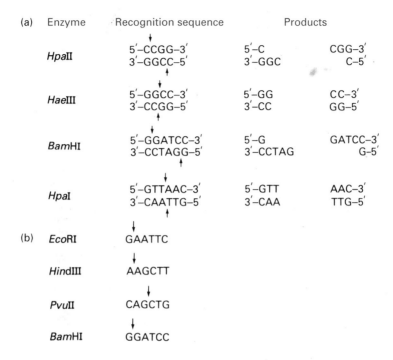

Fig. 5.20. Recognition sequences of some restriction enzymes showing (a) full descriptions and (b) conventional representations. Arrows indicate positions of cleavage. Note that all the information in (a) can be derived from knowledge of a single strand of the DNA, whereas in (b) only one strand is shown, drawn 5′ to 3′; this is the conventional way of representing restriction sites.

strands may be brought about by the enzyme DNA ligase (Section 6.2.2). This is widely exploited in molecular biology to enable the construction of recombinant DNA, i.e. the joining of DNA fragments from different sources. Approximately 500 restriction enzymes have been characterised that recognise over 100 different target sequences. A number of these, termed isoschizomers, recognise different target sequences but produce the same staggered ends or overhangs. A number of other enzymes have proved to be of value in the manipulation of DNA, as summarised in Table 5.3, and are indicated at appropriate points within the text.

5.7 ISOLATION AND SEPARATION OF NUCLEIC ACIDS

5.7.1 Isolation of DNA

The use of DNA for analysis or manipulation usually requires that it be isolated and purified to a certain extent. DNA is recovered from cells by the gentlest possible method of cell rupture to prevent the DNA from fragmenting by mechanical shearing. This is usually in the presence of EDTA, which chelates the Mg^{2+} needed for enzymes that degrade DNA (DNases). Ideally, cell walls, if present, should be digested enzymatically (e.g. lysozyme treatment of bacteria), and the cell

Table 5.3 **Types and examples of typical enzymes used in the manipulation of nucleic acids**

Enzyme	Specific example	Use in nucleic acid manipulation
	DNA pol I	DNA-dependent DNA polymerase $5' \rightarrow 3'/3' \rightarrow 5'$ exonuclease activity
DNA polymerases	Klenow	DNA pol I lacks $5' \rightarrow 3'$ exonuclease activity
	T4 DNA pol	Lacks $5' \rightarrow 3'$ exonuclease activity
	Taq DNA pol	Thermostable DNA polymerase used in PCR
	Tth DNA pol	Thermostable DNA polymerase with RT activity
	T7 DNA pol	Used in DNA sequencing
RNA polymerases	T7 RNA pol	DNA-dependent RNA polymerase
	T3 RNA pol	DNA-dependent RNA polymerase
	Qβ replicase	RNA-dependent RNA polymerase, used in RNA-amplification
Nucleases	DNase I	Non-specific endonuclease that cleaves DNA
	Exonuclease III	DNA-dependent $3' \rightarrow 5'$ stepwise removal of nucleotides
	RNase A	RNases used in mapping studies
	RNase H	Used in second strand cDNA synthesis
	S1 nuclease	Single-strand-specific nuclease
Reverse transcriptase	AMV-RT	RNA-dependent DNA polymerase, used in cDNA synthesis
Transferases	Terminal transferase (TdT)	Adds homopolymer tails to the 3′ end of DNA
Ligases	T4 DNA ligase	Links 5′-phosphate and 3′-hydroxyl ends via phosphodiester bond
Kinases	T4 polynucleotide kinase (PNK)	Transfers terminal phosphate groups from ATP to 5′-OH groups
Phosphatases	Alkaline phosphatase	Removes 5′-phosphates from DNA and RNA
Transferases	Terminal transferase	Adds homopolymer tails to the 3′ end of DNA
Methylases	*Eco*RI methylase	Methylates specific residues and protects from cleavage by restriction enzymes

PCR, polymerase chain reaction; RT, reverse transcriptase; cDNA, complementary DNA; AMV, avian myeloblastosis virus.

membrane should be solubilised using detergent. If physical disruption is necessary, it should be kept to a minimum, and should involve cutting or squashing of cells, rather than the use of shear forces. Cell disruption (and most subsequent steps) should be performed at 4 °C, using glassware and solutions that have been autoclaved to destroy DNase activity.

After release of nucleic acids from the cells, RNA can be removed by treatment with ribonuclease (RNase) that has been heat treated to inactivate any DNase contaminants; RNase is relatively stable to heat as a result of its disulphide bonds, which ensure rapid renaturation of the molecule on cooling. The other major contaminant, protein, is removed by shaking the solution gently with water-saturated phenol, or with a phenol/chloroform mixture, either of which will denature proteins but not nucleic acids. Centrifugation of the emulsion formed by this mixing produces a lower, organic phase, separated from the upper, aqueous phase by an interface of denatured protein. The aqueous solution is recovered and deproteinised repeatedly, until no more material is seen at the interface. Finally, the deproteinised DNA preparation is mixed with two volumes of absolute ethanol, and the DNA allowed to precipitate out of solution in a freezer. After centrifugation, the DNA pellet is redissolved in a buffer containing EDTA to inactivate any DNases present. This solution can be stored at 4 °C for at least a month. DNA solutions can be stored frozen, although repeated freezing and thawing tends to damage long DNA molecules by shearing. The procedure described above is suitable for total cellular DNA. If the DNA from a specific organelle or viral particle is needed, it is best to isolate the organelle or virus before extracting its DNA, since the recovery of a particular type of DNA from a mixture is usually rather difficult. Where a high degree of purity is required, DNA may be subjected to density gradient ultracentrifugation through caesium chloride, which is particularly useful for the preparation of plasmid DNA. A flowchart of DNA extraction is indicated in Fig. 5.21. It is possible to check the integrity of the DNA by agarose gel electrophoresis and determine the concentration of the DNA by using the fact that 1 absorbance unit equates to 50 μg cm^{-3} of DNA and so:

$$50 \times A_{260} = \text{concentration of DNA sample } (\mu\text{g cm}^{-3})$$

Contaminants may also be identified by scanning ultraviolet spectrophotometry from 200 nm to 300 nm. A ratio of 260 nm to 280 nm of approximately 1.8 indicates that the sample is free from protein contamination, which absorbs strongly at 280 nm.

5.7.2 Isolation of RNA

The methods used for RNA isolation are very similar to those described above for DNA; however, RNA molecules are relatively short, and therefore less easily damaged by shearing, so cell disruption can be rather more vigorous. RNA is, however, very vulnerable to digestion by RNases, which are present endogenously in various concentrations in certain cell types and exogenously on fingers. Gloves should therefore be worn, and a strong detergent should be included in the isolation medium to immediately denature any RNases. Subsequent deproteinisation should be particularly rigorous, since RNA is often tightly associated with proteins. DNase treatment can be used to remove DNA, and RNA can be precipitated by ethanol. One reagent in particular that is commonly used in RNA extraction is guanadinium thiocyanate, which is both a strong inhibitor of RNase and a protein denaturant. A flowchart of RNA extraction is indicated in Fig. 5.22. It is possible to check the integrity of an RNA extract by analysing it by agarose gel electrophoresis. The most abundant RNA species are the rRNA molecules, 23 S and 16 S for prokaryotes and 18 S and 28 S for eukaryotes. These appear as discrete bands on the agarose gel and indicate that the other RNA components are likely to be intact. This is usually carried out under denaturing conditions to prevent

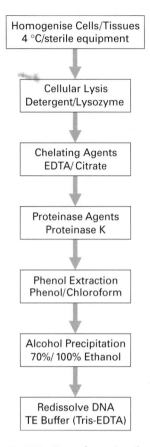

Fig. 5.21. General steps involved in extracting DNA from cells or tissues.

secondary structure formation in the RNA. The concentration of the RNA may be estimated by using ultraviolet spectrophotometry. At 260 nm 1 absorbance unit equates to 40 μg cm^{-3} of RNA and therefore:

$$40 \times A_{260} = \text{concentration of RNA sample μg cm}^{-3}$$

Contaminants may also be identified in the same way as for DNA by scanning ultraviolet spectrophotometry; however, in the case of RNA a 260 nm to 280 nm ratio of approximately 2 would be expected for a sample containing no protein (Section 5.7.1).

In many cases it is desirable to isolate eukaryotic mRNA, which constitutes only 2–5% of cellular RNA, from a mixture of total RNA molecules. This may be carried out by affinity chromatography on oligo(dT)-cellulose columns. At high salt concentrations, the mRNA containing poly(A) tails binds to the complementary oligo(dT) molecules of the affinity column, and so mRNA will be retained; all other RNA molecules can be washed through the column by further high salt solution. Finally, the bound mRNA can be eluted using a low concentration of salt (Fig 5.23). Nucleic acid species may also be subfractionated by more physical

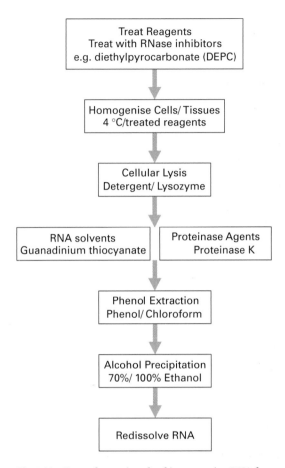

Fig. 5.22. General steps involved in extracting RNA from cells or tissues.

means such as electrophoretic or chromatographic separations based on differences in nucleic acid fragment sizes or physicochemical characteristics.

5.7.3 **Automated and kit-based extraction of nucleic acids**

Automation and kit-based manipulation in molecular biology is steadily increasing, and the extraction of nucleic acids by these means is no exception. There are many commercially available kits for nucleic acid extraction, although many rely on the methods described in Sections 5.8.1 and 5.8.2, their advantage lies in the fact that the reagents are standardised and quality control tested, providing a high degree of reliability. For example, the use of glass bead preparations for DNA purification has been used increasingly and with reliable results. Small compact column-type preparations are also used extensively in research and in routine DNA analysis such as QIAGEN columns. Essentially the same reagents for nucleic acid extraction may be used in a format that allows reliable and automated extraction. This is of particular use where a large number of DNA extractions are required.

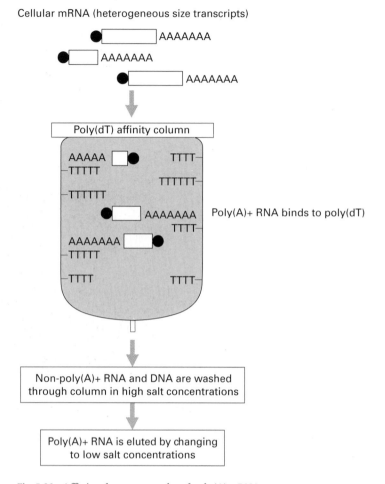

Fig. 5.23. Affinity chromatography of poly(A)+ RNA.

There are also many kit-based extraction methods for RNA, these in particular have overcome some of the problems of RNA extraction such as RNase contamination. A number of fully automated nucleic acid extraction machines are now employed in areas where high throughput is required, for example clinical diagnostic laboratories. Here, the raw samples such as blood specimens are placed in 96- or 384-well microtitre plates and these follow a set computer-controlled processing pattern carried out robotically. Thus the samples are rapidly manipulated and extracted in approximately 45 min without any manual operations being undertaken.

5.7.4 Electrophoresis of nucleic acids

Electrophoresis in agarose or polyacrylamide gels is the usual way to separate DNA molecules according to size. The technique can be used analytically or preparatively and can be qualitative or quantitative. Large fragments of DNA such as chromosomes may also be separated by a modification of electrophoresis termed

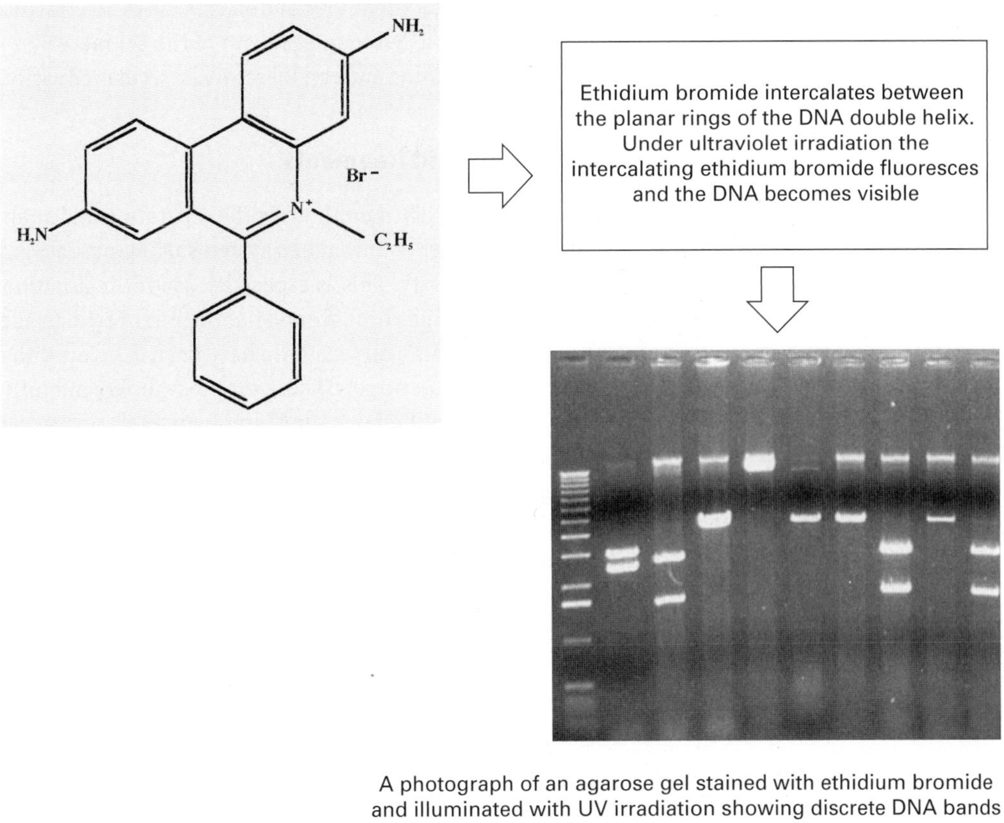

Ethidium bromide intercalates between the planar rings of the DNA double helix. Under ultraviolet irradiation the intercalating ethidium bromide fluoresces and the DNA becomes visible

A photograph of an agarose gel stained with ethidium bromide and illuminated with UV irradiation showing discrete DNA bands

Fig. 5.24. The use of ethidium bromide to detect DNA.

pulsed field gel electrophoresis (PFGE). The easiest and most widely applicable method is electrophoresis in horizontal agarose gels, followed by staining with ethidium bromide. This dye binds to DNA by insertion between stacked base-pairs (intercalation), and it exhibits a strong orange/red fluorescence when illuminated with ultraviolet light (Fig 5.24). Very often electrophoresis is used to check the purity and intactness of a DNA preparation or to assess the extent of an enzymatic reaction during, for example, the steps involved in the cloning of DNA. For such checks minigels are particularly convenient, since they need little preparation, use small samples and quickly give results. Agarose gels can be used to separate molecules larger than about 100 bp. For higher resolution or for the effective separation of shorter DNA molecules, polyacrylamide gels are the preferred method.

When electrophoresis is used preparatively, the piece of gel containing the desired DNA fragment is physically removed with a scalpel. The DNA may be recovered from the gel fragment in various ways. This may include crushing with a glass rod in a small volume of buffer, using agarase to digest the agarose, thus leaving the DNA, or by the process of electroelution. In this method the piece of gel is sealed in a length of dialysis tubing containing buffer and is then placed between two electrodes in a tank containing more buffer. Passage of an electrical current between the electrodes causes DNA to migrate out of the gel piece, but it remains trapped within the dialysis tubing and can therefore be recovered easily.

5.7.5 Automated analysis of nucleic acid fragments

Gel electrophoresis remains the established method for the separation and analysis of nucleic acids. However, a number of automated systems using pre-cast gels are available that are gaining popularity. This is especially useful in situations where a large number of samples or high throughput analysis is required. In addition, new technologies such as Agilents' Lab-on-a-chip have been developed that obviate the need to prepare electrophoretic gels. These systems employ microfluidic circuits where a small cassette unit that contains interconnected microreservoirs is used. The sample is applied in one area and driven through microchannels under computer-controlled electrophoresis. The channels lead to reservoirs allowing, for example, incubation with other reagents such as dyes for a specified time. Electrophoretic separation is thus carried out in a microscale format. The small sample size minimises sample and reagent consumption, and as such is useful for DNA and RNA sample analysis. In addition the units, being computer controlled, allow data to be captured within a very short time scale. More recently, alternative methods of analysis including high performance liquid chromatography-based approaches have gained in popularity, especially for mutation analysis (Section 6.8.6). Mass spectrometry is also becoming increasingly used for nucleic acid analysis (Section 9.2.4).

5.8 MOLECULAR BIOLOGY AND BIOINFORMATICS

5.8.1 Basic bioinformatics

Bioinformatics has become a vital resource for molecular biological research and is also increasingly used in the routine detection of DNA mutations. This growth of bioinformatics has been driven by the increase in genetic sequence information and the need to store, analyse and manipulate it. There are now a huge number of sequences stored in genetic databases from a variety of organisms, including the human genome. Indeed the genetic information from various organisms is an indispensable starting point for molecular biology research. The largest of the so-called primary databases include GenBank at the National Institutes of Health (NIH) in the USA, EMBL at the European Bioinformatics Institute (EBI) in Cambridge, UK, and the DNA database of Japan (DDBJ) at Mishima. These databases contain the nucleotide sequences that are annotated to allow easy identification. There are also many other databases such as secondary databases that contain information relating to sequence motifs, such as core sequences representing cytochrome P450 domains or DNA-binding domains. Importantly all of the databases may be accessed over the internet. A number of these important databases and internet resources are listed in Table 5.4.

Table 5.4 Nucleic acid and protein database resources available on the World Wide Web

Database or resource		URL (uniform resource locator)
General DNA sequence databases		
EMBL	European Bioinformatics Institute	\<http://www.ebi.ac.uk\>
GenBank	US genetic database resource	\<http://www.ncbi.nlm.nih.gov\>
DDBJ	Japanese genetic database	\<http://www.ddbj.nig.ac.jp\>
Protein sequence databases		
Swiss-Prot	European protein sequence database	\<http://www.expasy.org\>
UniProt TREMBL	European protein sequence database	\<http://www.ebi.ac.uk/trembl\>
Protein structure databases		
PDB	Protein structure database	\<http://www.rcsb.org\>
Genome project databases		
Human Genome Database, USA		\<http://gdbwww.gdb.org\>
dbEST (cDNA and partial sequences)		\<http://www.ncbi.nih.gov/dbEST/index.html\>
Généthon Genetic maps based on repeat markers		\<http://www.genethon.fr\>

DNA databases and other nucleic acid sequence and protein analysis software may all be accessed over the internet given the relevant software and authority. This is now relatively straightforward using web browsers that provide a user friendly graphical interface for data analysis and manipulation. Consequently the new expanding and exciting areas of bioscience research are those that analyse genome and cDNA sequence databases (genomics) and also their protein counterparts (proteomics). This is sometimes referred to as *in silico* research.

5.8.2 Analysing information using bioinformatics

One of the most useful bioinformatics resources is termed BLAST (basic local alignment search tool) located at the NCBI (\<www.ncbi.nlm.nih.gov\>). This allows a DNA sequence to be submitted via the World Wide Web in order to compare it to all the sequences contained within a DNA database. This is very useful, since it is possible once a nucleotide sequence has been deduced by, for example, Sanger sequencing, to identify sequences of similarity. Indeed if human sequences are used and have already been mapped it is possible to locate their position to a particular chromosome using NCBI, GenomeMap. A further resource such as an ORF (open reading frame) finder allows a search to be undertaken for ORFs, for example sequences beginning with a start codon (ATG) and continuing with a significant number of 'coding' triplets before a stop codon is reached. There are a number of other sequences that may be used to define coding sequences: these include ribosome binding sites, splice site junctions, poly(A) polymerase sequences and promoter sequences that lie outside the coding regions. These may

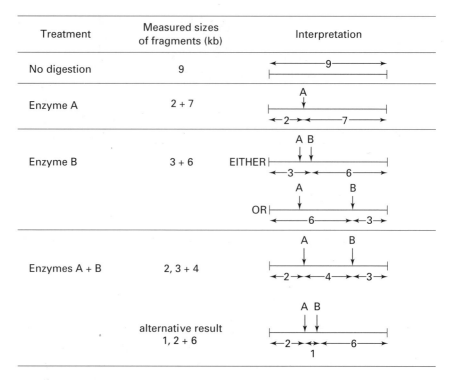

Treatment	Measured sizes of fragments (kb)	Interpretation
No digestion	9	
Enzyme A	2 + 7	
Enzyme B	3 + 6	EITHER / OR
Enzymes A + B	2, 3 + 4	
	alternative result 1, 2 + 6	

Fig. 5.25. Restriction mapping of DNA. Note that each experimental result and its interpretation should be considered in sequence, thus building up an increasingly unambiguous map.

also be identified using resources such as the nucleotide identification system (NIX). Here, secondary databases are queried with the unknown sequence and an output is generated indicating any potential promoter, exon/intron sequences, etc.

5.9 MOLECULAR ANALYSIS OF NUCLEIC ACID SEQUENCES

5.9.1 Restriction mapping of DNA fragments

Restriction mapping involves the size analysis of restriction fragments produced by several restriction enzymes individually and in combination (Section 5.6.1). The principle of this mapping is illustrated in Fig. 5.25, in which the restriction sites of two enzymes, A and B, are being mapped. Cleavage with A gives fragments 2 and 7 kilobases (kb) from a 9 kb molecule; hence we can position the single A site 2 kb from one end. Similarly, B gives fragments 3 and 6 kb away, so it has a single site 3 kb from one end; but it is not possible at this stage to say whether it is near to A's site or at the opposite end of the DNA. This can be resolved by a double digestion. If the resultant fragments are 2, 3 and 4 kb away, then A and B cut at opposite ends of the molecule; if they are 1, 2 and 6 kb away, the sites are near to each other. Not surprisingly, the mapping of real molecules is rarely as simple as

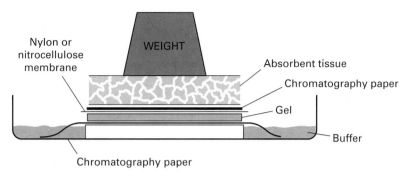

Fig. 5.26. Southern blot apparatus.

this, and bioinformatic analysis of the restriction fragment lengths is usually needed to construct a map.

5.9.2 Nucleic acid blotting methods

Electrophoresis of DNA restriction fragments allows separation based on size; however, it provides no indication as to the presence of a specific, desired fragment among the complex sample. This can be achieved by transferring the DNA from the intact gel onto a piece of nitrocellulose or nylon membrane placed in contact with it. This provides a more permanent record of the sample, since DNA begins to diffuse out of a gel that is left for a few hours. First the gel is soaked in alkali to render the DNA single stranded. It is then transferred to the membrane so that the DNA becomes bound to it in exactly the same pattern as that originally on the gel. This transfer, named a Southern blot after its inventor Ed Southern, can be performed electrophoretically or by drawing large volumes of buffer through both gel and membrane, thus transferring DNA from one to the other by capillary action (Fig. 5.26). The point of this operation is that the membrane can now be treated with a labelled DNA molecule, for example a gene probe (Section 5.9.3). This single-stranded DNA probe will hybridise under the right conditions to complementary fragments immobilised onto the membrane. The conditions of hybridisation, including the temperature and salt concentration, are critical for this process to take place effectively. This is usually referred to as the stringency of the hybridisation and it is particular for each individual gene probe and for each sample of DNA. A series of washing steps with buffer is then carried out to remove any unbound probe and the membrane is developed, like a photograph, after which the precise location of the probe and its target may be visualised. It is also possible to analyse DNA from different species or organisms by blotting the DNA and then using a gene probe representing a protein or enzyme from one of the organisms. In this way it is possible to search for related genes in different species. This technique is generally termed zoo blotting.

The same basic process of nucleic acid blotting can be used to transfer RNA from gels onto similar membranes. This allows the identification of specific mRNA sequences of a defined length by hybridisation to a labelled gene probe and is known as northern blotting. It is possible with this technique not only to detect specific mRNA molecules but also to quantify the relative amounts of the specific mRNA. It is usual to separate the mRNA transcripts by gel electrophoresis under denaturing conditions, since this improves resolution and allows a more accurate estimation of the sizes of the transcripts (Section 5.7.2). The format of the blotting may be altered from transfer from a gel to direct application to slots on a specific blotting apparatus containing the nylon membrane. This is termed slot or dot blotting and provides a convenient means of measuring the abundance of specific mRNA transcripts without the need for gel electrophoresis; however, it does not provide information regarding the size of the fragments.

5.9.3 Design and production of gene probes

The availability of a gene probe is essential in many molecular biological techniques yet in many cases is one of the most difficult steps. The information needed to produce a gene probe may come from many sources. However, the availability of bioinformatics resources and genetic databases has ensured that this is the usual starting point for gene probe design.

In some cases it is possible to use related genes, i.e. from the same gene family, to gain information on the most useful DNA sequence to use as a probe. Similar proteins or DNA sequences but from different species may also provide a starting point with which to produce a so-called heterologous gene probe. Although in some cases probes are already produced and cloned it is possible, armed with a DNA sequence from a DNA database, to chemically synthesise a single-stranded oligonucleotide probe. This is usually undertaken by computer-controlled gene synthesisers, which link dNTPs (deoxyribonucleoside triphosphates) together based on a desired sequence. It is essential to carry out certain checks before probe production to determine that the probe is unique, is not able to self-anneal or that it is self-complementary – all of which may compromise its use.

Where little information on the DNA is available to prepare a gene probe, it is possible in some cases to use the knowledge gained from analysis of the corresponding protein. Thus it is possible to isolate and purify proteins and sequence part of the N-terminal end or an internal region of the protein. From our knowledge of the genetic code, it is possible to predict the various DNA sequences that could code for the protein, and then to synthesise appropriate oligonucleotide sequences chemically. Owing to the degeneracy of the genetic code, most amino acids are coded for by more than one codon, therefore there will be more than one possible nucleotide sequence that could code for a given polypeptide (Fig. 5.27). The longer the polypeptide, the greater is the number of possible oligonucleotides that must be synthesised. Fortunately, there is no need to synthesise a sequence longer than about 20 bases, since this should hybridise efficiently with any complementary sequences and should be specific for one gene. Ideally, a section of the protein should be chosen that contains as many tryptophan and methionine residues as possible, since these have unique codons and there will therefore be

Polypeptide		Phe	Met	Pro	Trp	His	
Corresponding nucleotide sequences	5'	T TTC	ATC	T CCC A G	TGG	T CAC	3'

Fig. 5.27. Oligonucleotide probes. Note that only methionine and tryptophan have unique codons. It is impossible to predict which of the indicated codons for phenylalanine, proline and histidine will be present in the gene to be probed, so all possible combinations must be synthesised (16 in the example shown).

fewer possible base sequences that could code for that part of the protein. The synthetic oligonucleotides can then be used as probes in a number of molecular biological methods.

5.9.4 Labelling DNA gene probe molecules

An essential feature of a gene probe is that it can be visualised or labelled by some means. This allows any complementary sequence that the probe binds to be flagged up or identified.

There are two main types of label used for gene probes. Traditionally labelling has been carried out using radioactive labels, but non-radioactive labels are gaining in popularity.

Perhaps the most common radioactive label is 32-phosphorus (^{32}P), although for certain techniques 35-sulphur (^{35}S) and tritium (^{3}H) are used. These may be detected by the process of autoradiography (Section 14.2.3), where the labelled probe molecule, bound to sample DNA, located for example on a nylon membrane, is placed in contact with an X-ray-sensitive film. Following exposure the film is developed and fixed just as a black-and-white negative. The exposed film reveals the precise location of the labelled probe and therefore the DNA to which it has hybridised.

Non-radioactive labels are increasingly being used to label DNA gene probes. Until recently, radioactive labels were more sensitive than their non-radioactive counterparts. However, recent developments have led to similar sensitivities, which, when combined with the improved safety of non-radioactive labels, have led to their greater acceptance.

The labelling systems are termed either direct or indirect. Direct labelling allows an enzyme reporter such as alkaline phosphatase to be coupled directly to the DNA. Although this may alter the characteristics of the DNA gene probe, it offers the advantage of rapid analysis, since no intermediate steps are needed. However, indirect labelling is at present more popular. This relies on the incorporation of a nucleotide that has a label attached. At present three of the main labels in use are biotin, fluorescein and digoxygenin. These molecules are linked covalently to nucleotides using a carbon spacer arm of 7, 14 or 21 atoms. Specific binding proteins may then be used as a bridge between the nucleotide and a

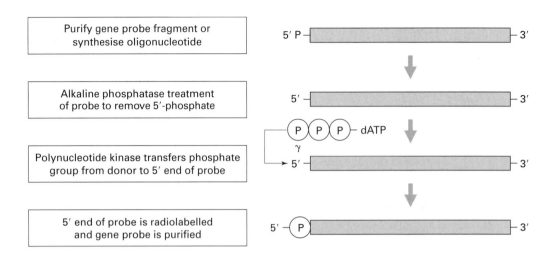

Fig. 5.28. End-labelling of a gene probe at the 5′ end with alkaline phosphatase and polynucleotide kinase.

reporter protein such as an enzyme. For example, biotin incorporated into a DNA fragment is recognised with a very high affinity by the protein streptavidin. This may be either coupled or conjugated to a reporter enzyme molecule such as alkaline phosphatase. This is able to convert a colourless substrate *p*-nitrophenol phosphate (PNPP) into a yellow-coloured compound *p*-nitrophenol (PNP) and also offers a means of signal amplification. Alternatively, labels such as digoxygenin incorporated into DNA sequences may be detected by monoclonal antibodies, again conjugated to reporter molecules such as alkaline phosphatase. Thus, rather than the detection system relying on autoradiography, which is necessary for radiolabels, a series of reactions resulting in the production of a colour, light, or the product of a chemiluminescence reaction take place. This has important practical implications, since autoradiography may take 1–3 days whereas colour and chemiluminescent reactions take minutes.

5.9.5 End-labelling of DNA molecules

The simplest form of labelling DNA is by 5′ or 3′ end-labelling. 5′ End-labelling involves a phosphate transfer or exchange reaction where the 5′ phosphate of the DNA to be used as the probe is removed and in its place a labelled phosphate, usually using ^{32}P, is added. This is carried out using two enzymes: the first, alkaline phosphatase, is used to remove the existing phosphate group from the DNA. After removal of the phosphate from the DNA, a second enzyme, polynucleotide kinase, is added, which catalyses the transfer of a phosphate group (^{32}P-labelled) to the 5′ end of the DNA. The newly labelled probe is then purified, usually by chromatography through a Sephadex column and may be used directly (Fig. 5.28).

Using the other end of the DNA molecule, the 3′ end, is slightly less complex. Here a new, labelled dNTP (e.g. ^{32}P-αdATP or biotin-labelled dNTP) is added to the

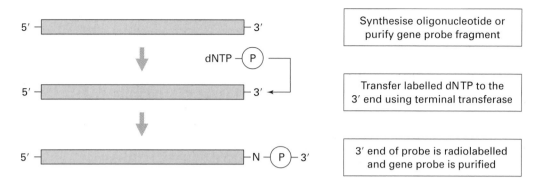

Fig. 5.29. End-labelling of a gene probe at the 3' end using terminal transferase. Note that the addition of a labelled dNTP at the 3' end alters the sequence of the gene probe.

3' end of the DNA by the enzyme terminal transferase. Although this is a simpler reaction, a potential problem exists because a new nucleotide is added to the existing sequence and so the complete sequence of the DNA is altered, which may affect its hybridisation to its target sequence. End-labelling methods also suffer from the fact that only one label is added to the DNA so they are of a lower activity in comparison with methods that incorporate label along the length of the DNA (Fig. 5.29).

5.9.6 Random primer labelling and nick translation

The DNA to be labelled is first denatured and then placed under renaturing conditions in the presence of a mixture of many different random sequences of hexamers or hexanucleotides. These hexamers will, by chance, bind to the DNA sample wherever they encounter a complementary sequence and so the DNA will rapidly acquire an approximately random sprinkling of hexanucleotides annealed to it. Each of the hexamers can act as a primer for the synthesis of a fresh strand of DNA catalysed by DNA polymerase, since it has an exposed 3'-hydroxyl group. The Klenow fragment of DNA polymerase is used for random primer labelling because it lacks a 5' to 3' exonuclease activity. This is prepared by cleavage of DNA polymerase with subtilisin, giving a large enzyme fragment that has no 5' to 3' exonuclease activity, but which still acts as a 5' to 3' polymerase. Thus, when the Klenow enzyme is mixed with the annealed DNA sample in the presence of dNTPs, including at least one that is labelled, many short stretches of labelled DNA will be generated (Fig. 5.30). In a similar way to random primer labelling, the polymerase chain reaction may also be used to incorporate radioactive or non-radioactive labels (Section 5.10.5).

A further traditional method of labelling DNA is by the process of nick translation. Low concentrations of DNase I are used to make occasional single-strand nicks in the double-stranded DNA that is to be used as the gene probe. DNA polymerase then fills in the nicks, using an appropriate dNTP, at the same time making a new nick to the 3' side of the previous one (Fig. 5.31). In this way the nick

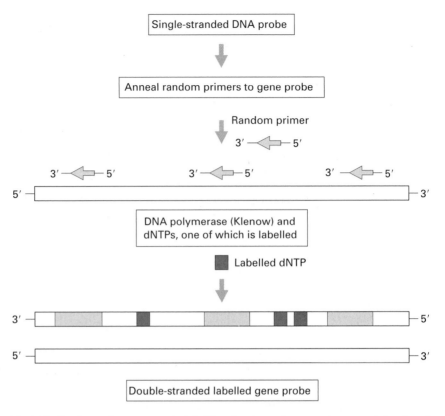

Fig. 5.30. Random primer gene probe labelling. Random primers are incorporated and used as a start point for Klenow DNA polymerase to synthesise a complementary strand of DNA whilst incorporating a labelled dNTP at complementary sites.

is translated along the DNA. If labelled dNTPs are added to the reaction mixture, they will be used to fill in the nicks, and so the DNA can be labelled to a very high specific activity.

5.9.7 Molecular beacon-based probes

A more recent development in the design of labelled oligonucleotide hybridisation probes is that of molecular beacons. These probes contain a fluorophore at one end of the probe and a quencher molecule at the other. The oligonucleotide has a stem–loop structure, where the stem places the fluorophore and quencher in close proximity. The loop structure is designed to be complementary to the target sequence. When the stem–loop structure is formed, the fluorophore is quenched by fluorescence resonance energy transfer (FRET), i.e. the energy is transferred from the fluorophore to the quencher and given off as heat. The elegance of these types of probe lies in the fact that, upon hybridisation to a target sequence, the stem and loop move apart, the quenching is then lost and emission of light occurs from the fluorophore upon excitation. These types of probe have also been used to

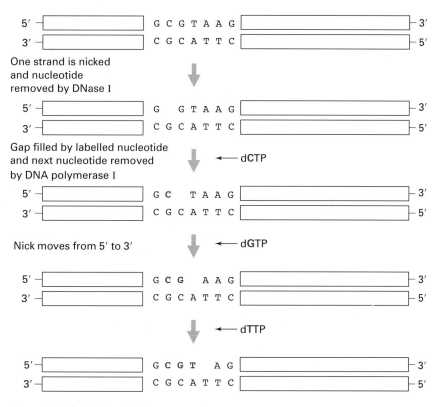

Fig. 5.31. Nick translation. The removal of nucleotides and their subsequent replacement with labelled nucleotides by DNA polymerase I increase the label in the gene probe as nick translation proceeds.

detect nucleic acid amplification systems products such as the polymerase chain reaction (PCR) and have the advantage that it is unnecessary to remove the unhybridised probes.

5.10 THE POLYMERASE CHAIN REACTION

5.10.1 Basic concept of the PCR

The polymerase chain reaction, or PCR, is one of the mainstays of molecular biology. One of the reasons for the wide adoption of the PCR is the elegant simplicity of the reaction and relative ease of the practical manipulation steps. Indeed, combined with the relevant bioinformatics resources for its design and for determination of the required experimental conditions, it provides a rapid means for DNA identification and analysis. It has opened up the investigation of cellular and molecular processes to those outside the field of molecular biology.

The PCR is used to amplify a precise fragment of DNA from a complex mixture of starting material usually termed the template DNA and in many cases requires little purification of the DNA. It does require the knowledge of some DNA

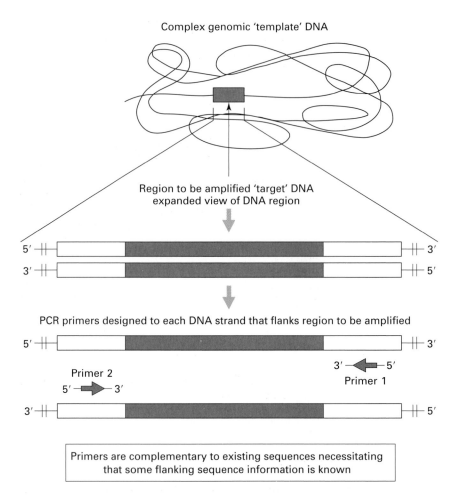

Fig. 5.32. The location of polymerase chain reaction (PCR) primers. PCR primers designed for sequences adjacent to the region to be amplified allowing a region of DNA (e.g. a gene) to be amplified from a complex starting material of genomic template DNA.

sequences which flank the fragment of DNA to be amplified (target DNA). From this information two oligonucleotide primers may be chemically synthesised, each complementary to a stretch of DNA to the 3′ side of the target DNA, one oligonucleotide for each of the two DNA strands (Fig. 5.32). It may be thought of as a technique analogous to the DNA replication process that takes place in cells, since the outcome is the same – the generation of new complementary DNA stretches based upon the existing ones. It is also a technique that has replaced, in many cases, the traditional DNA cloning methods, since it fulfils the same function, the production of large amounts of DNA from limited starting material. However, this is achieved in a fraction of the time needed to clone a DNA fragment (Chapter 6). Although not without its drawbacks, the PCR is a remarkable development that is changing the approach of many scientists to the analysis of nucleic acids and continues to have a profound impact on core biosciences and biotechnology.

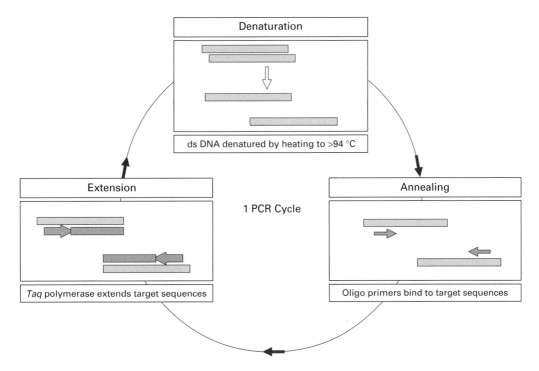

Fig. 5.33. A simplified scheme of one PCR cycle that involves denaturation, annealing and extension. ds, double-stranded.

5.10.2 **Stages in the PCR**

The PCR consists of three defined sets of times and temperatures termed steps: (i) denaturation, (ii) annealing and (iii) extension. Each of these steps is repeated 30–40 times, termed cycles (Fig. 5.33). In the first cycle the double-stranded template DNA is (i) denatured by heating the reaction to above 90 °C. Within the complex DNA the region to be specifically amplified (target) is made accessible. The temperature is then cooled to between 40 °C and 60 °C. The precise temperature is critical and each PCR system has to be defined and optimised. One useful technique for optimisation is touchdown PCR where a programmable cycler is used to incrementally decrease the annealing temperature until the optimum is derived. Reactions that are not optimised may give rise to other DNA products in addition to the specific target or may not produce any amplified products at all. The annealing step allows the hybridisation of the two oligonucleotide primers, which are present in excess, to bind to their complementary sites that flank the target DNA. The annealed oligonucleotides act as primers for DNA synthesis, since they provide a free 3′-hydroxyl group for DNA polymerase. The DNA synthesis step is termed extension and is carried out by a thermostable DNA polymerase, most commonly *Taq* DNA polymerase.

DNA synthesis proceeds from both of the primers until the new strands have been extended along and beyond the target DNA to be amplified. It is important to note that, since the new strands extend beyond the target DNA they will contain a region near their 3′ ends that is complementary to the other primer. Thus, if another round of DNA synthesis is allowed to take place, not only will the original strands be used as templates but also the new strands. Most interestingly, the products obtained from the new strands will have a precise length, delimited exactly by the two regions complementary to the primers. As the system is taken through successive cycles of denaturation, annealing and extension, all the new strands will act as templates and so there will be an exponential increase in the amount of DNA produced. The net effect is to selectively amplify the target DNA and the primer regions flanking it (Fig. 5.34).

One problem with early PCR reactions was that the temperature needed to denature the DNA also denatured the DNA polymerase. However, the availability of a thermostable DNA polymerase enzyme isolated from the thermophilic bacterium *Thermus aquaticus* found in hot springs provided the means to automate the reaction. *Taq* DNA polymerase has a temperature optimum of 72 °C and survives prolonged exposure to temperatures as high as 96 °C and so is still active after each of the denaturation steps. The widespread utility of the technique is also due to the ability to automate the reaction and, as such, many thermal cyclers have been produced in which it is possible to program in the temperatures and times for a particular PCR reaction.

5.10.3   PCR primer design and bioinformatics

The specificity of the PCR lies in the design of the two oligonucleotide primers. These must not only be complementary to sequences flanking the target DNA but not be self-complementary or bind to each other to form dimers, since both actions prevent DNA amplification. They also have to be matched in their G + C content and have similar annealing temperatures. The increasing use of bioinformatics resources such as Oligo, Generunner and Genefisher in the design of primers makes the design and the selection of reaction conditions much more straightforward. These resources allow the sequences to be specified; primer length, product size, G + C content etc. to be input; and following analysis provide a choice of matched primer sequences. Indeed the initial selection and design of primers without the aid of bioinformatics would now be unnecessarily time-consuming.

It is also possible to design primers with additional sequences at their 5′ end, such as restriction endonuclease target sites or promoter sequences. However, modifications such as these require that the annealing conditions be altered to compensate for the areas of non-homology in the primers. A number of PCR methods have been developed where either one primer or both are random. This gives rise to arbitrary priming in genomic templates but interestingly may give rise to discrete banding patterns when analysed by gel electrophoresis. In many cases this technique may be used reproducibly to identify a particular organism

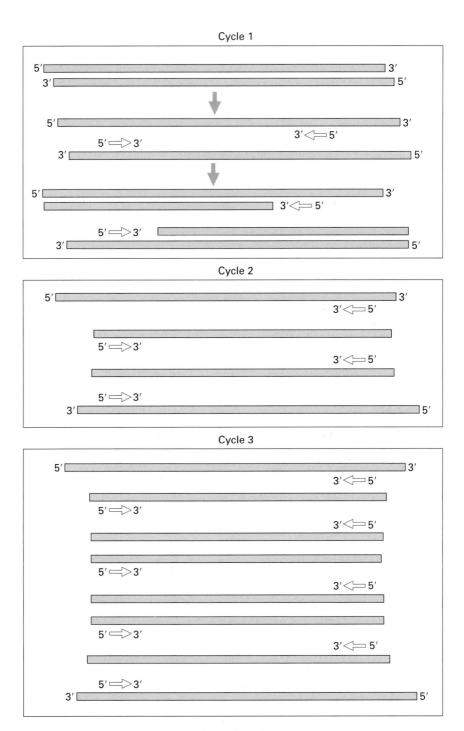

Fig. 5.34. Three cycles in the PCR. As the number of cycles in the PCR increases, the DNA strands that are synthesised and become available as templates are delimited by the ends of the primers. Thus specific amplification of the desired target sequence flanked by the primers is achieved. Primers are denoted as 5′ to 3′.

or species. This is sometimes referred to as rapid amplification of polymorphic DNA (RAPD) and has been used successfully in the detection and differentiation of a number of pathogenic strains of bacteria. In addition, primers can now be synthesised with a variety of labels such as fluorophores bound to them allowing easier detection and quantitation (Section 5.9.4).

5.10.4 **PCR amplification templates**

DNA from a variety of sources may be used as the initial source of amplification templates. It is also a highly sensitive technique and requires only one or two molecules for successful amplification. Unlike many manipulation methods used in molecular biology, the PCR technique is sensitive enough to require very little template preparation. The extraction from many prokaryotic and eukaryotic cells may involve a simple boiling step. Indeed the components of many extraction techniques such as SDS and proteinase K may adversely affect the PCR. The PCR may also be used to amplify RNA, a process termed RT–PCR (reverse transcriptase–PCR). Initially a reverse transcription reaction that converts the RNA to complementary DNA is carried out (Section 6.2.5). This reaction normally involves the use of the enzyme reverse transcriptase, although some thermostable DNA polymerases used in the PCR such as *Tth* from *Thermus thermophilus*, have a reverse transcriptase activity under certain buffer conditions. This allows mRNA transcription products to be effectively analysed. It may be also be used to differentiate latent viruses (detected by standard PCR) or active viruses that replicate and produce transcription products and are thus detectable by RT–PCR (Fig. 5.35). In addition the PCR may be extended to determine relative amounts of a transcription product.

5.10.5 **Sensitivity of the PCR**

The enormous sensitivity of the PCR system is also one of its main drawbacks, since the very large degree of amplification makes the system vulnerable to contamination. Even a trace of foreign DNA, such as that contained in dust particles, may be amplified to significant levels and may give misleading results. Hence cleanliness is paramount when carrying out PCR, and dedicated equipment, and in some cases dedicated laboratories, are used. It is possible that amplified products may also contaminate the PCR, although this may be overcome by ultraviolet irradiation to damage already amplified products so that they cannot be used as templates. A further interesting solution is to incorporate uracil into the PCR and then treat the products with the enzyme uracil *N*-glycosylase (UNG), which degrades any PCR amplified DNA products or amplicons with incorporated uracil, rendering them useless as templates. In addition, most PCRs are now undertaken using hotstart. Here, the reaction mixture is physically separated from the template or the enzyme. When the reaction begins, mixing occurs and thus avoids any mispriming that may have arisen.

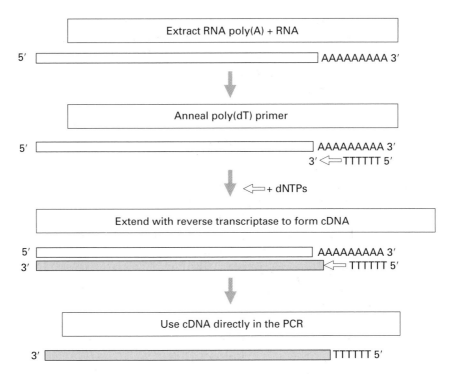

Fig. 5.35. Reverse transcriptase–PCR (RT–PCR), mRNA is converted to complementary DNA (cDNA) using the enzyme reverse transcriptase. The cDNA is then used directly in the PCR.

5.10.6 **Applications of the PCR**

Many traditional methods in molecular biology have now been superseded by the PCR and the applications for the technique appear to be unlimited. Some of the main techniques derived from the PCR are introduced in Chapter 6, whilst some of the main areas to which the PCR has been put to use are summarised in Table 5.5. The success of the PCR process has given impetus to the development of other amplification techniques that are based on either thermal cycling or non-thermal cycling (isothermal) methods. The most popular alternative to the PCR is termed the ligase chain reaction or LCR. This operates in a similar fashion to the PCR but a thermostable DNA ligase joins sets of primers together that are complementary to the target DNA. Following this, a similar exponential amplification reaction takes place producing amounts of DNA that are similar to the PCR. A number of alternative amplification techniques are listed in Table 5.6.

5.10.7 **Quantitative and real time PCR**

One of the most useful PCR applications is quantitative PCR or Q-PCR. This allows the PCR to be used as a means of identifying the initial concentrations of template

Table 5.5 Selected applications of the PCR. A number of the techniques are described in the text of Chapters 5 and 6

Field or area of study	Application	Specific examples or uses
General molecular biology	DNA amplification	Screening gene libraries
Gene probe production	Production/labelling	Use with blots/hybridisations
RNA analysis	RT–PCR	Active latent viral infections
Forensic science	Scenes of crime	Analysis of DNA from blood
Infection/disease monitoring	Microbial detection	Strain typing/analysis RAPDs
Sequence analysis	DNA sequencing	Rapid sequencing possible
Genome mapping studies	Referencing points in genome	Sequence-tagged sites (STS)
Gene discovery	mRNA analysis	Expressed sequence tags (EST)
Genetic mutation analysis	Detection of known mutations	Screening for cystic fibrosis
Quantification analysis	Quantitative PCR	5′ Nuclease (TaqMan assay)
Genetic mutation analysis	Detection of unknown mutations	Gel-based PCR methods (DGGE)
Protein engineering	Production of novel proteins	PCR mutagenesis
Molecular archaeology	Retrospective studies	Dinosaur DNA analysis
Single-cell analysis	Sexing or cell mutation sites	Sex determination of unborn
In situ analysis	Studies on frozen sections	Localisation of DNA/RNA

RT, reverse transcriptase; RAPDs, rapid amplification polymorphic DNA; DDGE, denaturing gradient gel electrophoresis.

Table 5.6 Selected alternative amplification techniques to the PCR. Two broad methodologies exist that either amplify the target molecules such as DNA and RNA or detect the target and amplify a signal molecule bound to it

Technique	Type of assay	Specific examples or uses
Target amplification methods		
Ligase chain reaction (LCR)	Non-isothermal, employs thermostable DNA ligase	Mutation detection
Nucleic acid sequence based amplification (NASBA)	Isothermal, involving use of RNA, RNase H/reverse transcriptase, and T7 DNA polymerase	Viral detection, e.g. HIV
Signal amplification methods		
Branched DNA amplification (b-DNA)	Isothermal microwell format using hybridisation or target/capture probe and signal amplification	Mutation detection

HIV, human immunodeficiency virus.

DNA and is very useful for the measurement of, for example, a virus or an mRNA representing a protein expressed in abnormal amounts in a disease process. Early quantitative PCR methods involved the comparison of a standard or control DNA template amplified with separate primers at the same time as the specific target DNA. These types of quantification rely on the reaction being exponential and

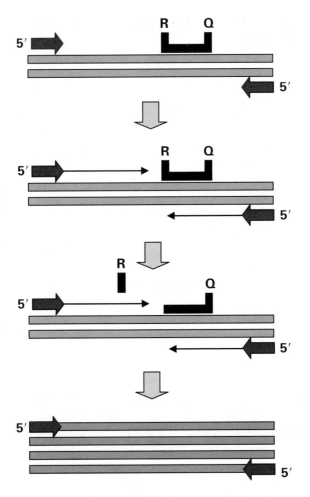

Fig. 5.36. 5′ Nuclease assay (TaqMan assay). PCR is undertaken with RQ probe (reporter/quencher dye). As R–Q are in close proximity, fluorescence is quenched. During extension by *Taq* polymerase the probe is cleaved as a result of *Taq* having 5′ nuclease activity. This cleaves R–Q probe and the reporter is released. This results in detectable increase in fluorescence and allows real time PCR detection.

so any factors affecting this may also affect the result. Other methods involve the incorporation of a radiolabel through the primers or nucleotides and their subsequent detection following purification of the amplicon. An alternative automated real time PCR method is the 5′ fluorogenic exonuclease detection system or TaqMan assay (Fig. 5.36). In its simplest form, a DNA binding dye such as SYBR Green is included in the reaction. As amplicons accumulate, SYBR green binds the double-stranded DNA proportionally. Fluorescence emission of the dye is detected after excitation. The binding of SYBR Green is non-specific. Therefore in order to detect specific amplicons an oligonucleotide probe labelled with a fluorescent reporter and quencher molecule, respectively, at either end is included in the reaction in place of SYBR Green. When the oligonucleotide probe binds to the target sequence the 5′ exonuclease activity of *Taq* polymerase degrades and releases the reporter from the quencher. A signal is thus generated that increases in direct proportion to the number of starting molecules. Thus a detection system is able to induce and detect fluorescence in real time as the PCR proceeds. Part of the system relies on the capillary-based thermal cycling using a specialised thermal cycler, for example the Roche light cycler. Although relatively expensive in comparison with other methods for determining expression levels, it is simple, rapid and reliable. In addition to quantification, real time PCR systems may also be used for genotyping and for accurate determination of amplicon melting temperature using melting curve analysis.

This allows accurate amplicon identification and also offers the potential to detect mutations and SNPs. Further developments in probe-based PCR systems have also been used and include scorpion probe systems, amplifluor and real time LUX probes.

5.11 NUCLEOTIDE SEQUENCING OF DNA

5.11.1 Concepts of nucleic acid sequencing

The determination of the order or sequence of bases along a length of DNA is one of the central techniques in molecular biology. Although it is now possible to derive amino acid sequence information with a degree of reliability, it is frequently more convenient and rapid to analyse the DNA coding information. Knowledge of the precise usage of codons, information regarding mutations and polymorphisms and the identification of gene regulatory control sequences are also possible only by analysing DNA sequences. Two techniques have been developed for this, one based on an enzymatic method frequently termed Sanger sequencing, after its developer, and a chemical method called Maxam and Gilbert, named for the same reason. At present, Sanger sequencing is by far the most popular method and many commercial kits are available for its use. However, there are certain occasions such as the sequencing of short oligonucleotides where the Maxam–Gilbert method is more appropriate.

One absolute requirement for Sanger sequencing is that the DNA to be sequenced is in a single-stranded form. Traditionally this demanded that the DNA fragment of interest be inserted and cloned into a specialised bacteriophage vector termed M13, which is naturally single stranded (Section 6.3.3). Although M13 is still universally used, the advent of the PCR has provided the means not only to amplify a region of any genome or cDNA but also very quickly to generate the corresponding nucleotide sequence. This has led to an explosion in the accumulation of DNA sequence information and has provided much impetus for gene discovery and genome mapping (Section 6.9).

The Sanger method is simple and elegant and mimics in many ways the natural ability of DNA polymerase to extend a growing nucleotide chain from an existing template. Initially the DNA to be sequenced is allowed to hybridise with an oligonucleotide primer that is complementary to a sequence adjacent to the 3′

Fragment to be sequenced, cloned in M13 phage

3′ – – – AG – – – CTGCTCGCAT – – – 5′
        TC – – – GA
       ‿‿‿‿‿‿‿‿
         Primer

| DNA polymerase
| 4 dNTPs (radioactive)
↓ ddGTP

Synthesis of complementary second strands:

5′ TC – – – GAC**ddG** 3′
5′ TC – – – GACGA**ddG** 3′
5′ TC – – – GACGAGC**ddG** 3′

Denature to give single strands

Run on sequencing gel alongside products of
ddCTP, ddATP and ddTTP reactions

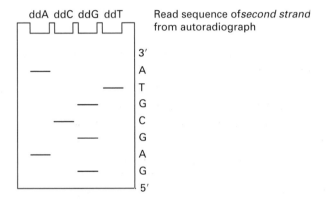

ddA ddC ddG ddT   Read sequence of *second strand*
                   from autoradiograph

Fig. 5.37. Sanger sequencing of DNA.

side of the DNA within a vector such as M13 or in an amplicon. The oligonucleotide will then act as a primer for synthesis of a second strand of DNA, catalysed by DNA polymerase (Fig. 5.37). Since the new strand is synthesised from its 5′
end, virtually the first DNA to be made will be complementary to the DNA to be
sequenced. One of the dNTPs that must be provided for DNA synthesis is labelled
with ^{32}P or ^{35}S, and so the newly synthesised strand will be radioactively labelled.
This reaction mixture is left to incubate at room temperature for a few minutes.

5.11.2 Dideoxynucleotide chain terminators

The reaction mixture is then divided into four aliquots, representing the four
dNTPs, A, C, G and T. In addition to all of the dNTPs being present in the A tube an
analogue of dATP is added (2′,3′-dideoxyadenosine triphosphate (ddATP)) that is
similar to A but has no 3′ hydroxyl group and so will terminate the growing chain

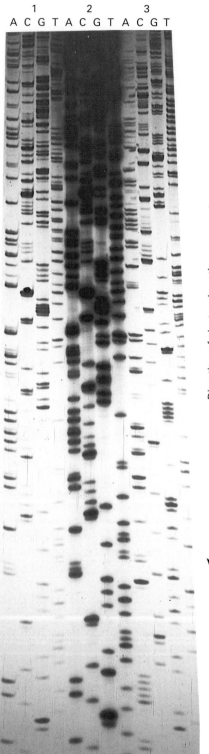

Fig. 5.38. Autoradiograph of a DNA sequencing gel. Samples were prepared using the Sanger dideoxy method of DNA sequencing. Each set of four samples was loaded into adjacent tracks, indicated by A,C, G and T, depending on the identity of the dideoxyribonucleotide used for that sample. Two sets of samples were labelled with ^{35}S(1 and 3) and one was labelled with ^{32}P(2). It is evident that ^{32}P generates darker but more diffuse bands than does ^{35}S, making the bands nearer the bottom of the autoradiograph easy to see. However, the broad bands produced by ^{32}P cannot be resolved near the top of the autoradiograph, making it impossible to read a sequence from this region. The much sharper bands produced by ^{35}S allow sequences to be read with confidence along most of the autoradiograph and so a longer sequence of DNA can be obtained from a single gel.

since a 5′ to 3′ phosphodiester linkage cannot be formed without a 3′-hydroxyl group. The situation for tube C is identical, except that ddCTP is added; similarly the G and T tubes contain ddGTP and ddTTP, respectively.

Since the incorporation of ddNTP rather than dNTP is a random event, the reaction will produce new molecules varying widely in length, but all terminating in the same type of base. Thus four sets of DNA sequences are generated, each terminating in a different type of base, but all having a common 5′ end (the primer). The four labelled and chain-terminated samples are then denatured by heating and loaded next to each other on a polyacrylamide gel for electrophoresis. Electrophoresis is performed at approximately 70 °C in the presence of urea, to prevent renaturation of the DNA, since even partial renaturation alters the rates of migration of DNA fragments. Very thin, long gels are used for maximum resolution over a wide range of fragment lengths. After electrophoresis, the positions of radioactive DNA bands on the gel are determined by autoradiography. Since every band in the track from the ddATP sample must contain molecules that terminate at adenine, and those in the ddCTP terminate in cytosine, etc., it is possible to read the sequence of the newly synthesised strand from the autoradiograph, provided that the gel can resolve differences in length equal to a single nucleotide (Fig. 5.38). Under ideal conditions, sequences up to about 300 bases in length can be read from one gel.

5.11.3 Direct PCR pyrosequencing

Rapid PCR sequencing has also been made possible by the use of pyrosequencing. This is a sequencing by synthesis whereby a PCR template is hybridised to an oligonucleotide and incubated with DNA polymerase, ATP sulphurylase, luciferase and apyrase. During the reaction, the first of the four dNTPs are added and, if incorporated, release pyrophosphate (PP_i). The ATP sulphurylase converts the PP_i to ATP, which drives the luciferase-mediated conversion of luciferin to oxyluciferin to generate light. Apyrase degrades the resulting component dNTPs and ATP. This is followed by another round of dNTP addition. A resulting pyrogram provides an output of the sequence. The method provides short reads very quickly and is especially useful for the determination of mutations or SNPs.

It is also possible to undertake nucleotide sequencing directly from double-stranded molecules such as plasmid cloning vectors and PCR amplicons. The double-stranded DNA must be denatured prior to annealing with primer. In the case of plasmids an alkaline denaturation step is sufficient; however, for amplicons this is more problematic and a focus of much research. Unlike plasmids, amplicons are short and reanneal rapidly, therefore preventing the reannealing process or biasing the amplification towards one strand by using a primer ratio of 100:1 overcomes this problem to a certain extent. Denaturants such as formamide or DMSO have also been used with some success in preventing the reannealing of PCR strands following their separation.

It is possible to physically separate and retain one PCR strand by incorporating a molecule such as biotin into one of the primers. Following PCR, one strand with an affinity molecule may be removed by affinity chromatography with strepavidin,

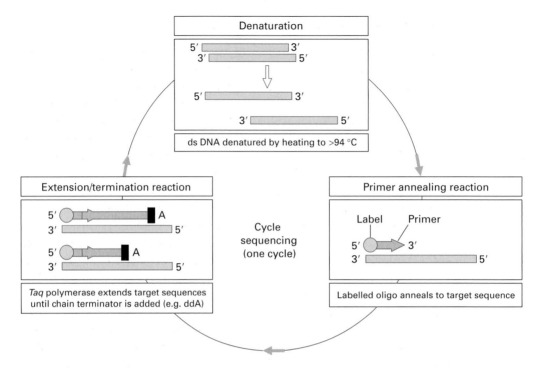

Fig. 5.39. Simplified scheme of cycle sequencing. Linear amplification takes place with the use of labelled primers. During the extension and termination reaction, the chain terminator dideoxynucleotides are incorporated into the growing chain. This takes place in four separate reactions (A, C, G and T). The products are then run on a polyacrylamide gel and the sequence analysed. The scheme indicates the events that take place in the A reaction only. ds, double-stranded.

leaving the complementary PCR strand. This affinity purification provides single-stranded DNA derived from the PCR amplicon and, although it is somewhat time consuming, does provide high quality single-stranded DNA for sequencing.

5.11.4 PCR cycle sequencing

One of the most useful methods of sequencing PCR amplicons is termed PCR cycle sequencing. This is not strictly a PCR, since it involves linear amplification with a single primer. Approximately 20 cycles of denaturation, annealing and extension take place. Radiolabelled or fluorescently labelled dideoxynucleotides are then introduced into the final stages of the reaction to generate the chain terminated extension products (Fig. 5.39). Automated direct PCR sequencing is increasingly being refined, allowing greater lengths of DNA to be analysed in one sequencing run, and provides a very rapid means of analysing DNA sequences.

5.11.5 **Automated fluorescent DNA sequencing**

Advances in fluorescent dye terminator and labelling chemistry has led to the development of high throughput automated sequencing techniques. Essentially most systems involve the use of dideoxynucleotides labelled with different fluoro-chromes. Thus the label is incorporated into the ddNTP and this is used to carry out chain termination as in the standard reaction indicated in Section 5.11.1. The advantage of this modification is that, since a different label is incorporated with each ddNTP, it is unnecessary to perform four separate reactions. Therefore the four chain-terminated products are run on the same track of a denaturing electrophoresis gel. Each product with their base-specific dye is excited by a laser and the dye then emits light at its characteristic wavelength. A diffraction grating separates the emissions, which are detected by a charge-coupled device and the sequence interpreted by a computer. The advantages of the technique include real time detection of the sequence. In addition the lengths of sequence that may be analysed are in excess of 500 bp (Fig. 5.40). Capillary electrophoresis is increasingly being used for the detection of sequencing products. This is where liquid polymers in thin capillary tubes are used, obviating the need to pour sequencing gels and requiring little manual operation. This substantially reduces the electrophoresis run times and allows high throughput to be achieved. A number of large-scale sequence facilities are now fully automated using 96-well microtitre-based formats. The derived sequences can be downloaded automatically to databases and manipulated using a variety of bioinformatics resources. Developments in the technology of DNA sequencing have made whole-genome sequencing projects a realistic proposition within achievable time scales, and a number of these have been completed or are nearing completion.

5.11.6 **Maxam and Gilbert sequencing**

Sanger sequencing is by far the most popular technique for DNA sequencing; however, an alternative technique developed at the same time may also be used. The chemical cleavage method of DNA sequencing developed by A. M. Maxam and W. Gilbert is often used for sequencing small fragments of DNA such as oligonucleotides, where Sanger sequencing is problematic. A radioactive label is added to either the 3′ or the 5′ end of a double-stranded DNA sample (Fig 5.41). The strands are then separated by electrophoresis under denaturing conditions, and analysed separately. DNA labelled at one end is divided into four aliquots and each is treated with chemicals that act on specific bases by methylation or removal of the base. Conditions are chosen so that, on average, each molecule is modified at only one position along its length; every base in the DNA strand has an equal chance of being modified. After the modification reactions, the separate samples are cleaved by piperidine, which breaks phosphodiester bonds exclusively at the 5′ side of nucleotides whose base has been modified. The result is similar to that produced by the Sanger method, since each sample now contains radioactively labelled molecules of various lengths, all with one end in common (the labelled

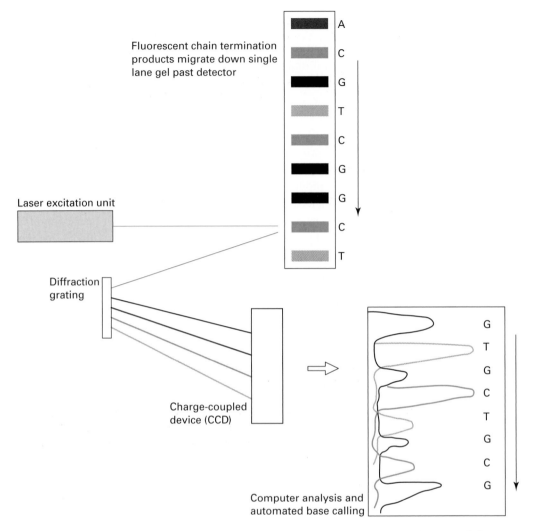

Fig. 5.40. Automated fluorescent sequencing detection using single-lane gel and charge-coupled device.

end), and with the other end cut at the same type of base. Analysis of the reaction products by electrophoresis is as described for the Sanger method.

The developments in DNA sequencing and techniques such as the PCR have allowed a means of rapidly identifying and analysing biological molecules. This, coupled with the rapid advancements in bioinformatics and the increasingly sophisticated methods of protein structure prediction, has led to the generalised scheme of work flow indicated in Fig. 5.42. These new methods of *in silico* methods will no doubt accelerate the understanding of molecular structure–function interactions in the coming years and be a central focus of bioscience research.

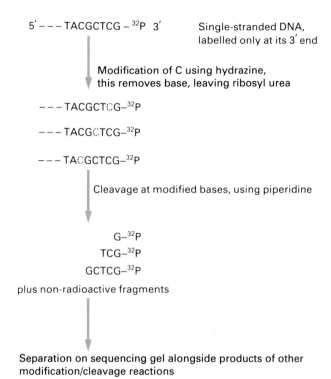

Fig. 5.41. Maxam and Gilbert sequencing of DNA. Only modification and cleavage of deoxycytidine is shown, but three more portions of the end-labelled DNA would be modified and cleaved at G, G + A, and T + C, and the products would be separated on the sequencing gel alongside those from the C reactions.

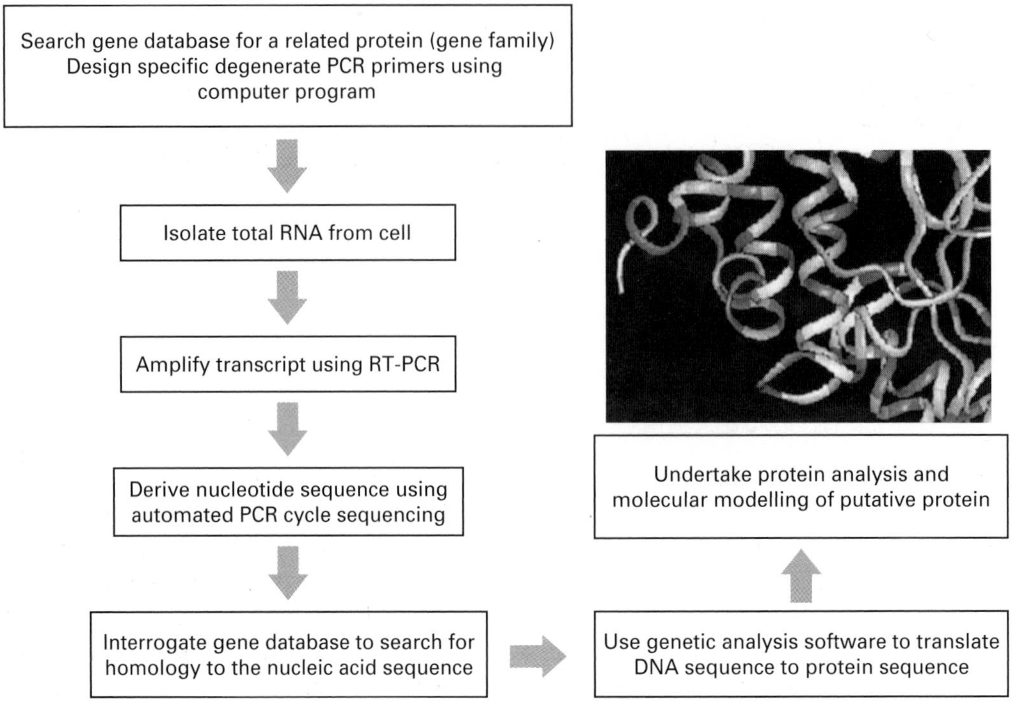

Fig. 5.42. Possible generalised scheme of work using bioinformatics to generate protein information.

5.12 SUGGESTIONS FOR FURTHER READING

ALBERTS, B., JOHNSON, A., LEWIS. J., RAFF, M., ROBERTS, K. and WALTER. P. (2002). *Molecular Biology of the Cell*, 4th edn. Garland Publishing, New York (A comprehensive all round text.)

BROWN, T. A. (2001). *Gene Cloning and DNA Analysis: An Introduction*. Blackwell Science, Oxford. (A very good introduction to genetics and molecular biology.)

CAMPBELL, A. M. and HEYER, L. J. (2002). *Discovering Genomics, Proteomics and Bioinformatics*. Addison Wesley, Boston, MA. (A very useful resource for genomics and bioinformatics.)

NEWTON, C. R. and GRAHAM, A. (1997). *PCR*, 2nd edn. Bios Scientific Publishers Ltd, Oxford. (An excellent introduction to the methods and application of the PCR.)

RAPLEY, R. and HARBRON, S. (2004). *Molecular Analysis and Genome Discovery*. John Wiley & Sons, Chichester. (An up-to-date collection of key nucleic acid and proteins techniques in analysis and drug discovery.)

READ, A. P. and STRACHEN, T. (2004). *Human Molecular Genetics*. Garland Science, London. (An excellent and very comprehensive textbook with excellent illustrations.)

Chapter 6

Recombinant DNA and genetic analysis

6.1 INTRODUCTION

The genomics era has provided a new approach to understanding and discovering biological processes. Indeed the many genome mapping and sequencing projects completed or under way now require new methods of analysis such as automated microarray technology and bioinformatics. New areas have recently been developed, such as pharmacogenomics, metabolomics and systems biology, all of which aim to analyse large numbers of samples simultaneously. This type of massive parallel analysis is set to be the main driving force of discovery and analysis in the coming years. However, developing techniques of molecular biology and genetic analysis have their foundations in methods developed decades ago. One of the main cornerstones on which molecular biology analysis was developed was the discovery of restriction endonucleases in the early 1970s, which led not only to the possibility of analysing DNA more effectively but also to the ability to cut different DNA molecules so that they could later be joined together to create new recombinant DNA fragments. The newly created DNA molecules heralded a new era in the manipulation, analysis and exploitation of biological molecules. This process, termed gene cloning, has led to numerous discoveries and insights into gene structure, function and regulation. Since their initial use, methods for the production of gene libraries have been steadily refined and developed. Although the polymerase chain reaction (PCR; Section 5.10) has provided shortcuts to gene analysis, there are still many cases where gene cloning methods are not only useful but an absolute requirement. The following provides an account of the process of gene cloning and other methods based on recombinant DNA technology.

6.2 CONSTRUCTING GENE LIBRARIES

6.2.1 Digesting genomic DNA molecules

Following the isolation and purification of genomic DNA, it is possible to specifically fragment it with enzymes termed restriction endonucleases. These enzymes are the key to molecular cloning because of the specificity they have for particular DNA sequences. It is important to note that every copy of a given DNA molecule from a specific organism will give the same set of fragments when digested with a

Table 6.1 Numbers of clones required for representation of DNA in a genome library

Species	Genome size (kb)	No. of clones required	
		17 kb fragments	35 kb fragments
Bacteria (*E. coli*)	4000	700	340
Yeast	20 000	3500	1700
Fruit fly	165 000	29 000	14 500
Man	3 000 000	535 000	258 250
Maize	15 000 000	2 700 000	1 350 000

particular enzyme. DNA from different organisms will, in general, give different sets of fragments when treated with the same enzyme. By digesting complex genomic DNA from an organism it is possible to reproducibly divide its genome into a large number of small fragments, each approximately the size of a single gene. Some enzymes cut straight across the DNA to give flush or blunt ends. Other restriction enzymes make staggered single-strand cuts, producing short single-stranded projections at each end of the digested DNA. These ends are not only identical, but complementary, and will base-pair with each other; they are therefore known as cohesive or sticky ends. In addition the 5′ end projection of the DNA always retains the phosphate groups.

Over 600 enzymes, recognising more than 200 different restriction sites, have been characterised. The choice of which enzyme to use depends on a number of factors. For example, the recognition sequence of 6 bp will occur, on average, every 4096 (4^6) bases, assuming a random sequence of each of the four bases. This means that digesting genomic DNA with *Eco*R1, which recognises the sequence 5′-GAATTC-3′, will produce fragments each of which is on average just over 4 kb. Enzymes with 8 bp recognition sequences produce much longer fragments. Therefore very large genomes, such as human DNA, are usually digested with enzymes that produce long DNA fragments. This makes subsequent steps more manageable, since a smaller number of those fragments need to be cloned and subsequently analysed (Table 6.1).

6.2.2 Ligating DNA molecules

The DNA products resulting from restriction digestion to form sticky ends may be joined to any other DNA fragments treated with the same restriction enzyme. Thus, when the two sets of fragments are mixed, base-pairing between sticky ends will result in the annealing together of fragments that were derived from different starting DNA. There will, of course, also be pairing of fragments derived from the same starting DNA molecules, termed reannealing. All these pairings are transient, owing to the weakness of hydrogen bonding between the few bases in the sticky ends, but they can be stabilised by use of an enzyme, called DNA ligase, in a process termed ligation. This enzyme, usually isolated from bacteriophage T4 and called T4 DNA ligase, forms a covalent bond between the 5′-phosphate group at

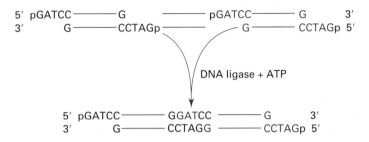

Fig. 6.1. Ligation molecules with cohesive ends. Complementary cohesive ends base-pair, forming a temporary link between two DNA fragments. This asscociation of fragments is stabilised by the formation of 3' to 5' phosphodiester linkages between cohesive ends, a reaction catalysed by DNA ligase.

the end of one strand and the 3'-hydroxyl group of the adjacent strand (Fig. 6.1). The reaction, which is ATP dependent, is often carried out at 10°C to lower the kinetic energy of molecules, and so reduce the chances of base-paired sticky ends parting before they have been stabilised by ligation. However, long reaction times are needed to compensate for the low activity of DNA ligase in the cold. It is also possible to join blunt ends of DNA molecules, although the efficiency of this reaction is much lower than that of sticky ended ligations.

Since ligation reconstructs the site of cleavage, recombinant molecules produced by ligation of sticky ends can be cleaved again at the 'joins', using the same restriction enzyme that was used to generate the fragments initially. In order to propagate digested DNA from an organism it is necessary to join or ligate that DNA with a specialised DNA carrier molecule termed a vector (Section 6.3). Thus each DNA fragment is inserted by ligation into the vector DNA molecule, which then allows the whole recombined DNA to be replicated indefinitely within microbial cells (Fig. 6.2). In this way a DNA fragment can be cloned to provide sufficient material for further detailed analysis, or for further manipulation. Thus all of the DNA extracted from an organism and digested with a restriction enzyme will result in a collection of clones. This collection of clones is known as a gene library.

6.2.3 Aspects of gene libraries

There are two general types of gene library. A genome library, which consists of the total chromosomal DNA of an organism, and a cDNA library, which represents the mRNA from a cell or tissue at a specific point in time (Fig. 6.3). The choice of the particular type of gene library depends on a number of factors, the most important being the final application of any DNA fragment derived from the library. If the ultimate aim is understanding the control of protein production for a particular gene or its architecture, then genome libraries must be used. However, if the goal is the production of new or modified proteins, or the determination of the tissue-specific expression and timing patterns, cDNA libraries are more appropriate. The main

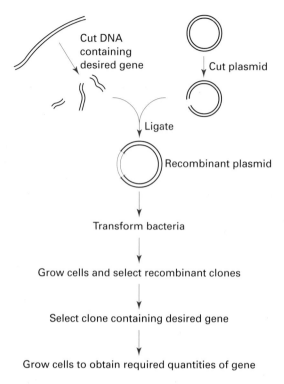

Fig. 6.2. Outline of gene cloning.

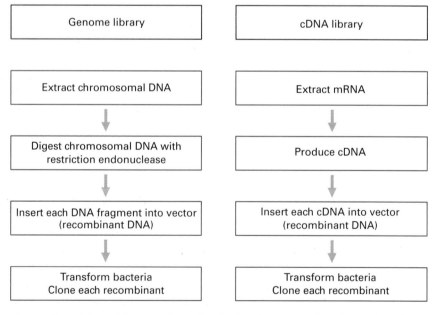

Fig. 6.3. Comparison of the general steps involved in the construction of genomic and complementary DNA (cDNA) libraries.

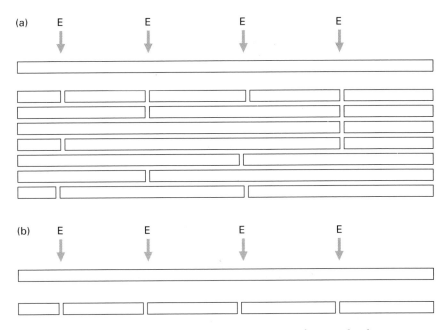

Fig. 6.4. Comparison of (a) partial and (b) complete digestion of DNA molecules at restriction enzymes sites (E).

consideration in the construction of genome or cDNA libraries is therefore the nucleic acid starting material. Since the genome of an organism is fixed, chromosomal DNA may be isolated from almost any cell type in order to prepare a genome library. In contrast, however, cDNA libraries represent only the mRNA being produced from a specific cell type at a particular time in the cell's development. Thus it is important to consider carefully the cell or tissue type from which the mRNA is to be derived in the construction of cDNA libraries.

There are a variety of cloning vectors available, many based on naturally occurring molecules such as bacterial plasmids or bacteria-infecting viruses. The choice of vector also depends on whether a genomic library or cDNA library is constructed. The various types of vectors are explained in more detail in Section 6.3.

6.2.4 Genome DNA libraries

Genomic libraries are constructed by isolating the complete chromosomal DNA from a cell and digesting it into fragments of the desired average length with restriction endonucleases. This can be achieved by partial restriction digestion with an enzyme that recognises tetranucleotide sequences. Complete digestion with such an enzyme would produce a large number of very short fragments, but, if the enzyme is allowed to cleave only a few of its potential restriction sites before the reaction is stopped, each DNA molecule will be cut into relatively large fragments. Average fragment size will depend on the relative concentrations of DNA and restriction enzyme, and, in particular, on the conditions and duration of incubation (Fig. 6.4). It is also possible to produce fragments of DNA by physical shearing, although the ends of the fragments may need to be repaired to make them flush ended. This is achieved by using a modified DNA polymerase termed Klenow poly- merase. The enzyme is prepared by cleavage of DNA polymerase with subtilisin, giving a large fragment that has no 5′ to 3′ exonuclease activity, but which still acts as a 5′ to 3′ polymerase. This will fill in any recessed 3′ ends on the sheared DNA using the appropriate deoxyribonucleoside triphosphates (dNTPs).

The mixture of DNA fragments is then ligated with a vector and subsequently cloned. If enough clones are produced there will be a very high chance that any par- ticular DNA fragment such as a gene will be present in at least one of the clones. To keep the number of clones to a manageable size, fragments about 10 kb in length are needed for prokaryotic libraries, but the length must be increased to about 40 kb for mammalian libraries. It is possible to calculate the number of clones that must be present in a gene library to give a probability of obtaining a particular DNA sequence. This formula is:

$$N = \frac{\ln(1 - P)}{\ln(1 - f)}$$

where N is the number of recombinants, P is the probability and f is the fraction of the genome in one insert. Thus, for the *Escherichia coli* DNA chromosome of 5×10^6 bp and with an insert size of 20 kb the number of clones needed (N) would be 1×10^3, with a probability of 0.99.

6.2.5 cDNA libraries

There may be several thousand different proteins being produced in a cell at any one time, all of which have associated mRNA molecules. To identify any one of those mRNA molecules, clones of each individual mRNA have to be synthesised. Libraries that represent the mRNA in a particular cell or tissue are termed cDNA libraries. mRNA cannot be used directly in cloning, since it is too unstable. However, it is possible to synthesise cDNA molecules to all the mRNAs from the selected tissue. The cDNA may be inserted into vectors and then cloned. The pro- duction of cDNA is carried out using an enzyme termed reverse transcriptase, which is isolated from RNA-containing retroviruses.

Reverse transcriptase is an RNA-dependent DNA polymerase and will synthe- sise a first-strand DNA complementary to an mRNA template, using a mixture of the four dNTPs. There is also a requirement (as with all polymerase enzymes) for a short oligonucleotide primer to be present (Fig. 6.5). With eukaryotic mRNA bearing a poly(A) tail, a complementary oligo(dT) primer may be used. Alter- natively random hexamers may be used, which anneal randomly to the mRNAs in the complex. Such primers provide a free 3′-hydroxyl group, which is used as the starting point for the reverse transcriptase. Regardless of the method used to prepare the first strand of cDNA one absolute requirement is high quality unde- graded mRNA (Section 5.7.2). It is usual to check the integrity of the RNA by gel elec- trophoresis (Section 5.7.4). Alternatively, a fraction of the extract may be used in a

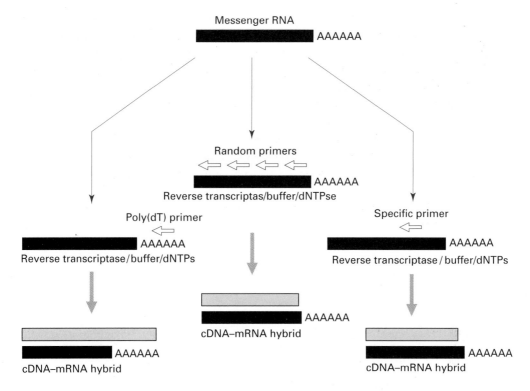

Fig. 6.5. Strategies for producing first-strand cDNA from mRNA.

cell-free translation system, which, if intact mRNA is present, will direct the synthesis of proteins represented by the mRNA molecules in the sample (Section 6.7).

Following the synthesis of the first DNA strand, a poly(dC) tail is added to its 3′ end, using terminal transferase and dCTP. This will also, incidentally, put a poly(dC) tail on the poly(A) of mRNA. Alkaline hydrolysis is then used to remove the RNA strand, leaving single-stranded DNA that can be used, like the mRNA, to direct the synthesis of a complementary DNA strand. The second-strand synthesis requires an oligo(dG) primer, base-paired with the poly(dC) tail, which is catalysed by the Klenow fragment of DNA polymerase I. The final product is double-stranded DNA, one of the strands being complementary to the mRNA. One further method of cDNA synthesis involves the use of RNase H. Here the first-strand cDNA is prepared as above with reverse transcriptase but the resulting mRNA–cDNA hybrid is retained. RNase H is then used at low concentrations to nick the RNA strand. The resulting nicks expose 3′-hydroxyl groups that are used by DNA polymerase as a primer to replace the RNA with a second strand of cDNA (Fig. 6.6).

6.2.6 Treatment of blunt cDNA ends

Ligation of blunt-ended DNA fragments is not as efficient as ligation of sticky ends, therefore with cDNA molecules additional procedures are undertaken before ligation with cloning vectors. One approach is to add small double-stranded

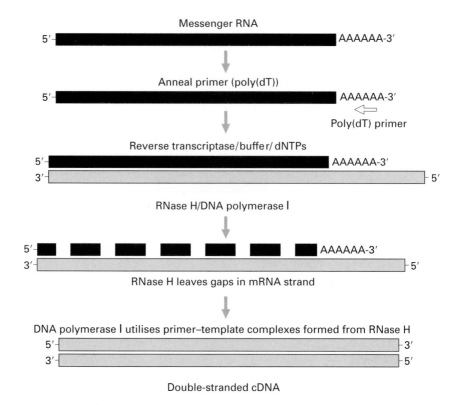

Fig. 6.6. Second-strand cDNA synthesis using the RNase H method.

molecules with one internal site for a restriction endonuclease, termed nucleic acid linkers, to the cDNA. Numerous linkers are commercially available with internal restriction sites for many of the most commonly used restriction enzymes. Linkers are blunt-end ligated to the cDNA but, since they are added much in excess of the cDNA, the ligation process is reasonably successful. Subsequently the linkers are digested with the appropriate restriction enzyme, which provides the sticky ends for efficient ligation to a vector digested with the same enzyme. This process may be made easier by the addition of adaptors rather than linkers, which are identical except that the sticky ends are pre-formed and so there is no need for restriction digestion following ligation (Fig. 6.7).

6.2.7 **Enrichment methods for RNA**

Frequently an attempt is made to isolate the mRNA transcribed from a desired gene within a particular cell or tissue that produces the protein in high amounts. Thus, if the cell or tissue produces a major protein of the cell, a large fraction of the total mRNA will code for the protein. An example of this is the B cells of the pancreas, which contain high levels of pro-insulin mRNA. In such cases it is possible to precipitate polysomes, which are actively translating the mRNA, by using antibodies to the ribosomal proteins; mRNA can then be dissociated from the precipitated ribosomes. More usually the mRNA required is only a minor component of the

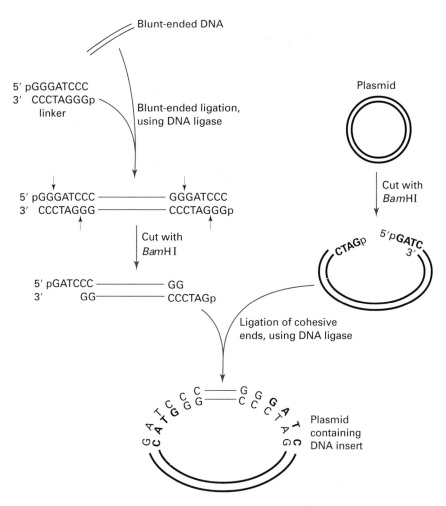

Fig. 6.7. Use of linkers. In this example, blunt-ended DNA is inserted into a specific restriction site on a plasmid, after ligation to a linker containing the same restriction site.

total cellular mRNA. In such cases total mRNA may be fractionated by size using sucrose density gradient centrifugation. Then each fraction is used to direct the synthesis of proteins using an *in vitro* translation system (Section 6.7).

6.2.8 Subtractive hybridisation

It is often the case that genes are transcribed in a specific cell type or differentially activated during a particular stage of cellular growth, often at very low levels. It is possible to isolate those mRNA transcripts by subtractive hybridisation. Usually the mRNA species common to the different cell types are removed, leaving the cell type or tissue-specific mRNAs for analysis (Fig. 6.8). This may be undertaken by isolating the mRNA from the so-called subtractor cells and producing a first-strand cDNA (Section 6.2.5). The original mRNA from the subtractor cells is then degraded and the mRNA from the target cells isolated and mixed with the cDNA.

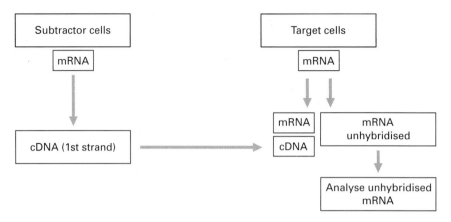

Fig. 6.8. Scheme of analysing specific mRNA molecules by subtractive hybridisation.

All the complementary mRNA–cDNA molecules common to both cell types will hybridise, leaving the unbound mRNA, which may be isolated and further analysed. A more rapid approach to analysing the differential expression of genes has been developed using the polymerase chain reaction (PCR). This technique, termed differential display, is explained in greater detail in Section 6.8.1.

6.2.9 Cloning PCR products

Whilst PCR has to some extent replaced cloning as a method for the generation of large quantities of a desired DNA fragment, there is, under certain circumstances, still a requirement for the cloning of PCR-amplified DNA. For example, certain techniques such as *in vitro* protein synthesis are best achieved with the DNA fragment inserted into an appropriate plasmid or phage cloning vector (Section 6.7.1). Cloning methods for PCR follow closely the cloning of DNA fragments derived from the conventional manipulation of DNA. The techniques by which this may be achieved are blunt-ended and cohesive-ended cloning. Certain thermostable DNA polymerases such as *Taq* DNA polymerase and *Tth* DNA polymerase give rise to PCR products having a 3′ overhanging A residue. It is possible to clone the PCR product into dT vectors termed dA:dT cloning. This makes use of the fact that the terminal additions of A residues may be successfully ligated to vectors prepared with T residue overhangs to allow efficient ligation of the PCR product (Fig. 6.9). The reaction is catalysed by DNA ligase as in conventional ligation reactions (Section 6.2.2).

It is also possible to carry out cohesive-ended cloning with PCR products. In this case oligonucleotide primers are designed with a restriction endonuclease site incorporated into them. Since the complementarity of the primers needs to be absolute at the 3′ end the 5′ end of the primer is usually the region for the location of the restriction site. This needs to be designed with care, since the efficiency of digestion with certain restriction endonucleases decreases if extra nucleotides not involved in recognition are absent at the 5′ end. In this case the digestion and ligation reactions are the same as those undertaken for conventional reactions (Sections 6.2.1 and 6.2.2).

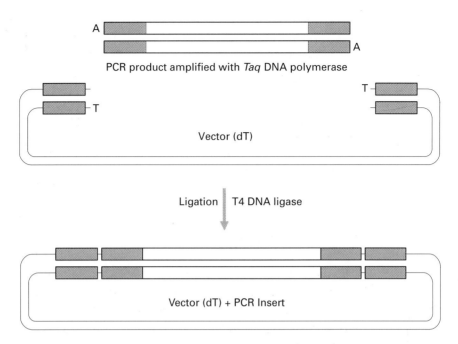

Fig. 6.9. Cloning of PCR products using dA:dT cloning.

6.3 **CLONING VECTORS**

For the cloning of any molecule of DNA it is necessary for that DNA to be incorporated into a cloning vector. These are DNA elements that may be stably maintained and propagated in a host organism for which the vector has replication
functions. A typical host organism is a bacterium such as *E. coli*, which grows and
divides rapidly. Thus any vector with a replication origin in *E. coli* will replicate
(together with any incorporated DNA) efficiently. Also any DNA cloned into a
vector will permit the amplification of the inserted foreign DNA fragment and also
allow any subsequent analysis to be undertaken. In this way the cloning process
resembles the PCR, although there are some major differences between the two
techniques. By cloning, it is possible not only to store a copy of any particular fragment of DNA but also to produce unlimited amounts of it (Fig. 6.10).

The vectors used for cloning vary in their complexity, ease of manipulation, their
selection and the amount of DNA sequence they can accommodate (the insert
capacity). Vectors have, in general, been developed from naturally occurring molecules such as bacterial plasmids, bacteriophages or combinations of the elements
that make them up, such as cosmids (Section 6.3.4). For gene library constructions
there is a choice and trade-off between various vector types, usually related to ease
of the manipulations needed to construct the library and the maximum size of
foreign DNA insert of the vector (Table 6.2). Thus vectors with the advantage of
large insert capacities are usually more difficult to manipulate, although there are
many more factors to be considered, which are indicated in the following treatment of vector systems.

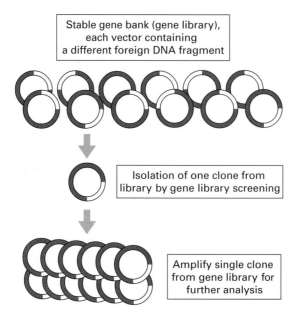

Fig. 6.10. Production of multiple copies of a single clone from a stable gene bank or library.

Table 6.2 **Comparison of vectors generally available for cloning DNA fragments**

Vector	Host cell	Vector structure	Insert range (kb)
M13	*E. coli*	Circular virus	1–4
Plasmid	*E. coli*	Circular plasmid	1–5
Phage λ	*E. coli*	Linear virus	2–25
Cosmids	*E. coli*	Circular plasmid	35–45
BACs	*E. coli*	Circular plasmid	50–300
YACs	*S. cerevisiae*	Linear chromosome	100–2000

BAC, bacterial artificial chromosome; YAC, yeast artificial chromosome.

6.3.1 Plasmids

Many bacteria contain an extrachromosomal element of DNA, termed a plasmid, which is a relatively small, covalently closed circular molecule carrying genes for antibiotic resistance, conjugation or the metabolism of 'unusual' substrates. Some plasmids are replicated at a high rate by bacteria such as *E. coli* and so are excellent potential vectors. In the early 1970s a number of natural plasmids were artificially modified and constructed as cloning vectors, by a complex series of digestion and ligation reactions. One of the most notable plasmids, termed pBR322 after its developers F. Bolivar and R. Rodriguez (pBR), was widely adopted and illustrates the desirable features of a cloning vector as indicated below (Fig. 6.11).

● The plasmid is much smaller than a natural plasmid, which makes it more resistant to damage by shearing, and increases the efficiency of uptake by bacteria, a process termed transformation.

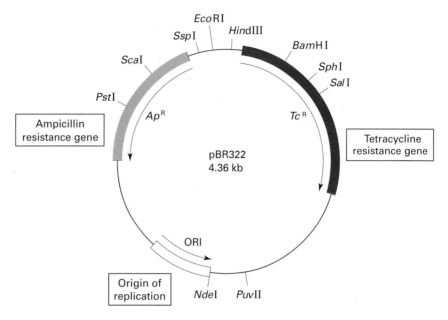

Fig. 6.11. Map and important features of pBR322.

- A bacterial origin of DNA replication ensures that the plasmid will be replicated by the host cell. Some replication origins display stringent regulation of replication, in which rounds of replication are initiated at the same frequency as cell division. Most plasmids, including pBR322, have a relaxed origin of replication, whose activity is not tightly linked to cell division, and so plasmid replication will be initiated far more frequently than chromosomal replication. Hence a large number of plasmid molecules will be produced per cell.
- Two genes coding for resistance to antibiotics have been introduced. One of these allows the selection of cells that contain plasmid: if cells are plated on a medium containing an appropriate antibiotic, only those that contain plasmid will grow to form colonies. The other resistance gene can be used, as described below, for detection of those plasmids that contain inserted DNA.
- There are single recognition sites for a number of restriction enzymes at various points around the plasmid that can be used to open or linearise the circular plasmid. Linearising a plasmid allows a fragment of DNA to be inserted and the circle then closed again. The variety of sites not only makes it easier to find a restriction enzyme suitable for both the vector and the foreign DNA to be inserted but, since some of the sites are placed within an antibiotic resistance gene, the presence of an insert can be detected by loss of resistance to that antibiotic. This is termed insertional inactivation.

Insertional inactivation is a useful selection method for identifying recombinant vectors with inserts. For example, a fragment of chromosomal DNA digested with

*Bam*HI would be isolated and purified. The plasmid pBR322 would also be digested at a single site, using *Bam*HI, and both samples would then be deproteinised to inactivate the restriction enzyme. *Bam*HI cleaves to give sticky ends, and so it is possible to obtain ligation between the plasmid and digested DNA fragments in the presence of T4 DNA ligase. The products of this ligation will include plasmid containing a single fragment of the DNA as an insert, but there will also be unwanted products, such as plasmid that has recircularised without an insert, dimers of plasmid, fragments joined to each other, and plasmid with an insert composed of more than one fragment. Most of these unwanted molecules can be eliminated during subsequent steps. The products of such reactions are usually identified by agarose gel electrophoresis (Section 5.7.4).

The ligated DNA must now be used to transform *E. coli*. Bacteria do not normally take up DNA from their surroundings but can be induced to do so by prior treatment with Ca^{2+} at 4 °C. They are then termed competent, since DNA added to the suspension of competent cells will be taken up during a brief increase in temperature termed heat shock. Small, circular molecules are taken up most efficiently, whereas long, linear molecules will not enter the bacteria.

After a brief incubation to allow expression of the antibiotic resistance genes the cells are plated onto medium containing an antibiotic, for example ampicillin. Colonies that grow on these plates must be derived from cells that contain plasmid, since this carries the gene for resistance to ampicillin. It is not, at this stage, possible to distinguish between those colonies containing plasmids with inserts and those that contain simply recircularised plasmids. To do this, the colonies are replica plated, using a sterile velvet pad, onto plates containing tetracycline in their medium. Since the *Bam*HI site lies within the tetracycline resistance gene, this gene will be inactivated by the presence of insert, but will be intact in those plasmids that have merely recircularised (Fig. 6.12). Thus colonies that grow on ampicillin but not on tetracycline must contain plasmids with inserts. Since replica plating gives an identical pattern of colonies on both sets of plates, it is straightforward to recognise the colonies with inserts, and to recover them from the ampicillin plate for further growth. This illustrates the importance of a second gene for antibiotic resistance in a vector.

Although recircularised plasmid can be selected against, its presence decreases the yield of recombinant plasmid containing inserts. If the digested plasmid is treated with the enzyme alkaline phosphatase prior to ligation, recircularisation will be prevented, since this enzyme removes the 5′-phosphate groups, which are essential for ligation. Links can still be made between the 5′-phosphate of insert and the 3′-hydroxyl of plasmid, so only recombinant plasmids and chains of linked DNA fragments will be formed. It does not matter that only one strand of the recombinant DNA is ligated, since the nick will be repaired by bacteria transformed with these molecules.

The valuable features of pBR322 have been enhanced by the construction of a series of plasmids termed pUC (produced at the University of California) (Fig. 6.13). There is an antibiotic resistance gene for tetracycline and origin of replication for *E. coli*. In addition the most popular restriction sites are concentrated

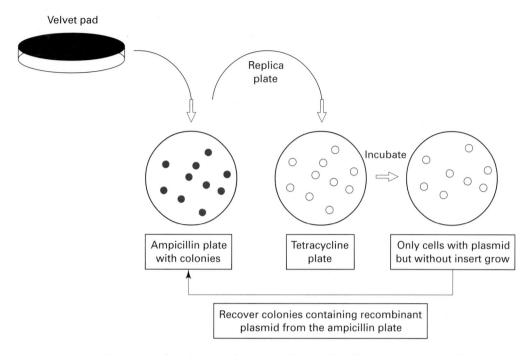

Fig. 6.12. Replica plating to detect recombinant plasmids. A sterile velvet pad is pressed onto the surface of an agar plate, picking up some cells from each colony growing on that plate. The pad is then pressed on to a fresh agar plate, thus inoculating it with cells in a pattern identical with that of the original colonies. Clones of cells that fail to grow on the second plate (e.g. owing to the loss of antibiotic resistance) can be recovered from their corresponding colonies on the first plate.

into a region termed the multiple cloning site or MCS. In addition the MCS is part of a gene in its own right and codes for a portion of a polypeptide called β-galactosidase. When the pUC plasmid has been used to transform the host cell *E. coli*, the gene may be switched on by adding the inducer IPTG (isopropyl β-D-thiogalactopyranoside). Its presence causes the enzyme β-galactosidase to be produced. The functional enzyme is able to hydrolyse a colourless substance called X-gal (5-bromo-4-chloro-3-indolyl-β-galactopyranoside) into a blue insoluble material (Fig. 6.14). However, if the gene is disrupted by the insertion of a foreign fragment of DNA, a non-functional enzyme results that is unable to carry out hydrolysis of X-gal. Thus a recombinant pUC plasmid may be easily detected, since it is white or colourless in the presence of X-gal, whereas an intact non-recombinant pUC plasmid will be blue, since its gene is fully functional and not disrupted. This elegant system, termed blue/white selection, allows the initial identification of recombinants to be undertaken very quickly and has been included in a number of subsequent vector systems. This selection method and insertional inactivation of antibiotic resistance genes do not, however, provide any information on the character of the DNA insert, merely the status of the vector. To screen gene libraries for a desired insert, hybridisation to gene probes is required and this is explained in Section 6.5.

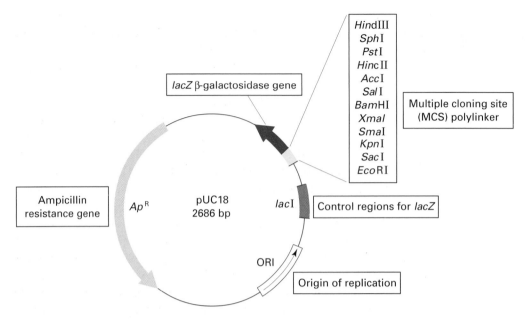

Fig. 6.13. Map and important features of pUC18.

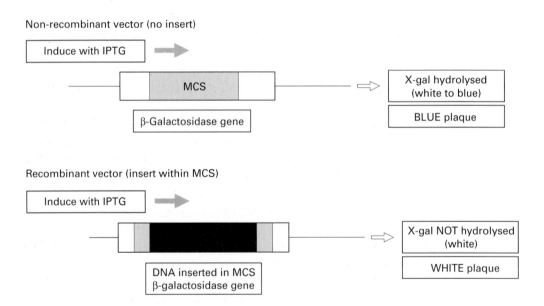

Fig. 6.14. Principle of blue/white selection for the detection of recombinant vectors.

6.3.2 **Virus-based vectors**

A useful feature of any cloning vector is the amount of DNA it may accept or have inserted before it becomes unviable. Inserts greater than 5 kb increase plasmid size to the point at which efficient transformation of bacterial cells decreases markedly, and so bacteriophages (phages or bacterial viruses) have been adapted as vectors in order to propagate larger fragments of DNA in bacterial cells. Cloning vectors derived from phage λ are commonly used since they offer an approximately 16-fold advantage in cloning efficiency by comparison with the most efficient plasmid cloning vectors.

Phage λ is a linear double-stranded phage approximately 49 kb in length (Fig. 6.15). It infects *E. coli* with great efficiency by injecting its DNA through the cell membrane. In the wild-type phage λ the DNA follows one of two possible modes of replication. First, the DNA may either become stably integrated into the *E. coli* chromosome, where it lies dormant until a signal triggers its excision. This is termed the lysogenic life cycle. Alternatively, it may follow a lytic life cycle where the DNA is replicated upon entry to the cell, phage head and tail proteins synthesised rapidly and new functional phage assembled. The phage are subsequently released from the cell by lysing the cell membrane to infect further *E. coli* cells nearby. At the extreme ends of the phage λ are 12 bp sequences termed cos (cohesive) sites. Although they are asymmetric, they are similar to restriction sites and allow the phage DNA to be circularised. Phage may be replicated very efficiently in this way, the result of which is concatemers of many phage genomes, which are cleaved at the cos sites and inserted into newly formed phage protein heads.

Much use of phage λ has been made in the production of gene libraries mainly because of its efficient entry into the *E. coli* cell and the fact that larger fragments of DNA may by stably integrated. For the cloning of long DNA fragments, up to approximately 25 kb, much of the non-essential λ DNA that codes for the lysogenic life cycle is removed and replaced by the foreign DNA insert. The recombinant phage is then assembled into pre-formed viral protein particles, a process termed *in vitro* packaging. These newly formed phage are used to infect bacterial cells that have been plated out on agar (Fig. 6.16).

Once inside the host cells, the recombinant viral DNA is replicated. All the genes needed for normal lytic growth are still present in the phage DNA, and so multiplication of the virus takes place by cycles of cell lysis and infection of surrounding cells, giving rise to plaques of lysed cells on a background, or lawn, of bacterial cells. The viral DNA including the cloned foreign DNA can be recovered from the viruses from these plaques and analysed further by restriction mapping (Section 5.9.1) and agarose gel electrophoresis (Section 5.7.4).

In general, two types of phage λ vectors have been developed, λ insertion vectors and λ replacement vectors (Fig. 6.17). The λ insertion vectors accept less DNA than the replacement type, since the foreign DNA is merely inserted into a region of the phage genome with appropriate restriction sites, common examples being λgt10 and λcharon16A. With a replacement vector, a central region of DNA not essential for lytic growth is removed (a stuffer fragment) by a double digestion with, for example, *Eco*RI and *Bam*HI. This leaves two DNA fragments termed right and left arms. The central stuffer fragment is replaced by inserting foreign DNA between the arms to form a functional recombinant phage λ. The most notable examples of λ replacement vectors are λEMBL and λZap.

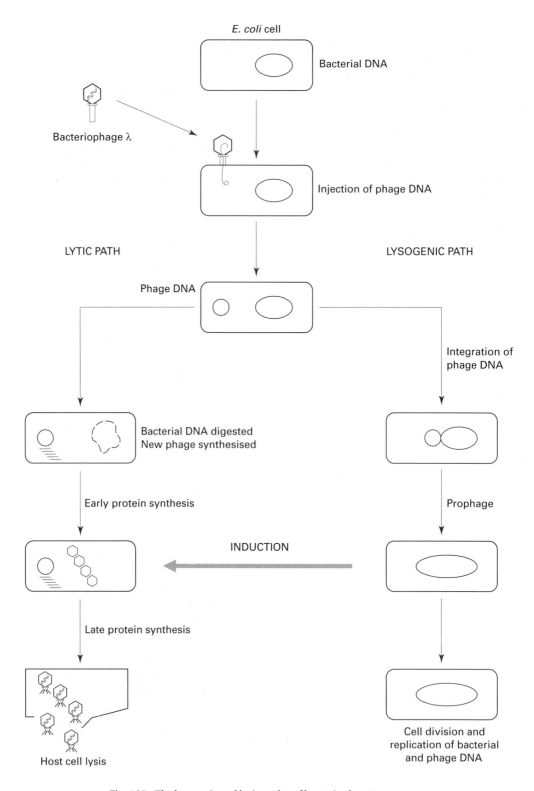

Fig. 6.15. The lysogenic and lytic cycles of bacteriophage λ.

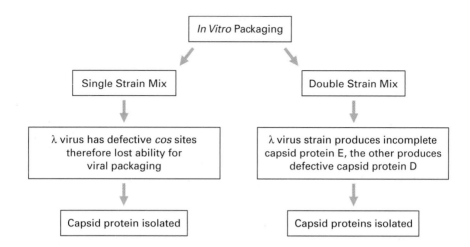

Fig. 6.16. Two strategies for producing *in vitro* packaging extracts for bacteriophage λ.

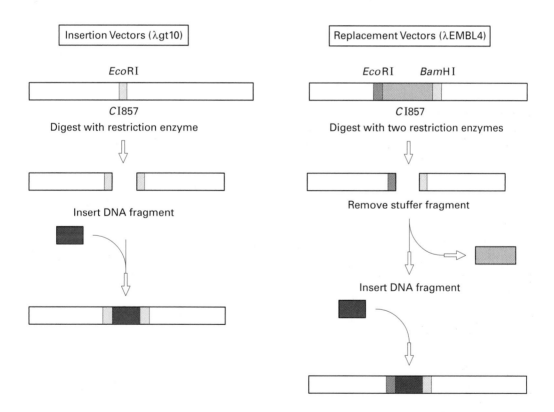

Fig. 6.17. General schemes used for cloning in λ insertion and λ replacement vectors. *C*I857 is a temperature-sensitive mutation that promotes lysis at 42 °C after incubation at 37 °C.

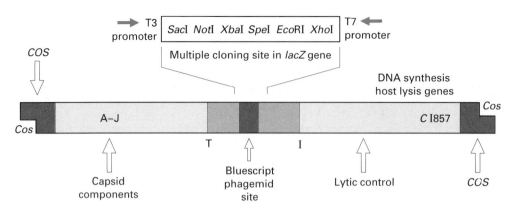

Fig. 6.18. General map of λZap cloning vector, indicating important areas of the vector. The multiple cloning site is based on the *lacZ* gene, providing blue/white selection based on the β-galactosidase gene. In between the initiator (I) site and terminator (T) site lie sequences encoding the phagemid Bluescript.

λZap is a commercially produced cloning vector that includes unique cloning sites clustered into a MCS (Fig. 6.18). Furthermore the MCS is located within a *lacZ* region providing a blue/white selection system based on insertional inactivation (Fig. 6.14). It is also possible to express foreign cloned DNA from this vector. This is a very useful feature of some λ vectors, since it is then possible to screen for protein product rather than the DNA inserted into the vector. This screening is therefore undertaken with antibody probes directed against the protein of interest (Section 6.5.4). Another feature that makes this a useful cloning vector is the ability to produce RNA transcripts, termed cRNA or riboprobes. This is possible because two promoters for RNA polymerase enzymes exist in the vector, a T7 and a T3 promoter, which flank the MCS (Section 6.4.2).

One of the most useful features of λZap is that it has been designed to allow automatic excision *in vivo* of a small 2.9 kb colony-producing vector termed a phagemid, pBluescript SK (Section 6.3.3). This technique is sometimes termed single-stranded DNA rescue and occurs as the result of a process termed superinfection, where helper phage are added to the cells, which are grown for an additional period of approximately 4 h (Fig. 6.19).

The helper phage displace a strand within the λZap that contains the foreign DNA insert. This is circularised and packaged as a filamentous phage similar to M13 (Section 6.3.3). The packaged phagemid is secreted from the *E. coli* cell and may be recovered from the supernatant. Thus the λZap vector allows a number of diverse manipulations to be undertaken without the necessity of recloning or subcloning foreign DNA fragments. The process of subcloning is sometimes necessary when the manipulation of gene fragment that has been cloned into a general purpose vector needs to be inserted into a more specialised vector for the application of techniques such as *in vitro* mutagenesis or protein production (Section 6.6).

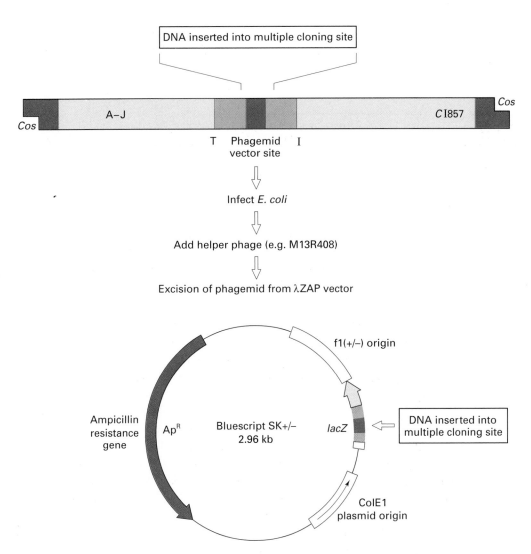

Fig. 6.19. Single-stranded DNA rescue of phagemid from λZap. The single-stranded phagemid pBluescript SK may be excised from λZap by addition of helper phage. This provides the necessary proteins and factors for transcription between the I and T sites in the parent phage to produce the phagemid with the DNA cloned into the parent vector.

6.3.3 M13 and phagemid-based vectors

Much use has been made of single-stranded bacteriophage vectors such as M13 and vectors that have the combined properties of phage and plasmids, termed phagemids. M13 is a filamentous coliphage with a single-stranded circular DNA genome (Fig. 6.20). Upon infection of *E. coli*, the DNA replicates initially as a double-stranded molecule but subsequently produces single-stranded virus particles or virions for infection of further bacterial cells (lytic growth). The nature of these vectors makes them ideal for techniques such as chain termination sequencing

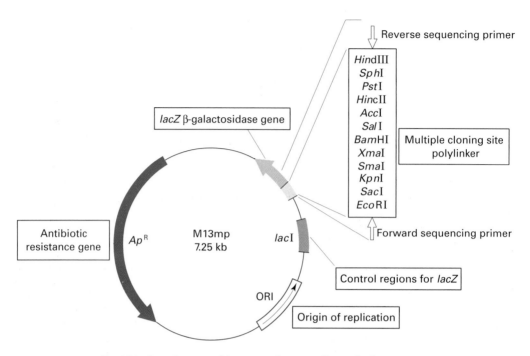

Fig. 6.20. Genetic map and important features of bacteriophage vector M13.

(Section 6.6.1) and *in vitro* mutagenesis (Section 6.6.2), since both require single-stranded DNA.

M13 or phagemids such as pBluescript SK infect *E. coli* harbouring a male-specific structure termed the F-pilus (Fig. 6.21). They enter the cell by adsorption to this structure and, once inside, the phage DNA is converted to a double-stranded replicative form or RF DNA. Replication then proceeds rapidly until some 100 RF molecules are produced within the *E. coli* cell. DNA synthesis then switches to the production of single strands and the DNA is assembled and packaged into the capsid at the bacterial periplasm. The bacteriophage DNA is then encapsulated by the major coat protein, gene VIII protein, of which there are approximately 2800 copies, with three to six copies of the gene III protein at one end of the particle. The extrusion of the bacteriophage through the bacterial periplasm results in a decreased growth rate of the *E. coli* cell rather than host cell lysis and is visible on a bacterial lawn as an area of clearing. Approximately 1000 packaged phage particles may be released into the medium in one cell division.

In addition to producing single-stranded DNA, the coliphage vectors have a number of other features that make them attractive as cloning vectors. Since the bacteriophage DNA is replicated as a double-stranded RF DNA intermediate, a number of regular DNA manipulations may be performed such as restriction digestion, mapping and DNA ligation. RF DNA is prepared by lysing infected *E. coli* cells and purifying the supercoiled circular phage DNA with the same methods used for plasmid isolation. Intact single-stranded DNA packaged in the phage protein coat located in the supernatant may be precipitated with reagents

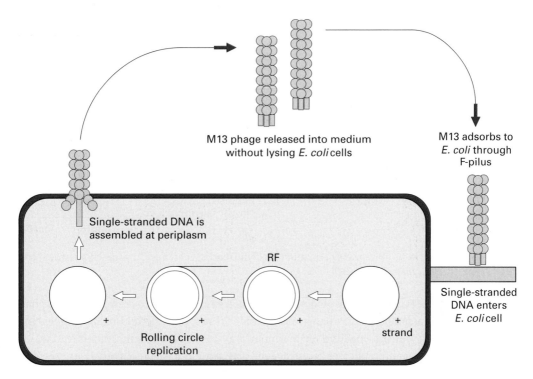

M13 phage released into medium
without lysing *E. coli* cells

M13 adsorbs to
E. coli through
F-pilus

Single-stranded DNA is
assembled at periplasm

RF

Rolling circle
replication

strand

Single-stranded
DNA enters
E. coli cell

Fig. 6.21. Life cycle of bacteriophage M13. The bacteriophage virus enters the *E. coli* cell through the F-pilus. It then enters a stage where the circular single strands are converted to double strands. Rolling-circle replication then produces single strands, which are packaged and extruded through the *E. coli* cell membrane.

such as polyethylene glycol, and the DNA purified with phenol/chloroform (Section 5.7.1). Thus the phage may act as a plasmid under certain circumstances and at other times produce DNA in the fashion of a virus. A family of vectors derived from M13, termed M13mp8/9, mp18/19 etc., are currently widely used all of which have a number of highly useful features. All contain a synthetic MCS, which is located in the *lacZ* gene without disruption of the reading frame of the gene. This allows efficient selection to be undertaken on the basis of the technique of blue/white selection (Section 6.3.1). As the series of vectors was developed, the number of restriction sites was increased in an asymmetric fashion. Thus M13mp8, mp12, mp18 and sister vectors that have the same MCS but in reverse orientation (M13mp9, mp13 and mp19, respectively) and have more restriction sites in the MCS, making the vector more useful as a greater choice of restriction enzymes is available (Fig. 6.22). However, one problem frequently encountered with M13 is the instability and spontaneous loss of inserts that are greater than 6 kb.

Phagemids are very similar to M13 and replicate in a similar fashion. One of the first phagemid vectors, pEMBL, was constructed by inserting a fragment of another phage termed f1 containing a phage origin of replication and elements for its morphogenesis into a pUC8 plasmid. After superinfection with helper phage,

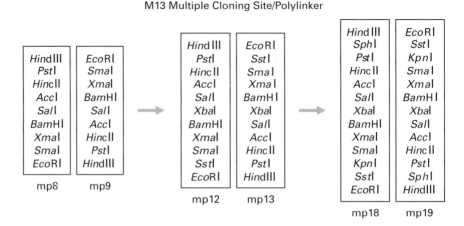

Fig. 6.22. Design and orientation of polylinkers in M13 series. Only the main restriction enzymes are indicated.

the f1 origin is activated, allowing single-stranded DNA to be produced. The phage is assembled into a phage coat extruded through the periplasm and secreted into the culture medium in a similar way to M13. Without superinfection, the phagemid replicates as a pUC-type plasmid and in the replicative form the DNA isolated is double stranded. This allows further manipulations such as restriction digestion, ligation and mapping analysis to be performed. The pBluescript SK vector is also a phagemid and can be used in its own right as a cloning vector and manipulated as if it were a plasmid. It may, like M13, be used in nucleotide sequencing and site-directed mutagenesis and it is also possible to produce RNA transcripts that may be used in the production of labelled complementary RNA probes or riboprobes (Section 6.4.2).

6.3.4 Cosmid-based vectors

The way in which the phage λ DNA is replicated is of particular interest in the development of larger insert cloning vectors termed cosmids (Fig. 6.23). These are especially useful for the analysis of highly complex genomes and are an important part of various genome mapping projects (Section 6.9).

The upper limit of the insert capacity of phage λ is approximately 21 kb. This is because of the requirement for essential genes and the fact that the maximum length between the *cos* sites is 52 kb. Consequently cosmid vectors have been constructed that incorporate the *cos* sites from phage λ and also the essential features of a plasmid, such as the plasmid origin of replication, a gene for drug resistance, and several unique restriction sites for insertion of the DNA to be cloned. When a cosmid preparation is linearised by restriction digestion and ligated to DNA for cloning, the products will include concatamers of alternating cosmid vector and insert. Thus the only requirement for a length of DNA to be packaged into viral heads is that it should contain *cos* sites spaced the correct distance apart; in practice this spacing can range between 37 and 52 kb. Such DNA can be packaged *in vitro* if

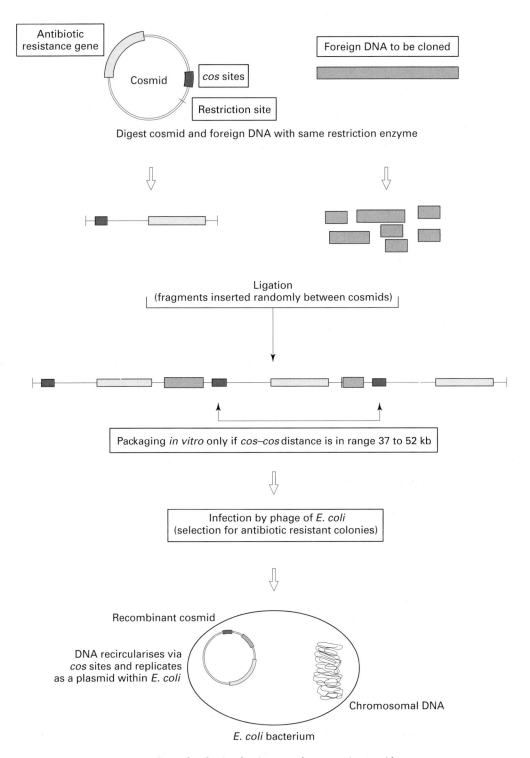

Fig. 6.23. Scheme for cloning foreign DNA fragments in cosmid vectors.

phage head precursors, tails and packaging proteins are provided. Since the cosmid is very small, inserts of about 40 kb in length will be most readily packaged. Once inside the cell, the DNA recircularizes through its *cos* sites and from then on behaves exactly like a plasmid.

6.3.5 Large insert capacity vectors

The advantage of vectors that accept larger fragments of DNA than phage λ or cosmids is that fewer clones need to be screened when one is searching for the foreign DNA of interest. They have also had an enormous impact on the mapping of the genomes of organisms such as the mouse and are used extensively in the Human Genome Mapping Project (Section 6.9.3). Recent developments have allowed the production of large insert capacity vectors based on bacterial artificial chromosomes (BACs), mammalian artificial chromosomes (MACs) and on the virus P1 artificial chromosomes (PACs). However, perhaps the most significant development is vectors based on yeast artificial chromosomes.

6.3.6 Yeast artificial chromosome vectors

Yeast artificial chromosomes (YACs) are linear molecules composed of a centromere, telomere and a replication origin termed an ARS (autonomous replicating sequence) element. The YAC is digested with restriction enzymes at the SUP4 site (a suppressor tRNA gene marker) and *Bam*HI sites separating the telomere sequences (Fig. 6.24). This produces two arms and the foreign genomic DNA is ligated to produce a functional YAC construct. YACs are replicated in yeast cells; however, the external cell wall of the yeast needs to be removed to leave a spheroplast. These are osmotically unstable and need to be embedded in a solid matrix such as agar. Once the yeast cells are transformed, only correctly constructed YACs with associated selectable markers are replicated in the yeast strains. DNA fragments with repeated sequences that are sometimes difficult to clone in bacterial-based vectors may also be cloned in YAC systems. The main advantage of YAC-based vectors, however, is the ability to clone very large fragments of DNA. Thus the stable maintenance and replication of foreign DNA fragments of up to 2000 kb have been carried out in YAC vectors and they are the main vector of choice in the various genome mapping and sequencing projects (Section 6.9).

6.3.7 Vectors used in eukaryotes

The use of *E. coli* for general cloning and manipulation of DNA is well established; however, numerous developments have been made for cloning in eukaryotic cells. Plasmids used for cloning DNA in eukaryotic cells require a eukaryotic origin of replication and marker genes that will be expressed by eukaryotic cells. At present the two most important applications of plasmids to eukaryotic cells are for cloning in yeast and in plants.

Although yeast has a natural plasmid, called the 2μ circle, this is too large for use in cloning. Plasmids such as the the yeast episomal plasmid (YEp) have been

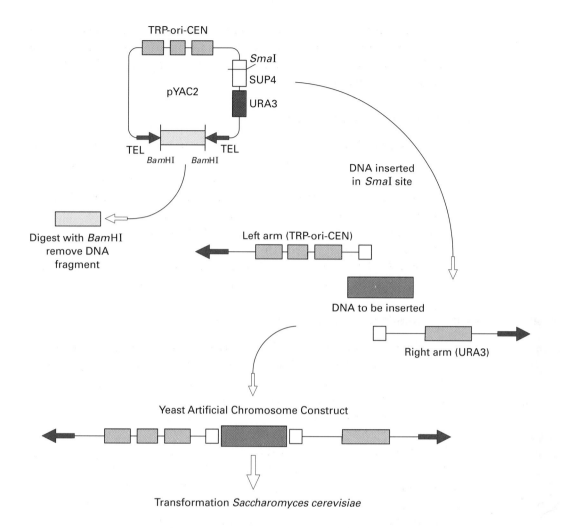

Fig. 6.24. Scheme for cloning large fragments of DNA into YAC vectors.

created by genetic manipulation using replication origins from the 2μ circle, and by incorporating a gene that will complement a defective gene in the host yeast cell. If, for example, a strain of yeast is used that has a defective gene for the biosynthesis of an amino acid, an active copy of that gene on a yeast plasmid can be used as a selectable marker for the presence of that plasmid. Yeast, like bacteria, can be grown rapidly and is therefore well suited for use in cloning. Of particular use has been the creation of shuttle vectors that have origins of replication for yeast and bacteria such as *E. coli*. This means that constructs may be prepared rapidly in the bacteria and delivered into yeast for expression studies.

The bacterium *Agrobacterium tumefaciens* infects plants that have been damaged near soil level, and this infection is often followed by the formation of plant tumours in the vicinity of the infected region. It is now known that *A. tumefaciens* contains a plasmid called Ti, part of which is transferred into the nuclei of plant cells infected by the bacterium. Once in the nucleus, this DNA is maintained by integrating with the chromosomal DNA. The integrated DNA carries genes for the synthesis of opines (which are metabolised by the bacteria but not by the plants) and for tumour induction (hence Ti). DNA inserted into the correct region of the Ti plasmid will be transferred to infected plant cells, and in this way it has been possible to clone and express foreign genes in plants (Fig. 6.25). This is a prerequisite for the genetic engineering of crops.

6.3.8 Delivery of vectors into eukaryotes

Following the production of a recombinant molecule, the so-called construct is subsequently introduced into cells to enable it to be replicated a large number of times as the cells replicate. Initial recombinant DNA experiments were performed in bacterial cells, because of their ease of growth and short doubling time. Gram-negative bacteria such as *E. coli* can be made competent for the introduction of extraneous plasmid DNA into cells (Section 6.3.1). The natural ability of phage to introduce DNA into *E. coli* has also been well exploited and results in 10- to 100-fold higher efficiency for the introduction of recombinant DNA as compared with transformation of competent bacteria with plasmids. These well-established and traditional approaches are the reason why so many cloning vectors have been developed for *E. coli*. The delivery of cloning vectors into eukaryotic cells is, however, not as straightforward as that for *E. coli*.

It is possible to deliver recombinant molecules into animal cells by transfection, the efficiency of which can be increased by first precipitating the DNA with Ca^{2+} or making the membrane permeable with divalent cations or high molecular weight polymers such as DEAE-dextran or polyethylene glycol (PEG). The technique is rather inefficient, although a selectable marker that provides resistance to a toxic compound such as neomycin can be used to monitor the success. Alternatively, DNA can be introduced into animal cells by electroporation. In this process the cells are subjected to pulses of a high voltage gradient, causing many of them to take up DNA from the surrounding solution. This technique has proved to be useful with cells from a range of animal, plant and microbial sources. More recently the technique of lipofection has been used as the delivery method. The recombinant DNA is encapsulated by a core of lipid-coated particles that fuse with the lipid membrane of cells and release the DNA into the cell. Microinjection of DNA into cell nuclei of eggs or embryos has also been performed successfully in many mammalian cells.

The ability to deliver recombinant molecules into plant cells is not without its problems. Generally the outer cell wall of the plant must be stripped, usually by enzymatic digestion, to leave a protoplast. The cells are then able to take up recombinants from the supernatant. The cell wall can be regenerated by providing appropriate media. In cases where protoplasts have been generated, transformation may also be achieved by electroporation. An even more dramatic transformation procedure involves propelling microscopically small titanium or gold pellet microprojectiles, coated with the recombinant DNA molecule, into plant cells in

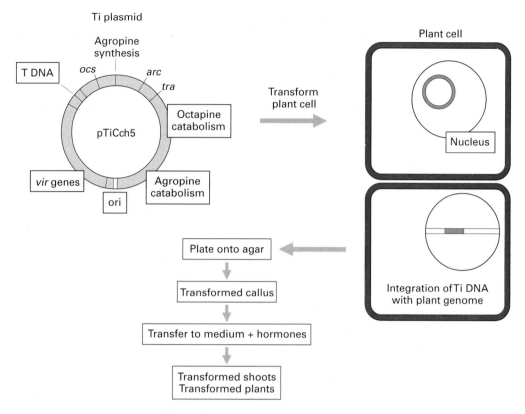

Fig. 6.25. Scheme for cloning in plant cells using the Ti plasmid.

intact tissues. This biolistic technique involves the detonation of an explosive charge, which is used to propel the microprojectiles into the cells at a high velocity. The cells then appear to reseal themselves after the delivery of the recombinant molecule. This is a particularly promising technique for use with plants whose protoplasts will not regenerate whole plants.

6.4 **HYBRIDISATION AND GENE PROBES**

6.4.1 **Cloned DNA probes**

The increasing accumulation of nucleic acid database entries and availability of custom synthesis of oligonucleotides has provided a relatively straightforward means for designing and producing gene probes and primers for PCR. Gene probes and primers are usually designed using bioinformatics software and nucleic acid databases or gene family-related sequences as indicated in Section 5.9.3. However, there are many gene probes that have traditionally been derived from cDNA or from genomic sequences and which have been cloned into plasmid and phage vectors. These require manipulation before they may be labelled and used in

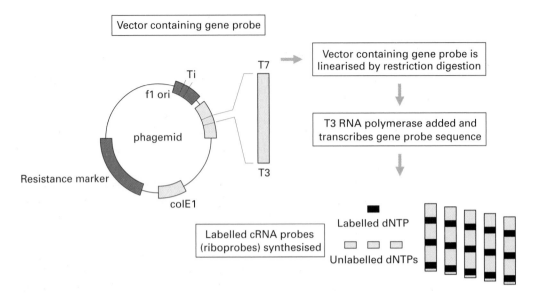

Fig. 6.26. Production of cDNA (riboprobes) using T3 RNA polymerase and phagemid vectors.

hybridisation experiments. Gene probes may vary in length from 100 bp to a number of kilobases, although this is dependent on their origin. Many are short enough to be cloned into plasmid vectors and are useful in that they may be manipulated easily and are relatively stable both in transit and in the laboratory. The DNA sequences representing the gene probe are usually excised from the cloning vector by digestion with restriction enzymes and purified. In this way vector sequences that may hybridise non-specifically and cause high background signals in hybridisation experiments are removed. There are various ways of labelling DNA probes and these are described in Section 5.9.4.

6.4.2 RNA gene probes

It is also possible to prepare cRNA probes or riboprobes by *in vitro* transcription of gene probes cloned into a suitable vector. A good example of such a vector is the phagemid pBluescript SK, since at each end of the multiple cloning site where the cloned DNA fragment resides are promoters for T3 or T7 RNA polymerase (Section 6.3.3). The vector is then made linear with a restriction enzyme and T3 or T7 RNA polymerase is used to transcribe the cloned DNA fragment. Provided a labelled NTP is added in the reaction a riboprobe labelled to a high specific activity will be produced (Fig. 6.26). One advantage of riboprobes is that they are single stranded and their sensitivity is generally regarded as superior to the cloned double-stranded probes mentioned in Section 6.4.1. They are used extensively in *in situ* hybridisation and for identifying and analysing mRNA and are described in more detail in Section 6.8.

6.5 **SCREENING GENE LIBRARIES**

6.5.1 **Colony and plaque hybridisation**

Once a cDNA or genomic library has been prepared, the next task is the identification of the specific fragment of interest. In many cases this may be more problematic than the library construction itself, since many hundreds of thousands of clones may be in the library. One clone containing the desired fragment needs to be isolated from the library and therefore a number of techniques based mainly on hybridisation have been developed.

Colony hybridisation is one method used to identify a particular DNA fragment from a plasmid gene library (Fig. 6.27). A large number of clones are grown up to form colonies on one or more plates, and these are then replica plated onto a nylon membrane placed on solid agar medium. Nutrients diffuse through the membranes and allow colonies to grow on them. The colonies are then lysed, and liberated DNA is denatured and bound to the membranes, so that the pattern of colonies is replaced by an identical pattern of bound DNA. The membranes are then incubated with a prehybridisation mix containing non-labelled non-specific DNA such as salmon sperm DNA to block non-specific sites. Following this, denatured labelled gene probe is added. Under hybridising conditions the probe will bind only to cloned fragments containing at least part of its corresponding gene (Section 5.9.2). The membranes are then washed to remove any unbound probe and the binding detected by autoradiography of the membranes. If non-radioactive labels have been used then alternative methods of detection must be employed (Section 5.9.4). By comparison of the patterns on the autoradiograph with the original plates of colonies, those that contain the desired gene (or part of it) can be identified and isolated for further analysis. A similar procedure is used to identify desired genes cloned into bacteriophage vectors. In this case the process is termed plaque hybridisation. It is the DNA contained in the bacteriophage particles found in each plaque that is immobilised onto the nylon membrane. This is then probed with an appropriately labelled complementary gene probe and the detection undertaken as for colony hybridisation.

6.5.2 **PCR screening of gene libraries**

In many cases it is now possible to use the PCR to screen cDNA or genomic libraries constructed in plasmids or bacteriophage vectors. This is usually undertaken with primers that anneal to the vector rather than the foreign DNA insert. The size of an amplified product may be used to characterise the cloned DNA and subsequent restriction mapping is then carried out (Fig. 6.28). The main advantage of the PCR over traditional hybridisation-based screening is the rapidity of the technique: PCR screening may be undertaken in 3–4 h whereas it may be several days before detection by hybridisation is achieved. The PCR screening technique gives an indication of the size of the cloned inserts rather than the sequence of the insert; however, PCR primers that are specific for a foreign DNA insert may also be used. This allows a more rigorous characterisation of clones from cDNA and genome libraries.

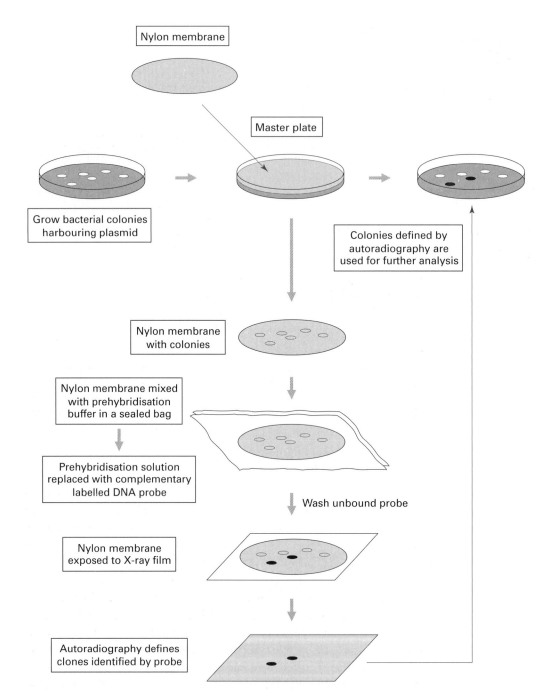

Fig. 6.27. Colony hybridisation technique for locating specific bacterial colonies harbouring recombinant plasmid vectors containing desired DNA fragments. This is achieved by hybridisation to a complementary labelled DNA probe and autoradiography.

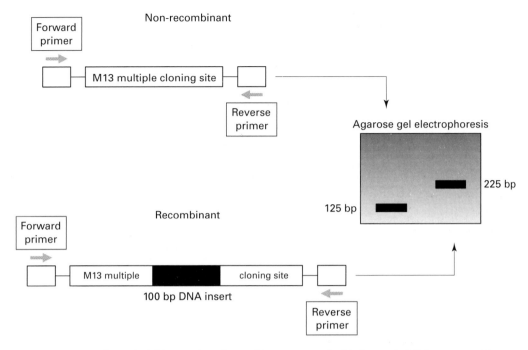

Fig. 6.28. PCR screening of recombinant vectors. In this figure, the M13 non-recombinant has no insert and so the PCR undertaken with forward and reverse sequencing primers gives rise to a product 125 bp in length. The M13 recombinant with an insert of 100 bp will give rise to a PCR product of 125 bp + 100 bp = 225 bp and thus may be distinguished from the non-recombinant by analysis on agarose gel electrophoresis.

6.5.3 Hybrid select/arrest translation

The difficulty of characterising clones and detecting a desired DNA fragment from a mixed cDNA library may be made simpler by two useful techniques termed hybrid select (release) translation or hybrid arrest translation. Following the preparation of a cDNA library in a plasmid vector the plasmid is extracted from part of each colony, and each preparation is then denatured and immobilised onto a nylon membrane (Fig. 6.29). The membranes are soaked in total cellular mRNA, under stringency conditions, i.e. usually at a temperature only a few degrees below the T_m at which hybridisation will occur only between complementary strands of nucleic acid. Hence each membrane will bind just one species of mRNA, since it has only one type of cDNA immobilised onto it. Unbound mRNA is washed off the membranes, and then the bound mRNA is eluted and used to direct *in vitro* translation (Section 6.7). By immunoprecipitation or electrophoresis of the protein, the mRNA coding for a particular protein can be detected, and the clone containing its corresponding cDNA isolated. This technique is known as hybrid release translation. In a related method called hybrid arrest translation, a positive result is indicated by the absence of a particular translation product when total mRNA is hybridised with excess cDNA. This is a consequence of the fact that mRNA cannot be translated when it is hybridised to another molecule.

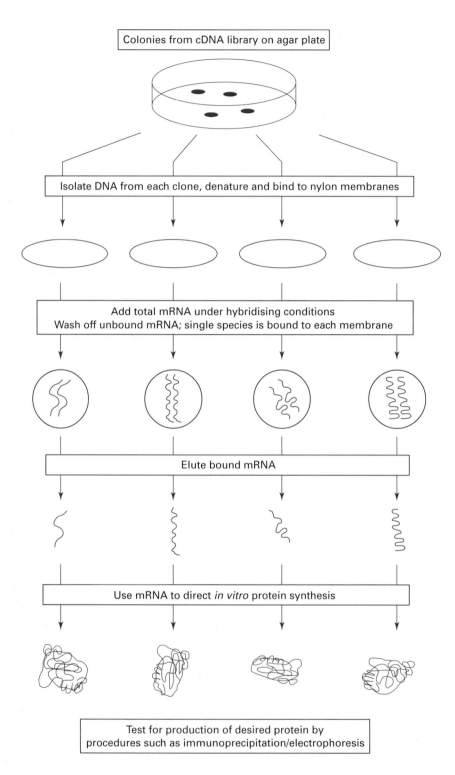

Fig. 6.29. General principles involved in the technique of a hybrid select translation.

6.5.4 Screening expression cDNA libraries

In some cases the protein for which the gene sequence is required is partially characterised and in these cases it may be possible to produce antibodies to that protein. This allows immunological screening to be undertaken rather than gene hybridisation. Such antibodies are useful, since they may be used as the probe if little or no gene sequence is available. In these cases it is possible to prepare a cDNA library in a specially adapted vector termed an expression vector, which transcribes and translates any cDNA inserted into it. The protein is usually synthesised as a fusion with another protein such as β-galactosidase. Common examples of expression vectors are those based on bacteriophage such as λgt11 and λZap or plasmids such as pEX. The precise requirements for such vectors are identical with vectors that are dedicated to producing proteins *in vitro* and are described in Section 6.7.1. In some cases, expression vectors incorporate inducible promoters that may be activated by, for example, increasing the temperature, thus allowing stringent control of expression of the cloned cDNA molecules (Fig. 6.30).

The cDNA library is plated out and nylon membrane filters prepared as for colony/plaque hybridisation. A solution containing the antibody to the desired protein is then added to the membrane. The membrane is then washed to remove any unbound protein and a further labelled antibody that is directed to the first antibody is applied. This allows visualisation of the plaque or colony that contains the cloned cDNA for that protein and this may then be picked from the agar plate and pure preparations grown for further analysis.

6.6 APPLICATIONS OF GENE CLONING

6.6.1 Sequencing cloned DNA

DNA fragments cloned into plasmid vectors may be subjected to the Sanger chain termination sequencing method detailed in Section 5.11.1. However, since plasmids are double stranded, further manipulation needs to be undertaken before this may be attempted. In these cases the plasmids are denatured usually by alkali treatment. Although the plasmids containing the foreign DNA inserts may reanneal, the kinetics of the reaction are such that the strands are single stranded for a long enough period to allow the sequencing method to succeed. It is also possible to include denaturants such as formamide to the reaction to further prevent reannealing. In general, however, the superior results gained with sequencing single-stranded DNA from M13 or single-stranded phagemids means that cloned DNA of interest is usually subcloned into such vectors.

M13 vectors are the traditional choice for chain termination sequencing because of the single-stranded nature of their DNA. A further modification that makes M13 useful in chain termination sequencing is the placement of universal priming sites at −20 or −40 bases from the start of the MCS. This allows any gene to be sequenced by using one universal primer, since annealing of the primer prior to sequencing occurs outside the MCS and so is M13 specific rather than gene

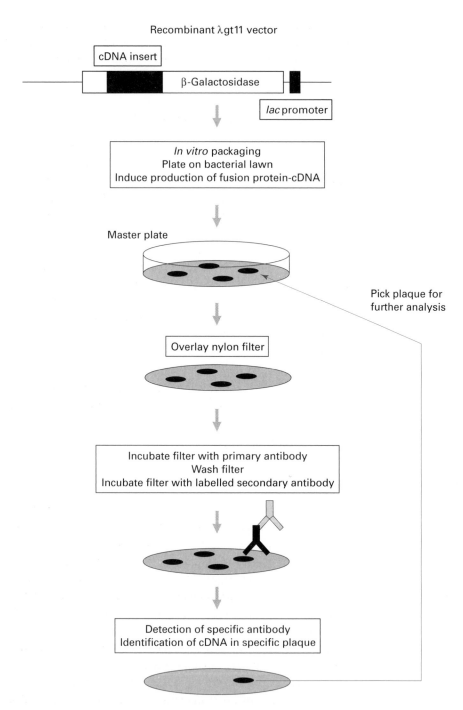

Fig. 6.30. Screening of cDNA libraries in expression vector λgt11. The cDNA inserted upstream from the gene for β-galactosidase will give rise to a fusion protein under induction (e.g. with IPTG). The plaques are then blotted onto a nylon membrane filter and probed with an antibody specific for the protein coded for by the cDNA. A secondary labelled antibody directed to the specific antibody can then be used to identify the location (plaque) of the cDNA.

specific. This obviates the need to synthesise new oligonucleotide primers for each new foreign DNA insert. A further, reverse priming site is also located at the opposite end of the polylinker, allowing sequencing in the opposite orientation to be undertaken.

6.6.2 *In vitro* mutagenesis and rational design

One of the most powerful developments in molecular biology has been the ability to artificially create defined mutations in a gene and analyse the resulting protein following *in vitro* expression. Numerous methods are now available for producing site-directed mutations, many of which now involve the PCR. Commonly termed protein engineering, this process undertakes a logical sequence of analytical and computational techniques centred around a design cycle. This involves the biochemical preparation and analysis of proteins, the subsequent identification of the gene encoding the protein and its modification. The production of the modified protein and its further biochemical analysis completes the concept of rational redesign to improve a protein's structure and function (Fig. 6.31).

The use of design cycles and rational design systems are exemplified by the study and manipulation of subtilisin. This is a serine protease of broad specificity and of considerable industrial importance as it is used in soap powder and in the food and leather industries. Protein engineering has been used to alter the specificity, pH profile and stability to oxidative, thermal and alkaline inactivation. Analysis of homologous thermophiles and their resistance to oxidation has also been improved. Engineered subtilisins of improved bleach resistance and wash performance are now used in many brands of washing powders.

6.6.3 Oligonucleotide-directed mutagenesis

The traditional method of site-directed mutagenesis demands that the gene be already cloned or subcloned into a single-stranded vector such as M13. Complete sequencing of the gene is essential to identify a potential region for mutation. Once the precise base change has been identified, an oligonucleotide is designed that is complementary to part of the gene but has one base difference. This difference is designed to alter a particular codon, which, after translation, gives rise to a different amino acid and hence may alter the properties of the protein.

The oligonucleotide and the single-stranded DNA are annealed and DNA polymerase is added together with the dNTPs. The primer for the reaction is the 3′ end of the oligonucleotide. The DNA polymerase produces a new DNA strand which is complementary to the existing one but incorporates the oligonucleotide with the base mutation. The subsequent cloning of the recombinant produces multiple copies, half of which contain a sequence with the mutation and the other half contain the wild-type sequence. Plaque hybridisation using the oligonucleotide as the probe is then used at a stringency that allows only those plaques containing a mutated sequence to be identified (Fig. 6.32). Further methods have also been developed that simplify the process of detecting the strands with the mutations.

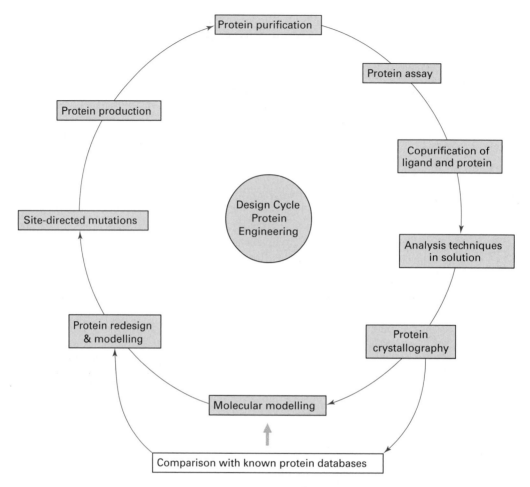

Fig. 6.31. Protein design cycle used in the rational redesign of proteins and enzymes.

6.6.4 **PCR-based mutagenesis**

The PCR has been adapted to allow mutagenesis to be undertaken and this relies on single bases mismatched between one of the PCR primers and the target DNA to become incorporated into the amplified product following thermal cycling.

The basic PCR mutagenesis system involves the use of two primary PCR reactions to produce two overlapping DNA fragments both bearing the same mutation in the overlap region. The technique is termed overlap extension PCR. The two separate PCR products are made single stranded and the overlap in sequence allows the products from each reaction to hybridise. Following this, one of the two hybrids bearing a free 3′-hydroxyl group is extended to produce a new duplex fragment. The other hybrid with a 5′-hydroxyl group cannot act as substrate in the reaction. Thus the overlapped and extended product will now contain the directed mutation (Fig. 6.33). Deletions and insertions may also be created with this method, although the requirements of four primers and three PCR reactions limits

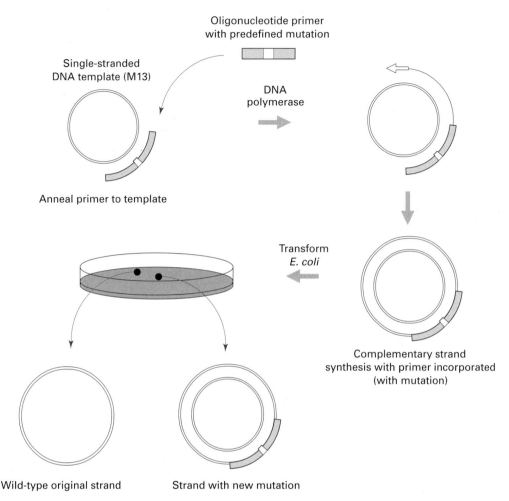

Fig. 6.32. Oligonucleotide-directed mutagenesis. This technique requires a knowledge of nucleotide sequence, since an oligonucleotide may then be synthesised with the base mutation. Annealing of the oligonucleotide to complementary (except for the mutation) single-stranded DNA provides a primer for DNA polymerase to produce a new strand and thus incorporates the primer with the mutation.

the general applicability of the technique. A modification of the overlap extension PCR may also be used to construct directed mutations; this is termed megaprimer PCR. This method utilises three oligonucleotide primers to perform two rounds of PCR. A complete PCR product, the megaprimer is made single stranded and this is used as a large primer in a further PCR reaction with an additional primer.

The above are all methods for creating rational defined mutations as part of a design cycle system. However, it is also possible to introduce random mutations into a gene and select for enhanced or new activities of the protein or enzyme that it encodes. This accelerated form of artificial molecular evolution may be undertaken using error-prone PCR, where deliberate and random mutations are introduced by a low fidelity PCR amplification reaction. The resulting amplified gene is

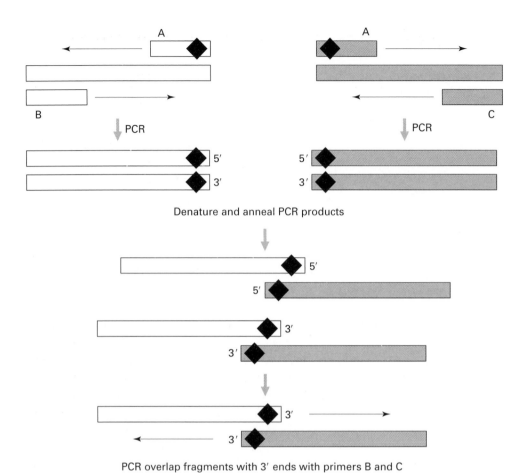

A

B

PCR

A

C

PCR

5′
3′

5′
3′

Denature and anneal PCR products

5′
5′

3′
3′

3′
3′

PCR overlap fragments with 3′ ends with primers B and C

Fig. 6.33. Construction of a synthetic DNA fragment with a predefined mutation using overlap PCR mutagenesis.

then translated and its activity assayed. This has already provided novel evolved enzymes such as a *p*-nitrobenzyl esterase, which exhibits an unusual and surprising affinity for organic solvents. This accelerated evolutionary approach to protein engineering has been useful in the production of novel phage-displayed antibodies (Section 6.7.2) and in the development of antibodies with enzymatic activities (catalytic antibodies) (Section 15.3.5).

6.7 EXPRESSION OF FOREIGN GENES

One of the most useful applications of recombinant DNA technology is the ability to artificially synthesise large quantities of natural or modified proteins in a host cell such as bacteria or yeast. The benefits of these techniques have been enjoyed for many years since the first insulin molecules were cloned and expressed in 1982 (Table 6.3). Contamination of other proteins, such as the blood product factor VIII, with infectious agents has also increased the need to develop effective vectors for

Table 6.3 A number of recombinant DNA-derived human therapeutic reagents

Therapeutic area	Recombinant product
Drugs	Erythropoietin
	Insulin
	Growth hormone
	Coagulation factors (e.g. factor VIII)
	Plasminogen activator
Vaccines	Hepatitis B
Cytokines/growth factors	GM-CSF
	G-CSF
	Interleukins
	Interferons

GM-CSF, granulocyte–macrophage colony-stimulating factor; G-CSF, granulocyte colony-stimulating factor.

in vitro expression of foreign genes. In general, the expression of foreign genes is carried out in specialised cloning vectors (Fig. 6.34). However, it is possible to use cell-free transcription and translation systems that direct the synthesis of proteins without the need to grow and maintain cells. *In vitro* translation is carried out with the appropriate amino acids, ribosomes, tRNA molecules and isolated mRNA fractions. Wheat germ extracts or rabbit reticulocyte lysates are usually the systems of choice for *in vitro* translation. The resulting proteins may be detected by polyacrylamide gel electrophoresis or by immunological detection using western blotting. Recently oligonucleotide PCR primers have been designed to incorporate a promoter for RNA polymerase and a ribosome binding site. When the so-called expression PCR (E-PCR) is carried out, the amplified products are denatured and transcribed by RNA polymerase, after which they are translated *in vitro*. The advantage of this system is that large amounts of specific RNA are synthesised, thus increasing the yield of specific proteins (Fig. 6.35).

6.7.1 Production of fusion proteins

For a foreign gene to be expressed in a bacterial cell, it must have particular promoter sequences upstream from the coding region, to which the RNA polymerase will bind prior to transcription of the gene. The choice of promoter is vital for correct and efficient transcription, since the sequence and position of promoters are specific to a particular host such as bacteria (Section 5.5.5). It must also contain a ribosome binding site, placed just before the coding region. Unless a cloned gene contains both of these sequences, it will not be expressed in a bacterial host cell. If the gene has been produced via cDNA from a eukaryotic cell, then it will certainly not have any such sequences. Consequently, expression vectors have been developed that contain promoter and ribosome binding sites positioned just before one or more restriction sites for the insertion of foreign DNA. These

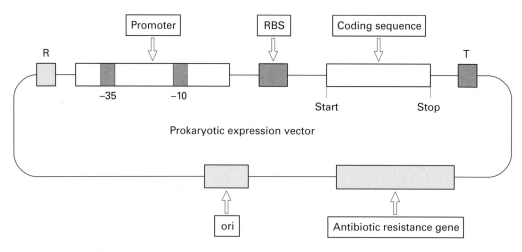

Fig. 6.34. Components of a typical prokaryotic expression vector. To produce a transcript (coding sequence) and translate it, a number of sequences in the vector are required. These include the promoter and ribosome-binding site (RBS). The activity of the promoter may be modulated by a regulatory gene (R), which acts in a way similar to that of the regulatory gene in the *lac* operon. T indicates a transcription terminator.

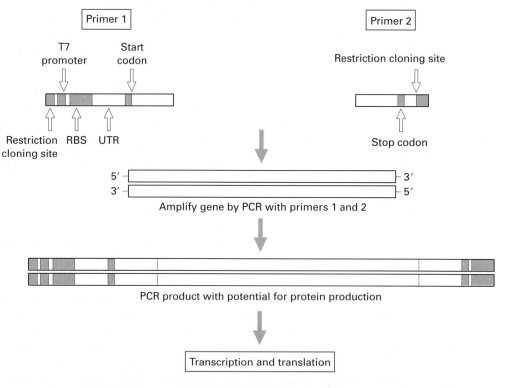

Fig. 6.35. Expression PCR (E-PCR). This technique amplifies a target sequence with one promoter that contains a transcriptional promoter, ribosome binding site (RBS), untranslated leader region (UTR) and start codon. The other primer contains a stop codon. The amplified PCR products may be used in transcription and translation to produce a protein.

regulatory sequences, such as that from the *lac* operon of *E. coli*, are usually derived from genes that, when induced, are strongly expressed in bacteria. Since the mRNA produced from the gene is read as triplet codons, the inserted sequence must be placed so that its reading frame is in phase with the regulatory sequence. This can be ensured by the use of three vectors that differ only in the number of bases between promoter and insertion site, the second and third vectors being, respectively, one and two bases longer than the first. If an insert is cloned in all three vectors then, in general, it will subsequently be in the correct reading frame in one of them. The resulting clones can be screened for the production of a functional foreign protein (Section 6.5.4).

In some cases the protein is expressed as a fusion with a general protein such as β-galactosidase or glutathione *S*-transferase (GST) to facilitate its recovery. It may also be tagged with a moiety such as a polyhistidine (6×His-Tag), which binds strongly to a nickel-chelate-nitrilotriacetate (Ni-NTA) chromatography column. The usefulness of this method is that the binding is independent of the three-dimensional structure of the 6×His-Tag and so recovery is efficient even under the strong denaturing conditions often required for membrane proteins and inclusion bodies (Fig. 6.36). The tags are subsequently removed by cleavage with a reagent such as cyanogen bromide and the protein of interest purified by protein biochemical methods such as chromatography and polyacrylamide gel electrophoresis.

It is not only possible but usually essential to use cDNA instead of a eukaryotic genomic DNA to direct the production of a functional protein by bacteria. This is because bacteria are not capable of processing RNA to remove introns, and so any foreign genes must be pre-processed as cDNA if they contain introns. A further problem arises if the protein must be glycosylated, by the addition of oligosaccharides at specific sites, in order to become functional. Although the use of bacterial expression systems is somewhat limited for eukaryotic systems there are a number of eukaryotic expression systems based on plant, mammalian, insect and yeast cells. These types of cell can perform such post-translational modifications, producing a correct glycosylation pattern and in some cases the correct removal of introns. It is also possible to include a signal or address sequence at the 5′ end of the mRNA that directs the protein to a particular cellular compartment or even out of the cell altogether into the supernatant. This makes the recovery of expressed recombinant proteins much easier, since the supernatant may be drawn off whilst the cells are still producing protein.

One useful eukaryotic expression system is based on the monkey COS cell line. These cells each contain a region derived from a mammalian monkey virus termed simian virus 40 (SV40). A defective region of the SV40 genome has been stably integrated into the COS cell genome. This allows the expression of a protein, termed the large T antigen, that is required for viral replication. When a recombinant vector having the SV40 origin of replication and carrying foreign DNA is inserted into the COS cells, viral replication takes place. This results in a high level of expression of foreign proteins. The disadvantages of this system are the ultimate lysis of the COS cells and the limited insert capacity of the vector. Much interest is also currently focused on other modified viruses: vaccinia virus and baculovirus.

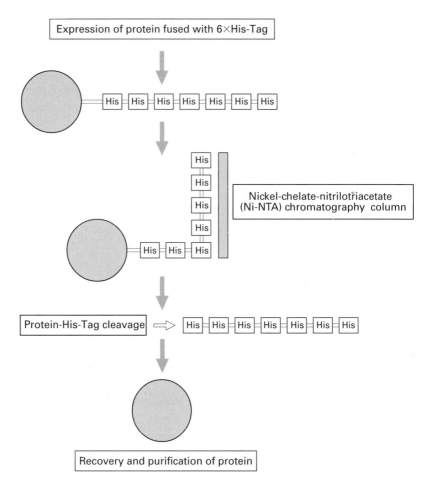

Fig. 6.36. Recovery of proteins using (6×His-Tag) and (Ni-NTA) chromatography columns.

These have been developed for high level expression in mammalian cells and insect cells, respectively. The vaccinia virus in particular has been used to correct the defective ion transport by introducing a wild-type cystic fibrosis gene into cells bearing a mutated cystic fibrosis transmember regulator (CFTR) gene. There is no doubt that the further development of these vector systems will enhance eukaryotic protein expression in the future.

6.7.2 Phage display techniques

As a result of the production of phagemid vectors and as a means of overcoming the problems of screening large numbers of clones generated from genomic libraries of antibody genes, a method for linking the phenotype or expressed protein with the genotype has been devised. This is termed phage display, since a functional protein is linked to a major coat protein of a coliphage whilst the single-stranded gene encoding the protein is packaged within the virion. The initial steps of the

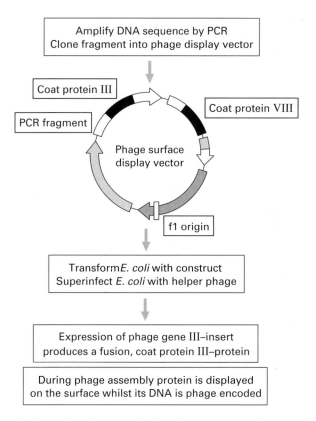

Fig. 6.37. Flow diagram indicating the main steps in the phage display technique.

method rely on the PCR to amplify gene fragments that represent functional domains or subunits of a protein such as an antibody. These are then cloned into a phage display vector that is an adapted phagemid vector (Section 6.3.3) and used to transform *E. coli*. A helper phage is then added to provide accessory proteins for new phage molecules to be constructed. The DNA fragments representing the protein or polypeptide of interest are also transcribed and translated, but linked to the major coat protein gIII. Thus, when the phage is assembled, the protein or polypeptide of interest is incorporated into the coat of the phage and displayed, whilst the corresponding DNA is encapsulated (Fig. 6.37).

There are numerous applications for the display of proteins on the surface of phage, viruses, bacteria and other organisms, and commercial organisations have been quick to exploit this technology. One major application is the analysis and production of the engineered antibodies from which the technology was mainly developed. Screening of novel recombinants may be carried out by techniques such as affinity chromatography. In this way it is possible to generate large numbers of antibody heavy and light chain genes by PCR amplification and mix them in a random fashion. This recombinatorial library approach may provide new or novel partners to be formed as well as naturally existing ones. This strategy is not restricted to antibodies and vast libraries of peptides may be used in this combinatorial chemistry approach to identify novel compounds for use in biotechnology and medicine.

Phage-based cloning methods also offer the advantage of allowing mutagenesis to be performed with relative ease. This may allow the production of antibodies with affinities approaching that derived from the human or mouse immune system. This may be brought about by using an error-prone DNA polymerase in the initial steps of constructing a phage display library. It is possible that these types of library may provide a route to high-affinity recombinant antibody fragments that are difficult to produce by more conventional hybridoma fusion techniques (Section 7.2.4). Surface display libraries have also been prepared for the selection of ligands, hormones and other polypeptides in addition to allowing studies on protein–protein or protein–DNA interactions, or determining the precise binding domains in these receptor–ligand interactions.

6.8 ANALYSING GENES AND GENE EXPRESSION

6.8.1 Identifying and analysing mRNA

The levels and expression patterns of mRNA dictate many cellular processes and therefore there is much interest in the ability to analyse and determine levels of a particular mRNA. Technologies such as real time or quantative PCR and microchip expression arrays are currently being employed and refined for high throughput analysis. A number of other informative techniques have been developed that allow the fine structure of a particular mRNA to be analysed and the relative amounts of an RNA quantified by non-PCR based methods. This is not only important for gene regulation studies but may also be used as a marker for certain clinical disorders. Traditionally the northern blot has been used for detection of particular RNA transcripts by blotting extracted mRNA and immobilising it onto a nylon membrane (Section 5.9.2). Subsequent hybridisation with labelled gene probes allows precise determination of the size and nature of a transcript. However, recently much use has been made of a number of nucleases that digest only single-stranded nucleic acids and not double-stranded molecules. In particular the ribonuclease protection assay (RPA) has allowed much information to be gained regarding the nature of mRNA transcripts (Fig. 6.38). In the RPA, single-stranded mRNA is hybridised in solution to a labelled, single-stranded RNA probe that is in excess. The hybridised part of the complex becomes protected whereas the unhybridised part of the probe made from RNA is digested with RNase A and RNase T1. The protected fragment may then be analysed on a high resolution polyacrylamide gel. This method may give valuable information regarding the mRNA in terms of the precise structure of the transcript (transcription start site, intron/exon junctions, etc.). It is also quantitative and requires less RNA than a northern blot. A related technique, S1 nuclease mapping, is similar, although the unhybridised part of a DNA probe, rather than an RNA probe, is digested, this time with the enzyme S1 nuclease.

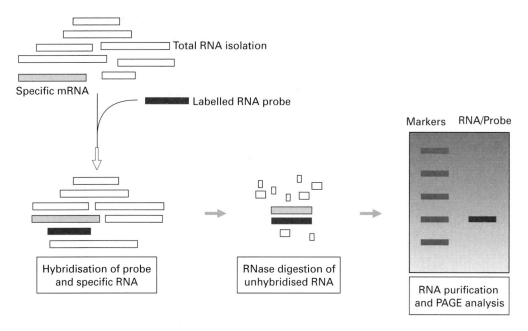

Fig. 6.38. Steps involved in the ribonuclease protection assay (RPA).

The PCR has also had an impact on the analysis of RNA via the development of a technique known as reverse transcriptase–PCR (RT–PCR). Here the RNA is isolated and a first strand cDNA synthesis undertaken with reverse transcriptase, the cDNA is then used in a conventional PCR (Section 6.2.5). Under certain circumstances a number of thermostable DNA polymerases have reverse transcriptase activity that obviates the need to separate the two reactions and allows the RT–PCR to be carried out in one tube. One of the main benefits of RT–PCR is the ability to identify rare or low levels of mRNA transcripts with great sensitivity. This is especially useful when detecting, for example, viral gene expression and furthermore allows the means of differentiating between latent and active virus (Fig. 6.39). The level of mRNA production may also be determined by using a PCR-based method, termed quantitative PCR (Section 5.10.7).

In many cases the analysis of tissue-specific gene expression is required and again the PCR has been adapted to provide a solution. This technique termed differential display is also an RT–PCR based system requiring that isolated mRNA be first converted into cDNA. Following this, one of the PCR primers designed to anneal to a general mRNA element such as the poly(A) tail in eukaryotic cells is used in conjunction with a combination of arbitrary 6–7 bp primers that bind to the 5′ end of the transcripts. Consequently this results in the generation of multiple PCR products with reproducible patterns (Fig. 6.40). Comparative analysis by gel electrophoresis of PCR products generated from different cell types therefore allows the identification and isolation of those transcripts that are differentially expressed. As with many PCR-based techniques the time to identify such genes is dramatically reduced from the weeks that are required to construct and screen cDNA libraries to a few days.

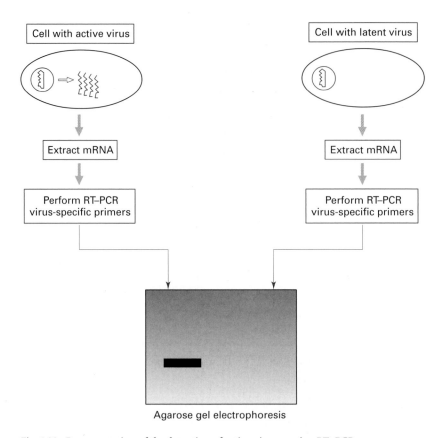

Fig. 6.39. Representation of the detection of active viruses using RT–PCR.

6.8.2 **Analysing genes *in situ***

Gross chromosomal changes are often detectable by microscopic examination of the chromosomes within a karyotype (Section 5.3.3). Single or restricted numbers of base substitutions, deletions, rearrangements or insertions are far less easily detectable but may induce similarly profound effects on normal cellular biochemistry. *In situ* hybridisation makes it possible to determine the chromosomal location of a particular gene fragment or gene mutation. This is carried out by preparing a radiolabelled DNA or RNA probe and applying this to a tissue or chromosomal preparation fixed to a microscope slide. Any probe that does not hybridise to complementary sequences is washed off and an image of the distribution or location of the bound probe is viewed by autoradiography (Fig. 6.41). Using tissue or cells fixed to slides it is also possible to carry out *in situ* PCR. This is a highly sensitive technique where PCR is carried out directly on the tissue slide with the standard PCR reagents. Specially adapted thermal cycling machines are required to hold the slide preparations and allow the PCR to proceed. This allows the localisation and identification of, for example, single copies of intracellular viruses.

An alternative labelling strategy used in karyotyping and gene localisation is fluorescence *in situ* hybridisation (FISH). This method, sometimes termed

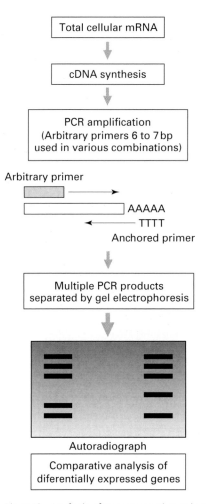

Fig. 6.40. Analysis of gene expression using differential display PCR.

chromosome painting, is based on *in situ* hybridisation but different gene probes are labelled with different fluorochromes, each specific for a particular chromosome. The advantage of this method is that separate gene regions may be identified and comparisons made within the same chromosome preparation. The technique is also likely to be highly useful in genome mapping for ordering DNA probes along a chromosomal segment (Section 6.9).

6.8.3 Analysing promoter–protein interactions

To determine potential transcriptional regulatory sequences, genomic DNA fragments may be cloned into specially devised promoter probe vectors. These contain sites for insertion of foreign DNA that lies upstream from a reporter gene. A number of reporter genes are currently used including the *lacZ* gene encoding β-galactosidase, the *CAT* gene encoding chloramphenicol acetyl transferase (CAT)

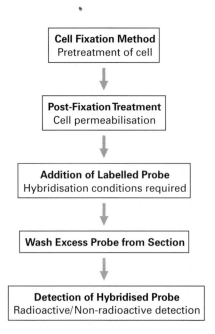

Fig. 6.41. General scheme for *in situ* hybridisation.

and the *lux* gene, which produces luciferase and is determined in a bioluminescent assay. Fragments of DNA, potentially containing a promoter region, are cloned into the vector and the constructs transfected into eukaryotic cells. Any expression of the reporter gene will be driven by the foreign DNA, which must therefore contain promoter sequences (Fig. 6.42). These plasmids and other reporter genes such as those using green fluorescent protein (GFP) or the firefly luciferase gene allow quantification of gene transcription in response to transcriptional activators.

The binding of a regulatory protein or transcription factor to a specific DNA site results in a complex that may be analysed by the technique gel retardation. Under gel electrophoresis, the migration of a DNA fragment bound to a protein of a relatively large mass will be retarded by comparison with the DNA fragment alone. For gel retardation to be useful, the region containing the promoter DNA element must be digested or mapped with a restriction endonuclease before it is complexed with the protein. The location of the promoter may then be defined by finding, on the restriction map, the position of the fragment that binds to the regulatory protein and therefore retards it during electrophoresis. One potential problem with gel retardation is the ability to define the precise nucleotide-binding region of the protein, since this depends on the accuracy and detail of the restriction map and the convenience of the restriction sites. However, it is a useful first step in determining the interaction of a regulatory protein with a DNA-binding site.

DNA footprinting relies on the fact that the interaction of a DNA-binding protein with a regulatory DNA sequence will protect that DNA sequence from degradation by an enzyme such as DNase I. The DNA regulatory sequence is first

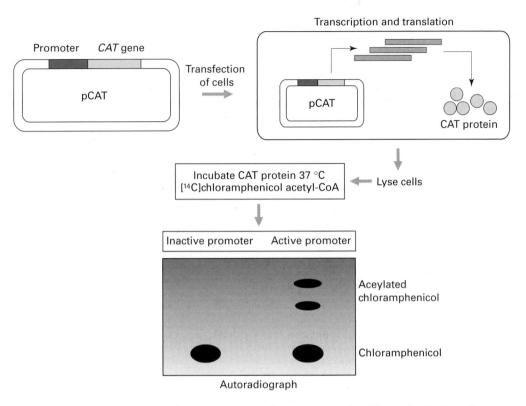

Fig. 6.42. Assay for promoters using the reporter gene for chloramphenicol acetyl transferase (CAT).

labelled at one end with a radioactive label and then mixed with the DNA-binding protein (Fig. 6.43). DNase I is added and partial digestion is then carried out. This limited digestion ensures that a number of fragments are produced where the DNA is not protected by the DNA-binding protein. The region protected by the DNA-binding protein will remain undigested. All the fragments are then separated on a high resolution polyacrylamide gel alongside a control digestion where no DNA-binding protein is present. The autoradiograph of a gel will contain a ladder of bands representing the partially digested fragments. Where DNA has been protected no bands appear, this region or hole is termed the DNA footprint. The position of the protein-binding sequence within the DNA may be elucidated from the size of the fragments either side of the footprint region. Footprinting is a more precise method of locating a DNA–protein interaction than gel retardation; however, it also is unable to give any information as to the precise interaction with or the contribution from individual nucleotides.

In addition to the detection of DNA sequences that contribute to the regulation of gene expression, an ingenious way of detecting the protein transcription factors has been developed. This is termed the yeast two-hybrid system. Transcription factors have two domains, one for DNA binding and the other to allow binding to further proteins (activation domain). These occur as part of the

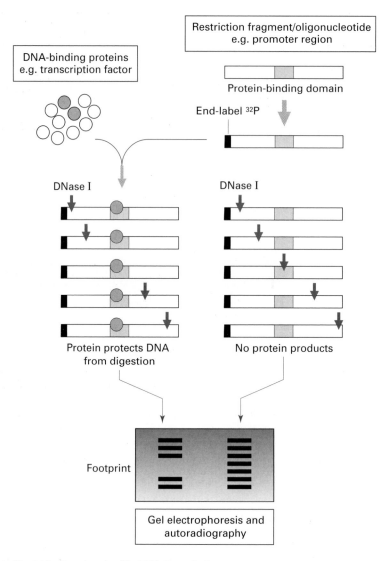

Fig. 6.43. Steps involved in DNA footprinting.

same molecule in natural transcription factors, for example TFIID (Section 5.5.4). However, they may also be formed from two separate domains. Thus a recombinant molecule is formed encoding the protein under study as a fusion with the DNA-binding domain. It cannot, however, activate transcription. Genes from a cDNA library are expressed as a fusion with the activator domain; this also cannot initiate transcription. But when the two fractions are mixed together transcription is initiated if the domains are complementary (Fig. 6.44). This is indicated by the transcription of a reporter gene such as the *CAT* gene. The technique is not confined only to transcription factors and may be applied to any protein system where interaction occurs.

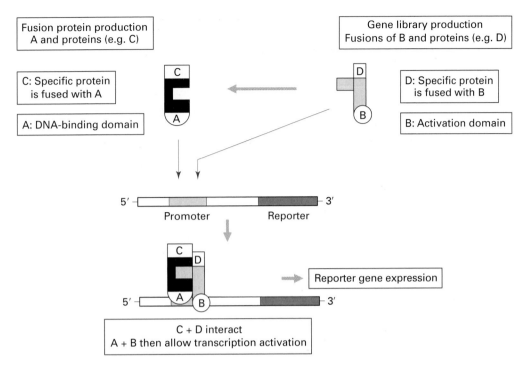

Fig. 6.44. Yeast two-hybrid system (interaction trapping technique). Transcription factors have two domains, one for DNA biding (A) and the other to allow binding to further proteins (B). Thus a recombinant molecule is formed from a protein (C) as a fusion with the DNA-binding domain. It cannot, however, activate transcription alone. Genes from a cDNA library (D) are expressed as a fusion with the activator domain (B) but also cannot initiate transcription alone. When the two fractions are mixed together, transcription is initiated if the domains are complementary and expression of a reporter gene takes place.

6.8.4 **Transgenics and gene targeting**

In many cases it is desirable to analyse the effect of certain genes and proteins in an organism rather than in the laboratory. Furthermore the production of pharmaceutical products and therapeutic proteins is also desirable in a whole organism (Table 6.4). This also has important consequences for the biotechnology and agricultural industries (see Table 6.10) (Section 6.11). The introduction of foreign genes into germ line cells and the production of an altered organism is termed transgenics. There are two broad strategies for transgenesis. The first is direct transgenesis in mammals, whereby recombinant DNA is injected directly into the male pronucleus of a recently fertilised egg. This zygote is then raised in a foster mother animal resulting in an offspring that is all transgenic. Selective transgenesis is where the recombinant DNA is transferred into embryo stem (ES) cells. The cells are then cultured in the laboratory and those expressing the desired protein selected and incorporated into the inner cell mass of an early embryo. The resulting transgenic animal is raised in a foster mother, but in this case the transgenic animal is a mosaic

Table 6.4 Use of transgenic mice for investigation of selected human disorders

Gene/protein	Genetic lesion	Disorder in humans
Tyrosine kinase (TK)	Constitutive expression of gene	Cardiac hypertrophy
HIV transactivator	Expression of HIV *tat* gene	Kaposi's sarcoma
Angiotensinogen	Expression of rat angiotensinogen gene	Hypertension
Cholesterol ester transfer protein (CET protein)	Expression of *CET* gene	Atherosclerosis
Hypoxanthine-guanine phosphoribosyl transferase (HPRT)	Inactivation of *HPRT* gene	HPRT deficiency

or chimeric, since only a small proportion of the cells will be expressing the protein. The initial problem with both approaches is the random nature of the integration of the recombinant DNA into the genome of the egg or embryo stem cells. This may produce proteins in cells where it is not required or disrupt genes necessary for correct growth and development.

A refinement of this is gene targeting, which involves the production of an altered gene in an intact cell, a form of *in vivo* mutagenesis as opposed to *in vitro* mutagenesis (Section 6.6.2). The gene is inserted into the genome of, for example, an ES cell by specialised virus-based vectors. The insertion is non-random, however, since homologous sequences exist on the vector to the gene and on the gene to be targeted. Thus homologous recombination may introduce a new genetic property on the cell, or inactivate an existing one, termed gene knockout. Perhaps the most important aspect of these techniques is that they allow animal models of human diseases to be created. This is useful, since the physiological and biochemical consequences of a disease are often complex and difficult to study, impeding the development of diagnostic and therapeutic strategies.

6.8.5 Modulating gene expression by RNAi

There are a number of ways of experimentally changing the expression of genes. Traditionally methods have focused on altering the levels of mRNA by manipulation of promoter sequences or levels of accessory proteins involved in the control of expression. In addition, post-mRNA production methods have also been employed such as antisense RNA, where a nucleic acid sequence complementary to an expressed mRNA is delivered into the cell. This antisense sequence binds to the mRNA and prevents its translation. A development of this theme and a process that is found in a variety of normal cellular processes is termed RNA interference or RNAi and uses micro RNA. Here, a number of techniques have been developed that allow the modulation of gene expression in certain cells. This type of cell-based gene expression modulation will no doubt extend to many organisms in the next few years.

6.8.6 **Analysing genetic mutations**

There are several types of mutation that can occur in nucleic acids, either transiently or by being stably incorporated into the genome. During evolution, mutations may be inherited in one or both copies of a chromosome, resulting in polymorphisms within the population (Section 5.3). Mutations may occur potentially at any site within the genome; however, there are several instances whereby mutations occur in limited regions. This is particularly obvious in prokaryotes, where elements of the genome (termed hypervariable regions) undergo extensive mutations to generate large numbers of variants, by virtue of the high rate of replication of the organisms. Similar hypervariable sequences are generated in the normal antibody immune response in eukaryotes. Mutations may have several effects upon the structure and function of the genome. Some mutations may lead to undetectable effects upon normal cellular functions, termed conservative mutations. Examples of these are mutations that occur in intron sequences and therefore play no part in the final structure and function of the protein or its regulation. Alternatively, mutations may result in profound effects upon normal cell function such as altered transcription rates or on the sequence of mRNAs necessary for normal cellular processes.

Mutations occurring within exons may alter the amino acid composition of the encoded protein by causing amino acid substitution or by changing the reading frame used during translation. These point mutations have traditionally been detected by Southern blotting or, if a convenient restriction site is available, by restriction fragment length polymorphism (RFLP) (Section 5.9.1). However, the PCR has been used to great effect in mutation detection, since it is possible to use allele-specific oligonucleotide PCR (ASO–PCR) where two competing primers and one general primer are used in the reaction (Fig. 6.45). One of the primers is directly complementary to the known point mutation whereas the other is a wild-type primer; that is, the primers are identical except for the terminal 3′ end base. Thus, if the DNA contains the point mutation, only the primer with the complementary sequence will bind and be incorporated into the amplified DNA, whereas, if the DNA is normal, the wild-type primer is incorporated. The results of the PCR are analysed by agarose gel electrophoresis. A further modification of ASO-PCR has been developed where the primers are each labelled with a different fluorochrome. Since the primers are labelled differently, a positive or negative result is produced directly without the need to examine the PCRs by gel electrophoresis.

Various modifications now allow more than one PCR to be carried out at a time (multiplex PCR), and hence the simultaneous detection of more than one mutation is possible. Where the mutation is unknown, it is also possible to use a PCR system with a gel-based detection method termed denaturing gradient gel electrophoresis (DGGE). In this technique a sample DNA heteroduplex containing a mutation is amplified by the PCR, which is also used to attach a G + C rich sequence to one end of the heteroduplex. The mutated heteroduplex is identified by its altered melting properties through a polyacrylamide gel that contains a gradient of denaturant

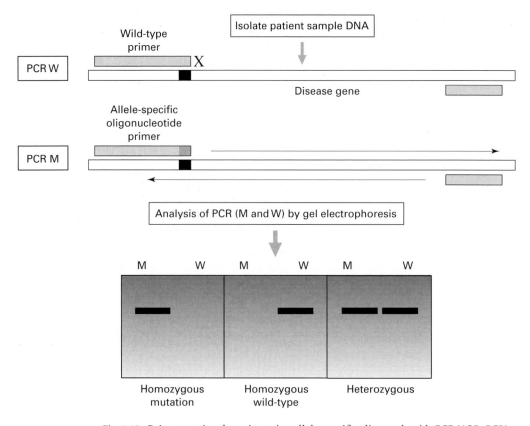

Fig. 6.45. Point mutation detection using allele-specific oligonucleotide PCR (ASO–PCR).

such as urea. At a certain point in the gradient the heteroduplex will denature relative to a perfectly matched homoduplex and thus may be identified. The GC 'clamp' maintains the integrity of the end of the duplex on passage through the gel (Fig. 6.46). The sensitivity of this and other mutation detection methods has been substantially increased by the use of PCR, and further mutation techniques, used to detect known or unknown mutations, are indicated in Table 6.5. An extension of this principle is used in a number of detection methods employing denaturing high performance liquid chromatography (dHPLC). Commonly known as wave technology, the detection of denatured single strands containing mismatches is rapid, allowing a high throughput analysis of samples to be achieved.

6.8.7 Detecting DNA polymorphisms

Polymorphisms are particularly interesting elements of the human genome and as such may be used as the basis for differentiating between individuals. All humans carry repeats of sequences known as minisatellite DNA, of which the number of repeats varies between unrelated individuals. Hybridisation of probes that anneal to these sequences using Southern blotting provides the means to type and identify those individuals (Section 5.3.1).

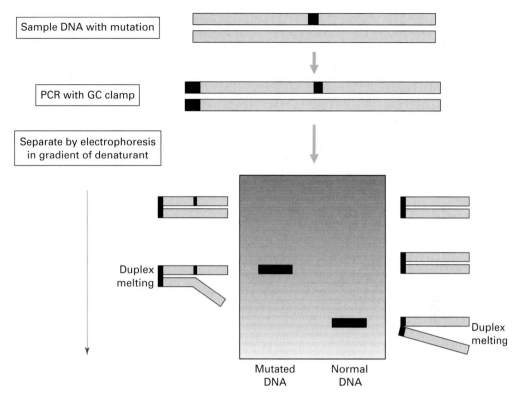

Sample DNA with mutation

PCR with GC clamp

Separate by electrophoresis in gradient of denaturant

Duplex melting

Duplex melting

Mutated DNA   Normal DNA

Fig. 6.46. Detection of mutations using denaturing gradient gel electrophoresis (DGGE).

Table 6.5 **Main methods of detecting mutations in DNA samples**

Technique	Basis of method	Main characteristics of detection
Southern blotting	Gel based	Labelled probe hybridisation to DNA
Dot/slot blotting	Sample application	Labelled probe hybridisation to DNA
Allele-specific oligo-PCR (ASO–PCR)	PCR based	Oligonucleotide matching to DNA sample
Denaturing gradient gel electrophoresis (DGGE)	Gel/PCR based	Melting temperature of DNA strands
Single-stranded conformation polymorphism (SSCP)	Gel/PCR based	Conformation difference of DNA strands
Ligase chain reaction (LCR)	Gel/automated	Oligonucleotide matching to DNA sample
DNA sequencing	Gel based	Nucleotide sequence analysis of DNA
DNA microchips	Glass chip based	Sample DNA hybridisation to oligo arrays

DNA fingerprinting is a collective term for two distinct genetic testing systems that use either 'multilocus' probes or 'single-locus' probes. Initially described DNA fingerprinting probes were multilocus probes, so termed because they detect hypervariable minisatellites throughout the genome (i.e. at multiple locations within the genome). In contrast, several single-locus probes were discovered that under specific conditions detect only the two alleles at a single locus and generate what have been termed DNA profiles because, unlike multilocus probes, the two-band pattern result is in itself insufficient to uniquely identify an individual.

Techniques based on the PCR have been coupled to the detection of minisatellite loci. The inherent larger size of such DNA regions was not best suited to PCR amplification; however, new PCR developments are beginning to allow this to take place. The discovery of polymorphisms within the repeating sequences of minisatellites has led to the development of a PCR-based method that distinguishes an individual on the basis of the random distribution of repeat types along the length of that person's two alleles for one such minisatellite. Known as minisatellite variant repeat (MVR) analysis or digital DNA typing, this technique can lead to a simple numerical coding of the repeat variation detected. Potentially this combines the advantages of PCR sensitivity and rapidity with the discriminating power of minisatellite alleles. Thus, for the future, there are a number of interesting identification systems under development and evaluation. The genetic detection of polymorphisms has been used in many cases of paternity testing and immigration control, and is becoming the central factor in many criminal investigations. It is also a valuable tool in plant biotechnology for cereal typing and in the fields of pedigree analysis and animal breeding.

6.8.8 Microarrays and DNA microchips

One exciting area of current development in molecular biology is in the development and refinement of microarrays or DNA microchips (Section 8.5). These provide a radically different approach to current laboratory molecular biological research strategies in that large-scale analysis and quantification of genes and gene expression are possible simultaneously. A microarray consists of an ordered arrangement of thousands of DNA sequences such as oligonucleotides or cDNAs deposited onto a solid surface approximately 1.2 cm $\times$ 1.2 cm. The solid support is usually glass, although silicon wafers have also been used successfully. Currently the arrays are synthesised on or off the glass and require complex fabrication methods similar to that used in producing microchips. They may also be spotted by robotic ultrafine microarray deposition instruments that dispense volumes as low as 30 pl. Alternatively on-chip fabrication as used by Affymetrix builds up layers of nucleotides using a process, borrowed from the microchip industry, termed photolithography. Here, wafer-thin masks with holes allow photoactivation of specific dNTPs, which are linked together at specific regions on the chip. The whole process allows layers of oligonucleotides to be built up, with each nucleotide at each position being defined by computer.

The arrays themselves may represent a variety of nucleic acid material. This may be mRNA produced in a particular cell type, termed cDNA expression arrays, or may alternatively represent coding and regulatory regions of a particular gene or group of genes. One commercial example uses a 50 000 oligonucleotide array that represents known mutations in a tumour suppressor gene called *p53*, a protein known to be mutated in many human cancers. Thus patient sample DNA is incubated on the array and any unhybridised DNA washed off. The array is then analysed and scanned for patterns of hybridisation by detection of a fluorescence signal. Any mutations in the *p53* gene may be rapidly analysed by computer interpretation of the resulting hybridisation pattern and mutation defined. Indeed the collation and manipulation of data from microarrays presents as big a problem as fabricating the chips in the first place. The potential of microarrays appears to be limitless and a number of arrays have been developed for the detection of various genetic mutations including the cystic fibrosis CFTR gene, the breast cancer gene *BRCA1* and in the study of the human immunodefficiency virus (HIV).

At present, microarrays require DNA to be highly purified, which limits their applicability. However, as DNA purification becomes automated and microarray technology develops it is not difficult to envisage numerous laboratory tests on a single DNA microchip. This could be used for analysing not only single genes but large numbers of genes or DNA representing microorganisms, viruses, etc. Since the potential for quantification of gene transcription exists, expression arrays could also be used in defining a particular disease status. This technique may be very significant, since it will allow large amounts of sequence information to be gathered very rapidly and assist in many fields of molecular biology, especially in large genome sequencing projects or in so-called re-sequencing projects where gene regions such as those containing potentially important polymorphisms require analysis in a number of samples.

One current application of microarray technology is the generation of a catalogue of SNPs across the human genome. Estimates indicate that there are approximately 10 million SNPs and importantly 200 000 coding or cSNPs that lie within genes and may point to the development of certain diseases. SNPs are therefore clearly a candidate for microarray analysis and developments such as the Affymetrix HuSNP chip enables the simultaneous analysis of more than 10 000 SNPs on one gene chip. In order to simplify the problem of the vast numbers of SNPs that need to be analysed a haplotype mapping or HapMap project is underway to analyse SNPs that are inherited as a block; in theory as few as 500 000 SNPs will be required to genotype an individual.

An extension of microarray technology may also be used to analyse tissue sections. This process, termed tissue microarrays (TMA), uses tissue cores or biopsies from conventional paraffin-embedded tissues. Thousands of tissue cores are sliced and placed on a solid support such as glass where they may all be subjected to the same immunohistochemical staining process or analysis with gene probes using *in situ* hybridisation. As with DNA microarrays, many samples may be analysed simultaneously, less tissue is required and greater standardisation is possible.

6.9 ANALYSING WHOLE GENOMES

Perhaps the most ambitious project in the biosciences is the initiative to map and completely sequence a number of genomes from various organisms. The mapping

Table 6.6	Current selected genome-sequencing projects	Genome size (Mb)
Organism		
Bacteria	*Escherichia coli*	4.6
Yeast	*Saccharomyces cerevisiae*	14
Roundworm	*Caenorhabditis elegans*	100
Fruit fly	*Drosophila melanogaster*	165
Puffer fish	*Fugu rubripes rubripes*	400
Mouse	*Mus musculus*	3000

and sequencing of a number of organisms indicated in Table 6.6 has been completed and many more are due for completion. Some have been completed already such as the bacterium *E. coli*. The demands of such large-scale mapping and sequencing have provided the impetus for the development and refinement of even the most standard of molecular biological techniques such as DNA sequencing. It has also led to new methods of identifying the important coding sequences that represent proteins and enzymes. The use of bioinformatics to collate, annotate and publish the information on the World Wide Web has also been an enormous undertaking. The availability of an informative map of the human genome, such as the Genome Web (NCBI), that may be analysed and studied in detail chromosome by chromosome is just one of the rapid developments in the field of genome analysis and bioinformatics. Such is the power and ease of use of resources such as this that it is now inconceivable to work without them.

6.9.1 Physical genome mapping

In terms of genome mapping a physical map is the primary goal. Genetic linkage maps have also been produced by determining the recombination frequency between two particular loci. YAC-based vectors essential for large-scale cloning contain DNA inserts that are on average 300 000 bp in length, which is longer by a factor of 10 than the longest inserts in the clones used in early mapping studies. The development of vectors with large insert capacity has enable the production of contigs. These are continuous overlapping cloned fragments that have been positioned relative to one another. Using these maps any cloned fragment may be identified and aligned to an area in one of the contig maps. In order to position cloned DNA fragments resulting from the construction of a library in a YAC or cosmid it is necessary to detect overlaps between the cloned DNA fragments. Overlaps are created because of the use of partial digestion conditions with a particular restriction endonuclease when constructing the libraries. This ensures that when each DNA fragment is cloned into a vector it has overlapping ends that theoretically may be identified and the clones positioned or ordered so that a physical map may be produced (Fig. 6.47).

In order to position the overlapping ends it is preferable to undertake DNA sequencing; however, owing to the impracticality of this approach a fingerprint of

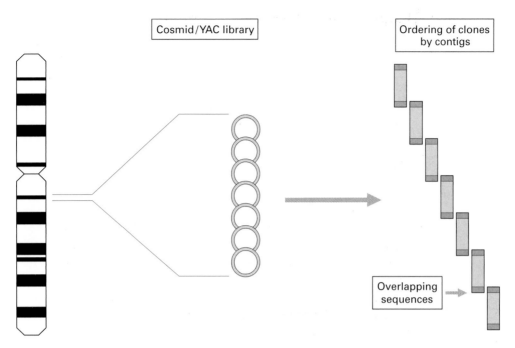

Fig. 6.47. Physical mapping using continuous overlapping cloned fragments (contigs). In order to assign the position of cloned DNA fragments resulting from the construction of a library in a YAC or cosmid vector, overlaps are detected between the clone fragments. These are created because of the use of partial digestion conditions when the libraries are constructed.

each clone is made by using restriction enzyme mapping. Although this is not an unambiguous method of ordering clones, it is useful when also applying statistical probabilities of the overlap between clones. In order to link the contigs, techniques such as *in situ* hybridisation may be used or a probe generated from one end of a contig in order to screen a different disconnected contig. This method of probe production and identification is termed walking, and has been used successfully in the production of physical maps of *E. coli* and yeast genomes. This cycle of clone to fingerprint to contig is amenable to automation; however, the problem of closing the gaps between contigs remains very difficult.

In order to define a common way for all research laboratories to order clones and connect physical maps together an arbitrary molecular technique based on the PCR has been developed based on sequence-tagged sites (STS). This is a small unique sequence of between 200 and 300 bp that is amplified by PCR (Fig. 6.48). The uniqueness of the STS is defined by the PCR primers that flank it. A PCR with those primers is performed and if the PCR results in selected amplification of the target region it may be defined as a potential STS marker. In this way, defining STS markers that lie approximately 100 000 bases apart along a contig map allows the ordering of those contigs. Thus all groups working with clones have definable landmarks with which to order clones produced in their libraries.

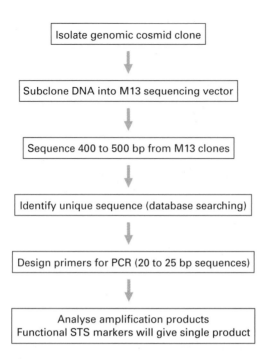

Fig. 6.48. General scheme of the production of a functional STS marker.

The same STS that occurs in two clones may be used to order the clones in a contig. Clones containing the STS are usually detected by Southern blotting where the clones have been immobilised onto a nylon membrane.

Alternatively a library of clones may be divided into pools and and each pool PCR screened. This is usually a more rapid method of identifying an STS within a clone and further refinements of the PCR-based screening method allows the identification of a particular clone within a pool (Fig. 6.49). STS elements may also be generated from variable regions of the genome to produce a polymorphic marker that may be traced through families, along with other DNA markers, and located on a genetic linkage map. These polymorphic STSs are useful, since they may serve as markers on both a physical map and a genetic linkage map for each chromosome and therefore provide a useful marker for aligning the two types of map.

6.9.2 Gene discovery and localisation

A number of disease loci have been identified and located to certain chromosomes. This has been facilitated by the use of *in situ* mapping techniques such as FISH (Section 6.8.2). In fact a number of genes have been identified and their proteins determined where little was initially known about the genes except for their location. This method of gene discovery is known as positional cloning and was instrumental in the isolation of the *CFTR* gene (Fig. 6.50).

The number of genes that are actively expressed in a cell at any one time is estimated to be as little as 10% of the total. The remaining DNA is packaged and serves

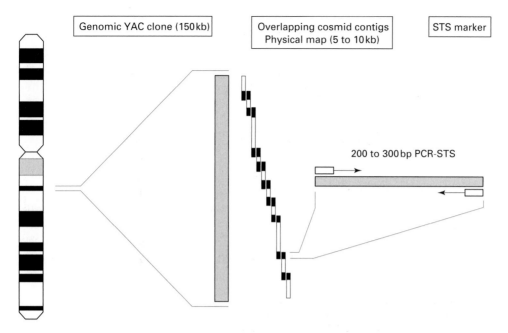

Fig. 6.49. The derivation of an STS marker. An STS is small unique sequence of between 200 and 300 bp that is amplified by PCR and allows ordering along a contig map. Such sequences are definable landmarks with which to order clones produced in genome libraries and usually lie approximately 100 000 bp apart.

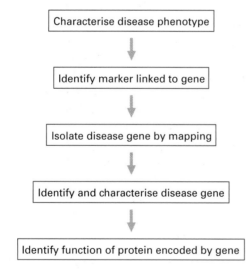

Fig. 6.50. The scheme of identification of a disease gene by positional cloning.

an as-yet unknown function. Recent investigations have found that certain active genes may be identified by the presence of so-called HTF (*Hpa*II tiny fragments) islands often found at the 5′ end of genes. These are CpG-rich sequences that are not methylated and form tiny fragments on digestion with the restriction enzyme *Hpa*II. A further gene discovery method that has been used extensively in the past few years is a PCR-based technique giving rise to a product termed an expressed-sequence tag (EST). This represents part of a putative gene for which a function has yet to be assigned. It is carried out on cDNA by using primers that bind to an anchor sequence such as a poly(A) tail and primers that bind to sequences at the 5′ end of the gene. Such PCRs may subsequently be used to map the putative gene to a chromosomal region or be used as probes to search a genomic DNA library for the remaining parts of the gene. Much interest currently lies in ESTs, since they may represent a shortcut to gene discovery.

A further gene isolation system that uses adapted vectors, termed exon trapping or exon amplification, may be used to identify exon sequences. Exon trapping requires the use of a specialised expression vector that will accept fragments of genomic DNA containing sequences for splicing reactions to take place. Following transfection of a eukaryotic cell line, a transcript is produced that may be detected by using specific primers in a RT–PCR. This indicates the nature of the foreign DNA by virtue of the splicing sequences present. A list of further techniques that aid in the identification of a potential gene-encoding sequence is indicated in Table 6.7.

6.9.3 **Human Genome Project**

There is no doubt that the mapping and sequencing of the human genome was one of the most ambitious projects in contemporary science. Completed ahead of schedule, it has provided many new insights into gene function and gene regulation. It was also a multicollaborative effort that has engaged scientific research groups around the world and given rise to many scientific, technical, financial and ethical debates. One interesting issue is the sequencing of the whole genome in relation to the coding sequences. Much of the human genome appears to be non-coding and composed of repetitive sequences. Estimates indicate that as little as 10% of the genome appears to encode enzymes and proteins. Nevertheless this still corresponds to approximately 22 000 genes, although the understanding of the complete function of many remains a challenge. There is an extensive use of alternative splicing, where exons are essentially mixed and matched to form different mRNAs and thus different proteins. The study further aims to understand and possibly provide the eventual means of treating some of the 4000 known genetic diseases in addition to other diseases whose inheritance is multifactorial. In this respect there are a number of specific genome projects such as the Cancer Genome Anatomy Project that aim to understand the mutations that arise in the development of tumours.

6.10 **PHARMACOGENOMICS**

As a result of the developments in genomics, new methods of providing targeted drug treatment are beginning to be developed. This area is linked to the proposal that it is possible to identify those people that react in a specific way to drug treatment by identifying their genetic make-up. In particular SNPs (single nucleotide polymorphisms) may provide a key marker of potential disease development and

Table 6.7 Techniques used to determine putative gene-encoding sequences

Identification method	Main details
Zoo blotting (cross-hybridisation)	Evolutionary conservation of DNA sequences that suggest functional significance
Homology searching	Gene database searching to gene family-related sequences
Identification of CpG islands	Regions of hypomethylated CpG frequently found 5′ to genes in vertebrate animals
Identification of open reading frames (ORF) promoters/splice sites/RBS	DNA sequences scanned for consensus sequences by computer
Northern blot hybridisation	mRNA detection by binding to labelled gene probes
Exon trapping technique	Artificial RNA splicing assay for exon identification
Expressed sequence tags (ESTs)	cDNAs amplified by PCR that represent part of a gene

RBS, ribosome binding site; cDNA, complementary DNA.

reaction to a particular treatment. A simple example that has been known for some time is the reaction to a drug used to treat childhood acute lymphoblastic leukaemia. Successful treatment of the majority of patients may be achieved with 6-mercaptopurine. A number of patients do not respond well, but in some cases it may be fatal to administer this drug. This is now known to be due to a mutation in the gene encoding the enzyme that metabolises the drug. Thus it is possible to analyse patient DNA prior to administration of a drug to determine what the likely response will be. The technology to deduce a patient's genotype is already developed as indicated in Section 6.8.7. It is also now possible to analyse SNPs that may also correlate with certain disease processes in a microarray type format. This opens up the possibility that it may be possible to assign a pharmacogenetic profile at birth, in much the same way as blood typing for later treatment. A further possibility is the determination of likely susceptibility to a disease based on genetic information. This is available at present, although in a limited form, and commercial operations such as the Icelandic genetics company deCode may provide information based on analysis of disease genes in large population studies.

6.11 MOLECULAR BIOTECHNOLOGY AND ITS APPLICATIONS

It is a relatively short time since the early 1970s, when the first recombinant DNA experiments were carried out. However, huge strides have been made not only in the development of molecular biology techniques but also in their practical

Table 6.8 **General classification of oncogenes and their cellular and biochemical functions**

Oncogene	Example	Main details
G-proteins	H-K- and N-*ras*	GTP-binding protein/GTPase
Growth factors	*sis, nt-2, hst*	β-chain of PDGF (platelet-derived growth factor)
Growth factor receptors	*erbB*	Epidermal growth factor receptor (EGFR)
	fms	Colony-stimulating factor-1 receptor
Protein kinases	*abl, src*	Protein tyrosine kinases
	mos, ras	Protein serine kinases
Nucleus-located transcription factors	*myc*	DNA-binding protein
	myb	DNA-binding protein
	jun, fos	DNA-binding protein

Table 6.9 **A number of selected examples of targets for gene therapy**

Disorder	Defect	Gene target	Target cell
Emphysema	Deficiency (α1-AT)	α1-Antitrypsin (α1-AT)	Liver cells
Gaucher disease (storage disorder)	GC deficiency	Glucocerebrosidase	GC fibroblasts
Haemoglobinopathies	Thalassaemia	β-Globin	Fibroblasts
Lesch–Nyhan syndrome	Metabolic deficiency	Hypoxanthine guanine phosphoribosyl transferase (HPRT)	HPRT cells
Immune system disorder	Adenosine deaminase deficiency	Adenosine deaminase (ADA)	T and B cells

Table 6.10 **Current selected plant/crops modified by genetic manipulation**

Crop or plant	Genetic modification
Canola (oil seed rape)	Insect resistance, seed oil modification
Maize	Herbicide tolerance, resistance to insects
Rice	Modified seed storage protein, insect resistance
Soybean	Tolerance to herbicide, modified seed storage protein
Tomato	Modified ripening, resistance to insects and viruses
Sunflower	Modified seed storage protein

application. The molecular basis of disease and the new areas of genetic analysis and gene therapy hold great promise. In the past, medical science relied on the measurement of protein and enzyme markers that reflect disease states. It is possible now not only to detect such abnormalities at an earlier stage using mRNA techniques but also in some cases to predict such states using genome analysis. The complete mapping and sequencing of the human genome and the development of techniques such as DNA microchips will certainly accelerate such events. Perhaps even more difficult is the elucidation of diseases that are multifactorial and involve a significant contribution from environmental factors. One of the best-studied examples of this type of disease is cancer. Molecular genetic analysis has allowed a discrete set of cellular genes, termed oncogenes, to be defined that play key roles in such events. These genes and their proteins are also active at major points in the cell cycle and are intimately involved in cell regulation. A number of these are indicated in Table 6.8. In some cancers, well-defined molecular events have been correlated with mutations in oncogenes and therefore in the corresponding proteins. It is already possible to screen and predict the fate of some disease processes at an early stage, a point which itself raises significant ethical dilemmas. In addition to understanding cellular processes in both normal and disease states, great promise is also evident in drug discovery and molecular gene therapy. A number of genetically engineered therapeutic proteins and enzymes have been developed and are already having an impact on disease management. In addition, the correction of disorders at the gene level (gene therapy) is also under way and perhaps is one of the most startling applications of molecular biology to date. A number of these developments are indicated in Table 6.9.

The production of modified crops and animals for farming and as producers of important therapeutic proteins are also three of the most exciting developments of molecular biology. Genetic manipulation has allowed the production of modified crops, improving their resistance to environmental factors and their stability (Table 6.10). The production of transgenic animals also holds great promise for improved livestock quality, low cost production of pharmaceuticals and disease-free or disease-resistant strains. In the future this may overcome such factors as contamination with agents such as BSE. There is no doubt that improved methods of producing livestock by whole-animal cloning will also be of major benefit. All of these developments do, however, require debate and the many ethical considerations that arise from them require careful consideration.

6.12 **SUGGESTIONS FOR FURTHER READING**

ALBERTS, B., JOHNSON, A., LEWIS, J., RAFF, M., ROBERT, K. and WATER, P. (2002). *Molecular Biology of the Cell*, 4th edn. Garland Publishing, London. (A comprehensive all round text.)

BROWN, T. A. (2001). *Gene Cloning and DNA Analysis: An Introduction*. Blackwell Science, Oxford. (A very good introduction to genetics and molecular biology.)

BROWN, T. A. (2002). *Genomes 2*. Bios Scientific Publishers, Oxford. (A very good introduction to the concepts of the genome.)

RAPLEY, R. and HARBRON, S. (2004). *Molecular Analysis and Genome Discovery*. John Wiley & Sons, Chichester. (An up-to-date collection of key nucleic acid and proteins techniques in analysis and drug discovery.)

STRACHEN, T. and READ, A. P. (2004). *Human Molecular Genetics*. Garland Science, London. (An excellent and comprehensive textbook with very good illustrations.)

TURNER, P. C. C., BATES, A. D. and MCLENNAN, A. G. (2000). *Instant Notes in Molecular Biology*. Barnes and Noble/Bios Scientific Publishers Ltd, Oxford. (A clear treatment of key molecular biology concepts.)

Chapter 7

Immunochemical techniques

7.1 INTRODUCTION

7.1.1 The immune system

The immune system of animals is responsible for mounting immune responses against molecules recognised as being foreign (non-self). The science of immunology studies such responses and the immune system responsible for them.

The immune system provides protection for animals against infectious microorganisms (viruses, bacteria, mycoplasmas, fungi and protozoa) and also helps in the elimination of parasites and toxins. It combats tumours and neoplastic cells and can reject transfused cells and transplanted organs from genetically non-identical animals. Its physiological role is to ensure that the animal is free from life-threatening life forms and biological substances (the derivation of the word 'immunology' is from the Latin *immunitas* = freedom from). Inappropriate (i.e. undesirable) immune responses can cause clinical problems such as allergies, graft-versus-host disease and autoimmune disorders. Immune responses can be classified as either innate or aquired. Innate immunity does not require prior exposure to the foreign substance and is mediated mainly by cells of the monocytic lineage (e.g. macrophages) and polymorphonuclear leukocytes. Innate immunity is relatively non-specific, although it clearly normally distinguishes between self and non-self. It constitutes a potent, rapid-reacting, first-line defence against invasion and unwanted infection. Laboratory procedures based on innate immunity are limited in usefulness in general application to biochemical methodology.

Acquired immunity requires exposure ('priming') to the non-self material. It is mediated primarily by lymphocytes and may be further divided into cell-mediated and humoral immune responses. Cell-mediated immunity can be attributed mainly to the activity of T lymphocytes, which interact with foreign substances (antigens) in a specific manner and mediate a diverse array of immuno-biological processes; for example, cytotoxic T cells specifically 'kill' unwanted cells or microorganisms. Methodology based on cell-mediated immune mechanisms can be useful for the study of cellular immunology and some aspects of clinical immunology, but its application to biochemistry is neither easy nor (usually) useful.

Humoral immunity is mediated primarily by soluble proteins known as antibodies, which circulate in blood and permeate most body organs. They can also be present on cell surfaces, where they function as antigen receptors and binding proteins. Antibodies are produced and secreted by B lymphocytes, but this is influenced by the activity of cells of other types (especially lymphocytes of the T-helper type). Terminally differentiated B cells known as plasma cells are the most potent natural secretors of antibodies. The study of antibodies (and some other immunologically important molecules such as complement components) is known as immunochemistry. Such antibodies can show exquisite specificity and sensitivity for antigens, although this is not always the case, and many procedures and methods have been devised that exploit these properties. Such methods are known as immunochemical techniques. They are obviously very important for studying aspects of immunology itself but are invaluable methods for carrying out investigations in just about every biological science (especially biochemistry). Definitions of some commonly used immunochemical terms are given in Table 7.1.

7.1.2 Antibodies

Antibodies are a group of globular proteins known as immunoglobulins. These consist of monomers or multimers of a basic four-chain, bilaterally symmetrical structure containing two light and two heavy chains (Fig. 7.1). Five varieties of heavy chain (known as γ, μ, α, δ and ϵ chains) occur in higher vertebrates and these determine the class of the immunoglobulin (known as IgG, IgM, IgA, IgD and IgE, respectively; Table 7.2). All classes can bind antigen but the immunobiological functions mediated by the immunoglobulin molecules vary. In mammals, the IgG and IgA classes are divided into subclasses, which reflect different heavy chain amino acid sequences (but less different than the sequences of the different classes). The number of subclasses found differs between species. The light chains do not mediate significant immunobiological activity, but do contribute to antigen binding and the stability and higher structure of the immunoglobulin molecule. IgG, IgE and IgD are predominantly monomers of the basic four-chain structure, but IgA is often dimeric and IgM is pentameric, at least in mammals. Multimeric IgA and IgM contain an additional small protein known as the J chain, which is necessary for polymerisation, and IgA present in secretions also contains a protein known as the secretory component.

Immunoglobulin molecules can be cleaved by some proteolytic enzymes to yield fragments that are useful for immunochemical procedures and also reveal important aspects of antibody structure and function. The plant protease papain cleaves human IgG to yield three fragments of approximately the same size (about $50\,000\ M_r$). Two of the fragments are identical and one is different; the former can be separated from the latter using ion-exchange chromatography. The two identical fragments are able to bind antigen in a monovalent manner, but cannot precipitate antigen from solution or in gel. They are known as fragment–antigen binding or Fab in immunochemical terminology. The third

Table 7.1   Glossary of immunochemical terms

Antigen
A substance that is recognised and bound by an antibody.

Antigenic determinant
See Epitope.

Antiserum
Serum from an animal containing antibodies reacting with particular antigens. Sometimes known as an immune serum.

Autoantibodies
Antibodies that react with self antigen(s). These are not normally present in blood or body fluids, but, if present, are often associated with pathological conditions known as autoimmune diseases, e.g. rheumatoid arthritis, systemic lupus erythematosus, primary biliary cirrhosis, insulin-dependent diabetes mellitus.

Clone
A growing population of cells, derived from a single progenitor cell. The clone is derived asexually by continued division and all cells are genetically identical unless mutation occurs during growth.

Divalent
Able to bind two molecules of ligand. A divalent antibody is thus able to bind two molecules of antigen.

Epitope
A site on the antigen that is recognised and bound by an antibody. It is normally about six amino acid or carbohydrate residues in size. Epitopes on protein antigens may not be continuous in structure. Sometimes also called an antigenic determinant.

Lymphocytes
Cells associated with functions responsible for development and maintenance of specific immunity. They are a subdivision of leukocytes and are the main constituents of lymphoid tissues.

Immunogen
A substance or mixture of substances used to induce an immune response.

Microtitre plate
Plastic plate containing many (usually 96) wells in which many types of imunoassay may be carried out more conveniently than in individual tubes. The wells may be flat-bottomed for use in ELISA, U-shaped for use in RIA or V-shaped for haemagglutination tests. They may be flexible or rigid.

Monovalent
Able to bind only one molecule of ligand.

Multivalent
Able to bind more than one molecule of ligand.

Myeloma cells
Tumour cells of plasma cell lineage. Sometimes also called plasmacytoma cells.

Paraprotein
Monoclonal immunoglobulin secreted by myeloma cells (see above). Such molecules closely resemble immunoglobulins produced by 'normal' plasma cells/lymphocytes. They are sometimes called myeloma proteins.

Peptide
A molecule consisting of a number of amino acid residues linked by peptide bonds. Large peptides are sometimes called polypeptides and/or proteins.

Plasma
Fluid obtained from uncoagulated blood after removal of cellular components. Differs from serum (see below) in containing all components of the coagulation system. Its preparation necessitates the use of an anticoagulant, e.g. heparin, citrate.

Serum
Fluid derived from coagulated blood after removal of the clot and cell components.

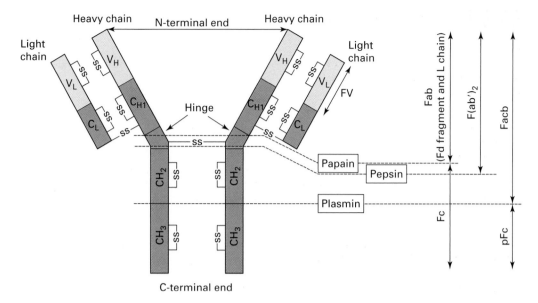

Fig. 7.1. General structure of IgG showing enzyme cleavage sites and resulting fragments. Note that the number of -S—S- bonds in the hinge area varies according to subclass and species.

fragment does not bind antigen, but early biochemical studies showed it to be more easy to crystallize than the Fab fragments (this reflects a greater homogeneity in structure). It is known as fragment crystallisable or Fc by immunochemists. The mammalian protease pepsin cleaves human IgG at low pH to produce one large fragment, a smaller fragment and some small peptides. The large fragment (100 000 M_r) can bind antigen divalently (as long as the antigen is relatively small), can cross-link antigen and can form antigen complexes that precipitate. It is structurally very similar to a dimer of the Fab fragment produced by papain digestion and is known as F(ab')$_2$. Similarly, the smaller fragment is a truncated version of the Fc fragment and is known as Fc'. Both papain and pepsin cleave the IgG molecule in the hinge region, but the former enzyme cuts next to the hinge on the N-terminal side whereas the latter enzyme acts on the C-terminal side of the hinge (see Fig. 7.1). This explains the production of monovalent Fab fragments by papain, but divalent dimeric antigen-binding F(ab')$_2$ fragments by pepsin; the two Fab' components comprising F(ab')$_2$ are linked via the disulphide bridges that make up the hinge region. Other enzymes can also be used to derive immunoglobulin fragments, but papain and pepsin are the most commonly used. Similar fragments can be produced from non-human IgG, but there is considerable species variation in susceptibility to digestion. Enzyme-derived fragments of other immunoglobulin classes can also be produced (see Suggestions for further reading, Section 7.11).

For most immunochemical procedures, IgG is by far the most useful immunoglobulin reagent.

Table 7.2 Polypeptide chain composition of human immunoglobulins

Class/ subclass	Normal serum concentration (mg ml⁻¹)	M_r (×10⁻³)	H chains domains	Chain compositions	M_r (×10⁻³) Total	M_r (×10⁻³) Peptide	% Carbohydrate of chains (no. of groups)	Hinge amino acids	Intra-heavy chain disulphide bonds
IgG1	5–10	146	4	2γ1	51	49	3–4 (1)	15	2
				2L(κ:λ 2:1)	23	23	<0.5		
IgG2	1.8–3.5	146	4	2γ2	51	49	3–4 (1)	12	4
				2L(κ:λ 2:1)	23	23	<0.5		
IgG3	0.6–1.2	170	4	2γ3	60	57	3–4 (1)	62	11
				2L(κ:λ 1:1)	23	23	<0.5		
IgG4	0.3–0.6	146	4	2γ4	51	49	3–4 (1)	12	2
				2L(κ:λ 1:1)	23	23	<0.5		
IgM	0.5–2.0	900	5	10μ	67	57	12–16 (5)	0	1[a]
				2L(κ:λ 3:1)	23	23	<0.5		
				1J[f]	15	14	7.5		
IgA1[b]	0.8–3.4	160	4	2α1	56	50	10–15 (5)	20	2[c]
				2L(κ:λ 1:1)	23	23	<0.5		
IgA2[b]	0.2–0.6	160	4	2α2	53	48	10–15 (2)	7	2[c]
				2L(κ:λ 1:1)	23	23	<0.5		
Secretory IgA1 or IgA2[d]	–	390	4	4α	53–56	48–50	10–15		
				4L	23	23	<0.5		
				1J	15	14	7.5		
				1SC[e]	75	63	15–16		
IgD	0.003–0.3	165	4	2δ	60	51	14–71 (3)	64	1
				2L(κ:λ 1:10)	23	23	<0.5		
IgE	0.0001–0.0007	185	5	2ε	70	59	13–16 (6)	0	2
				2L	23	23	<0.5		

[a] There is one intra-heavy chain disulphide bond linking cysteines between C_H2 and C_H3 domains; there are further disulphide bonds between monomer units.

[b] Data are given for the monomeric form, which predominates in human sera. Polymeric forms also exist (up to pentamer); these contain one molecule of J chain per polymer in addition to α and L chains.

[c] There is an additional disulphide bond from the cysteine in the tailpiece to either the corresponding cysteine in the other heavy chain or to a cysteine in J chain or secretory component in secretory IgA.

[d] Data are given for the dimer; a tetrameric form is also common in humans.

[e] SC, secretory component, derived from a membrane-bound poly(Ig)receptor used to transport the IgA through epithelial cells during its secretion.

Source: Reproduced from M. A. Kerr and R. Thorpe, *Immunochemistry Labfax* (1994), Bios Scientific, Oxford.

7.1.3 **Immunoglobulin structure, immunoglobulin genes and the generation of antibody diversity**

Immunoglobulin chains of particular classes or types contain distinct regions that are either very constant in sequence or more variable. The chains are built up of domains which exhibit a similar three-dimensional structure (Fig. 7.1). The heavy chains are made up of three (γ-, α- and δ-chains) or four (μ- and ϵ-chains) constant domains and one variable domain, whereas light chains have one constant and one variable domain (Fig. 7.1 and Table 7.2). The constant regions of antibodies are important for immunoglobulin three-dimensional structure, are responsible for most immunobiological functions such as complement fixation and interact with the immunoglobulin receptors found on many types of cells. The variable regions are responsible for binding antigen. Within the variable regions are relatively short sequences that show particularly high variability in sequence and these are responsible for direct interaction with the antigen. These are known as hypervariable regions or complementarity-determining regions (CDRs), and there are three of these per heavy or light chain. The less variable portions of the variable regions are important for maintenance of the appropriate structure of the antibody molecule, especially for efficient antigen binding.

Immunoglobulins are clear exceptions to the normal rule that one gene codes for one protein chain, and several germline genes are involved in coding for each of the heavy and light chains. The constant regions of heavy chains are coded for by single genes, one for each class or subclass, known as C_H genes, which are distinct in the germline from genes for the heavy chain variable region (V_H genes). Relatively large numbers of variable region genes occur in clusters (for human heavy chains there are about 100 V_H genes) and between these and the constant region genes there are additional short genes that code for joining (J; six for human heavy chain genes) and diversity-associated (D; four for human heavy chain genes) sequences. A similar gene organization exists for the light chains (known as V_L, J_L and C_L gene segments), except that D sequence light chain genes do not occur; there are about 70 V_L and 4 J genes for human κ light chains. Early in B cell maturation, translocation of the genes occurs such that a linear assembly of a particular V gene with a J gene, a D gene (only for heavy chains) and a C gene occurs; this codes for a complete immunoglobulin chain. This results in the ability of an animal to produce a range of immunoglobulin molecules that differ particularly in their hypervariable region sequences and thus the part of the molecule that binds antigen. This diversity can be increased by use of variable amounts of the D region (for heavy chains) and by somatic mutation during maturation of the immune response. All of these combinations are responsible for the ability of at least higher vertebrates to produce a very large number of different antibodies (theoretical considerations suggest that humans can produce an estimated 10^8 different antibodies), and accounts for the differing specificity and affinity of immunoglobulin molecules for antigen. It also allows production of antibodies that recognise virtually *any* foreign antigen of appropriate size. These properties of antibodies are exploited in immunochemical methods.

7.2 **PRODUCTION OF ANTIBODIES**

Virtually all immunochemical techniques rely on the use of antibodies and their effectiveness is dependent on the quality of the antibody or antibodies employed. The nature of the antibody affects both the specificity of the methods (i.e. the ability to discriminate between the desired analyte and other substances that may be present) and the sensitivity of the procedure (i.e. its ability to detect/measure low concentrations of the analyte). The avidity of the antibody for antigen is important for the latter (see Section 7.9). Although some antibodies that can be useful in immunochemical methods occur 'naturally', for example some autoanti-bodies, it is normally necessary to stimulate their production by immunising animals (but see Section 7.2.6 for an an important exception to this). Many different procedures for this have been developed.

7.2.1 **The immune response; polyclonal and monoclonal antibodies**

All vertebrates can produce antibodies against foreign antigens. However, responses in lower vertebrates are very limited (although even the most primi-tive animals, such as hagfish and lampreys, can mount immune responses against some non-self proteins) and normally antibodies derived from such species are not useful for immunochemical methods. Mammals mount the most useful humoral immune responses and mammalian antibodies are normally used in immunochemical techniques. However, avian antibodies can also be employed in special cases. In most cases IgG antibodies are the most useful for immunochemical techniques, but IgM and IgA can be used for some procedures. IgE is limited to studies relating to allergic and anaphylactic phenomena and IgD is not normally useful. No specific functions have been identified for secreted IgD.

It is now clear that each mature B lymphocyte secretes an antibody with a single immunoglobulin sequence. The humoral response to antigen results in activa-tion of a heterogeneous population of B cells that secretes different immuno-globulins. Maturation of the response results in clonal expansion of these initially primed cells to derive populations of plasma cells that secrete an array of antigen-binding immunoglobulins, often of different classes and subclasses. In the antigen-binding fraction of antibodies, immunoglobulins showing variable specificity and avidity for the immunogen will be present. Usually, many different antibodies, recognising several different epitopes on each antigen are present. Such a response is described as polyclonal, as antibody is derived from more than one clone of B lymphocytes and shows heterogeneity in the amino acid sequences of the antigen-binding immunoglobulins present. Preparations of such polyclonal antibodies, either unpurified as immune sera or purified (see Section 7.3) are often used for immunochemical techniques. However, more recently, methods have been developed for deriving monoclonal antibodies, which are derived from a single B cell clone and show identical amino acid sequence. Monoclonal antibody preparations show homogeneous characteristics (including specificity and avidity for antigen, i.e. they recognise a single epitope) and can be advantageous for immunochemical purposes, if carefully selected and characterised. Production of monoclonal antibodies is considered in Section 7.2.3.

7.2.2 Production of polyclonal antibodies (antisera)

It is possible to produce antibodies that bind to proteins, peptides, carbohydrates and nucleic acids, but the latter show little if any specificity for sequence and so are usually of little use for immunochemical techniques. Antibodies against carbohydrate can be used for analytical work, but can show limited specificity, except in some special cases. In general, most immunochemical methods are devised for use with antibodies that recognise proteins and peptides.

Most higher vertebrates will produce a humoral immune response against a 'foreign' protein. However, the magnitude of the antibody response depends on a number of variables. Of particular importance are the size of the protein/peptide and the phylogenetic distance between the source of the antigen and the animal used to produce antibody. For the latter it is generally the case that the greater the phylogenetic difference, the better. However, choice of species for antibody production also depends on the amount of antigen available, the amount of antiserum required and the quality of antiserum desired. In some cases use of closely related species or even different strains of a single species for derivation of antigen and production of antibodies can provide antibodies with particular properties/specificities. The most important consideration for immunogenicity is the difference in amino acid sequence (and therefore structure) of the antigen used as immunogen and the equivalent antigen (if present) in the animal used to produce antibody. It is generally the case that the greater this difference, the more immunogenic the antigen will be. In some cases, particular parts of the antigen produce very potent immune responses and such epitopes are known as immunodominant.

Peptides with an M_r of less than about 2000 are normally poorly immunogenic or non-immunogenic. Immunogenicity tends to increase with size; proteins with $M_r > 10\,000$ are usually immunogenic as long as they are recognised as foreign in responding animals.

Antibodies that bind small peptides (and other small, non-immunogenic molecules such as steroids and drugs) can be produced by linking (conjugating) these substances to larger proteins (known as carrier proteins). The antisera produced will contain antibodies that recognise the carrier as well as others that bind to the small molecule. Some proteins are particularly effective as carriers (such as keyhole limpet haemocyanin and thyroglobulin) and some produce a restricted anti-carrier humoral response, such as purified protein derivative (PPD) from Bacille, Calmette, Guérin (BCG). Substances that are not immunogenic alone, but are when conjugated, are known as haptens.

For production of potent antibodies that perform well in immunochemical techniques, it is usually necessary to use an adjuvant as part of the immunogen.

Table 7.3 Some commonly used adjuvants

Adjuvant	Composition and use
Freund's complete adjuvant (FCA)	Mineral oil containing heat-killed mycobacteria (*Mycobacterium tuberculosis* or *M. butyricum*) Used as emulsion with aqueous antigen
Freund's incomplete adjuvant (FIA)	Mineral oil Used as emulsion with aqueous antigen
Alum	Complex aluminium salts. There are various versions of the adjuvant: some can be purchased ready for use (e.g. Alhydrogel); others can be prepared in the laboratory by mixing various salts, e.g. $NaHCO_3$, and aluminium potassium sulphate. Aqueous antigen is absorbed to gel
Bentonite	Wyoming sodium bentonite (Montmorillonite) as gel. Aqueous antigen adsorbed to surface
Quil A	Saponin derived from *Quillaja saponana* Molina (South American tree). Mixed to form a complex with aqueous antigen
Muramyl dipeptide (MDP)	*N*-Acetylmuramyl-L-alanyl-D-isoglutamine. Mixed with aqueous antigen. Various derivations of MDP are also used as adjuvants
Monophosphoryl lipid A (MPL)	Used in various formulations, often as an emulsion with oils. Antigen included in emulsion
Bacillus pertussis	Killed organisms mixed with aqueous antigen

FCA is probably the most potent adjuvant but may be inappropriate for some purposes.
Source: Reproduced from M. A. Kerr and R. Thorpe, *Immunochemistry Labfax* (1994), Bios Scientific, Oxford.

Such substances potentiate the immune reponse by forming a slow-release depot of antigen, by stimulating T cell help or by aiding antigen presentation. Some adjuvants function by more than one of these effects (see Table 7.3 for some adjuvants commonly used for immunochemical purposes). Although a single immunisation with antigen will usually result in production of antibodies, such antisera are usually suboptimal, containing antibodies of low avidity and a high proportion of IgM, which can be of limited use for immunochemical methods. It is usual practice to use several subsequent immunisations, spaced such that the immune response is boosted to produce a hyperimmune animal, with a high concentration of avid antibodies specific for antigen in its blood. Such 'hyperimmune sera' (really antisera from hyperimmunised animals) are usually the polyclonal reagents of choice for immunochemical techniques. Precise details of amount of antigen used and spacing of 'boosting' immunisations vary enormously according to antigen and species used; for some general principles see Table 7.4. In general, the larger the animal, the more antigen is required; however, larger animals

Table 7.4 Examples of immunisation protocols that have been used successfully

Species	Priming	Rest period (weeks)	First boost	Rest period (weeks)	Subsequent boosts
Mice, rats and guinea pigs	5–100 μg antigen in FCA (or other adjuvant), s.c. or i.m.	2–3	50–100 μg antigen in FIA, other adjuvant or PBS, i.m. or s.c.	3	5–100 μg antigen in FIA or PBS, i.p., s.c., i.m. or i.v.
Rabbits	50–250 μg antigen in FCA or other adjuvant, i.d., i.m. or s.c.	3–4	50–250 μg antigen in FIA or other adjuvant or PBS, i.m., or s.c.	4 or longer	50–250 μg antigen in FIA or PBS, i.m., s.c. or i.v.
Sheep and goats	250 μg–10 mg antigen in FCA or other adjuvant, i.m., s.c. or i.d.	4	250 μg–10 mg antigen in FIA or other adjuvant, i.m. or s.c.	4–8 or longer	250 μg–10 mg antigen in FIA or other adjuvant, i.m., s.c. or i.v.
Horses and donkeys	250 μg–50 mg antigen in FCA or other adjuvant, i.m., s.c. or i.d.	4	250 μg–50 mg antigen in FIA or other adjuvant, i.m. or s.c.	4–8 or longer	250 μg–50 mg antigen in FIA or other adjuvant, i.m. or s.c.
Primates	50 μg–1 mg antigen in adjuvant, i.m. or s.c.	4	50 μg–1 mg antigen in adjuvant, or PBS, i.m., s.c. or i.v.	4–8 or longer	50 μg–1 mg antigen in adjuvant or PBS, i.m., s.c. or i.d.
Chickens	30–200 μg antigen in FCA or other adjuvant, i.m.	2–3	30–200 μg antigen in FIA or other adjuvant, i.m.	3 or longer	30–200 μg in FIA or other adjuvant or PBS, i.m.

FCA Freund's complete adjuvant; FIA, Freund's incomplete adjuvant; PBS, phosphate-buffered saline; i.p., intraperitoneally; s.c., subcutaneously; i.m., intramuscularly; i.v., intravenously; i.d., intradermally.

Source: Reproduced from M. A. Kerr and R. Thorpe, *Imunochemistry Labfax* (1994), Bios Scientific, Oxford.

contain more blood (and therefore serum/plasma). Thus larger animals will require the availability of greater quantities of immunogen for antibody production but will generate larger amounts of antiserum (mice will produce only a few millilitres whereas sheep and horses can yield several litres).

7.2.3 Monoclonal antibodies

Monoclonal antibodies can be especially useful for immunochemical methods. Such antibodies are secreted by cloned, i.e. monoclonal cells. Mature, antibody-secreting lymphocytes from immunised animals can be cloned, but these survive for only a very short period in culture, and therefore do not provide useful amounts of antibody. However, procedures have been developed to allow production of large quantities of monoclonal antibodies by producing continuously growing (immortal) cell lines that secrete antibody efficiently. These involve generation of hybrid cells, transformation of lymphocytes with a virus, or recombinant DNA procedures.

7.2.4 Hybridoma production

In 1975, Köhler and Milstein devised a procedure for producing hybrid cells that secrete antibody and grow continuously in culture (Fig. 7.2). This involves fusing lymphocytes from immune mice with mouse myeloma cells. Such hybrid fused cells, known originally as fusomas but later as hybridomas inherit the ability to secrete antibody from the lymphocyte parent and the ability to grow continuously from the myeloma cell. Myeloma cell lines that no longer secrete immunoglobulin paraprotein have been derived and are advantageous for hybridoma technology (the hybridomas derived do not secrete the paraprotein).

Lymphocytes and myeloma cells are mixed together at high density and treated with a fusing agent (nowadays polyethylene glycol, although Sendai virus was originally used). Under such conditions, fused cells are produced but unfused lymphocytes and myeloma cells predominate and the latter will overgrow and overwhelm the hydridomas if they are not removed. This is normally achieved by the use of a selective medium in which the myeloma cells die, but hybridomas survive. The most widely used selective system involves the inclusion of the antibiotic aminopterin in growth medium. This inhibits the *de novo* nucleotide synthesis pathway, in which nucleotides (and thus eventually nucleic acids) are produced from small molecules. Normal cells survive in this medium as they are able to use the salvage pathway for nucleic acid synthesis, in which nucleotides produced by breakdown of nucleic acid are recycled. But, if cells are unable to produce the enzyme hypoxanthine–guanine phosphoribosyl transferase (HGPRT), they are unable to utilise the salvage pathway and therefore die in aminopterin-containing medium. Such cells can be produced by culture in 8-azaguanine and numerous HGPRT-negative mouse myeloma cell lines have been established.

After fusion of lymphocytes with HGPRT-negative myeloma cells, aminopterin-containing medium, supplemented with hypoxanthine and thymidine to ensure

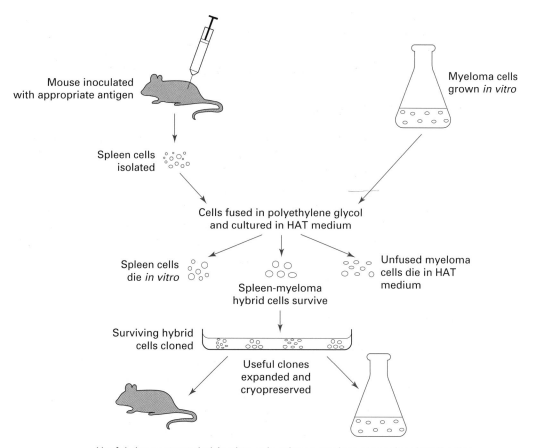

Useful clones expanded *in vitro* or in mice to produce monoclonal antibodies

Fig. 7.2. A schematic representation of a typical procedure for production of murine monoclonal antibodies.

an adequate supply of substrates for the salvage pathway (HAT medium) is added, which kills myeloma cells but allows hybridomas to survive as they inherit HGPRT from the lymphocyte parent. Residual unfused lymphocytes die after a short period in culture, which results in a pure preparation of hybridomas that can be cloned using one of three procedures:

- *Limiting dilution cloning:* A single hybridoma cell suspension is diluted and dispensed into culture plate wells to approximate one cell per well (and numbers surrounding this). Wells are inspected to assess clonality and, after culture, cell supernatant is assessed for the presence of appropriate antibody. This procedure is normally repeated (often more than once) to obtain a monoclonal hybridoma line.
- *Soft agar cloning:* A single cell suspension is diluted in approximately 0.25% molten agar, overlayed on solid 0.5% agar and allowed to set. Clones grow in culture as foci that can be located visually (using an inverted microscope).

When of appropriate size, the resulting clumps of cells are 'picked' from the agar using a fine Pasteur pipette, cultured in medium and the supernatant assessed for antibody content.

- *Cloning using fluorescence-activated cell sorting:*   Cells are fluorescently labelled for appropriate antibody secretion (e.g. using fluorescein isothiocyanate-labelled antigen) and then individually isolated using flow cytometry via a fluorescence-activated cell sorting (FACS) machine. Appropriate cells are cultured and supernatants screened for antibody content.

All cloning methods are designed to produce cultures of monoclonal hybridomas but do not guarantee this. Repeating the cloning techniques will obviously increase the chance of cells being monoclonal, but cloning checks need to be used if assurance of monoclonality is to be obtained. For this, 'subclones' of the hybrid-oma lines are prepared (as above) and the percentage of cells secreting antibody of appropriate defined specificity assessed. If the parental line is monoclonal, this should be close to 100%. If not, the hybridoma line either is not monoclonal or is unstable in respect to secretion of monoclonal antibody.

Such monoclonal cell lines can be grown in culture to produce supernatant containing monoclonal antibody (industrial-scale fermenters or hollow fibre culture supports can be used that yield kilograms of antibody) or grown in the peritoneal cavities of mice to produce ascitic fluid containing high concentrations (about 5–10 mg cm^{-3}) of antibody. The cell lines can be cryopreserved to provide an ever-lasting source of monoclonal antibody.

A similar approach can be used for the production of rat monoclonal antibodies, except that O-diazoacetyl-L-serine (azaserine) is sometimes substituted for amino-pterin in the selective medium. This inhibits a range of amination reactions, some of which are essential for *de novo* purine synthesis. Hamster heterohybridomas can also be produced by fusing hamster lymphocytes with mouse HGPRT-deficient myeloma cells. Hybridoma technology is generally less successful with higher mammals, owing to the lack of suitable myeloma cell lines for fusion and the instability of mouse/higher species lymphocyte heterohybridomas. A rabbit myeloma cell line suitable for production of rabbit hybridomas has been described.

7.2.5 Transformation of lymphocytes with virus; production of human monoclonal antibodies

In some cases, it it desirable or even essential to use human rather than rodent monoclonal antibodies. For example, human antibodies are generally better for *in vivo* therapeutic use in humans as they are much less immunogenic and mediate immunobiological functions, and it can be very difficult if not impossible to produce rodent monoclonal antibodies against some antigens, for example the human Rh D blood group antigen. A few hybridoma-derived human monoclonal antibodies have been produced (almost always from heterohybridomas), but this approach is difficult and inefficient. However, infection of human B lymphocytes with Epstein–Barr virus results in transformation of a subpopulation of cells and allows the production of continuously growing cell lines that can be cloned. Some of these clones secrete monoclonal antibody, which can be used for therapeutic and immunochemical purposes. A relatively high proportion of such cell lines secrete IgM antibody, but lines secreting immunoglobulin of all classes and subclasses can be produced. Some cell lines show instability and low level immunoglobulin secretion that can sometimes be resolved by fusion with stable non-antibody-secreting heterohybridomas or myeloma lines.

7.2.6 Engineered antibodies

Although mouse or rat monoclonal antibodies with the desired antigen-binding properties can be produced from deliberately immunised laboratory animals, a problem with their clinical use in humans, for example in cancer patients, is that they can elicit an immune response in the recipient as they are recognised as being 'foreign'. Also, some potential applications of monoclonal antibodies may require particular effector functions (mediated by the Fc portion of particular subclasses) combined with a particular specificity (determined by the variable portion), which may not be readily produced simply by immunisation. Small antibody fragments rather than the relatively large intact molecule may be preferable for other clinical applications, for example where tissue penetration is desired. Genetic engineering methods have therefore been developed to attempt to overcome these limitations. Genes encoding antibody heavy and light chains can be amplified using the polymerase chain reaction (PCR) and cloned into suitable vectors for expression and manipulation, for example splicing the variable region from one antibody to the constant region of another. Mammalian cells are usually used for expression of whole antibodies (to ensure glycosylation and correct chain folding and assembly) whereas antibody fragments can be expressed in *Escherichia coli*. It has also become possible to mimic the *in vivo* antibody response *in vitro* by expressing antibody fragments derived from gene repertoires on the surface of bacteriophage (phage display) to allow selection of particular specificities.

Polymerase chain reaction amplification of antibody genes

Antibody genes may be readily amplified by PCR. This amplification involves repeated cycles of extension between two oligonucleotide primers that hybridise to the 5′ and 3′ ends of the gene sequence. The steps involve:

- preparation of a cell lysate and extraction of the RNA (this fraction will contain the mRNA which encodes the antibody heavy and light chains);
- synthesis of single-stranded complementary DNA (cDNA) using the enzyme reverse transcriptase, the RNA/cDNA hybrid then being used as a template for the PCR;
- specific amplification of the antibody gene(s) present in the RNA/cDNA template using oligonucleotide primers that anneal to sequences outside the region for which sequence information is required (usually the variable region; Fig. 7.3).

(a)

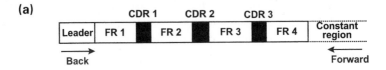

(b)

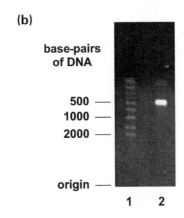

base-pairs
of DNA

500 —
1000 —
2000 —

origin —

1   2

Fig. 7.3. PCR amplification of a heavy chain variable region gene. (a) The position of
the forward and back primers relative to the variable region. FR, framework region;
CDR, complementarity-determining region. (b) Photograph showing agarose gel
electrophoretic analysis of the product of PCR amplification of the heavy chain variable
region gene (track 2). Track 1 shows DNA markers. The gel was stained with ethidium
bromide (a fluorescent dye that binds to nucleic acid) and viewed under ultraviolet
illumination.

Primers can be designed for PCR amplification of most families of variable region
genes as the nucleotide sequences flanking the variable region genes are relatively
conserved. The incorporation of restriction endonuclease sites in the primers
allows subsequent cloning of the amplified gene(s).

   The starting material may be a hybridoma secreting a monoclonal antibody to
allow, for example, genetic manipulations. Alternatively, RNA prepared from
human peripheral blood lymphocytes can be used to prepare repertoires of heavy
and light chain variable region genes to allow the creation of antibody fragment
gene repertoires and phage display (see below).

Gene repertoires and phage display

Amplified heavy and light variable region (V_H and V_L, respectively) gene repertoires can be spliced together using a stretch of synthetic DNA that encodes a
peptide 'linker' to form single-chain (sc) Fv antibody fragment gene repertoires (Fv
fragments are the smallest antibody fragments that still contain the intact antigen-
binding site; Fig. 7.4b). The use of a linker prevents the otherwise non-covalently
attached V_H and V_L portions from dissociating. The scFv repertoire is then ream-
plified with flanking primers containing appropriate restriction endonuclease

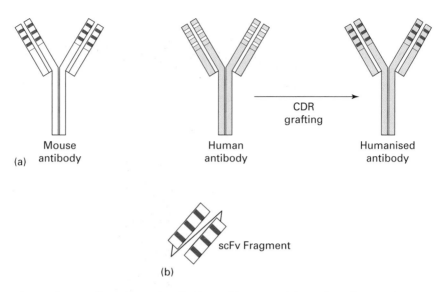

(a) Mouse antibody — Human antibody — CDR grafting → Humanised antibody

(b) scFv Fragment

Fig. 7.4. Genetically engineered antibodies and fragments. (a) CDR (complementarity-determining region) grafting to produce humanised antibody; (b) single-chain Fv fragment.

sites that allow subsequent digestion with the appropriate enzymes and ligation into a suitable phage display vector, for example pHEN-1, which is then expressed in *E. coli*. Thus a phage antibody 'library' can be created. The phage display vector allows the scFv fragments to be expressed at the surface of the phage as a fusion product with a phage coat protein. This allows phage-encoding fragments to be selected by screening against antigen bound to a solid support. Alternatively, soluble scFv fragments can be expressed (depending on the strain of *E. coli* used as host). A potential advantage of the above technology is the production of antibodies from non-immunised individuals. This depends on the creation of a vast number of antibody gene repertoires, phage display, and selection using the antigen of interest.

The use of antibody fragments may be advantageous for certain clinical applications, for example their small size should increase tumour penetration. However, their use in the laboratory as reagents can be problematical as they tend to have relatively low functional affinity.

Strategies for reducing immunogenicity

Several approaches have been developed to render antibodies less immunogenic, whilst retaining their antigen-binding properties. In chimeric antibodies, the constant domains of the mouse or rat antibody are substituted with those of human sequence. This also confers effective Fc-mediated properties for *in vivo* use in humans and human-based *in vitro* methods. The constant domains may even be substituted with a non-antibody protein such as a toxin or enzyme. An alternative approach is to humanise the mouse or rat antibody by grafting the mouse CDR into human variable region genes (Fig. 7.4a). These antibodies need to be expressed in mammalian cells. Amino acid residues may also have to be changed or added to ensure correct conformation of the variable region.

It is now possible to produce monoclonal antibodies that are entirely human sequence with a range of desirable specificities and immunological functions. For this, genes coding for antigen-binding fragments with appropriate specificities, usually derived using phage display, are spliced onto genes coding for appropriate immunoglobulin heavy and light chains. The constructed genes are expressed (normally in mammalian myeloma cells) to provide complete immunoglobulin molecules that are entirely derived from human gene sequences. As for 'conventional' phage display production of Fv fragments, the antigen-binding moieties can be derived from Fv libraries constructed from 'naïve' i.e. non-immunised individuals.

Sequencing monoclonal antibodies

PCR cloning of antibody variable region genes has greatly facilitated elucidation of the encoded amino acid sequences, since it is much easier to sequence the nucleic acid encoding the antibody, and then translate this into protein sequence, than to carry out amino acid sequencing by Edman degradation (see Section 8.4.3) of immunoglobulin protein. The latter method of sequencing requires relatively large amounts of pure antibody preparations and is limited to relatively short stretches of sequence, which necessitates sequencing many overlapping peptides to obtain a complete sequence. Determining the amino acid sequence of antibodies allows their structure to be correlated with their immunological properties, for example antigen-binding properties, and prediction of their three-dimensional shape. The nucleotide sequence also gives information on the use of germline genes in a given antibody response (remember that the antibody-encoding genes are formed from the joining of different germline gene segments during lymphocyte maturation; Section 7.1) and the process of affinity maturation (somatic mutation).

Amplified antibody genes can be sequenced directly; alternatively, to avoid any spurious sequences present in the PCR product, the amplified material can be cloned into a bacteriophage vector and used to transform *E. coli* to provide more reliable and reproducible sequence data. The chain termination method of sequencing is described in Section 5.11.

7.3 PURIFICATION AND FRAGMENTATION OF IMMUNOGLOBULINS

Many immunochemical techniques can be carried out using unpurified antibody in the form of antisera, monoclonal antibody-containing culture supernatant or rodent ascites, for example agar gel methods or immunohistochemistry (Sections 7.4 and 7.8). However, other methods require partial or complete purification of specific antibodies or at least isolation of the total immunoglobulin fraction, for example if they are to be labelled (Section 7.5), immobilised for use in immunoaffinity chromatography (Section 7.3.4), or analysed by isoelectric focusing (Section 10.3.4) or high performance liquid chromatography (HPLC)

(Section 11.3.2). There are a variety of procedures available for purifying immunoglobulins, the optimal method and experimental details depend on the class/subclass, the species in which the antibody was produced, the intended use, and the type of starting material, for example serum in the case of polyclonal antibodies or culture supernatant or ascites in the case of monoclonal antibodies. Methods of immunoglobulin purification from the mixtures of proteins found in serum, culture supernatant and ascites include precipitation techniques that exploit differential solubility characteristics of antibodies and other proteins: ion-exchange chromatography (exploits charge differences between immunoglobulins and other proteins), gel filtration (separates proteins according to size) and affinity chromatography (exploits a specific interaction between antibody and a molecule which it binds – termed the 'ligand' from the Latin *ligare* = to tie or bind). It may be necessary to combine two or more of these procedures to achieve the required purity. However, only affinity chromatography using immobilised antigen is normally capable of purifying antibodies of a single specificity unless the starting material contains a monoclonal antibody.

7.3.1 **Precipitation techniques**

Certain salts, organic solvents and organic polymers cause immunoglobulin molecules to precipitate from solution to form visible, insoluble aggregates that can be collected by centrifugation, and then resolubilised in an appropriate buffer (see Section 8.3.4). Immunoglobulin molecules in solution are surrounded by a tightly bound hydration shell, and precipitation techniques work by perturbing this hydration layer. Immunoglobulins are soluble within a certain salt concentration range, but become insoluble at both high and low extremes. High concentrations of salts attract the hydration layer away from the protein as the ions become solvated, encouraging hydrophobic areas on the immunoglobulin molcule to interact with similar areas on other molecules causing 'clumping' of molecules. This is called 'salting out' and results in reversible precipitation of the antibody. Multiply charged anions with monovalent cations are most effective at salting out; ammonium and sodium sulphate are most commonly used. However, the solubility of some immunoglobulins also decreases as the salt concentration is lowered because there are insufficient ions to maintain hydration of the immunoglobulin protein. This is called euglobulin precipitation, and is particularly useful for preliminary purification of IgM, although it usually does not work well for IgG. Water-miscible organic solvents can also be used to precipitate immunoglobulins by decreasing the solvating power of water. Ethanol precipitation is used on an industrial scale for fractionation of immunoglobulin from other plasma proteins. Polyethylene glycol is a high molecular weight, water-soluble organic polymer that can be used to separate immunoglobulins from other plasma proteins by precipitation, in a similar way to organic solvents.

Precipitation of immunoglobulin tends to be most effective at its isoelectric point (the pH at which the immunoglobulin has no net charge), since electrostatic repulsion between molecules is minimised. Precipitation techniques are cheap and easy to carry out but are often used only as a preliminary step in multistep purification schedules as the product is usually not sufficiently pure.

7.3.2 Gel filtration

Gel filtration separates molecules according to size (Section 11.7). Since IgM is considerably larger than other immunoglobulin subclasses and most other serum proteins, conventional or HPLC gel filtration is commonly used for IgM purification. Although gel filtration alone is not very good for IgG purification, it can be used in combination with other methods such as ion-exchange chromatography for IgG purification.

7.3.3 Ion-exchange chromatography

Conventional or HPLC or fast protein liquid chromatography (FPLC) ion-exchange chromatography systems make use of the surface charge of immunoglobulins to separate them from other components (Section 11.7). At neutral pH, most immunoglobulins are negatively charged and will bind to positively charged anion-exchange matrices. Increasing the salt concentration or changing the pH of the buffer will then elute the immunoglobulin from the matrix (Fig. 7.5).

7.3.4 Affinity chromatography

Affinity chromatography exploits a specific but reversible interaction between a ligand that is covalently attached to an inert support and the antibody to be purified (Section 11.8). The ligand may be, for example, an antigen for purification of antibodies of a particular specificity, an anti-immunoglobulin antibody for purification of antibodies from a particular species, class or subclass, or an immunoglobulin-binding protein: several strains of bacteria produce such proteins that bind immunoglobulin with high affinity (Table 7.5). The most commonly used bacterial immunoglobulin-binding proteins are called protein A and protein G; they bind the constant region of IgG (depending on species and subclass). A light-chain-binding protein has also been described (protein L), but this binds only some light chain types. Affinity chromatography using immobilised protein A or G is often the method of choice for purification of IgG monoclonal antibodies from culture supernatants. The inert support can be agarose, sepharose, polyacrylamide, polystyrene or high-pressure stable acrylic polymer for use in HPLC. Alternatively, ligand can be attached to magnetic beads, which can then be isolated using a magnetic attractor. Many different immobilised ligands are available commercially; alternatively, ligands can be coupled, via primary amine, carboxyl or thiol groups, to activated supports in the laboratory (for examples, see Fig. 7.6). When the solution containing the antibody is brought into contact with the immobilised ligand, the antibody binds to the ligand and is thus also immobilised (Fig. 7.7). The

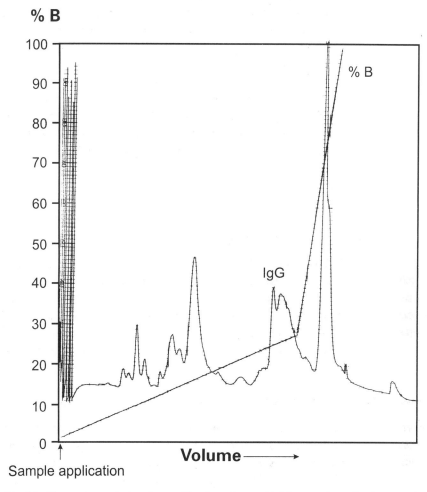

% B

Sample application

Fig. 7.5. Chromatograph showing purification of mouse IgG from ascites using fast protein liquid chromatography ion-exchange chromatography. A preliminary IgG purification step was carried out using ammonium sulphate precipitation from the ascites (Section 7.3.1). The precipitate was redissolved and equilibrated in 20 mM triethanolamine pH 7.7 (A). The anion-exchanger was also equilibrated in A. Following application of the sample, a salt gradient formed by using increasing amounts of B (A + 1 M NaCl) was used to elute the immunoglobulin. The peak corresponding to IgG is indicated.

non-bound material can then be washed away. The specific interaction between antibody and ligand is then disrupted to elute the antibody (see below), whilst the ligand remains immobilised. Conditions for dissociating the specific ligand–antibody interaction commonly disrupt the electrostatic interactions and/or hydrophobic bonding (due to van der Waals' interactions) involved in antibody–ligand binding (Table 7.6).

Lectins are glycoproteins of non-immune origin, isolated from plants and animals, which bind specific carbohydrates such as galactose or fucose. For

Table 7.5 Ligands for affinity chromatography		
Ligand type	Example(s)	Antibody purification
Hapten	DNP	Antibodies that bind hapten
Antigen	Haemoglobin, factor VIII	Antibodies of a single specificity
Bacterial immunoglobulin binding protein	Protein A, protein G	Most IgG subclasses from many species
	Protein L	Some κ chains from many species
Anti-immunoglobulin antibodies	Goat anti-human IgG antibodies	Class and/or species-specific immunoglobulin fraction
Lectins	Jacalin	Human IgA
	Mannan-binding protein	Mouse IgM

DNP, dinitrophenol.

example, mannan-binding protein (MBP) is a mannose- and N-acetylglucosamine-binding lectin found in mammalian sera. When coupled to an inert support, it can be used to purify mouse IgM, which contains 12–16% mannose-containing carbohydrate. Jacalin is a galactose-binding lectin that can be used to purify human IgA1.

Affinity chromatography techniques using immobilised antibodies are widely used to purify antigens.

7.3.5 Fragmentation and dissociation of immunoglobulins

Some applications of antibodies require the use of antibody fragments rather than the intact molecule (see Section 7.1.2). For example, removing the antibody Fc portion will prevent binding of antibodies to Fc receptors present on leukocytes and other cells. This may be necessary if cell surface antigens recognised by the antibody are to be evaluated by, for example, immunofluorescence microscopy. The preparation of antibody fragments normally involves the use of proteolytic enzymes to cleave peptide bonds. Different enzymes can be used to cleave the heavy chain in specific places to give rise to different fragments. The most commonly used fragments are those produced by papain, pepsin and plasmin; their cleavage sites on IgG are shown in Fig. 7.1, with fragment nomenclature. These enzymes are available commercially either in soluble form or covalently coupled to Sepharose (an inert support), which facilitates removal of the enzyme when digestion is completed (the Sepharose and immobilised enzyme can be removed simply by centrifugation). Antibodies can also be dissociated into their constitutive chains. The heavy and light chains are joined by disulphide bridges that can be easily broken by a reducing agent such as dithiothreitol under conditions that

(a) Mechanism of activation of Sepharose by CNBr to allow subsequent coupling of proteins via amine groups

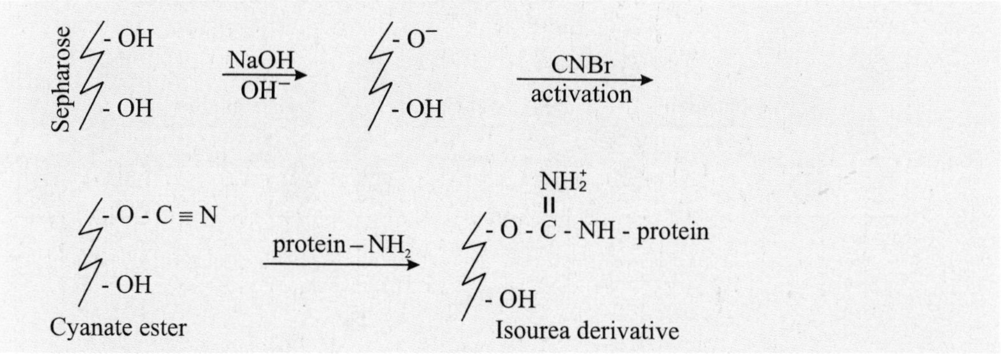

At high pH, CNBr reacts with hydroxyl groups on the Sepharose to form cyanate esters. These react with the amine groups of proteins to form covalent linkages.

(b) Mechanism of ligand immobilisation via commercially available *N*-hydroxy succinamide ester coupling

(i) Affi-Gel 10 (used for basic protein coupling)

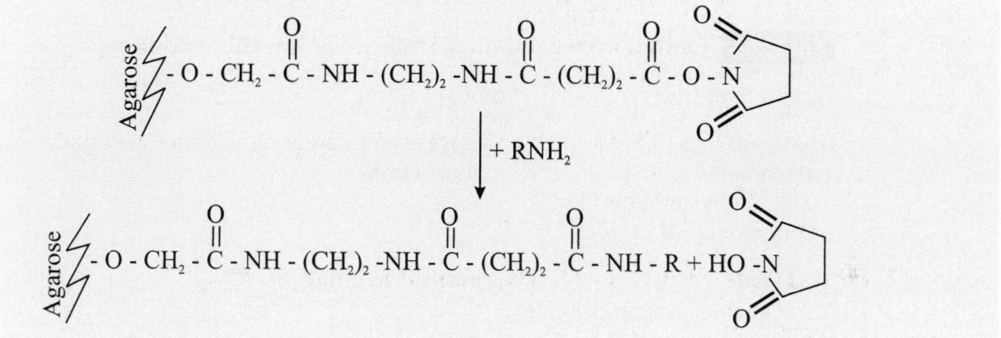

(ii) Affi-Gel 15 (used for acidic protein coupling)

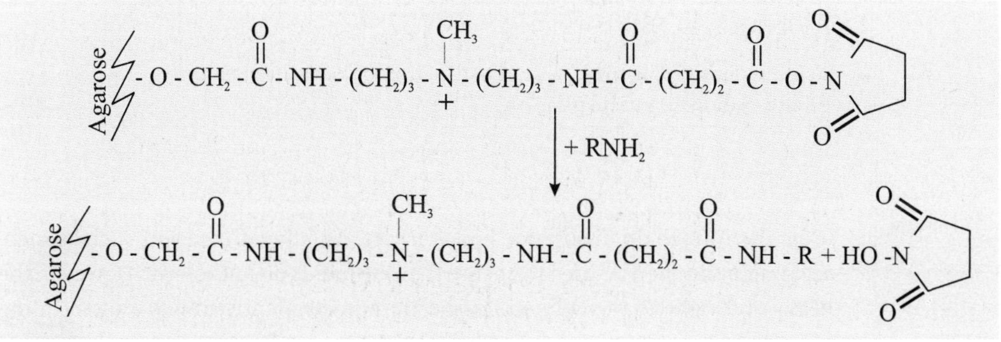

Fig. 7.6. Coupling of ligands to supports to prepare affinity columns.

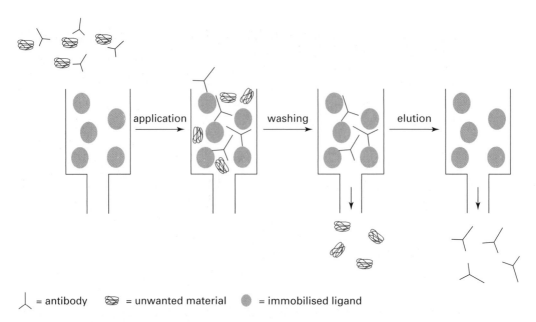

$\curlywedge$ = antibody   🦪 = unwanted material   ● = immobilised ligand

Fig. 7.7. Diagrammatic representation of antibody purification by affinity chromatography.

Table 7.6 **Conditions for elution of antibodies from affinity columns**

Elution conditions	Mode of action
Glycine-HC1, pH 2.2–2.8 1 M propionic acid 0.05 M diethylamine, pH 11.5 1 M ammonia, pH 11.0	Change conformation and disrupt electrostatic interactions
2–8 M urea 5–6 M guanidine hydrochloride	Strongly denaturing
3.5 M sodium thiocyanate 4 M potassium thiocyanate 2–5 M MgCl$_2$, KI, NaI	Chaotropic agents
50% ethylene glycol, pH 11.5 10% (v/v) dioxane at acid pH	Disrupt hydrophobic interactions

leave the intrachain disulphide bonds intact. An alkylating agent such as iodo-acetamide can then be used to ensure that the bonds do not reform. However, the heavy and light chains will still associate non-covalently unless a dissociating agent such as propionic acid is added. The chains can be separated on the basis of differing size by gel filtration (Fig. 7.8). Isolated immunoglobulin chains usually bind antigen less avidly than do the intact molecule and fragments such as Fab and F(ab')$_2$.

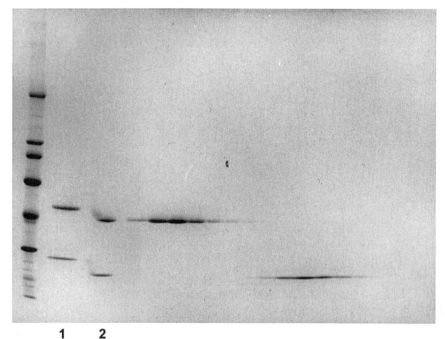

Fig. 7.8. Analysis of separated heavy and light chains of IgG using sodium dodecyl sulphate–polyacrylamide gel electrophoresis (SDS–PAGE). IgG was reduced and alkylated and the heavy and light chains were separated by gel filtration in propionic acid. The fractions were analysed by SDS–PAGE under non-reducing conditions. Lanes 1 and 2 show the reduced and alkylated IgG before gel filtration, analysed under reducing and non-reducing conditions, respectively. Note the apparent increase in size of the chains (lane 1) when analysed under conditions that reduce the intra-chain disulphide bonds. Molecular weight markers are on the left.

7.4 IMMUNOPRECIPITATION

An important property of many antibodies is their ability to precipitate antigens from solution. Antibodies are divalent (IgG) or multivalent (IgM), and if the antigen is also multivalent, the antibody–antigen interactions give rise to a molecular lattice that is too large to remain in solution, so precipitation occurs. The formation of an insoluble antibody–antigen complex is very dependent on antibody and antigen concentrations, and occurs within a narrow concentration range known as the zone of equivalence. This represents the conditions under which macromolecular antigen/antibody complexes are formed that are sufficiently large to be precipitated. Outside the equivalence concentration, conditions known as antigen or antibody excess occur, which result in the formation of small, soluble complexes (see Fig. 7.9). However, precipitation never occurs with some monoclonal antibodies that recognise a single epitope on an antigen (i.e. a monovalent antigen) because a lattice is not formed.

Immunoprecipitation can be exploited in both agar techniques and in solution.

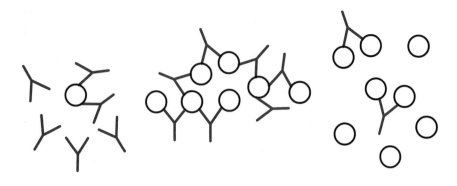

| Antibody excess | Equivalence | Antigen excess |

Fig. 7.9. Diagrammatic representation of immune complexes formed at varying antigen : antibody ratios. Immunoprecipitation occurs only when an insoluble antigen–antibody lattice is formed at the equivalence point.

7.4.1 Agar and agarose immunoprecipitation

Agar is a high molecular weight polysaccharide derived from seaweed; agarose is a purified linear galactan hydrocolloid isolated from the same substance. Both dissolve in aqueous solutions upon heating and, upon cooling, form gels with a large pore size that allow most proteins, including antibodies, to diffuse through. If antibody migrating through the gel encounters antigen, an insoluble precipitate is commonly formed at equivalence. The precipitate can often be visualised as an opaque line in the gel (precipitin line); the use of a protein stain such as Coomassie Brilliant Blue allows visualisation of weak (invisible) precipitin lines. Protein antigens that are insoluble in physiological buffers (e.g. membrane or cytoskeletal proteins) can be solubilised in non-ionic detergents for analysis in detergent-containing gels without adversely affecting the formation of the precipitin line.

Precipitation techniques in agar are typically carried out using gels 2–3 mm thick, cast on glass (e.g. microscope) slides (warm agar solution is simply poured onto the slide and allowed to set). Wells are then cut into the gel using, for example, a large-bore pipette. In diffusion techniques, antibody and/or antigen migrate through the gel by simple diffusion. In double diffusion, separate wells cut in the agar are filled with antibody and antigen, respectively (Fig. 7.10). Both diffuse into and through the agar, automatically forming concentration gradients. Provided these cover the equivalence concentrations, a precipitin line is formed at the equivalence point. The technique can be used to give information on antigenic (and hence structural) similarities or differences between antigens (Fig. 7.11).

In single radial immunodiffusion (SRID), antigen is loaded into wells cut in an agar gel containing a fixed concentration of antibody (Fig. 7.10). A precipitin ring around the well is formed at equivalence. The diameter of the ring at equivalence is related to the antigen concentration. Two relationships have been determined:

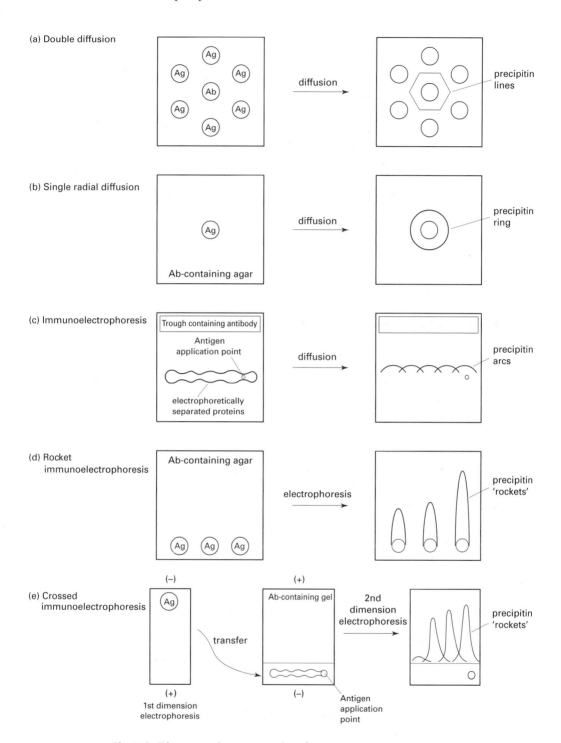

Fig. 7.10. Diagrammatic representation of immunoprecipitation techniques in agar. For details, see the text. Ag, antigen; Ab, antibody.

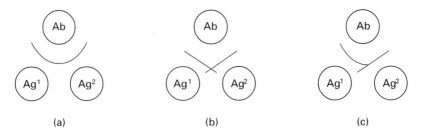

Fig. 7.11. Interpretation of precipitin lines following double immunodiffusion. Fusion of immunoprecipitin lines (a) infers immunochemical identity of antigens (Ag) 1 and 2, whereas crossing of the lines (b) shows their non-identity. Partial fusion or spur formation (c) suggests partial identity, i.e. antigen 2 has some determinants that are not shared by antigen 1, but all the determinants recognised by these antibodies (Ab) that are present on antigen 1 are also present on antigen 2.

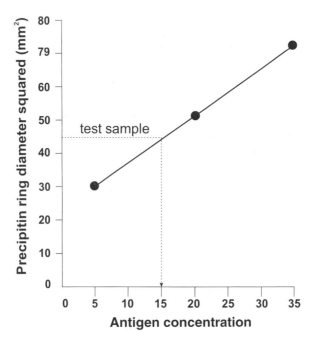

Fig. 7.12. The use of single radial immunodiffusion to measure antigen concentrations in test samples. The standard curve was constructed from the square of the precipitin ring diameters given by calibrator samples containing known amounts of antigen. The square of the precipitin ring diameters of the test samples can then be read from the standard curve to give the antigen concentration in the samples.

(i) the square of the ring diameter is proportional to the antigen concentration (Mancini method; Fig. 7.12); and (ii) the diameter of the ring is proportional to the log of the antigen concentration (Fahey and McKelvey method). This technique is useful for determining concentrations of antigens such as serum proteins. For example, if the agar contains specific antibodies against human IgG, and wells cut into the gel are loaded with test samples containing unknown quantities of human IgG (e.g. serum samples) together with calibrator samples containing known concentrations of human IgG, precipitin rings will form around the wells at equivalence. By measuring the ring diameters produced by the calibrator samples of known IgG concentration, a standard curve can be constructed by plotting the square of the diameter of the precipitin ring against the IgG concentration. The square of the ring diameters of the test samples can then be read off the standard curve to give the IgG concentration in the test samples (see Fig. 7.12).

In immunoelectrophoresis, a mixture of proteins containing the antigen are first separated by agar gel electrophoresis. Antibody is then allowed to diffuse through the gel from a trough cut in the gel parallel to the direction of electrophoresis (Fig. 7.10). Precipitin arcs are then formed where antibody meets antigen at equivalence. A disadvantage of this technique is the relatively poor resolution of antigen mixtures using agar gel electrophoresis, but it can be useful for detecting precipitating antibodies. Clinically, the technique is carried out on samples of patient's serum, concentrated urine or spinal fluid to detect abnormalities in concentrations of antigens and/or the presence of abnormal proteins relative to normal control samples analysed at the same time.

Rocket immunoelectrophoresis is an adaption of single radial immunodiffusion and involves electrophoretic migration of antigen from wells cut in antibody-containing gel (Fig. 7.10). At equivalence, rocket-shaped precipitin lines are formed, the area under which is proportional to the antigen concentration. The technique can be used to determine antigen concentrations in unknown samples (e.g. serum protein levels) by reference to a standard curve as in RID, or to investigate immunochemical relationships between different samples if these are placed in adjacent wells close together (see Fig. 7.11 for interpretation of precipitin line patterns).

In crossed immunoelectrophoresis, proteins are first separated by agar gel electrophoresis, after which they are electrophoresed into an antibody-containing gel at right angles to the direction of the first electrophoresis (Fig. 7.10). The technique can be used for analysis of serum proteins.

The sensitivity of precipitation techniques in agar varies enormously depending on the antibodies and antigens involved.

7.4.2 **Immunoprecipitation in solution**

An antibody can be used specifically to immunoprecipitate its antigen from a mixture of proteins in solution, for example a cell lysate. If the immunoprecipitate is insoluble, it can be sedimented by centrifugation for analysis; soluble antibody–antigen complexes can be isolated by precipitation with an immunoglobulin-binding protein such as protein A or G, or an anti-immunoglobulin antibody, or those reagents covalently bound to an insoluble support such as agarose (see Section 7.3.4). This basic method forms the basis of classical radioimmunoassays (RIA) (see Section 7.7.1). It also allows the isolation of an unknown antigen from a mixture of proteins. For the latter, it may be necessary to label the mixture of

Example 1 **SINGLE RADIAL DIFFUSION FOR ESTIMATING THE CONCENTRA-
TION OF ANTIGEN**

Question

The precipitin ring diameters of an antigen calibrator at three different concentrations were:

Concentration ($\mu g\,cm^{-3}$)	Ring diameter (mm)	Ring diameter squared (mm^2)
10	4	16
60	7	49
100	8.7	76

The ring diameter of the sample of unknown antigen concentration was 6 mm. What was the concentration of the antigen in the unknown?

Answer

To answer this question, a graph of the type shown in Fig. 7.12 must be plotted. The graph of the precipitin ring diameter squared (y-axis) against the antigen concentration (x-axis) is a straight line. Given that the unknown sample gave a ring diameter of 6 mm (i.e. 36 mm^2), the antigen concentration in the sample can be read off the calibration graph and seen to be 40 $\mu g\,cm^{-3}$.

proteins, for example cell lysate, with ^{125}I prior to immunoprecipitation. The immunoprecipitate can then be analysed by SDS–PAGE (Section 10.3.1) and autoradiography (Section 14.2.3) to give information on the antigen. Alternatively, non-radiolabelled immunoprecipitate can be analysed by SDS–PAGE and immunoblotting with antibodies of known specificity (Section 7.6), which can allow positive identification of immunoprecipitated proteins. Immunoprecipitation is commonly carried out on radiolabelled intact cells or cell membranes to give information on cell surface antigens (Fig. 7.13).

Although an antibody can be used to analyse individual proteins in a mixture separated by SDS–PAGE using immunoblotting procedures (Section 7.6), immunoprecipitation in solution has the advantage that the antibody is allowed to react with native rather than partially denatured antigen as is the case in immunoblots. Some antigens lose their immunoreactivity following electrophoresis and immunoblotting, or even (especially for cell surface antigens) solubilisation. This occurs when epitopes are conformation dependent or arise through the interaction of several protein subunits/components.

7.5 **LABELLING ANTIBODIES**

The specificity of antibodies makes them powerful analytical tools. Although immunoprecipitation techniques in agar (see Section 7.4) result in visible precipitated antibody–antigen complexes, in most immunochemical assays binding of antibody to antigen can be visualised only by labelling the antibody (or

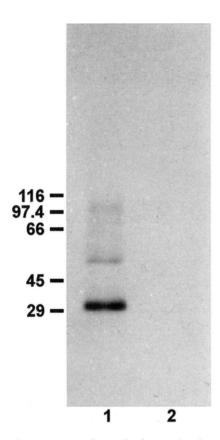

Fig. 7.13. Autoradiograph of monoclonal anti-Rh D immune precipitates from ^{125}I-labelled Rh D-positive and Rh D-negative erythrocyte membranes after analysis by SDS–PAGE. Human erythrocytes positive or negative for the Rh D blood group antigen were surface labelled with^{125} I. The cells were lysed by hypotonic shock and the membranes incubated with monoclonal anti-Rh D. After being washed to remove unbound antibody, the membranes were solubilised and the antibody–antigen complexes isolated using protein A–Sepharose. The antibody–antigen complexes were then analysed by SDS–PAGE and autoradiography. The molecular weight of the major protein immunoprecipitated from Rh D-positive membranes is approximately 31 000 (lane 1) and corresponds to the Rh D polypeptide. No protein was immunoprecipitated from the Rh D-negative membranes (lane 2). The relative positions of the molecular weight markers are shown ($M_r \times 10^{-3}$).

sometimes antigen) or (more commonly) an antibody against immunoglobulin (see Section 7.5.1) with a marker that can be qualitatively and sometimes quantitatively detected. Thus an antibody can be labelled with a radioactive isotope for use in radioimmunoassays, or an enzyme that gives a coloured product for use in enzyme-linked immunosorbent assay (ELISA), or a fluorochrome that emits visible fluorescence for use in immunohistochemistry (Table 7.7). Binding of unlabelled antibody to antigen in these techniques would be undetectable. Antibodies labelled with fluorochromes or enzymes are commonly referred to as conjugates

Table 7.7 Common antibody labels for immunochemical techniques

Label	Examples	Main use(s)
Fluorochromes	Fluorescein	Immunohisto/cytochemistry; flow cytofluorimetry; fluorimetric assays
	Rhodamine	Immunohisto/cytochemistry; flow cyotfluorimetry
	Phycoerythrin	Flow cytofluorimetry
	Texas Red	Flow cytofluorimetry
	7-Amino-4-methylcoumarin 3-acetate (AMCA)	Flow cytofluorimetry
	[a] BODIPY derivatives	Flow cytofluorimetry
	[a] Cascade Blue	Flow cytofluorimetry
Enzymes	AP	Immunohistochemistry; EIA; immunoblotting
	β-Galactosidase	As above
	HRP	As above; immunoelectron microscopy
	Glucose oxidase	Immunohistochemistry
	Urease	EIA
Radioisotope	^{125}I	Competitive and non-competitive RIA
Electron dense	Gold	Immunoelectron microscopy
	Ferritin	As above

BODIPY, 4,4-difluoro-4-bora-3a,4a-diaza-s-indacene; AP, alkaline phosphatase; EIA, enzyme immunometric assay; HRP, horseradish peroxidase.
[a] Trademark of Molecular Probes Inc.

7.5.1 Direct and indirect immunochemical procedures

In simple, direct immunochemical procedures, the antibody against the antigen of interest (the 'primary' antibody) is conjugated with the label. In the more commonly used indirect procedures, binding of unlabelled primary antibody to the antigen is detected using a labelled antibody against immunoglobulin (or less commonly, a labelled bacterial immunoglobulin-binding protein such as protein A or protein G). This secondary antibody is usually raised against the immunoglobulin from the animal species in which the primary antibody was produced, and may also be class or subclass specific. Direct and indirect procedures are illustrated diagrammatically in Fig. 7.14. Indirect methods utilising labelled anti-immunoglobulin antibodies have several advantages over direct procedures: they are more sensitive, since several labelled anti-immunoglobulin molecules can bind to each unlabelled primary antibody, resulting in a stronger signal; each primary antibody does not have to be labelled individually as, for example, labelled rabbit anti-mouse IgG antibodies will recognise all mouse IgG monoclonal antibodies; and there is no risk of loss of reactivity of the primary antibody as a result of direct labelling. However,

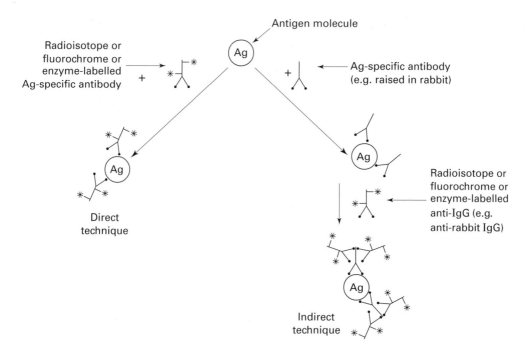

Fig. 7.14. Diagrammatic representation of direct and indirect immunochemical methodology. Ag, antigen.

there are cases that necessitate the use of directly labelled antibodies (see Sections 7.8.3 and 7.8.5). A semi-direct procedure takes advantage of the high-affinity specific interaction between biotin and avidin/streptavidin (see Section 7.5.5) and involves the use of biotinylated primary antibody and labelled avidin/streptavidin preparations.

7.5.2 **Radiolabelling**

Radioiodination

The most commonly used radioisotope for radiolabelling antibodies is ^{125}I. This isotope is readily available as Na^{125}I, is relatively inexpensive and has a high specific activity. It emits γ-radiation, which can be easily and directly detected and quantified using a γ-counter, and is good for autoradiography. However, suitable precautions must be taken to minimise exposure of workers to radiation and to prevent contact, contamination and ingestion (the thyroid is particularly susceptible). Covalent labelling of proteins directly with ^{125}I involves oxidative generation of cationic iodine (I^{+}) and its spontaneous electrophilic addition to tyrosine residues, and, to a lesser extent, to tryptophan and histidine residues. The major substitution is a monoiodotyrosyl residue, although di-iodotyrosyl residues may also be formed (Fig. 7.15). The concentrations of reagents should allow for only one or two tyrosine residues per antibody

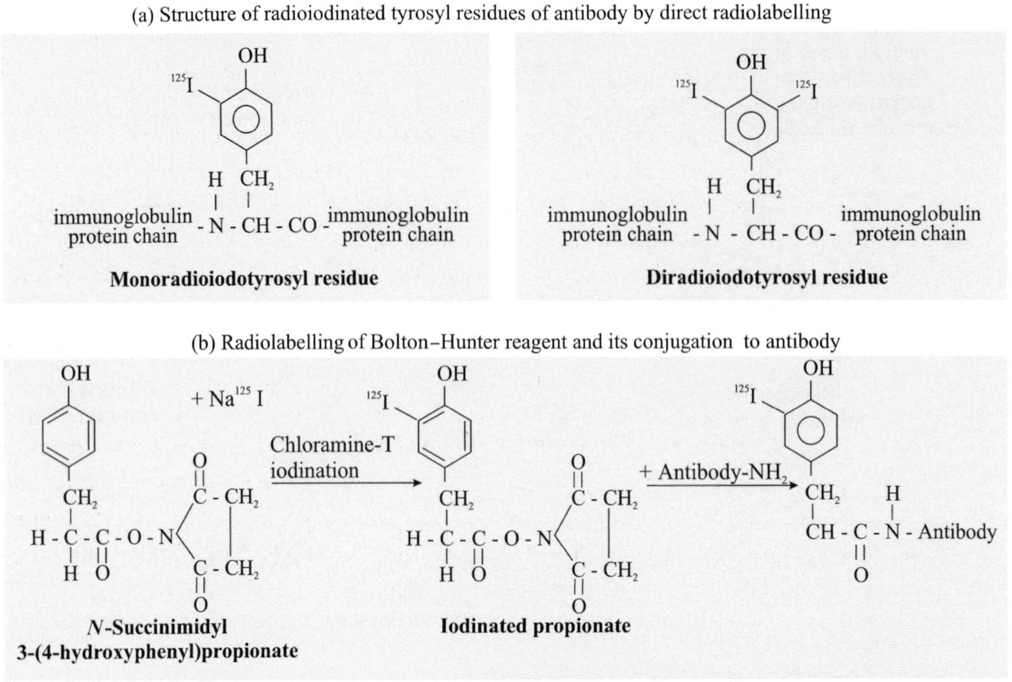

(a) Structure of radioiodinated tyrosyl residues of antibody by direct radiolabelling

Monoradioiodotyrosyl residue

Diradioiodotyrosyl residue

(b) Radiolabelling of Bolton–Hunter reagent and its conjugation to antibody

N-Succinimidyl
3-(4-hydroxyphenyl)propionate

Iodinated propionate

Fig. 7.15. Direct and indirect radiolabelling of antibodies with ^{125}I.

molecule to be ^{125}I-labelled otherwise loss of immunoreactivity and/or radiation damage may occur.

There are several established methods for radioiodination, which differ in the choice of oxidising agent used to generate I^+. Since strong oxidising agents can destroy the immunoreactivity of antibodies, there must be a compromise between efficient generation of I^+ and preservation of antigen-binding capacity.

Chloramine T (*N*-chloro-*p*-toluene sulphonamide) is an aromatic oxidising agent commonly used for high specific activity iodination of antibodies and other proteins. Chloramine T iodination is very rapid (45 s), but it can denature antibodies and lead to loss of antigen-binding capacity. The reaction must be stopped quickly after appropriate iodination, by adding a reducing agent such as sodium metabisulphite or an excess of tyrosine to 'mop up' iodine as iodotyrosine. Following radioiodination, the antibody needs to be separated from free (i.e. non-antibody bound) ^{125}I. This can be achieved either by gel filtration, or if IgG antibody has been radiolabelled, a strongly basic anion exchanger can be used to adsorb iodotyrosine. The use of chloramine T immobilised on beads offers a milder alternative, since the reaction can be stopped simply by removing the solid material.

Another oxidising agent commonly used for radioiodination is iodogen (1,3,4,6-tetrachloro-3α,6α-diphenylglycoluril), which is milder than chloramine T. Iodogen is insoluble in aqueous solvents, so its use necessitates dissolving it in chloroform or benzene, usually in a plastic tube, and then allowing the organic solvent to evaporate and leave the iodogen coated on the side of the tube. The radioiodination procedure is then carried out in the iodogen-coated tube and stopped by taking the solution out of the tube.

Radioiodination of antibodies using the enzyme lactoperoxidase is a very mild procedure that does minimal damage to antibodies, but does not produce radio-labelled antibodies of high specific activity. Lactoperoxidase-catalysed iodination is therefore usually used only for iodinating cell surface components, since it minimises diffusion of reactants across the cell membrane to label internal components.

Antibodies can also be conjugated with low molecular weight, previously radio-iodinated phenolic compounds. Commonly, N-succinimidyl 3-(4-hydroxyphenyl) propionate (the Bolton–Hunter reagent) is radioiodinated using chloramine T and the 5-[^{125}I]iodophenyl derivative is then conjugated to amino groups of the antibody (Fig. 7.15). The advantage of indirectly radiolabelling antibodies in this way is that there is no risk of oxidative damage, but, as with direct labelling, only one or two residues per antibody molecule should be conjugated with the iodophenyl derivative.

7.5.3 Labelling with fluorochromes

Fluorochromes emit fluorescent light under ultraviolet illumination. The fluorescence of fluorochrome-labelled antibody in solution can be quantified using a fluorimeter. However, the greatest use of fluorochrome-labelled antibodies is in immunohisto/cytochemistry where binding of fluorochrome-labelled antibodies to tissue sections or cells is visualised using a microscope equipped with fluorescence optics (Section 7.8.3). Antibodies labelled with fluorochromes are used extensively in flow cytometric techniques (Section 7.8.5).

Many fluorochromes are available with different excitation and emission spectra, but the ones most commonly used for microscopy are fluorescein, which emits green fluorescence, and tetramethylrhodamine, which emits red fluorescence. For conjugation, fluorescein and tetramethylrhodamine isothiocyanate are usually used, they readily form covalent linkages with primary amine groups on lysine residues in the antibody molecule (Fig. 7.16), although iodoacetamido derivatives of fluorescein and rhodamine are also available for coupling via sulphydryl groups. Other fluorochromes, mostly used in flow cytofluorimetry, and which can be coupled to amine (or sulphydryl groups) include Texas Red (sulpho-rhodamine; Fig. 7.16), 7-amino-4-methylcoumarin 3-acetate (AMCA; fluoresces blue) and BODIPY (4,4-difluoro-4-bora-3a,4a-diaza-s-indacene).

Phycobiliproteins are a group of intensely fluorescent proteins found in algae and cyanobacteria and widely used in flow cytofluorimetry. They include B- and R-phycoerythrin (M_r 240 000), C-phycocyanin (M_r 72 000) and allophycocyanin (M_r 110 000). Phycobiliproteins can be attached via their amine groups to the thiol groups of the antibody, using chemical heterobifunctional cross-linking agents (Section 7.5.4).

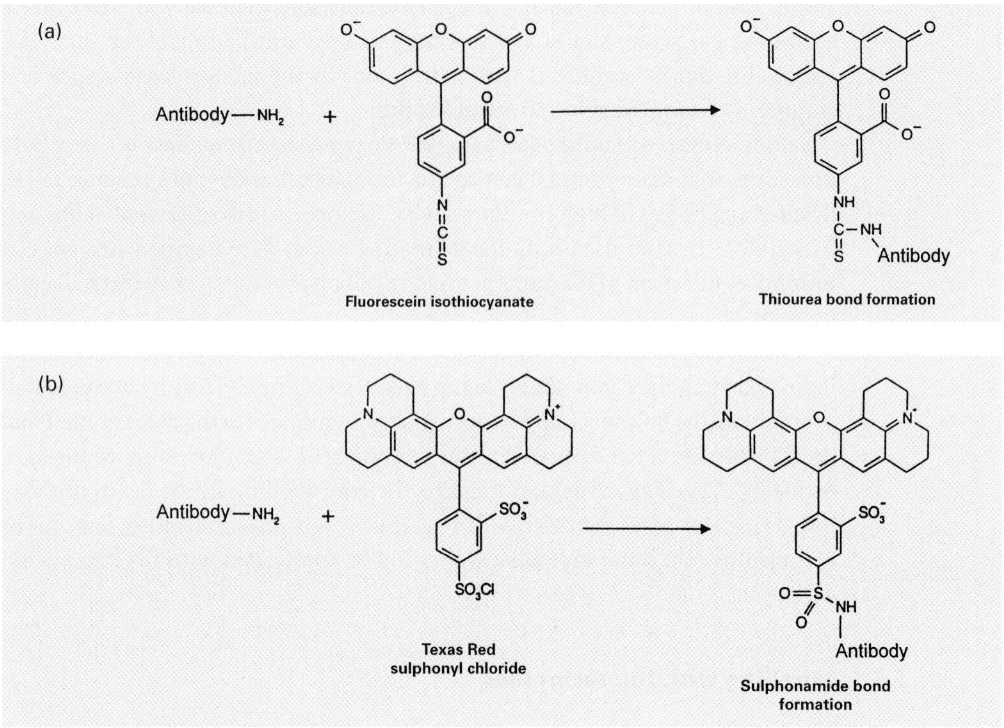

(a)

Antibody—NH$_2$ +

Fluorescein isothiocyanate

Thiourea bond formation

(b)

Antibody—NH$_2$ +

Texas Red
sulphonyl chloride

Sulphonamide bond
formation

Fig. 7.16. Conjugation of (a) fluorescein isothiocyanate and (b) Texas Red
(sulphorhodamine) to amine groups of antibody.

7.5.4 Labelling with enzymes

Enzyme-labelled antibodies are widely used in immunoassays (e.g. ELISA),
immunoblotting and immunohisto/cytochemistry. In each case, direct or indirect binding (Section 7.5.1) of the enzyme-labelled antibody to antigen (which
may be in tissue sections or on blots or on the wells of a microtitre plate) is visualised by carrying out the enzyme reaction in which a colourless substrate is
converted to a coloured product. In enzyme immunoassays, the product needs to
be soluble to allow spectrophotometric quantification; in immunoblotting and
immunohistochemical procedures, the product must be insoluble to allow
precise localisation of the initial antigen–antibody interaction and visible either
directly by eye or using microscopy. The use of enzyme-labelled antibodies allows
catalytic amplification of the signal, since each enzyme molecule can convert
many substrate molecules into coloured product. Properties of enzymes commonly used for conjugation are listed in Table 7.8. Since enzymes are proteins,
they have to be conjugated to antibody using chemical cross-linking reagents.
There are two types of cross-linker: homobifunctional reagents, which react with
the same chemical group on both the enzyme and the antibody, and heterobifunctional reagents, which react with different chemical groups on each protein.

Table 7.8 Properties of enzymes used for conjugation to antibodies

Enzyme	Source	Structure	Reaction catalysed
Peroxidase	Horseradish	Monomeric glycoprotein M_r 40 000	H_2O_2 + oxidisable substrate $\rightarrow$ oxidised product + $2H_2O$
Alkaline phosphatase	Calf intestine (usually)	Zn^{2+}-containing glycoprotein	R-O-P + H_2O $\rightarrow$ R-OH + P_i orthophosphoric alcohol inorganic monoester phosphate substrate
β-Galactosidase	E. coli	Multimeric protein (4 subunits) M_r 540 000	β-D-Galactoside + H_2O $\rightarrow$ galactose + alcohol
Glucose oxidase	Aspergillus niger	Flavo-glycoprotein	β-D-Glucose + O_2 $\rightarrow$ H_2O_2 + gluconic acid
Urease	Jack bean	M_r 480 000	$(NH_2)_2CO$ + $3H_2O$ $\rightarrow$ CO_2 + $2NH_4OH$

Glutaraldehyde is a simple homobifunctional cross-linker that cross-links the amine groups (e.g. of lysine; Fig. 7.17) of proteins. Conjugation can be carried out either in a one-step procedure in which the glutaraldehyde is added to a mixture of enzyme and protein (works for horseradish peroxidase (HRP), alkaline phosphatase and β-galactosidase), or, for HRP conjugation, in a two-step procedure in which glutaraldehyde is first reacted with enzyme, and the glutaraldehyde-coupled enzyme is then reacted with antibody. There is a wide range of heterobifunctional reagents available, consisting typically of an amine-reactive group and a thiol-reactive group separated by a spacer arm, which cross-links the amine groups of antibodies to the sulphydryl groups of enzymes. An example is succinimidyl-4-(N-maleimidomethyl)cyclohexane 1-carboxylate (SMCC; Fig. 7.17). Another method of conjugation involves the use of periodate to generate active aldehyde groups by cleavage of carbohydrate chains of glycoprotein enzymes. These groups then react with primary amine groups in the antibody to form Schiff bases, which are then reduced to produce stable bonds.

7.5.5 Biotinylation of antibodies

The very high affinity interaction (affinity constant $> 10^{15}$ M^{-1}) between biotin (vitamin H; M_r 244) and avidin (a protein from egg white) or streptavidin (a protein from the bacterium *Streptomyces avidinii*) can be exploited in immunochemical techniques by conjugating biotin to antibodies for use with fluorochrome- or enzyme-conjugated or radiolabelled avidin/streptavidin (Fig. 7.18). Antibodies can be conjugated easily with biotin derivatives, most commonly N-hydroxysuccinimidobiotin or analogues incorporating a spacer arm. The latter reduces steric hindrance by increasing the distance between the biotin and the antibody. Most of these biotin derivatives react with primary amine groups, although there are some that are reactive with thiol groups or carbohydrate residues on the immunoglobulin.

7.6 IMMUNOBLOTTING

In many cases it is informative to establish the specificity of antibodies by investigating their ability to recognise components present in complex mixtures. Specific antibodies can also be used to identify such components and establish cross-reactivities that may occur with immunochemically related molecular species. For such methods it is clearly necessary to separate the antigenic components using an analytical method. In theory, any biochemical technique can be used for this, but the high resolving power of polyacrylamide gel electrophoretic methods (especially SDS–PAGE and isoelectric focusing; see Sections 10.3.1 and 10.3.4) makes these ideal for such purposes. The most commonly used technique involves transferring separated proteins from polyacrylamide gels to a porous membrane and probing this 'blot' with antibody (antibody can be applied directly to the gel, but the very limited permeability of polyacrylamide gel makes this inefficient and time consuming). Antibody–antigen complexes are then detected either by the use of labelled anti-immunoglobulin reagent or by labelling the antibody directly

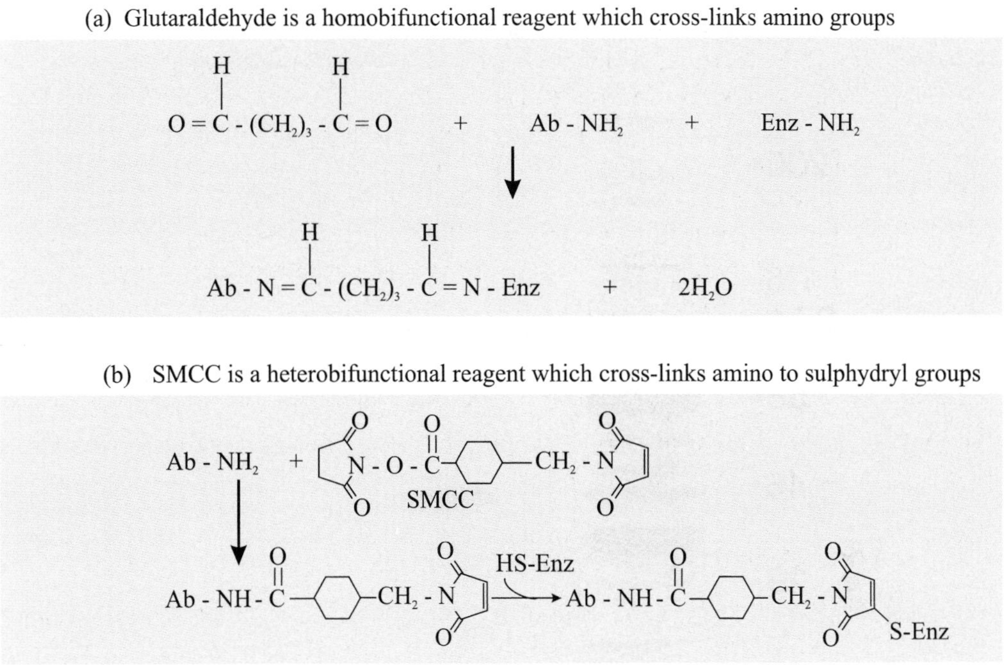

(a) Glutaraldehyde is a homobifunctional reagent which cross-links amino groups

$$\underset{\substack{|\\ O=C-(CH_2)_3-C=O}}{\overset{\substack{H \qquad\qquad H\\ |\qquad\qquad\;\;}}{}} \qquad + \qquad Ab - NH_2 \qquad + \qquad Enz - NH_2$$

$$\downarrow$$

$$\underset{Ab-N=C-(CH_2)_3-C=N-Enz}{\overset{H \qquad\qquad\;\; H}{}} \qquad + \qquad 2H_2O$$

(b) SMCC is a heterobifunctional reagent which cross-links amino to sulphydryl groups

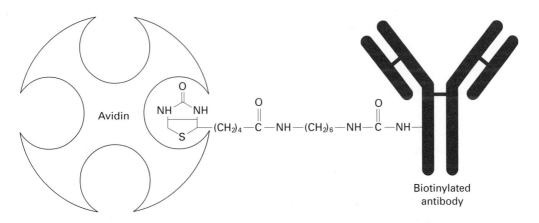

Fig. 7.17. (a and b) Structure and mode of action of cross-linking reagents. Ab, antibody; Enz, enzyme.

Fig. 7.18. The interaction of biotin-conjugated IgG with avidin. The binding is very strong and each avidin molecule has four biotin binding sites. For the structure shown, coupling of biotin to immunoglobulin has been carried out using biotinamidocaproate N-hydroxysuccinimide ester.

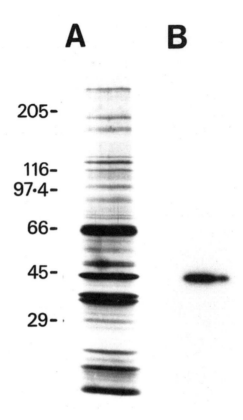

Fig. 7.19. Use of immunoblotting to show how specific antibodies can be used to identify their antigens in complex mixtures. Components of smooth muscle homogenate were separated using SDS-PAGE in duplicate tracks. One track was protein-stained to allow visualisation of all the components present in the homogenate (lane A); components in the second track were electrophoretically transferred to nitrocellulose and incubated with mouse monoclonal antibody against smooth muscle α-actin followed by ^{125}I-labelled anti-mouse IgG. After autoradiography, one protein band is immunostained (lane B) corresponding to smooth muscle α-actin. The relative positions of molecular weight markers ($\times 10^{-3}$) are shown.

with radioisotope (^{125}I is usually employed for this) or enzyme (see Section 7.5). Antigens recognised by antibody thus appear as 'bands' on autoradiographs or substrate-developed blots and comparison of these with protein-stained gels allows identification of antigens recognised by antibody (Fig. 7.19). This process shows some similarity to Southern and northern blotting used with nucleic acid and is known as immunoblotting or 'western' blotting (see also Section 10.3.8).

Nitrocellulose is normally employed as the porous membrane for immunoblotting, but other materials are also occasionally used. Increased sensitivity with immunoblotting can be obtained by the use of enhanced chemiluminescence (ECL) development. In ECL-linked immunoblotting, peroxidase-conjugated anti-immunoglobulin is used to detect antigen–antibody complexes (cf. ELISA; Section 7.7.3). This enzyme is used to generate a peracid by cleavage of hydrogen peroxide and this in turn oxidises a substrate to yield light, which is detected using X-ray film (as for autoradiography). The substrate is normally luminol, and phenolic 'enhancer' compounds are included to increase photon yield. Other ECL systems have been developed for use with alkaline phosphatase conjugates. ECL detection is sensitive and fast compared to direct use of enzyme or radioisotope conjugates. Other chemiluminescence amplification systems suitable for use in immunoblotting involving different enzymes, substrates and enhancers are also available.

7.7　IMMUNOASSAYS

Many immunochemical techniques provide quantitative assessment of the concentration of analyte in pure solutions or complex mixtures, for example single radial immunodiffusion and rocket immunoelectrophoresis (Section 7.4.1). However, the great potential of the application of immunochemistry to sensitive and specific assay of a diverse range of chemical and biological molecules has led to very considerable effort being focused in this area. Many versions of basic immunochemical assay principles now exist; such methodologies are termed immunoassays to emphasise their quantitative aspect.

Refinements to immunoassay methodology for research purposes have been driven mainly by the need for ever greater specificity and particularly sensitivity. Immunoassays are widely used for routine diagnostic/prognostic purposes and other applications (e.g. measuring levels of enviromental contaminants such as pesticides and toxic by-products of industrial processes); techniques that allow high sample throughput, ease of automation (robotic processing is often used), economy, robustness, precision and accuracy have been developed and are being sought. A thorough description of all alternative immunoassay techniques and formats would occupy several volumes, but the general principles and some of the more frequently employed options are described below.

7.7.1　Competitive binding immunoassays

In competitive binding immunoassays, antigen present in the samples to be assayed competes with a fixed amount of labelled antigen in the presence of a limiting quantity of antibody. When the system has reached equilibrium, free antigen is separated from antibody-bound antigen and the amount of labelled antigen present in the latter determined by scintillation (for β emission) or γ counting. This is inversely proportional to the concentration of antigen present in the samples (see Fig. 7.20). Inclusion of a number of dilutions of a standard solution of known antigen content allows the construction of a dose–response curve (often known as a standard curve), which can be used, by comparison, to derive antigen concentrations in samples. The earliest immunoassays were of this type, and the most common label used was a radioisotope (^{3}H, ^{125}I). Such assays are normally known as radioimmunoassays (RIAs), although they should be called competitive binding radioimmunoassays to distinguish them from radiobinding assays (Section 7.7.3). The first RIA described was for insulin, and similar approaches using binding

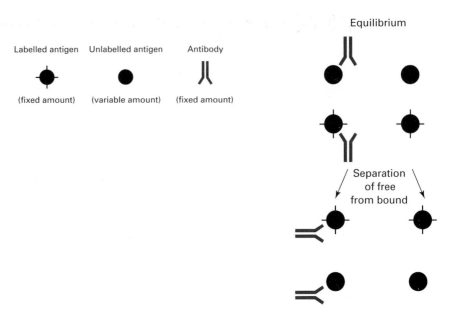

Fig. 7.20. Diagrammatic representation of competitive binding (inhibition) immunoassay.

proteins rather than antibodies were also developed at this time, for example for vitamin B12. The sensitivity of such assays varies considerably and depends on several factors, such as the label used. RIAs using ^{125}I labels can theoretically reach a sensitivity of 10^{-14} M, but in practice this is usually $\leq 10^{-12}$ M. In developing an RIA, it is initially necessary to derive an antibody versus labelled antigen binding curve to select appropriate antibody and labelled antigen concentrations for the assay. Normally, conditions at which 50–70% of the labelled antigen is bound by antibody are selected for the competitive RIA. Numerous procedures have been developed for separating free from bound antigen (see Table 7.9).

RIAs have been produced for a wide range of analytes from small molecules (e.g. steroids, peptide hormones in human or animal serum/plasma) to large proteins (e.g. serum levels of α_2-macroglobulin, immunoglobulins). They can be precise, accurate and economical (very small amounts of antibody are required). However, they are difficult to automate, take a relatively long time and the dose–response curve usually covers only a relatively narrow range of analyte concentration. They can be less sensitive than some other immunoassays. It is also necessary to establish systems for containment and disposal of radioactive reagents and for medical surveillance of staff involved in use of RIA methods. This bureaucracy has resulted in a reduction in use of RIA technology.

As the antibody concentrations used are limiting, competitive binding assays are sometimes called reagent (antigen) excess immunoassays (cf. immunometric assays; Section 7.7.2). Competitive immunoassays using non-radioisotope labels have been developed, but this approach is rather disappointing. Use of enzyme labels often results in insensitive assays and other labelling options can produce

Table 7.9 Methods for separating bound and free labelled ligand in radio-immunoassays

Method	Principle
Coated charcoal	Adsorption of bound or free fraction
Florisil	
S. aureus – protein A	
Polyethylene glycol	Fractional precipitation of bound fraction
Ethanol	
Ammonium sulphate	
Second antibody	Precipitation of bound fraction
soluble	
solid phase – cellulose	
– magnetic particles	
First antibody	Precipitation of bound fraction
solid phase – coated disks and tubes	
– cellulose	
– magnetic particles	

non-robust, imprecise and insensitive assays. The reason for this is not always clear, but labelling antigen with relatively bulky enzyme molecules (rather than the small atoms used in RIA) can alter antibody recognition of labelled compared with unlabelled antigen species, causing assay problems. This limitation has resulted in decreasing use of competitive immunoassay technology.

7.7.2 **Immunometric assays**

Immunometric assays differ from competitive immunoassays in several ways, although they provide similar quantitative information concerning antigen concentration. In the first-described immunometric assays, a fixed amount of labelled antibody was allowed to react with variable amounts of antigen. Unbound labelled antibody was then removed by washing and the labelled antibody remaining measured to provide an estimate of the antigen content (see Fig. 7.21). This approach is rarely used nowadays, but the concept of using an excess of labelled antibody, i.e. antibody excess immunoassays, rather than excess of labelled antigen (antigen excess immunoassays, i.e. competitive immunoassays) has numerous advantages and a few disadvantages (see below).

In most recently devised immunometric assays, antigen is allowed to react with insoluble or immobilised antibody, i.e. is 'captured' from solution, and the bound antigen is then detected using an excess of another (or in some special cases the same) antibody specific for the antigen. Captured antibody can be immobilised by covalent attachment to agarose microbeads, or by electrostatic binding to plastic or glass beads or the surfaces of plastic tubes or microtitre plates (see Fig. 7.22). The latter option is most often used, and special plates are available that have been treated to optimise antigen binding. Some methods use immobilised anti-Fc

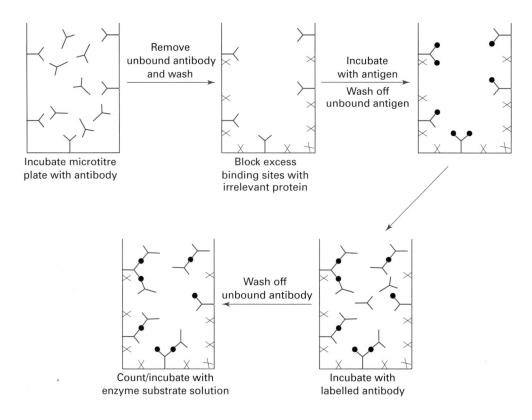

Fig. 7.21. Diagrammatic representation of a two-site immunometric assay (IRMA or two-site ELISA) for estimation of antigens. This particular format uses 96-well microtitre plates.

immunoglobulin to ensure that the captured antibody is immobilised in the correct orientation to interact optimally with antigen.

The detecting antibody can be directly labelled or can be indirectly measured using labelled anti-immunoglobulin reagent or other approaches, for example the avidin–biotin interaction (Section 7.5.5). Immunometric assays are usually relatively fast to carry out, can be very sensitive, and cover a wider range of analyte concentration than competitive assays. However, they require more antibody than competitive assays and normally two antibodies that recognise different determinants on the antigen are needed. Some immunometric assay formats (especially those employing microtitre plate layouts; see Fig. 7.21) can be automated and performed and controlled robotically to enable very high sample throughput.

Immunometric assays using radiolabelled antibody have been developed for a wide range of analytes and the first such assays were of this type. They are known as immunoradiometric assays (IRMAs). Even more immunometric assays using enzyme-labelled antibodies have been produced and these should be referred to as enzyme immunometric assays (EIAs or EIMAs). However, they are often unfortunately called ELISAs, which confuses them with enzyme-linked

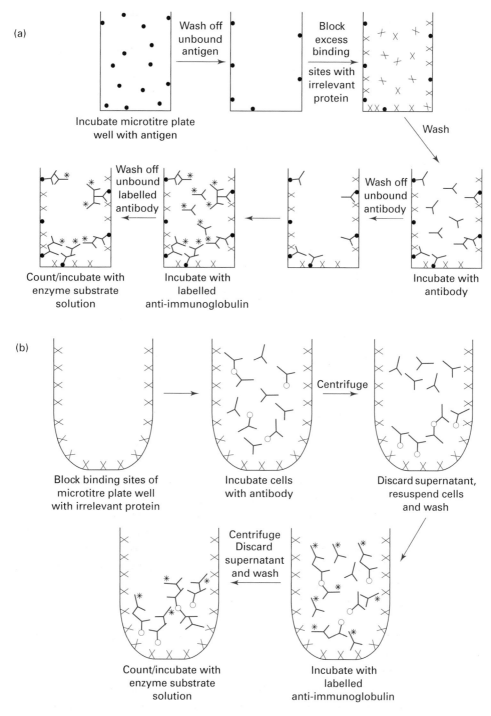

(a)

Incubate microtitre plate
well with antigen

Wash off
unbound
antigen

Block
excess
binding
sites with
irrelevant
protein

Wash

Wash off
unbound
labelled
antibody

Count/incubate with
enzyme substrate
solution

Incubate with
labelled
anti-immunoglobulin

Wash off
unbound
antibody

Incubate with
antibody

(b)

Block binding sites of
microtitre plate well
with irrelevant protein

Incubate cells
with antibody

Centrifuge

Discard supernatant,
resuspend cells
and wash

Centrifuge
Discard
supernatant
and wash

Count/incubate with
enzyme substrate
solution

Incubate with
labelled
anti-immunoglobulin

Fig. 7.22. Diagrammatic representation of microtitre plate format solid-phase binding immunoassays: (a) for antibodies directed against soluble antigens; (b) for antibodies directed against cell surface antigens.

immunobinding assays (Section 7.7.3). To try to distinguish them from 'real' ELISAs, they are often called sandwich ELISAs or two-site ELISAs. Most enzyme immunometric assays use a colorimetric substrate that is measured spectro-photometrically to determine antigen concentration. However, fluorescent sub-strates can be used for some enzymes (such as β-galactosidase) that have been claimed to increase assay sensitivity. An ever-increasing range of other labelling systems have been devised for immunometric assays and some of these are described in Section 7.7.4. All immunometric assays require calibration using dilutions of a standard solution of analyte of known concentration (cf. competitive immunoassays). The requirement that immunometric assay theory requires antibodies recognising different epitopes on antigen limited their application until the advent of monoclonal antibody technology (Section 7.2). Polyclonal antibodies can be used for immunometric assays, but unless the antigen is polymeric this approach is of limited use owing to occupation, by the capture antibody, of the antibody-binding sites recognised by the detecting antibody. The use of two monoclonal antibodies recognising different antigenic epitopes that do not display steric hindrance for binding of either antibody allows optimisation of immunometric assays. Combination of the use of a monoclonal antibody (for capture) with polyclonal detecting antibody can provide sensitive and specific immunoassays. Selection of appropriate antibodies and producing antibody preparations of appropriate quality are crucial for successful immunometric assays.

7.7.3 Solid-phase immunobinding assays (for estimation of antibody)

Immunobinding assays are solid-phase assays using immobilised antigen for assessing the antibody content of samples. They are often regarded as immuno-assays, although their value for accurate quantification of antibody concentration can be questioned (if accuracy is important it is usually better to use an immunometric or competitive binding assay; Sections 7.7.1 and 7.7.2). However, immunobinding assays are very easy, quick, cheap and simple, and are ideal for checking the comparative antibody content of sera and other biological fluids and especially for screening sera from immunised animals, hybridoma culture supernatants, ascitic fluid and pathological samples. Antigen-containing solution is simply incubated in plastic tubes or (more often) in the wells of plastic microtitre plates, which allows a (small) proportion of the protein to coat the surfaces of the tubes or wells. After unbound antigen(s) has been washed away, the samples of known or unknown antibody content are incubated in the antigen-coated tubes/wells. Antibody (if present) binds to the immobilised antigen(s) and, after washing, can be detected using labelled anti-immunoglobulin or immunoglobulin-binding protein (see Fig. 7.22). Such assays, which use radio-labelled antibody or antibody-binding protein are nomally called solid-phase radiobinding assays, but most assays used nowadays employ enzyme-labelled detecting reagent. They are usually called enzyme-linked immunosorbent assays (ELISAs) but can be referred to as solid-phase enzyme immunobinding assays.

Unfortunately, enzyme immunometric assays are also often called ELISAs (Section 7.7.2) and to try to avoid confusion, the immunometric version is sometimes called two-site ELISA whereas the binding assay type is known as one-site ELISA. As antigen is simply captured onto tube or well surfaces by non-specific binding, such assays are occasionally known as sticky plate assays or (especially when complex impure antigen solution is used) as dirty plate techniques.

Quantification can be achieved by comparison with a standard solution of known antibody content, but this can be difficult largely due to the heterogeneity of immunoglobulin molecules present. It is very common to express comparative results as a titre derived from dose–response curves generated using different samples. Mid-point titres, i.e. the dilution at which 50% maximal binding is achieved, are the usual way of calculating the titre, but this requires the maximal value of the dose–response curve to be the same for all samples. The use of end-point titres, i.e. the minimal dilution at which no signal is generated, is unreliable and very often invalid.

A variant of conventional solid-phase immunobinding assays, usually known as dot blot assays are occasionally encountered. For these techniques, antigen-containing solution is spotted, dried onto nitrocellulose filters and then incubated with samples with suspected antibody content. Any antigen-specific antibodies are then detected by using an enzyme-labelled or radiolabelled anti-immunoglobulin or antibody-binding protein. Advantages of the method are that antigen can be concentrated by repeat spotting at a single location on the filter, and that many antigen samples can be incubated with a single antibody sample. A major disadvantage is that valid quantification of results is virtually impossible. The name of the technique is misleading as no blotting actually occurs at any stage of the assay; it probably relates to many technical similarities with immunoblotting (see Section 7.6). A possibly better name is dot immunobinding assay, but this is not often used.

7.7.4 Enhanced immunoassays

The quest for evermore sensitive immunoassays has resulted in the design of amplification systems to enhance the signal derived from the immunoassay (cf. immunoblotting; Section 7.6). Most of these are based on the enzyme immunometric assay (two-site ELISA) format and are carried out in microtitre plates. Several different amplification systems have been developed but a commonly encountered system is enzyme-linked, and is added as a 'cassette' to a conventional alkaline phosphatase-based two-site immunometric assay. In this, the alkaline phosphatase is used to dephosphorylate $NADP^+$ to produce NAD^+. The NAD^+ comprises the limiting concentration reagent of an alcohol dehydrogenase catalysed loop in which the NAD^+ is reduced to NADH and this in turn generates a coloured formazan by reduction from the oxidised leukoformazan (see Fig. 7.23). The additional enzyme-catalysed loop amplifies the original signal considerably as compared with that which could be produced from the alkaline phosphatase conjugate alone. Another popular amplification system, known

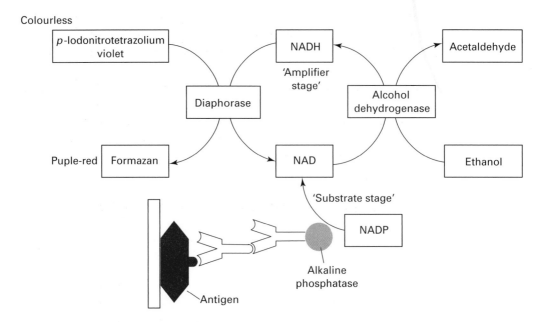

Fig. 7.23. Substrate amplification system for the detection of alkaline phosphatase.

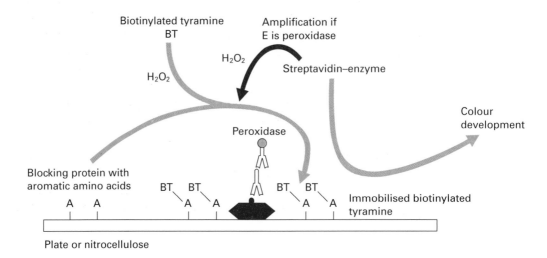

Fig. 7.24. Principles of the ELAST amplification system.

as the ELISA amplification system or ELAST (see Fig. 7.24) uses a standard peroxidase-based immunometric assay, but involves incorporation of a biotinylated tyramine reagent that, when oxidised (by the peroxidase conjugate), binds covalently to tyrosine or tryptophan residues present on the excess of blocking protein used to coat antigen-unoccupied sites on the microtitre plate surface.

The immobilised biotin is then detected using labelled streptavidin (Section 7.5.5). The amplification system results in a far greater number of immobilised biotin molecules than would arise from the use of a simple biotin-labelled antibody.

Amplification systems almost always result in enhanced signal, but this often affects both the 'real' analyte-derived output and the assay background. At worst, this can simply increase the total assay signal but not improve sensitivity. Unless care is shown, use of potent amplification systems can result in less robust assays, with increased chance of assay artefacts.

7.7.5 Peptide-based immunobinding assays (peptide mapping, epitope mapping)

Synthetic peptides can be substituted for antigen in solid-phase immunobinding assays. This allows detection of antibodies with known epitope specificity and also the determination of the epitope specificity of new antibodies (peptide mapping or epitope mapping). For the latter, a series of overlapping sequence peptides are made, covering the entire primary structure of the antigen and used sequentially to coat the wells of microtitre plates. Incubation with either labelled antibody or antibody followed by labelled anti-immunoglobulin allows the identification of peptides recognised by the antibody and therefore elucidation of the epitope(s) recognised by the antibody(s). This approach is especially useful with monoclonal antibodies. Usually peptides of 10 to 18 residues length are used, with an overlap of about 5 to 8 residues. The procedure is simple and valuable, but is limited to detection of 'linear' antigenic determinants and care must be taken to ensure that all the peptides bind efficiently to microtitre plate well surfaces. Coating the wells with polylysine can improve peptide binding (it produces a relatively strong positively charged surface) or they can be synthesised with biotin end-residues and captured with streptavidin-coated plates (this also optimises orientation on binding). It is also possible to synthesise peptides on 'pins' formed in the wells of special plates and use these for mapping (the pepscan procedure). The 'pin' heads are chemically activated to ensure binding of activated amino acid residues to be added sequentially thus building the required peptide sequence.

7.7.6 Fluorescence- and photoluminescence-based immunoassays

In attempts to increase assay sensitivity and ease, a variety of adaptions of the basic competitive and especially immunometric immunoassay methods have been developed and involve fluorescence or luminescence readouts. At their simplest, these substitute fluorescent or luminescent substrates for the colorimetric substrates normally used for two-site ELISAs. These are called fluorimetric EIAs or enzyme-linked fluorescence immunoassays (ELFIAs) and luminoimmunoassays (LIAs) or enzyme-linked chemiluminescence immunoassays (ECLIAs),

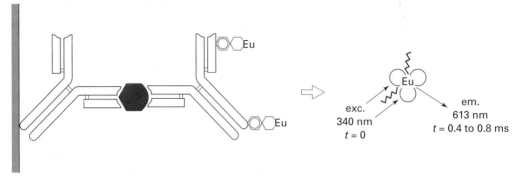

1	2	3	4
Solid-phase immunoassay	Eu-labelled immunoreagents	Dissociative fluorescence enhancement	Time-related fluorimetry

Fig. 7.25. The dissociative fluorescence enhancement principle exemplified in a two-site sandwich assay. exc., excitation; em., emission.

respectively. However, some assays use sufficiently different approaches to be considered separately (see below).

7.7.7 Delayed enhanced lanthanide fluorescence immunoassay

Most delayed enhanced lanthanide fluorescence immunoassays (DELFIAs) (see Section 12.5.3) use the standard two-site immunometric assay principle and are carried out in microtitre plates. The detecting antibody (see Fig. 7.25) is labelled directly with a lanthanide (these are 4f transition metals – europium is usually used in DELFIA) that is non-covalently coupled via a chelating agent such as diethylenetriaminepenta-acetic anhydride (DTPA) or diethylenetriaminetetra-acetic anhydride (DTTA). After the immunometric assay has been carried out, the lanthanide is released from the antibody by lowering the pH to about 3.2 (the chelates are unstable at this pH) and free lanthanide is then captured using a soluble diketone. This is complexed into micelles, which prevents subsequent quenching of fluorescence (the so-called enhancer step). The antibody–lanthanide chelates are not fluorescent, but the captured, micelle-bound lanthanide ion is, and this permits its detection. The peak fluorescence emission of miscelle-complexed lanthanides is relatively slow and this allows delayed measurement of light output after addition of the enhancing reagents. By this means, artefactual immediate autofluorescence due to sample components etc. can be distinguished from the later 'real' lanthanide signal. Because of this, such assays are often called time-resolved immunofluorimetric assays (TRIFMA). In such assays, the fluorescence is proportional to the amount of antigen present in samples. DELFIAs can be sensitive, fast, accurate, robust, cover a relatively wide analyte concentration range and run using robots to allow very high sample throughput.

7.7.8 **Homogeneous substrate-labelled fluorescence immunoassay**

Substrate-labelled fluorescence immunoassays (SLFIAs) use principles similar to those of competitive immunoassays, but do not require separation of free from bound antigen. They require the synthesis of antigen conjugates containing a chemical structure that is not fluorescent per se, but is cleaved by an enzyme to yield an intensely fluorescent compound. They also need an antibody that binds the antigen conjugate such that the enzyme is prevented from cleaving it and liberating the fluorochrome. In SLFIA, samples containing known and unknown amounts of antigen are incubated with a fixed amount of antigen conjugate in the presence of a limiting concentration of antibody. Under such conditions, the antigen in the samples competes for antibody with the conjugated antigen. After equilibrium has been reached, enzyme is added to liberate the fluorochrome from non-antibody-bound antigen conjugate. The fluorescence measured is therefore proportional to the amount of antigen in the samples. A combination of the enzyme β-galactosidase and conjugates prepared by coupling antigen to a galactosyl 4-methylumbelliferyl residue is often employed for SLFIA. The β-galactosidase hydrolyses the conjugate to liberate free 4-methylumbelliferone, which is readily measured using fluorimetry. A major difficulty encountered with the general application of this type of assay is producing the appropriate antibody, i.e. an antibody that effectively inhibits the enzyme-catalysed reaction. It is usually successful only for relatively small analytes, for example morphine and other opiates.

7.8 **IMMUNOHISTO/CYTOCHEMISTRY**

To understand cell structure, organisation and function, and cell or tissue development and differentiation in health and disease, it is often necessary to be able to determine the distribution of an antigen *in situ*. Immunohistochemical and immunocytochemical techniques exploit the specific interaction of an antibody with its antigen to locate or to determine the distribution of the antigen *in situ* in tissues or cells, respectively. Alternatively, these procedures can be carried out using tissues or cells known to contain a particular antigen to investigate the specificity of antibodies or antisera. The principle of immunohisto/cytochemistry is analogous to those of solid-phase immunobinding (Section 7.7.3) and immunoblotting (Section 7.6), except that the antibody is incubated with thin sections of solid tissue mounted on glass slides or cell preparations containing the antigen rather than with antigen immobilised on microtitre plates or nitrocellulose membranes. In immunohisto/cytochemistry, the antibody (or anti-immunoglobulin antibody; Section 7.5.1) must be conjugated with a fluorescent or enzyme label that gives an intense signal to allow visualisation when the sections or cells are examined using immunoenzyme microscopy. The location of the label reveals the site of the antibody–antigen interaction, which can be localised to, for example, particular cell types or cellular organelles (an example is shown in Fig. 7.26).

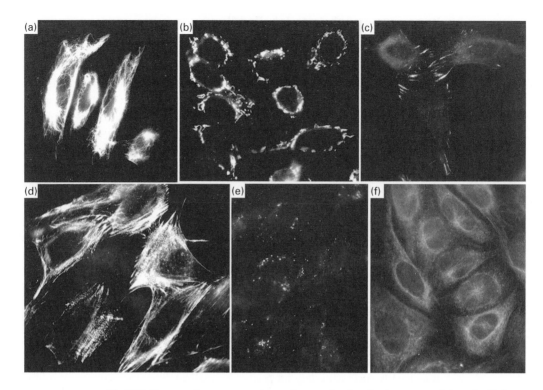

Fig. 7.26. Immunofluorescence photomicrographs showing immunostaining of cellular organelles: (a) intermediate filaments; (b) mitochondria; (c) microspikes; (d) stress fibres; (e) granules; (f) cytoplasmic component(s). Monolayers of the rat glioma cell line C6 were incubated with human IgM monoclonal antibodies and then fluorescein-labelled anti-human IgM.

All immunohisto/cytochemical procedures need stringent positive and negative control antibodies for comparison with the test antibody to ensure that the immunostaining is specific. Although it is common for the binding of labelled antibody to a specific tissue or cellular antigen to be referred to as immunostaining, this term should not be confused with the differential staining of tissue constituents by routine chemical stains such as haematoxylin and eosin for histology and pathology.

7.8.1 Immunoenzyme microscopy

The main advantage of enzyme labels (usually horseradish peroxidase (HRP) or alkaline phosphatase (AP); Section 7.5.4) for immunohisto/cytochemical procedures is that an ordinary white light microscope can be used for viewing the sections or cells, and the use of chemical counterstains such as haematoxylin (stains nuclei blue) aids in identification of morphology. The main disadvantages are the presence of endogenous tissue enzymes (which can give high background staining) and the extra step involved in carrying out the enzyme reaction.

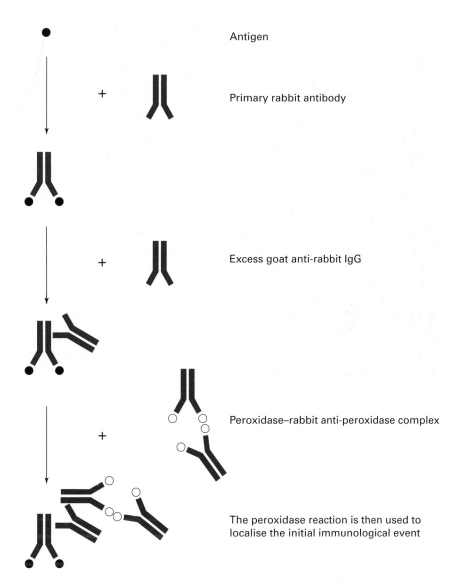

Antigen

Primary rabbit antibody

Excess goat anti-rabbit IgG

Peroxidase–rabbit anti-peroxidase complex

The peroxidase reaction is then used to localise the initial immunological event

Fig. 7.27. Diagrammatic representation of the peroxidase–anti-peroxidase technique. ●, antigen; ○, peroxidase.

7.8.2 **The peroxidase–anti-peroxidase technique**

The PAP (peroxidase–anti-peroxidase) technique is a modification of the indirect enzyme immunohisto/cytochemical procedure for amplifying the signal (Fig. 7.27). In this method, unlabelled anti-rabbit or anti-mouse immunoglobulin forms a bridge between rabbit or mouse primary antibody, respectively, and a peroxidase–(rabbit or mouse)–anti-peroxidase complex. Alkaline phosphatase–anti-alkaline phosphatase complexes are also available. An advantage of this procedure is that no possible destruction of antibody and/or enzyme can occur during chemical coupling. Specially developed commercial systems that exploit both anti-immunoglobulin and biotin–avidin reactions are also available. Such amplification systems are many times more sensitive than standard indirect procedures.

7.8.3 **Immunofluorescence techniques**

Immunohistochemistry was originally developed using fluorochrome-labelled antibodies (see Section 7.5.3). Their use has dramatically increased in recent years with the expansion of flow cytofluorimetric techniques (Section 16.3.2), which allow analysis of single cells in suspension according to the expression of cell surface antigens (Section 7.8.5), and the advent of confocal microscropy in which laser light sources replace the standard light sources to allow analysis of images at different depths through the tissue section or cell to build up a three-dimensional picture. A unique application of fluorochrome-labelled antibodies for immuno-histo/cytochemistry is that, because different fluorochromes emit different wavelengths of ultraviolet light, the use of appropriate filters on a fluorescence microscope allows the same tissue section or cell sample to be immunostained with two, three or even four different antibodies, each of which is used in conjunction with a different fluorochrome. Such double or triple staining procedures sometimes necessitate the use of directly conjugated primary antibodies, as, for example, fluorescein conjugated rabbit anti-mouse immunoglobulin antibodies will not distinguish between primary mouse monoclonal antibodies of differing specificity.

The choice of fluorochrome depends on the light source, detection system available and personal preference. Light sources include tungsten, quartz-halogen or mercury arc lamps for fluorescence microscopes, argon ion or krypton–argon lasers for flow cytometry.

Fluorochrome-labelled antibodies are quick and easy to use, and offer good sensitivity. Their main disadvantage is the requirement for a microscope equipped with fluorescence optics, and that the fluorescence, particularly that of fluorescein, fades during prolonged viewing of individual microscopic fields unless a powerful reducing agent such as 1,4-bicyclo-2,2,2-octane is included in the mountant. Such agents are thought to suppress a destructive reaction of the fluorescein in its excited state with protein. Autofluorescence of some tissue components, i.e. their intrinsic fluorescence, can also be a problem.

7.8.4 **Capping**

An important feature of immunostaining viable cells, particularly lymphocytes, is the aggregation of cell surface antigens due to cross-linkage by intact antibodies. Such patches eventually form a cap over one pole of the cell, which is subsequently shed or endocytosed. Capping can be visualised using fluorochrome-labelled antibodies and provides information on the association of molecules carrying different antigenic markers if double or triple immunofluorescence labelling is carried out. It can be prevented by immunostaining at 4 °C or in the presence of sodium azide, which prevents modulation of cell surface molecules, or by the use of monovalent Fab fragments, in order to study the initial binding of antibody to cell surface antigen.

7.8.5 **Flow cytometry**

A disadvantage of assessment of immunocytochemical staining using conventional microscopy is that it is very difficult to quantify the intensity of the immunostaining. Although it is possible to estimate the proportion of cells that are immunostained in a population by performing manual cell counts, the accuracy of the estimate is dependent on the total number of cells that are counted and the proportion of positive cells.

These limitations are overcome in flow cytofluorimetric analysis. In this technique, cells that have been labelled with fluorochrome-conjugated antibody in suspension are introduced into a liquid jet and passed individually through the beam of a laser. As each cell passes through it emits a flash of fluorescence and scattered light. The signals are collected and converted by the flow cytofluorimeter to give quantitative information on the intensity of fluorescence and the light-scattering properties of each cell. Forward light scatter is related to cell size; the amount of side scatter is related to the granularity of the cell (presence of intracellular granules, pronounced organelles and/or nucleus). Examples of data displays are shown in Fig. 7.28. Many thousands of cells can be quickly analysed in this way, for example with respect to the proportion of cells that are immunostained or the intensity of fluorescence. Flow cytofluorimeters are also able to sort cells according to specified parameters such as intensity of fluorescence and size (cells usually remain viable after immunostaining with fluorochrome-labelled antibody). Many fluorochromes are available for flow cytofluorimetric analysis that allow simultaneous monitoring for several colours, provided the emission spectra do not overlap. This allows the use of several antibodies, conjugated with different fluorochromes, at the same time. Directly conjugated monoclonal antibodies are often used in flow cytofluorimetric techniques. This permits simultaneous labelling with several fluorochromes (see Sections 7.8.3 and 7.5.3). Also the anti-immunoglobulin conjugates used in indirect immunocytochemical techniques can either bind directly to lymphocytes that express cell surface immunoglobulin or bring about agglutination of primary antibody-coated cells. (IgG is divalent and can bind two primary antibody molecules, each of which is bound to a separate cell, thus bringing the cells together.) A wide range of directly conjugated monoclonal antibodies against different cell surface markers such as the CD (cluster of differentiation) series of antigens, which are characteristic of different populations of blood cells, are available commercially. These allow analysis of cell sets and subsets involved in biological systems to be evaluated, for example T and B lymphocyte populations. If immunostaining of surface antigens of viable cells for flow cytometric analysis is being carried out, steps may have to be taken to prevent non-antigen-specific binding of antibody to Fc receptors that are present on, for example, leukocytes. This can be achieved

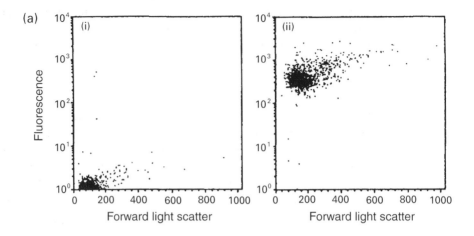

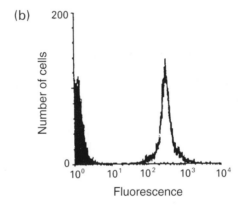

Fig. 7.28. Examples of flow cytometry displays. (a) Dot plots of erythrocytes (red blood cells) stained with a fluorescently labelled mouse monoclonal anti-haemoglobin antibody (ii) or a fluorescently labelled irrelevant mouse monoclonal antibody (i). Each dot represents an erythrocyte. The intensity of fluorescence is on the *y*-axis; forward light scatter (i.e. size) is on the *x*-axis. The erythrocytes are not fluorescently stained with the irrelevant antibody (i), but virtually all the cells are stained with the anti-haemoglobin antibody (ii). (b) The same data displayed as a profile histogram with number of cells on the *y*-axis and intensity of fluorescence on the *x*-axis.

either by blocking these sites with non-immune serum that contains high levels of immunoglobulin, or by the use of antibody F(ab')$_2$ fragments.

7.8.6 Immunoelectron microscopy

Subcellular detail that is not discernible by conventional microscopy can be resolved using electron microscopy, since electrons have a shorter wavelength than white or ultraviolet light. Antibodies labelled with electron-dense reagents such as gold or ferritin (an iron-containing protein) or with HRP, which can yield an electron-dense product with an appropriate substrate, are used in immunoelectron microscopy to immunostain ultrathin sections of tissue or cells.

7.9 AFFINITY AND AVIDITY

Determining the affinity of an antibody can be important for predicting and/or explaining its immunochemical characteristics. Affinity is defined as the equilibrium constant when 'a monovalent antibody reacts with (binds) a monovalent antigen, i.e. an antigenic determinant'. As antibodies are usually di- or multivalent, and antigens usually have more than one antigenic determinant, this concept is relatively rarely encountered. The term avidity is normally used to describe the equilibrium constant applicable to whole antibody–antigen interactions and this includes the affinity component plus additive factors due to multiple valency of binding and other considerations. The terms affinity and avidity are sometimes replaced by intrinsic affinity and functional affinity, respectively, and these are certainly more descriptive.

7.9.1 Measurement of affinity and avidity

The affinity of monovalent antibody for its epitope can be expressed arithmetically as the equilibrium association constant using the following relationship:

$$K_a = \frac{[AgAb]}{[Ag][Ab]}$$

where K_a is the equilibrium association constant, [Ag] is the concentration of antigen, [Ab] is the concentration of antibody, and [AgAb] is the concentration of the antigen–antibody complex.

Practically, this requires that all components are absolutely pure and relate to equilibrium in homogeneous solution. Such conditions rarely apply to most immunochemical techniques as applied to biochemical methodology. However, calculating the relative affinity of antibodies can be useful in predicting their use in immunochemical techniques (see also Section 16.2.1).

7.10 IMMUNOCHEMICAL USE OF SURFACE PLASMON RESONANCE

Surface plasmon resonance (Section 16.3.2) uses the optical properties at the surface of a thin gold-film-coated glass 'chip' to study binding phenomena. The physical principles of the method are as follows. A beam of polarised light will be internally reflected by the chip (mounted on a glass prism). The angle of reflection is changed if material binds to the surface of the chip and the alteration in the angle of reflection is proportional to the *mass* of substance bound to the chip surface. Instruments for the application of surface plasmon resonance technology to immunochemistry are commercially available. The Biacore™ biosensor system is probably most appropriate for general immunochemical use, can be programmed for a variety of differing applications and is automated. In this system, the chip is coated with a dextran matrix to which antigen or antibody can be chemically coupled, and thus immobilised. Samples to be analysed for antigen (if antibody has been immobilised) or antibody (if antigen has been immobilised) are allowed to flow over the chip surface, and binding is continuously detected by measuring the alteration in the angle of reflection of light incident on the prism side of the chip. The measurements are directly proportional to the mass of substance binding and can be used to compare the antigen or antibody content of samples and also for calculation of kinetic parameters related to antigen–antibody interaction, for example association and dissociation affinity constants.

Surface plasmon resonance is a rapid procedure (measurements are made in a few minutes), does not require labelling of antibodies or antigens or the use of anti-immunoglobulin reagents and can be adapted for a wide range of purposes. It is not usually particularly sensitive, for example compared with immunoassays, but can be used to allow detection of very low affinity interactions.

7.11 SUGGESTIONS FOR FURTHER READING

DABBS, D. J. (2002). *Diagnostic Immunohistochemistry.* Churchill Livingstone, New York. (Good coverage of the clinical applications of this technique.)

HAYAT, M. A. (2002). *Microscopy, Immunohistochemistry and Antigen Retrieval Methods: For Light and Electron Microscopy.* Plenum Press, London. (An authoritative text on all aspects of the application of immunological techniques to microscopic and histochemical analytical methods.)

HERMANSON, G. T. (1996). *Bioconjugate Techniques.* Academic Press Inc., London and New York. (A very comprehensive, detailed account of just about every procedure for conjugating labels to biological molecules. Includes a large number of methods used to produce conjugates employed in immunochemical techniques.)

JOHNSTONE, A. P. and THORPE, R. (1996). *Immunochemistry in Practice,* 3rd edn. Blackwell Science, Oxford. (Contains detailed protocols for many immunochemical techniques plus a resumé of their underlying scientific basis.)

JOHNSTONE, A. P. and TURNER, M. W. (eds.) (1997). *Immunochemistry – A Practical Approach.* IRL Press, Oxford. (Chapters devoted to many immunochemical procedures.)

LACHMANN, P. J., PETERS, D. K. AND ROSENS, F. S. (eds.) (1992). *Clinical Aspects Of Immunology,* 5th edn. Blackwell Science, Oxford. (A large three-volume work describing most aspects of clinical immunology and much theoretical immunology.)

ROITT, I. M. (2001). *Essential Immunology,* 10th edn. Blackwell Science, Oxford. (An excellent general textbook on immunology.)

Chapter 8

Protein structure, purification, characterisation and function analysis

8.1 IONIC PROPERTIES OF AMINO ACIDS AND PROTEINS

Twenty amino acids varying in size, shape, charge and chemical reactivity are found in proteins and each has at least one codon in the genetic code (Section 5.3.5). Nineteen of the amino acids are α-amino acids (i.e. the amino and carboxyl groups are attached to the carbon atom that is adjacent to the carboxyl group) with the general formula $RCH(NH_2)COOH$, where R is an aliphatic, aromatic or hetero-cyclic group. The only exception to this general formula is proline, which is an imino acid in which the $-NH_2$ group is incorporated into a five-membered ring. With the exception of the simplest amino acid glycine (R = H), all the amino acids found in proteins contain one asymmetric carbon atom and hence are optically active and have been found to have the L configuration.

For convenience, each amino acid found in proteins is designated by either a three-letter abbreviation, generally based on the first three letters of their name, or a one-letter symbol, some of which are the first letter of the name. Details are given in Table 8.1.

Since they possess both an amino group and a carboxyl group, amino acids are ionised at all pH values, i.e. a neutral species represented by the general formula does not exist in solution irrespective of the pH. This can be seen as follows:

$$
\begin{array}{ccc}
R & R & R \\
| & | & | \\
{}^{\alpha}CH-\overset{+}{N}H_3 \underset{}{\overset{pK_{a_1}}{\rightleftharpoons}} & {}^{\alpha}CH-\overset{+}{N}H_3 \underset{}{\overset{pK_{a_2}}{\rightleftharpoons}} & {}^{\alpha}CH-NH_2 \\
| & | & | \\
COOH & COO^- & COO^- \\
\text{Net positive} & \text{Zero net} & \text{Net negative} \\
\text{charge} & \text{charge} & \text{charge} \\
& \text{'zwitterion'} &
\end{array}
$$

Increasing pH
⟶

Thus at low pH values an amino acid exists as a cation and at high pH values as an anion. At a particular intermediate pH the amino acid carries no net charge, although it is still ionised, and is called a zwitterion. It has been shown that, in the

Table 8.1 Abbreviations for amino acids

Amino acid	Three-letter symbol	One-letter symbol
Alanine	Ala	A
Arginine	Arg	R
Asparagine	Asn	N
Aspartic acid	Asp	D
Asparagine or aspartic acid	Asx	B
Cysteine	Cys	C
Glutamine	Gln	Q
Glutamic acid	Glu	E
Glutamine or glutamic acid	Glx	Z
Glycine	Gly	G
Histidine	His	H
Isoleucine	Ile	I
Leucine	Leu	L
Lysine	Lys	K
Methionine	Met	M
Phenylalanine	Phe	F
Proline	Pro	P
Serine	Ser	S
Threonine	Thr	T
Tryptophan	Trp	W
Tyrosine	Tyr	Y
Valine	Val	V

crystalline state and in solution in water, amino acids exist predominantly as this zwitterionic form. This confers upon them physical properties characteristic of ionic compounds, i.e. high melting point and boiling point, water solubility and low solubility in organic solvents such as ether and chloroform. The pH at which the zwitterion predominates in aqueous solution is referred to as the isoionic point, because it is the pH at which the number of negative charges on the molecule produced by ionisation of the carboxyl group is equal to the number of positive charges acquired by proton acceptance by the amino group. In the case of amino acids this is equal to the isoelectric point (pI), since the molecule carries no net charge and is therefore electrophoretically immobile. The numerical value of this pH for a given amino acid is related to its acid strength (pK_a values) by the equation:

$$pI = \frac{pK_{a_1} + pK_{a_2}}{2} \tag{8.1}$$

where pK_{a_1} and pK_{a_2} are equal to the negative logarithm of the acid dissociation constants, K_{a_1} and K_{a_2} (Section 1.4.2).

In the case of glycine, pK_{a_1} and pK_{a_2} are 2, 3 and 9.6, respectively, so that the isoionic point is 6.0. At pH values below this, the cation and zwitterion will coexist in equilibrium in a ratio determined by the Henderson–Hasselbalch equation (Section 1.4.2), whereas at higher pH values the zwitterion and anion will coexist in equilibrium.

For acidic amino acids such as aspartic acid, the ionisation pattern is different owing to the presence of a second carboxyl group:

$$
\begin{array}{llll}
\text{COOH} & \text{COOH} & \text{COO}^- & \text{COO}^- \\
| & | & | & | \\
\text{CH}_2 & \text{CH}_2 & \text{CH}_2 & \text{CH}_2 \\
| \qquad\ \ \ \text{p}K_{a_1} & | \qquad\ \ \ \text{p}K_{a_2} & | \qquad\ \ \ \text{p}K_{a_3} & | \\
\text{CH}-\overset{+}{\text{N}}\text{H}_3 \rightleftharpoons \text{CH}-\overset{+}{\text{N}}\text{H}_3 \rightleftharpoons \text{CH}-\overset{+}{\text{N}}\text{H}_3 \rightleftharpoons \text{CH}-\text{NH}_2 \\
| \qquad 2.1 \quad | \qquad 3.9 \quad | \qquad 9.8 \quad | \\
\text{COOH} & \text{COO}^- & \text{COO}^- & \text{COO}^-
\end{array}
$$

Cation   Zwitterion   Anion   Anion

(1 net   pH 3.0   (1 net   (2 net

positive   (isoionic   negative   negative

charge)   point)   charge)   charges)

In this case, the zwitterion will predominate in aqueous solution at a pH determined by $\text{p}K_{a_1}$ and $\text{p}K_{a_2}$, and the isoelectric point is the mean of $\text{p}K_{a_1}$ and $\text{p}K_{a_2}$.

In the case of lysine, which is a basic amino acid, the ionisation pattern is different again and its isoionic point is the mean of $\text{p}K_{a_2}$ and $\text{p}K_{a_3}$:

$$
\begin{array}{llll}
\overset{+}{\text{N}}\text{H}_3 & \overset{+}{\text{N}}\text{H}_3 & \overset{+}{\text{N}}\text{H}_3 & \text{NH}_2 \\
| & | & | & | \\
(\text{CH}_2)_4 & (\text{CH}_2)_4 & (\text{CH}_2)_4 & (\text{CH}_2)_4 \\
| \qquad\ \ \ \text{p}K_{a_1} & | \qquad\ \ \ \text{p}K_{a_2} & | \qquad\ \ \ \text{p}K_{a_3} & | \\
\text{CH}-\overset{+}{\text{N}}\text{H}_3 \rightleftharpoons \text{CH}-\overset{+}{\text{N}}\text{H}_3 \rightleftharpoons \text{CH}-\text{NH}_2 \rightleftharpoons \text{CH}-\text{NH}_2 \\
| \qquad 2.2 \quad | \qquad 9.0 \quad | \qquad 10.5 \quad | \\
\text{COOH} & \text{COO}^- & \text{COO}^- & \text{COO}^-
\end{array}
$$

Cation   Cation   Zwitterion   Anion

(2 net   (1 net   pH 3.0   (1 net

positive   positive   (isoionic   negative

charges)   charge)   point)   charge)

As an alternative to possessing a second amino or carboxyl group, an amino acid side chain may contain in the R of the general formula a quite different chemical group that is also capable of ionising at a characteristic pH. Such groups include a phenolic group (tyrosine), guanidino group (arginine), imidazolyl group (histidine) and sulphydryl group (cysteine) (Table 8.2). It is clear that the state of ionisation of the main groups of amino acids (acidic, basic, neutral) will be grossly different at a particular pH. Moreover, even within a given group there will be minor differences due to the precise nature of the R group. These differences are exploited in the electrophoretic and ion-exchange chromatographic separation of mixtures of amino acids such as those present in a protein hydrolysate (Section 8.4.2).

Proteins are formed by the condensation of the α-amino group of one amino acid with the α-carboxyl of the adjacent amino acid (Section 8.2). With the exception of the two terminal amino acids, therefore, the α-amino and carboxyl groups are all involved in peptide bonds and are no longer ionisable in the protein. Amino, carboxyl, imidazolyl, guanidino, phenolic and sulphydryl groups in the side chains are, however, free to ionise and of course there may be many of these.

Table 8.2   Ionisable groups found in proteins

Amino acid group	pH-dependent ionisation	Approx. pK_a
N-terminal α-amino	$-NH_3 \rightleftharpoons NH_2 + H^+$	8.0
C-terminal α-carboxyl	$-COOH \rightleftharpoons COO^- + H^+$	3.0
Asp-β-carboxyl	$-CH_2COOH \rightleftharpoons CH_2COO^- + H^+$	3.9
Glu-γ-carboxyl	$-(CH_2)_2COOH \rightleftharpoons (CH_2)_2COO^- + H^+$	4.1
His-imidazolyl		6.0
Cys-sulphydryl	$-CH_2SH \rightleftharpoons -CH_2S^- + H^+$	8.4
Tyr-phenolic		10.1
Lys-ε-amino	$-(CH_2)_4\overset{+}{N}H_3 \rightleftharpoons -(CH_2)_4NH_2 + H^+$	10.3
Arg-guanidino		12.5

Proteins fold in such a manner that the majority of these ionisable groups are on the outside of the molecule, where they can interact with the surrounding aqueous medium. Some of these groups are located within the structure and may be involved in electrostatic attractions that help to stabilise the three-dimensional structure of the protein molecule. The relative numbers of positive and negative groups in a protein molecule influence aspects of its physical behaviour, such as solubility and electrophoretic mobility.

    The isoionic point of a protein and its isoelectric point, unlike that of an amino acid, are generally not identical. This is because, by definition, the isoionic point is the pH at which the protein molecule possesses an equal number of positive and negative groups formed by the association of basic groups with protons and dissociation of acidic groups, respectively. In contrast, the isoelectric point is the pH at which the protein is electrophoretically immobile. In order to determine electrophoretic mobility experimentally, the protein must be dissolved in a buffered medium containing anions and cations, of low relative molecular mass, that are capable of binding to the multi-ionised protein. Hence the observed balance of charges at the isoelectric point could be due in part to there being more bound mobile anions (or cations) than bound cations (anions) at this pH. This could mask an imbalance of charges on the actual protein.

    In practice, protein molecules are always studied in buffered solutions, so it is the isoelectric point that is important. It is the pH at which, for example, the protein has minimum solubility, since it is the point at which there is the greatest opportunity for attraction between oppositely charged groups of neighbouring molecules and consequent aggregation and easy precipitation.

8.2 **PROTEIN STRUCTURE**

Proteins are formed by condensing the α-amino group of one amino acid or the imino group of proline with the α-carboxyl group of another, with the concomitant loss of a molecule of water and the formation of a peptide bond.

$$\overset{+}{N}H_3-\underset{\underset{R}{|}}{C}H-COO^- + \overset{+}{N}H_3-\underset{\underset{R'}{|}}{C}H-COO^- \underset{-H_2O}{\rightleftharpoons} \overset{+}{N}H_3-\underset{\underset{R}{|}}{C}H-CO-NH-\underset{\underset{R'}{|}}{C}H-COO^-$$

Peptide bond

The progressive condensation of many molecules of amino acids gives rise to an unbranched polypeptide chain. By convention, the N-terminal amino acid is taken as the beginning of the chain and the C-terminal amino acid the end of the chain (proteins are biosynthesised in this direction). Polypeptide chains contain between 20 and 2000 amino acids residues and hence have a relative molecular mass ranging between about 2000 and 200 000. Many proteins have a relative molecular mass in the range 20 000 to 100 000. The distinction between a large peptide and a small protein is not clear. Generally, chains of amino acids containing fewer than 50 residues are referred to as peptides, and those with more than 50 are referred to as proteins. Most proteins contain many hundreds of amino acids (ribonuclease is an extremely small protein with only 103 amino acid residues) and many biologically active peptides contain 20 or fewer amino acids, for example oxytocin (9 amino acid residues), vasopressin (9), enkephalins (5), gastrin (17), somatostatin (14) and lutenising hormone (10).

The primary structure of a protein defines the sequence of the amino acid residues and is dictated by the base sequence of the corresponding gene(s). Indirectly, the primary structure also defines the amino acid composition (which of the possible 20 amino acids are actually present) and content (the relative proportions of the amino acids present).

The peptide bonds linking the individual amino acid residues in a protein are both rigid and planar, with no opportunity for rotation about the carbon–nitrogen bond, as it has considerable double bond character due to the delocalisation of the lone pair of electrons on the nitrogen atom; this, coupled with the tetrahedral geometry around each α-carbon atom, profoundly influences the three-dimensional arrangement which the polypeptide chain adopts.

Secondary structure defines the localised folding of a polypeptide chain due to hydrogen bonding. It includes structures such as the α-helix and β-pleated sheet. Certain of the 20 amino acids found in proteins, including proline, isoleucine, tryptophan and asparagine, disrupt α-helical structures. Some proteins have up to 70% secondary structure but others have none.

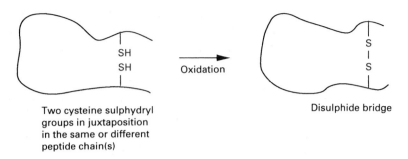

Two cysteine sulphydryl
groups in juxtaposition
in the same or different
peptide chain(s)

Disulphide bridge

Fig. 8.1. The formation of a disulphide bridge.

Tertiary structure defines the overall folding of a polypeptide chain. It is stabilised by electrostatic attractions between oppositely charged ionic groups ($-\overset{+}{N}H_3$, COO^-), by weak van der Waals forces, by hydrogen bonding, hydrophobic interactions and, in some proteins, by disulphide ($-S-S-$) bridges formed by the oxidation of spatially adjacent sulphydryl groups (-SH) of cysteine residues (Fig. 8.1). The three-dimensional folding of polypeptide chains is such that the interior consists predominantly of non-polar, hydrophobic amino acid residues such as valine, leucine and phenylalanine. The polar, ionised, hydrophilic residues are found on the outside of the molecule, where they are compatible with the aqueous environment. However, some proteins also have hydrophobic residues on their outside and the presence of these residues is important in the processes of ammonium sulphate fractionation (Section 8.3.4) and hydrophobic interaction chromatography (Sections 8.3.4 and 11.4.3).

Quaternary structure is restricted to oligomeric proteins, which consist of the association of two or more polypeptide chains held together by electrostatic attractions, hydrogen bonding, van der Waals forces and occasionally disulphide bridges. Thus disulphide bridges may exist within a given polypeptide chain (intra-chain) or linking different chains (inter-chain). An individual polypeptide chain in an oligomeric protein is referred to as a subunit. The subunits in a protein may be identical or different: for example, haemoglobin consists of two α- and two β-chains, and lactate dehydrogenase of four (virtually) identical chains.

Traditionally, proteins are classified into two groups – globular and fibrous. The former are approximately spherical in shape, are generally water soluble and may contain a mixture of α-helix, β-pleated sheet and random structures. Globular proteins include enzymes, transport proteins and immunoglobulins. Fibrous proteins are structural proteins, generally insoluble in water, consisting of long cable-like structures built entirely of either helical or sheet arrangements. Examples include hair keratin, silk fibroin and collagen. The native state of a protein is its biologically active form.

The process of protein denaturation results in the loss of biological activity, decreased aqueous solubility and increased susceptibility to proteolytic degradation. It can be brought about by heat and by treatment with reagents such as acids and alkalis, detergents, organic solvents and heavy-metal cations such as mercury and lead. It is associated with the loss of organised (tertiary) three-dimensional structure and exposure to the aqueous environment of numerous hydrophobic groups previously located within the folded structure.

In enzymes, the specific three-dimensional folding of the polypeptide chain(s) results in the juxtaposition of certain amino acid residues that constitute the active site or catalytic site. Oligomeric enzymes may possess several such sites. Many enzymes also possess one or more regulatory site(s). X-ray crystallography studies have revealed that the active site is often located in a cleft that is lined with hydrophobic amino acid residues but which contains some polar residues. The binding of the substrate at the catalytic site and the subsequent conversion of substrate to product involves different amino acid residues.

Some oligomeric enzymes exist in multiple forms called isoenzymes or isozymes (Section 15.1). Their existence relies on the presence of two genes that give similar but not identical subunits. One of the best-known examples of isoenzymes is lactate dehydrogenase, which reversibly interconverts pyruvate and lactate. It is a tetramer and exists in five forms (LDH1 to 5) corresponding to the five permutations of arranging the two types of subunits (H and M), which differ only in a single amino acid substitution, into a tetramer:

H_4 LDH1
H_3M LDH2
H_2M_2 LDH3
HM_3 LDH4
M_4 LDH5

Each isoenzyme promotes the same reaction but has different kinetic constants (K_m, V_{max}), thermal stability and electrophoretic mobility. The tissue distribution of isoenzymes within an organism is frequently different, for example, in humans LDH1 is the dominant isoenzyme in heart muscle but LDH5 is the most abundant form in liver and muscle. These differences are exploited in diagnostic enzymology to identify specific organ damage, for example following myocardial infarction, and thereby aiding clinical diagnosis and prognosis.

8.2.1 Post-translational modifications

Proteins are synthesised at the ribosome and as the growing polypeptide chain emerges from the ribosome it folds up into its native three-dimensional structure. However, this is often not the final active form of the protein. Many proteins undergo modifications once they leave the ribosome, where one or more amino acid side chains are modified by the addition of a further chemical group; this is referred to as post-translational modification. Such changes include extensive modifications of the protein structure, for example the addition of chains of carbohydrates to form glycoproteins (see Section 8.4.4), where in some cases the final protein consists of as much as over 40% carbohydrate. Less dramatic, but equally important modifications include the addition of a hydroxyl group to proline to produce hydroxyproline (found in the structure of collagen), or the phosphorylation of one or more amino acids (tyrosine, serine and threonine residues are all capable of being phosphorylated). Many cases are known, for example, where the addition of a single phosphate group (by enzymes known as kinases) can activate a protein molecule, and the subsequent removal of the phosphate group (by a phosphatase) can inactivate the molecule; protein phosphorylation reactions are a central part of intracellular signalling (Sections 16.5 and 16.6). Another example can be found in the post-translational modification of proline residues in the transcription factor HIF (the α subunit of the hypoxia-inducible factor), which is a key oxygen-sensing mechanism in cells. Many proteins therefore are not in their final active, biological form until post-translational modifications have taken place. Over 200 different post-translational modifications have been reported for proteins from microbial, plant and animal sources. Mass spectrometry is used to determine such modifications (see Section 9.5.6).

8.3 PROTEIN PURIFICATION

8.3.1 Introduction

At first sight, the purification of *one* protein from a cell and tissue homogenate that will typically contain 10 000–20 000 different proteins, seems a daunting task. However, in practice, on average, only four different fractionation steps are needed to purify a given protein. Indeed, in exceptional circumstances proteins have been purified in a single chromatographic step. Since the reason for purifying a protein is normally to provide material for structural or functional studies, the final degree of purity required depends on the purposes for which the protein will be used, i.e. you may not need a protein sample that is 100% pure for your studies. Indeed, to define what is meant by a 'a pure protein' is not easy. Theoretically, a protein is pure when a sample contains only a single protein species, although in practice it is more or less impossible to achieve 100% purity. Fortunately, many studies on proteins can be carried out on samples that contain as much as 5–10% or more contamination with other proteins. This is an important point, since each purification step necessarily involves loss of some of the protein you are trying to purify. An extra (and unnecessary) purification step that increases the purity of your sample from, say, 90% to 98% may mean that you now have a more pure protein, but insufficient protein for your studies. Better to have studied the sample that was 90% pure and have enough to work on!

For example, a 90% pure protein is sufficient for amino acid sequence determination studies as long as the sequence is analysed quantitatively to ensure that the deduced sequence does not arise from a contaminant protein. Similarly, immunisation of a rodent to provide spleen cells for monoclonal antibody production (Section 7.2.3) can be carried out with a sample that is considerably less than 50% pure. As long as your protein of interest raises an immune response it matters not at all that antibodies are also produced against the contaminating proteins. For kinetic studies on an enzyme, a relatively impure sample can be used provided it does not contain any competing activities. On the other hand, if you are raising a monospecific polyclonal antibody in an animal (see Section 7.2.3), it is necessary to have a highly purified protein as antigen, otherwise immunogenic contaminating proteins will give rise to additional antibodies. Equally, proteins that are to have a therapeutic use must be extremely pure to satisfy regulatory (safety) requirements. Clearly, therefore, the degree of purity required depends on the purpose for which the protein is needed.

8.3.2 The determination of protein concentration

The need to determine protein concentration in solution is a routine requirement during protein purification. The only truly accurate method for determining protein concentration is to acid hydrolyse a portion of the sample and then carry out amino acid analysis on the hydrolysate (see Section 8.4.2). However, this is relatively time-consuming, particularly if multiple samples are to be analysed. Fortunately, in practice, one rarely needs decimal place accuracy and other, quicker methods that give a reasonably accurate assessment of protein concentrations of a solution are acceptable. Most of these (see below) are colorimetric methods, where a portion of the protein solution is reacted with a reagent that produces a coloured product. The amount of this coloured product is then measured spectrophotometrically and the amount of colour related to the amount of protein present by appropriate calibration. However, none of these methods is absolute, since, as will be seen below, the development of colour is often at least partly dependent on the amino acid composition of the protein(s). The presence of prosthetic groups (e.g. carbohydrate) also influences colorimetric assays. Many workers prepare a standard calibration curve using bovine serum albumin (BSA), chosen because of its low cost, high purity and ready availability. However, it should be understood that, since the amino acid composition of BSA will differ from the composition of the sample being tested, any concentration values deduced from the calibration graph can only be approximate.

Ultraviolet absorption

The aromatic amino acid residues tyrosine and tryptophan in a protein exhibit an absorption maximum at a wavelength of 280 nm. Since the proportions of these aromatic amino acids in proteins vary, so too do extinction coefficients for individual proteins. However, for most proteins the extinction coefficient lies in the range 0.4–1.5; so for a complex mixture of proteins it is a fair approximation to say that a solution with an absorbance at 280 nm (A_{280}) of 1.0, using a 1 cm pathlength, has a protein concentration of approximately 1 mg cm^{-3}. The method is relatively sensitive, being able to measure protein concentrations as low as 10 μg cm^{-3}, and, unlike colorimetric methods, is non-destructive, i.e. having made the measurement, the sample in the cuvette can be recovered and used further. This is particularly useful when one is working with small amounts of protein and cannot afford to waste any. However, the method is subject to interference by the presence of other compounds that absorb at 280 nm. Nucleic acids fall into this category having an absorbance as much as 10 times that of protein at this wavelength. Hence the presence of only a small percentage of nucleic acid can greatly influence the absorbance at this wavelength. However, if the absorbances (A) at 280 and 260 nm wavelengths are measured it is possible to apply a correction factor:

$$\text{Protein (mg cm}^{-3}) = 1.55\,A_{280} - 0.76\,A_{260}$$

The great advantage of this protein assay is that it is non-destructive and can be measured continuously, for example in chromatographic column effluents.

Even greater sensitivity can be obtained by measuring the absorbance of ultraviolet light by peptide bonds. The peptide bond absorbs strongly in the far ultraviolet, with a maximum at about 190 nm. However, because of the difficulties caused by the absorption by oxygen and the low output of conventional spectrophotometers at this wavelength, measurements are usually made at 205 or 210 nm. Most proteins have an extinction coefficient for a 1 µg cm^{-3} solution of about 30 at 205 nm and about 20 at 210 nm. Clearly therefore measuring at these wavelengths is 20 to 30 times more sensitive than measuring at 280 nm, and protein concentration can be measured to less than 1 µg cm^{-3}. However, one disadvantage of working at these lower wavelengths is that a number of buffers and other buffer components commonly used in protein studies also absorb strongly at this wavelength, so it is not always practical to work at this lower wavelength.

Nowadays all purpose-built column chromatography systems (e.g. fast protein liquid chromatography and high-performance liquid chromatography (HPLC)) have in-line variable wavelength ultraviolet light detectors that monitor protein elution from columns.

Lowry (Folin–Ciocalteau) method

In the past this has been the most commonly used method for determining protein concentration, although it is tending to be replaced by the more sensitive methods described below. The Lowry method is reasonably sensitive, detecting down to 10 µg cm^{-3} of protein, and the sensitivity is moderately constant from one protein to another. When the Folin reagent (a mixture of sodium tungstate, molybdate and phosphate), together with a copper sulphate solution, is mixed with a protein solution, a blue-purple colour is produced which can be quantified by its absorbance at 660 nm. As with most colorimetric assays, care must be taken that other compounds that interfere with the assay are not present. For the Lowry method this includes Tris, zwitterionic buffers such as Pipes and Hepes, and EDTA. The method is based on both the Biuret reaction, where the peptide bonds of proteins react with Cu^{2+} under alkaline conditions producing Cu^{+}, which reacts with the Folin reagent, and the Folin–Ciocalteau reaction, which is poorly understood but essentially involves the reduction of phosphomolybdotungstate to heteropolymolybdenum blue by the copper-catalysed oxidation of aromatic amino acids. The resultant strong blue colour is therefore partly dependent on the tyrosine and tryptophan content of the protein sample.

The bicinchoninic acid method

This method is similar to the Lowry method in that it also depends on the conversion of Cu^{2+} to Cu^+ under alkaline conditions. The Cu^+ is then detected by reaction with bicinchoninic acid (BCA) to give an intense purple colour with an absorbance maximum at 562 nm. The method is more sensitive than the Lowry method, being able to detect down to 0.5 µg protein cm^{-3}, but perhaps more importantly it is generally more tolerant of the presence of compounds that interfere with the Lowry assay, hence the increasing popularity of the method.

The Bradford method

This method relies on the binding of the dye Coomassie Brilliant Blue to protein. At low pH the free dye has absorption maxima at 470 and 650 nm, but when bound to protein has an absorption maximum at 595 nm. The practical advantages of the method are that the reagent is simple to prepare and that the colour develops rapidly and is stable. Although it is sensitive down to 20 µg protein cm^{-3}, it is only a relative method, as the amount of dye binding appears to vary with the content of the basic amino acids arginine and lysine in the protein. This makes the choice of a standard difficult. In addition, many proteins will not dissolve properly in the acidic reaction medium.

Example 1 PROTEIN ASSAY

Question

A series of dilutions of bovine serum albumin (BSA) was prepared and 0.1 cm^3 of each solution subjected to a Bradford assay. The increase in absorbance at 595 nm relative to an appropriate blank was determined in each case, and the results are shown in the table.

Concentration of BSA (mg cm^{-3})	A_{595}
1.5	1.40
1.0	0.97
0.8	0.79
0.6	0.59
0.4	0.37
0.2	0.17

A sample (0.1 cm^3) of a protein extract from E. coli gave an A_{595} of 0.84 in the same assay. What was the concentration of protein in the E. coli extract?

Answer

If a graph of BSA concentration against A_{595} is plotted it is seen to be linear. From the graph, at an A_{595} of 0.84 it can be seen that the protein concentration of the E. coli extracted is 0.85 mg cm^{-3}.

Kjeldahl analysis

This is a general chemical method for determining the nitrogen content of any compound. It is not normally used for the analysis of purified proteins or for monitoring column fractions but is frequently used for analysing complex solid samples and microbiological samples for protein content. The sample is digested by boiling with concentrated sulphuric acid in the presence of sodium sulphate (to raise the boiling point) and a copper and/or selenium catalyst. The digestion converts all the organic nitrogen to ammonia, which is trapped as ammonium sulphate. Completion of the digestion stage is generally recognised by the formation of a clear solution. The ammonia is released by the addition of excess sodium hydroxide and removed by steam distillation in a Markham still. It is collected in boric acid and titrated with standard hydrochloric acid using methyl red–methylene blue as indicator. It is possible to carry out the analysis automatically in an autokjeldahl apparatus. Alternatively, a selective ammonium ion electrode (Section 1.5.2) may be used to directly determine the content of ammonium ion in the digest. Although Kjeldahl analysis is a precise and reproducible method for the determination of nitrogen, the determination of the protein content of the original sample is complicated by the variation of the nitrogen content of individual proteins and by the presence of nitrogen in contaminants such as DNA. In practice, the nitrogen content of proteins is generally assumed to be 16% by weight.

8.3.3 Cell disruption and production of initial crude extract

The initial step of any purification procedure must, of course, be to disrupt the starting tissue to release proteins from within the cell. The means of disrupting the tissue will depend on the cell type (see Cell disruption, below), but thought must first be given to the composition of the buffer used to extract the proteins.

Extraction buffer

Normally extraction buffers are at an ionic strength (0.1–0.2 M) and pH (7.0–8.0) that is considered to be compatible with that found inside the cell. Tris or phosphate buffers are most commonly used. However, in addition a range of other reagents may be included in the buffer for specific purposes. These include:

- *An anti-oxidant:* Within the cell the protein is in a highly reducing environment, but when released into the buffer it is exposed to a more oxidising environment. Since most proteins contain a number of free sulphydryl groups (from the amino acid cysteine) these can undergo oxidation to give inter- and intramolecular disulphide bridges. To prevent this, reducing agents such as dithiothreitol, β-mercaptoethanol, cysteine or reduced glutathione are often included in the buffer.
- *Enzyme inhibitors:* Once the cell is disrupted the organisational integrity of the cell is lost, and proteolytic enzymes that were carefully packaged and controlled within the intact cells are released, for example from lysosomes. Such enzymes will of course start to degrade proteins in the extract, including the protein of interest. To slow down unwanted proteolysis, all extraction and purification steps are carried out at 4 °C, and in addition a range of protease

inhibitors is included in the buffer. Each inhibitor is specific for a particular type of protease, for example serine proteases, thiol proteases, aspartic proteases and metalloproteases. Common examples of inhibitors include: di-isopropylphosphofluoridate (DFP), phenylmethyl sulphonylfluoride (PMSF) and tosylphenylalanyl-chloromethylketone (TPCK) (all serine protease inhibitors); iodoacetate and cystatin (thiol protease inhibitors); pepstatin (aspartic protease inhibitor); EDTA and 1,10-phenanthroline (metalloprotease inhibitors); and amastatin and bestatin (exopeptidase inhibitors).

- *Enzyme substrate and cofactors:*   Low levels of substrate are often included in extraction buffers when an enzyme is purified, since binding of substrate to the enzyme active site can stabilise the enzyme during purification processes. Where relevant, cofactors that otherwise might be lost during purification are also included to maintain enzyme activity so that activity can be detected when column fractions, etc. are screened.

- *EDTA:*   This can be present to remove divalent metal ions that can react with thiol groups in proteins giving *mercaptids*.

$$R - SH + Me^{2+} \rightarrow R - S - Me^+ + H^+$$

- *Polyvinylpyrrolidone (PVP):*   This is often added to extraction buffers for plant tissue. Plant tissues contain considerable amounts of phenolic compounds (both monomeric, such as *p*-hydroxybenzoic acid, and polymeric, such as tannins) that can bind to enzymes and other proteins by non-covalent forces, including hydrophobic, ionic and hydrogen bonds, causing protein precipitation. These phenolic compounds are also easily oxidised, predominantly by endogenous phenol oxidases, to form quinones, which are highly reactive and can combine with reactive groups in proteins causing cross-linking, and further aggregation and precipitation. Insoluble PVP (which mimics the polypeptide backbone) is therefore added to adsorb the phenolic compounds which can then be removed by centrifugation. Thiol compounds (reducing agents) are also added to minimise the activity of phenol oxidases, and thus prevent the formation of quinones.

- *Sodium azide:*   For buffers that are going to be stored for long periods of time, antibacterial and/or antifungal agents are sometimes added at low concentrations. Sodium azide is frequently used as a bacteriostatic agent

Membrane proteins

Membrane-bound proteins (normally glycoproteins) require special conditions for extraction as they are not released by simple cell disruption procedures alone. Two classes of membrane proteins are identified. Extrinsic (or peripheral) membrane proteins are bound only to the surface of the cell, normally via electrostatic and hydrogen bonds. These proteins are predominantly hydrophilic in nature and are relatively easily extracted either by raising the ionic concentration of the extraction buffer (e.g. to 1 M NaCl) or by changes of pH (e.g. to pH 3–5 or pH 9–12). Once extracted, they can be purified by conventional chromatographic procedures. Intrinsic membrane proteins are those that are embedded in the membrane (integrated membrane proteins). These invariably have significant regions of hydrophobic amino acids (those regions of the protein that are embedded in the membrane, and associated with lipids) and have low solubility in aqueous buffer systems. Hence, once extracted into an aqueous polar environment, appropriate conditions must be used to retain their solubility. Intrinsic proteins are usually extracted with buffer containing detergents. The choice of detergent is mainly one of trial and error but can include ionic detergents such as sodium dodecyl sulphate (SDS), sodium deoxycholate, cetyl trimethylammonium bromide (CTAB) and CHAPS, and non-ionic detergents such as Triton X-100 and Nonidet P-40.

Once extracted, intrinsic membrane proteins can be purified using conventional chromatographic techniques such as gel filtration, ion-exchange chromatography or affinity chromatography (using lectins). However, in each case it is necessary to include detergent in all buffers to maintain protein solubility. The level of detergent used is normally 10- to 100-fold less than that used to extract the protein, in order to minimise any interference of the detergent with the chromatographic process.

Cell disruption

Unless one is isolating proteins from extracellular fluids such as blood, protein purification procedures necessarily start with the disruption of cells or tissue to release the protein content of the cells into an appropriate buffer. This initial extract is therefore the starting point for protein purification. Clearly one chooses, where possible, a starting material that has a high level of the protein of interest. Depending on the protein being isolated one might therefore start with a microbial culture, plant tissue, or mammalian tissue. The last of these has generally been the tissue of choice where possible, owing to the relatively large amounts of starting material available. However, the ability to clone and overexpress genes for proteins from any source, in both bacteria and yeast, means that nowadays more and more protein purification protocols are starting with a microbial lysate. The different methods available for disrupting cells are described below. Which method one uses depends on the nature of the cell wall/membrane being disrupted.

Mammalian cells   Mammalian cells are of the order of 10 μm in diameter and enclosed by a plasma membrane, weakly supported by a cytoskeleton. These cells therefore lack any great rigidity and are easy to disrupt by shear forces.

Plant cells   Plant cells are of the order of 100 μm in diameter and have a fairly rigid cell wall, comprising carbohydrate complexes and lignin or wax that surround the plasma membrane. Although the plasma membrane is protected by this outer layer, the large size of the cell still makes it susceptible to shear forces.

Bacteria   Bacteria have cell diameters of the order of 1 to 4 μm and generally have extremely rigid cell walls. Bacteria can be classified as either Gram positive or Gram negative depending on whether or not they are stained by the Gram stain (crystal violet and iodine). In Gram-positive bacteria (Fig. 8.2) the plasma

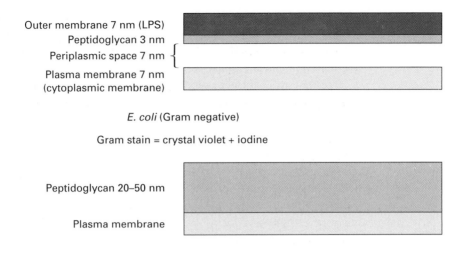

Outer membrane 7 nm (LPS)
Peptidoglycan 3 nm
Periplasmic space 7 nm
Plasma membrane 7 nm
(cytoplasmic membrane)

E. coli (Gram negative)

Gram stain = crystal violet + iodine

Peptidoglycan 20–50 nm

Plasma membrane

Gram positive

Fig. 8.2. The structure of the cell wall of Gram-positive and of Gram-negative bacteria. LPS, lipopolysaccharide.

membrane is surrounded by a thick shell of peptidoglycan (20–50 nm), which stains with the Gram stain. In Gram-negative bacteria (e.g. *Escherichia coli*) the plasma membrane is surrounded by a thin (2–3 nm) layer of peptidoglycan but this is compensated for by having a second outer membrane of lipopolysaccharide. The negatively charged lipopolysaccharide polymers interact laterally, being linked by divalent cations such as Mg^{2+}. A number of Gram-negative bacteria secrete proteins into the periplasmic space

Fungi and yeast   Filamentous fungi and yeasts have a rigid cell wall that is composed mainly of polysaccharide (80–90%). In lower fungi and yeast the polysaccharides are mannan and glucan. In filamentous fungi it is chitin cross-linked with glucans. Yeasts also have a small percentage of glycoprotein in the cell wall, and there is a periplasmic space between the cell wall and cell membrane. If the cell wall is removed the cell content, surrounded by a membrane, is referred to as a spheroplast.

Cell disruption methods

Blenders   These are commercially available, although a typical domestic kitchen blender will suffice. This method is ideal for disrupting mammalian or plant tissue by shear force. Tissue is cut into small pieces and blended, in the presence of buffer, for about 1 min to disrupt the tissue, and then centrifuged to remove debris. This method is inappropriate for bacteria and yeast, but a blender can be used for these microorganisms if small glass beads are introduced to produce a bead mill. Cells are trapped between colliding beads and physically disrupted by shear forces.

Grinding with abrasives   Grinding in a pestle and mortar, in the presence of sand or alumina and a small amount of buffer, is a useful method for disrupting bacterial or plant cells; cell walls are physically ripped off by the abrasive. However, the method is appropriate for handling only relatively small samples. The Dynomill is a large-scale mechanical version of this approach. The Dynomill comprises a chamber containing glass beads and a number of rotating impeller discs. Cells are ruptured when caught between colliding beads. A 600 cm^3 laboratory scale model can process 5 kg of bacteria per hour.

Presses   The use of a press such as a French Press, or the Manton–Gaulin Press, which is a larger-scale version, is an excellent means for disrupting microbial cells. A cell suspension ($\sim$ 50 cm^3) is forced by a piston-type pump, under high pressure (10 000 PSI = lbf in.$^{-2}$ $\approx$ 1450 kPa) through a small orifice. Breakage occurs due to shear forces as the cells are forced through the small orifice, and also by the rapid drop in pressure as the cells emerge from the orifice, which allows the previously compressed cells to expand rapidly and effectively burst. Multiple passes are usually needed to lyse all the cells, but under carefully controlled conditions it can be possible to selectively release proteins from the periplasmic space. The X-Press and Hughes Press are variations on this method; the cells are forced through the orifice as a frozen paste, often mixed with an abrasive. Both the ice crystal and abrasive aid in disrupting the cell walls.

Enzymatic methods   The enzyme lysozyme, isolated from hen egg whites, cleaves peptidoglycan. The peptidoglycan cell wall can therefore be removed from Gram-positive bacteria (see Fig. 8.2) by treatment with lysozyme, and if carried out in a suitable buffer, once the cell wall has been digested the cell membrane will rupture owing to the osmotic effect of the suspending buffer.

Gram-negative bacteria can similarly be disrupted by lysozyme but treatment with EDTA (to remove Ca^{2+}, thus destabilising the outer lipopolysaccharide layer) and the inclusion of a non-ionic detergent to solubilise the cell membrane are also needed. This effectively permeabilises the outer membrane, allowing access of the lysozyme to the peptidoglycan layer. If carried out in an isotonic medium so that the cell membrane is not ruptured, it is possible to selectively release proteins from the periplasmic space.

Yeast can be similarly disrupted using enzymes to degrade the cell wall and either osmotic shock or mild physical force to disrupt the cell membrane. Enzyme digestion alone allows the selective release of proteins from the periplasmic space. The two most commonly used enzyme preparations for yeast are zymolyase or lyticase, both of which have β-1,3-glucanase activity as their major activity, together with a proteolytic activity specific for the yeast cell wall. Chitinase is commonly used to disrupt filamentous fungi. Enzymic methods tend to be used for laboratory-scale work, since for large-scale work their use is limited by cost.

Sonication   This method is ideal for a suspension of cultured cells or microbial cells. A sonicator probe is lowered into the suspension of cells and high frequency sound waves (>20 kHz) generated for 30–60 s. These sound waves cause disruption of cells by shear force and cavitation. Cavitation refers to areas where there is alternate compression and rarefaction, which rapidly interchange. The gas bubbles in the buffer are initially under pressure but, as they decompress, shock waves are released and disrupt the cells. This method is suitable for relatively small volumes (50–100 cm³). Since considerable heat is generated by this method, samples must be kept on ice during treatment.

8.3.4 Fractionation methods

Monitoring protein purification

As will be seen below, the purification of a protein invariably involves the application of one or more column chromatographic steps, each of which generates a relatively large number of test tubes (fractions) containing buffer and protein eluted from the column. It is necessary to determine how much protein is present in each tube so that an elution profile (a plot of protein concentration versus tube number) can be produced. Appropriate methods for detecting and quantifying protein in solution are described in Section 8.3.2. A method is also required for determining which tubes contain the protein of interest so that their contents can be pooled and the pooled sample progressed to the next purification step. If one is purifying an enzyme, this is relatively easy as each tube simply has to be assayed for the presence of enzyme activity (Section 15.2.2).

For proteins that have no easily measured biological activity, other approaches have to be used. If an antibody to the protein of interest is available then samples from each tube can be dried onto nitrocellulose and the antibody used to detect the protein-containing fractions using the dot blot method (Section 5.9.2). Alternatively, an immunoassay such as ELISA or radioimmunoassay (Section 7.7) can be used to detect the protein. If an antibody is not available, then portions from each fraction can be run on a sodium dodecyl sulphate–polyacrylamide gel and the protein-containing fraction identified from the appearance of the protein band of interest on the gel (Section 10.3.1).

An alternative approach that can be used for cloned genes that are expressed in cells is to express the protein as a fusion protein, i.e. one that is linked via a short peptide sequence to a second protein. This can have advantages for protein purification (see Section 8.3.5). However, it can also prove extremely useful for monitoring the purification of a protein that has no easily measurable activity. If the second protein is an enzyme that can be easily assayed (e.g. using a simple colorimetric assay), such as β-galactosidase, then the presence of the protein of interest can be detected by the presence of the linked β-galactosidase activity.

A successful fractionation step is recognised by an increase in the specific activity of the sample, where the specific activity of the enzyme relates its total activity to the total amount of protein present in the preparation:

$$\text{specific activity} = \frac{\text{total units of enzyme in fraction}}{\text{total amount of protein in fraction}}$$

The measurement of units of an enzyme relies on an appreciation of certain basic kinetic concepts and upon the availability of a suitable analytical procedure. These are discussed in Section 15.2.2.

The amount of enzyme present in a particular fraction is expressed conventionally not in terms of units of mass or moles but in terms of units based upon the rate of the reaction that the enzyme promotes. The international unit (IU) of an enzyme is defined as the amount of enzyme that will convert 1 μmole of substrate to product in 1 minute under defined conditions (generally 25 or 30°C at the optimum pH). The SI unit of enzyme activity is defined as the amount of enzyme that will convert 1 mole of substrate to product in 1 second. It has units of katal (kat) such that $1 \text{ kat} = 6 \times 10^7 \text{ IU}$ and $1 \text{ IU} = 1.7 \times 10^{-8} \text{ kat}$. For some enzymes, especially those where the substrate is a macromolecule of unknown relative molecular mass (e.g. amylase, pepsin, RNase, DNase), it is not possible to define either of these units. In such cases arbitrary units are used generally that are based upon some observable change in a chemical or physical property of the substrate.

For a purification step to be successful, therefore, the specific activity of the protein must be greater after the purification step than it was before. This increase is best represented as the fold purification:

$$\text{fold purification} = \frac{\text{specific activity of fraction}}{\text{original specific activity}}$$

A significant increase in specific activity is clearly necessary for a successful purification step. However, another important factor is the yield of the step. It is no use having an increased specific activity if you lose 95% of the protein you are trying to purify. Yield is defined as follows:

$$\text{yield} = \frac{\text{units of enzyme in fraction}}{\text{units of enzyme in original preparation}}$$

A yield of 70% or more in any purification step would normally be considered as acceptable. Table 8.3 shows how yield and specific activity vary during a purification schedule.

Preliminary purification steps

The initial extract, produced by the disruption of cells and tissue, and referred to at this stage as a homogenate, will invariably contain insoluble matter. For example, for mammalian tissue there will be incompletely homogenised connective and/or vascular tissue, and small fragments of non-homogenised tissue. This is most easily removed by filtering through a double layer of cheesecloth or by low speed (5000 **g**) centrifugation. Any fat floating on the surface can be removed by coarse filtration through glass wool or cheesecloth. However, the solution will still be cloudy with organelles and membrane fragments that are too small to be conveniently removed by filtration or low speed centrifugation. These may not be much of a problem as they will often be lost in the preliminary stages of protein purification, for example during salt fractionation. However, if necessary they can be removed first by

Table 8.3 Example of a protein purification schedule

Fraction	Volume (cm³)	Protein concentration (mg U cm⁻³)	Total protein (mg)	Activity[a] (mg U cm⁻³)	Total activity (U)	Specific activity (U mg⁻¹)	Purification factor[b]	Overall yield[c] (%)
Homogenate	8500	40	340 000	1.8	15 300	0.045	1	100
45%–70% (NH₄)₂SO₄	530	194	103 000	23.3	12 350	0.12	2.7	81
CM-cellulose	420	19.5	8 190	25	10 500	1.28	28.4	69
Affinity chromotography	48	2.2	105.6	198	9500	88.4	1964	62
DEAE-Sepharose	12	2.3	27.6	633	7600	275	6110	50

[a] The unit of enzyme activity (U) is defined as that amount which produces 1 μmole of product per minute under standard assay conditions.
[b] Defined as: purification factor = (specific activity of fraction/specific activity of homogenate).
[c] Defined as: overall yield = (total activity of fraction/total activity of homogenate).

Reproduced with permission from *Methods in Molecular Biology*, **59**, *Protein Purification Protocols*, ed. S. Doonan (1996), Humana Press Inc. Totowa, NJ.

Example 2 ENZYME FRACTIONATION

Question

A tissue homogenate was prepared from pig heart tissue as the first step in the preparation of the enzyme aspartate aminotransferase (AAT). Cell debris was removed by filtration and nucleic acids removed by treatment with polyethyleneimine, leaving a total extract (solution A) of 2 dm^3. A sample of this extract (50 mm^3) was added to 3 cm^3 of buffer in a 1 cm pathlength cuvette and the absorbance at 280 nm shown to be 1.7.

  (i) Determine the approximate protein concentration in the extract, and hence the total protein content of the extract.

  (ii) One unit of AAT enzyme activity is defined as the amount of enzyme in 3 cm^3 of substrate solution that causes an absorbance change at 260 nm of 0.1 min^{-1}. To determine enzyme activity, 100 mm^3 of extract was added to 3 cm^3 of substrate solution and an absorbance change of 0.08 min^{-1} was recorded. Determine the number of units of AAT actively present per cm^3 of extract A, and hence the total number of enzyme units in the extract.

  (iii) The initial extract (solution A) was then subjected to ammonium sulphate fractionation. The fraction precipitating betweeen 50% and 70% saturation was collected and redissolved in 120 cm^3 of buffer (solution B). Solution B (5 mm^3 (0.005 cm^3)) was added to 3 cm^3 of buffer and the absorbance at 280 nm determined to be 0.89 using a 1 cm pathlength cuvette. Determine the protein concentration, and hence total protein content, of solution B.

  (iv) Solution B 20 mm^3 was used to assay for AAT activities and an absorbance change of 0.21 per min at 260 nm was recorded. Determine the number of AAT units cm^{-3} in solution B and hence the total number of enzyme units in solution B.

  (v) From your answers to (i) to (iv), determine the specific activity of AAT in both solutions A and B.

  (vi) From your answers to question (v), determine the fold purification achieved by the ammonium sulphate fractionation step.

  (vii) Finally, determine the yield of AAT following the ammonium sulphate fractionation step.

Answer

  (i) Assuming the approximation that a 1 mg protein cm^{-3} solution has an absorbance of 1.0 at 280 nm using a 1 cm pathlength cell, then we can deduce that the protein concentration *in the cuvette* is approximately 1.7 mg cm^{-3}. Since 50 μl (0.05 cm^3) of the solution A was added to 3.0 cm^3 then the solution A sample had been diluted by a factor of 3.05/0.05 = 61.

Therefore the protein concentration of solution A is 61 × 1.7 mg cm^{-3} =~ 104 mg cm^{-3}. Since there is 2 dm^3 (2000 cm^3) of solution A, the *total* amount of protein in solution A is 2000 × 104 = 208 000 mg or 208 g.

  (ii) Since one enzyme unit causes an absorbance change of 0.1 per minute, there was 0.08/0.1 = 0.8 enzyme units in the cuvette. These 0.8 enzyme units came from the 100 mm^3 of solution A that was added to the cuvette.

Therefore in 100 mm^3 of solution A there is 0.8 enzyme unit.

Therefore in 1 cm^3 of solution A there are 8.0 enzyme units.

Since we have 2000 cm³ of solution A there is a total of $2000 \times 8.0 = 16\,000$ enzyme units in solution A.

(iii) Using the same approach as in Example 2(i), the protein concentration of solution B is $3.005/0.005 \times 0.89 = 601 \times 0.89 = 535$ mg cm^{-3}.

Therefore the total protein present in solution B $= 120 \times 535 = 64\,200$ mg.

i(iv) Using the same approach as in Example 2(ii), there are $0.21/0.1 = 2.1$ units of enzyme activity in the cuvette. These units came from the 20 mm³ that was added to the cell.

Therefore, 20 mm³ (0.020 cm³) of solution B contains 2.1 enzyme units.

Thus, 1 cm³ of solution B contains $1.0/0.02 \times 2.1 = 105$ units. Therefore, solution B has 105 units cm^{-3}.

Since there are 120 cm³ of solution B, total units in solution B $= 120 \times 105 = 12\,600$.

(v) For solution A, specific activity $= 16\,000/208\,000 = 0.077$ units mg^{-1}.

For solution B, specific activity $= 12\,600/64\,200 = 0.197$ units mg^{-1}.

(vi) Fold purification $= 0.197/0.077 = 2.6$ (approx.).

(vii) Yield $= (12\,600/16\,000) \times 100\% = 79\%$.

precipitation using materials such as Celite (a diatomaceous earth that provides a large surface area to trap the particles), Cell Debris Remover (CDR) a cellulose-based absorber, or any number of flocculants such as starch, gums, tannins or polyamines, the resultant precipitate being removed by centrifugation or filtration.

It is tempting to assume that the cell extract contains only protein, but of course a range of other molecules is present such as DNA, RNA, carbohydrate and lipid as well as any number of small molecular weight metabolites. Small molecules tend to be removed later on during dialysis steps or steps that involve fractionation based on size (e.g. gel filtration) and therefore are of little concern. However, specific attention has to be paid at this stage to macromolecules such as nucleic acids and polysaccharides. This is particularly true for bacterial extracts, which are particularly viscous owing to the presence of chromosomal DNA. Indeed microbial extracts can be extremely difficult to centrifuge to produce a supernatant extract. Some workers include DNase I in the extraction buffer to reduce viscosity, the small DNA fragments generated being removed at later dialysis/gel filtration steps. Likewise RNA can be removed by treatment with RNase. DNA and RNA can also be removed by precipitation with protamine sulphate. Protamine sulphate is a mixture of small, highly basic (i.e. positively charged) proteins, whose natural role is to bind to DNA in the sperm head. (Protamines are usually extracted from fish organs, which are obtained as a waste product at canning factories.) These positively charged proteins bind to negatively charged phosphate groups on nucleic acids, thus masking the charged groups on the nucleic acids and rendering them insoluble. The addition of a solution of protamine sulphate to the extract therefore precipitates most of the DNA and RNA, which can subsequently be removed by centrifugation. An alternative is to use polyethyleneimine, a synthetic long chain cationic (i.e. positively charged) polymer (molecular mass 24 kDa). This also binds to the phosphate groups in nucleic acids, and is very effective, precipitating DNA and RNA almost instantly. For bacterial extracts, carbohydrate capsular gum can also be a problem as this can interfere with protein precipitation methods. This is best removed by totally precipitating the protein with ammonium sulphate (see below) leaving the gum in solution. The protein can then be recovered by centrifugation and redissolved in buffer. However, if lysozyme (plus detergent) is used to lyse the cells (see Section 8.3.3) capsular gum will not be a problem as it is digested by the lysozyme.

The clarified extract is now ready for protein fractionation steps to be carried out. The concentration of the protein in this initial extract is normally quite low, and in fact the major contaminant at this stage is water! The initial purification step is frequently based on solubility methods. These methods have a high capacity, can therefore be easily applied to large volumes of initial extracts and also have the advantage of concentrating the protein sample. Essentially, proteins that differ considerably in their physical characteristics from the protein of interest are removed at this stage, leaving a more concentrated solution of proteins that have more closely similar physical characteristics. The next stages, therefore, involve higher resolution techniques that can separate proteins with similar characteristics. Invariably these high resolution techniques are chromatographic. Which technique to use, and in which order, is more often than not a matter of trial and error. The final research paper that describes in four pages a three-step, four-day protein purification procedure invariably belies the months of hard work that went into developing the final 'simple' purification protocol!

All purification techniques are based on exploiting those properties by which proteins differ from one another. These different properties, and the techniques that exploit these differences, are as follows.

Stability   Denaturation fractionation exploits differences in the heat sensitivity of proteins. The three-dimensional (tertiary) structure of proteins is maintained by a number of forces, mainly hydrophobic interactions, hydrogen bonds and sometimes disulphide bridges. When we say that a protein is denatured we mean that these bonds have by some means been disrupted and that the protein chain has unfolded to give the insoluble, 'denatured' protein. One of the easiest ways to denature proteins in solution is to heat them. However, different proteins will denature at different temperatures, depending on their different thermal stabilities; this, in turn, is a measure of the number of bonds holding the tertiary structure together. If the protein of interest is particularly heat stable, then heating the extract to a temperature at which the protein is stable yet other proteins denature can be a very useful preliminary step. The temperature at which the protein being purified is denatured is first determined by a small-scale experiment. Once this temperature is known, it is possible to remove more thermolabile contaminating proteins by heating the mixture to a temperature 5–10 deg.C below this critical temperature for a period of 15–30 min. The denatured, unwanted protein is then removed by centrifugation. The presence of the substrate, product or a competitive inhibitor of an enzyme often stabilises it and allows an even higher heat denaturation temperature to be employed. In a similar way, proteins differ in the ease with which they are denatured by extremes of pH (<3 and >10). The sensitivity of the protein under investigation to extreme pH is determined by a small-scale trial. The whole protein extract is then adjusted to a pH not less than 1 pH unit within that at which the test protein is preciptiated. More sensitive proteins will precipitate and are removed by centrifugation.

Solubility   Proteins differ in the balance of charged, polar and hydrophobic amino acids that they display on their surfaces. Charged and polar groups on the surface are solvated by water molecules, thus making the protein molecule soluble, whereas hydrophobic residues are masked by water molecules that are necessarily found adjacent to these regions. Since solubility is a consequence of solvation of charged and polar groups on the surfaces of the protein, it follows that, under a particular set of conditions, proteins will differ in their solubilities. In particular, one exploits the fact that proteins precipitate differentially from solution on the addition of species such as neutral salts or organic solvents. It should be stressed here that these methods precipitate native (i.e. active) protein that has become insoluble by aggregation; we have not denatured the protein.

Salt fractionation is frequently carried out using ammonium sulphate. As increasing salt is added to a protein solution, so the salt ions are solvated by water molecules in the solution. As the salt concentration increases, freely available water molecules that can solvate the ions become scarce. At this stage those water molecules that have been forced into contact with hydrophobic groups on the surface of the protein are the next most freely available water molecules (rather than those involved in solvating polar groups on the protein surface, which are bound by electrostatic interactions and are far less easily given up) and these are therefore removed to solvate the salt molecules, thus leaving the hydrophobic patches exposed. As the ammonium sulphate concentration increases, the hydrophobic surfaces on the protein are progressively exposed. Thus revealed, these hydrophobic patches cause proteins to aggregate by hydrophobic interaction, resulting in precipitation. The first proteins to aggregate are therefore those with most hydrophobic residues on the surface, followed by those with less hydrophobic residues. Clearly the aggregates formed are made of mixtures of more than one protein. Individual identical molecules do not seek out each other, but simply bind to another adjacent molecule with an exposed hydrophobic patch. However, many proteins are precipitated from solution over a narrow range of salt concentrations, making this a suitably simple procedure for enriching the proteins of interest.

Organic solvent fractionation is based on differences in the solubility of proteins in aqueous solutions containing water-miscible organic solvents such as ethanol, acetone and butanol. The addition of organic solvent effectively 'dilutes out' the water present (reduces the dielectric constant) and at the same time water molecules are used up in hydrating the organic solvent molecules. Water of solvation is therefore removed from the charged and polar groups on the surface of proteins, thus exposing their charged groups. Aggregation of proteins therefore occurs by charge (ionic) interactions between molecules. Proteins consequently precipitate in decreasing order of the number of charged groups on their surface as the organic solvent concentration is increased.

Organic polymers can also be used for the fractional precipitation of proteins. This method resembles organic solvent fractionation in its mechanism of action but requires lower concentrations to cause protein precipitation and is less likely to cause protein denaturation. The most commonly used polymer is polyethylene glycol (PEG), with a relative molecular mass in the range 6000–20 000.

The fractionation of a protein mixture using ammonium sulphate is given here as a practical example of fractional precipitation. As explained above, as increasing amounts of ammonium sulphate are dissolved in a protein solution, certain proteins start to aggregate and precipitate out of solution. Increasing the salt strength results in further, different proteins precipitating out. By carrying out a controlled pilot experiment where the percentage of ammonium sulphate is increased stepwise say from 10% to 20% to 30% etc., the resultant precipitate at each step being recovered by centrifugation, redissolved in buffer and analysed for the protein of interests, it is possible to determine a fractionation procedure that will give a significantly purified sample. In the example shown in Table 8.3, the original homogenate was made 45% in ammonium sulphate and the precipitate recovered and discarded. The supernatant was then made 70% in ammonium sulphate, the precipitate collected, redissolved in buffer, and kept, with the supernatant being discarded. This produced a purification factor of 2.7. As can be seen, a significant amount of protein has been removed at this step (237 000 mg of protein) while 81% of the total enzyme present was recovered, i.e. the yield was good. This step has clearly produced an enrichment of the protein of interest from a large volume of extract and at the same time has concentrated the sample.

Isoelectric precipitation fractionation is based upon the observations that proteins have their minimum solubility at their isoelectric point. At this pH there are equal numbers of positive and negative charges on the protein molecule; intermolecular repulsions are therefore minimised and protein molecules can approach each other. This therefore allows opposite charges on different molecules to interact, resulting in the formation of insoluble aggregates. The principle can be exploited either to remove unwanted protein, by adjusting the pH of the protein extract so as to cause the precipitation of these proteins but not that of the test protein, or to remove the test protein, by adjusting the pH of the extract to its pI. In practice, the former alternative is preferable, since some denaturation of the precipitation protein inevitably occurs.

Finally, an unusual solubility phenomenon can be utilised in some cases for protein purification from *E. coli*. Early workers who were overexpressing heterologous proteins in *E. coli* at high levels were alarmed to discover that, although their protein was expressed in high yield (up to 40% of the total cell protein), the protein aggregated to form insoluble particles that became known as inclusion bodies. Initially this was seen as a major impediment to the production of proteins in *E. coli*, the inclusion bodies effectively being a mixture of monomeric and polymeric denatured proteins formed by partial or incorrect folding, probably due to the reducing environment of the *E. coli* cytoplasm. However, it was soon realised that this phenomenon could be used to advantage in protein purification. The inclusion bodies can be separated from a large proportion of the bacterial cytoplasmic protein by centrifugation, giving an effective purification step. The recovered inclusion bodies must then be solubilised and denatured and subsequently allowed to refold slowly to their active, native configuration. This is normally achieved by heating in 6 M guanidinium hydrochloride (to denature the protein) in the presence of a reducing agent (to disrupt any disulphide bridges). The denatured protein is then either diluted in buffer or dialysed against buffer, at which time the protein slowly refolds. Although the refolding method is not always 100% successful, this approach can often produce protein that is 50% or more pure.

Having carried out an initial fractionation step such as that described above, one would then move towards using higher resolution chromatographic methods. Chromatographic techniques for purifying proteins are summarised in Table 8.4, and some of the more commonly used methods are outlined below. The precise practical details of each technique are discussed in Chapter 11.

Charge Proteins differ from one another in the proportions of the charged amino acids (aspartic and glutamic acids, lysine, arginine and histidine) that they contain. Hence proteins will differ in net charge at a particular pH. This difference is exploited in ion-exchange chromatography (Section 11.6), where the protein of interest is bound onto a solid support material bearing charged groups of the opposite sign (ion-exchange resin). Proteins with the same charge as the resin pass through the column to waste, after which bound proteins, containing the protein of interest, are selectively released from the column by gradually increasing the strength of salt ions in the buffer passing through the column or by gradually changing the pH of the eluting buffer. These ions compete with the protein for binding to the resin, the more weakly charged protein being eluted at the lower salt strength and the more strongly charged protein being eluted at higher salt strengths.

Another feature of the different charged groups found in proteins is the fact that most proteins will differ in their isoelectric points (Section 8.1), i.e. they will differ in the pH value at which they have zero overall charge. This difference in pI can be exploited using chromatofocusing (Section 11.6.3).

Size Size differences between proteins can be exploited in molecular exclusion (also known as gel filtration) chromatography. The gel filtration medium consists of a range of beads with slighly differing amounts of cross-linking and therefore slightly different pore sizes. The separation process depends on the different abilities of the various proteins to enter some, all or none of the beads, which in turn relates to the size of this protein (Section 11.7). The method has limited resolving power, but can be used to obtain a separation between large and small protein molecules and therefore be useful when the protein of interest is either particularly large or particularly small. This method can also be used to determine the relative molecular mass of a protein (Section 11.7.2) and for concentrating or desalting a protein solution (Section 11.7.2).

Table 8.4 Summary of chromatographic techniques commonly used in protein purification

Technique	Property exploited	Capacity	Resolution	Practical points	Further details
Hydrophobic interaction	Hydrophobicity	High	Medium	Can cope with high ionic strength samples, e.g. ammonium sulphate precipitates. Fractions are of varying pH and/or ionic strength. Medium yield. Commonly used in early stages of purification protocol. Unpredictable	Section 11.4.3
Ion exchange	Charge	High	Medium	Sample ionic strength must be low. Fractions are of varying pH and/or ionic strength. Medium yield. Commonly used in early stages of purification protocol	Section 11.6
Affinity	Biological function	Medium (cost limited)	High	Limited by availability of immobilised ligand. Elution may denature protein. Yield medium–low. Commonly used towards end of purification protocol	Section 11.8
Dye affinity	Structure and hydrophobicity	High	High	Necessary to carry out initial screening of a wide range of dye–ligand supports	Section 11.8.6
Chromatofocusing	Charge and pI	High–medium	High–medium	Sample ionic strength must be low. Fractions contaminated with ampholytes	Section 11.6.3
Covalent	Thiol groups	Medium–low	High	Specific for thiol-containing proteins. Limited by high cost and long (3 h) regeneration time	Section 11.8.7
Metal chelate	Imidazole, thiol, tryptophan groups	Medium–low	High	Relatively few examples in literature. Expensive	Section 11.8.5
Exclusion	Molecular size	Medium	Low	Commonly used as a final stage of purification. Can give information about protein molecular weight. Good for desalting protein samples	Section 11.7

Affinity   Certain proteins bind strongly to specific small molecules. One can take advantage of this by developing an affinity chromatography system where the small molecule (ligand) is bound to an insoluble support. When a crude mixture of proteins containing the protein of interest is passed through the column, the ligand binds the protein to the matrix whilst all other proteins pass through the column. The bound protein can then be eluted from the column by changing the pH, increasing salt strength or passing through a high concentration of unbound free ligand. For example, the protein concanavalin A (con A) binds strongly to glucose. An affinity column using glucose as the ligand can therefore be used to bind con A to the matrix, and the con A can be recovered by passing a high concentration of glucose through the column. Lectins (Section 11.8.3) are particularly useful ligands for purifying glycoproteins by affinity chromatography. Affinity chromatography is covered in detail in Section 11.8.

Hydrophobicity   Proteins differ in the amount of hydrophobic amino acids that are present on their surface. This difference can be exploited in salt fractionation (see above) but can also be used in a higher resolution method using hydrophobic interaction chromatography (HIC) (Section 11.4.3). A typical column material would be phenyl-Sepharose, where phenyl groups are bonded to the insoluble support Sepharose. The protein mixture is loaded on the column in high salt (to ensure hydrophobic patches are exposed) where hydrophobic interaction will occur between the phenyl groups on the resin and hydrophobic regions on the proteins. Proteins are then eluted by applying a decreasing salt gradient to the column and should emerge from the column in order of increasing hydrophobicity. However, some highly hydrophobic proteins may not even be eluted in the total absence of salt. In this case it is necessary to add a small amount of water-miscible organic solvent such as propanol or ethylene glycol to the column buffer solution. This will compete with the proteins for binding to the hydrophobic matrix and will elute any remaining proteins.

8.3.5 Engineering proteins for purification

With the ability to clone and overexpress genes for proteins using genetic engineering methodology has also come the ability to aid considerably the purification process by manipulation of the gene of interest prior to expression. These manipulations are carried out either to ensure secretion of the proteins from the cell or to aid protein purification.

Ensuring secretion from the cell

For cloned genes that are being expressed in microbial or eukaryotic cells, there are a number of advantages in manipulating the gene to ensure that the protein product is secreted from the cell:

- *To facilitate purification:*   Clearly if the protein is secreted into the growth medium, there will be far fewer contaminating proteins present than if the cells had to be ruptured to release the protein, when all the other intracellular proteins would also be present.

- *Prevention of intracellular degradation of the cloned protein:*   Many cloned proteins are recognised as 'foreign' by the cell in which they are produced and are therefore degraded by intracellular proteases. Secretion of the protein into the culture medium should minimise this degradation.

- *Reduction of the intracellular concentration of toxic proteins:*   Some cloned proteins are toxic to the cell in which they are produced and there is therefore a limit to the amount of protein the cell will produce before it dies. Protein secretion should prevent cell death and result in continued production of protein.

- *To allow post-translational modification of proteins:*   Most post-translational modifications of proteins occur as part of the secretory pathway, and these modifications, for example glycosylation (see Section 8.4.4), are a necessary process in producing the final protein structure. Since prokaryotic cells do not glycosylate their proteins, this explains why many proteins have to be expressed in eukaryotic cells (e.g. yeast) rather than in bacteria. The entry of a protein into a secretory pathway and its ultimate destination is determined by a short amino acid sequence (signal sequence) that is usually at the N terminus of the protein. For proteins going to the membrane or outside the cell the route is via the endoplasmic reticulum and Golgi apparatus, the signal sequence being cleaved-off by a protease prior to secretion. For example, human γ-interferon has been secreted from the yeast *Pichia pastoris* using the protein's native signal sequence. Also there are a number of well-characterised yeast signal sequences (e.g. the α-factor signal sequence) that can be used to ensure secretion of proteins cloned into yeast.

Fusion proteins to aid protein purification

This approach requires an additional gene to be joined to the gene of the protein of interest such that the protein is produced as a fusion protein (i.e. linked to this second protein, or tag). As will be seen below, the purpose of this tag is to provide a means whereby the fusion protein can be selectively removed from the cell extract. The fusion protein can then be cleaved to release the protein of interest from the tag protein. Clearly the amino acid sequence of the peptide linkage between tag and protein has to be carefully designed to allow chemical or enzymatic cleavage of this sequence. The following are just a few examples of different types of fusion proteins that have been used to aid protein purification.

Flag™   This is a short hydrophilic amino acid sequence that is attached to the N-terminal end of the protein, and is designed for purification by immunoaffinity chromatography.

Asp-Tyr-Lys-Asp-Asp-Asp-Asp-Lys-Protein

A monoclonal antibody against this Flag sequence is available on an immobilised support for use in affinity chromatography. The cell extract, which includes the Flag-labelled protein, is passed through the column where the antibody binds to the Flag-labelled protein, allowing all other proteins to pass through. This is carried out in the presence of Ca^{2+}, since the binding of the Flag sequence to the monoclonal antibody is Ca^{2+} dependent. Once all unbound protein has been eluted from the column, the Flag-linked protein is released by passing EDTA through the column, which chelates the Ca^{2+}. Finally the Flag sequence is removed by the enzyme enterokinase, which recognises the following amino acid sequence and cleaves C-terminal to the lysine residue

N-Asp-Asp-Asp-Lys-C

Using this approach, granulocyte–macrophage colony-stimulating factor (GMCSF) was cloned in and secreted from yeast, and purified in a single step. GMCSF was produced in the cell as signal peptide–Flag–gene. The signal sequence used was the signal sequence for the outer membrane protein OmpA. The Flag–gene protein was thus secreted into the periplasm, the fusion protein purified, and finally the Flag sequence removed, as described above.

Glutathione affinity agarose   In this method the protein of interest is expressed as a fusion protein with the enzyme glutathione S-transferase. The cell extract is passed through a column of glutathione-linked agarose beads, where the enzyme binds to the glutathione. Once all unbound protein has been washed through the column, the fusion protein is eluted by passing reduced glutathione through the column. Finally, cleavage of the fusion protein is achieved using human thrombin, which recognises a specific amino acid sequence in the linker region.

Protein A   As described in Section 7.3.4, protein A binds to the Fc region of the immunoglobulin G (IgG) molecule. The protein of interest is cloned fused to the protein A gene, and the fusion protein purified by affinity chromatography on a column of IgG–Sepharose. The bound fusion protein is then eluted using either high salt or low pH, to disrupt the binding between the IgG molecule and the protein A–protein fusion product. Protein A is then finally removed by treatment with 70% (v/v) formic acid for 2 days, which cleaves an acid-labile Asp-Pro bond in the linker region.

Poly(arginine)   This method requires the addition of a series of arginine residues to the C terminus of the protein to be purified. This makes the protein highly basic (positively charged at neutral pH). The cell extract can therefore be fractionated using cation-exchange chromatography. Bound proteins are sequentially released from the column by applying a salt gradient, with the poly(Arg)-containing protein, because of its high overall positive charge, being the last to be eluted. The poly(Arg) tail is then removed by incubation with the enzyme carboxypeptidase B. Carboxypeptidase B is an exoprotease that sequentially removes arginine or lysine residues from the C terminus of proteins. The arginine residues are therefore sequentially removed from the C terminus, the removal of amino acid residues stopping when the 'normal' (i.e. non-arginine) C-terminal amino acid residue of the protein is reached.

8.4 **PROTEIN STRUCTURE DETERMINATION**

8.4.1 **Relative molecular mass**

There are three methods available for determining protein relative molecular mass, M_r, frequently referred to as molecular weight. The first two described here are quick and easy methods that will give a value to $\pm$ 5–10%. For many purposes one simply needs a rough estimate of size and these methods are sufficient. The third method, mass spectrometry, requires expensive specialist instruments and can give accuracy to $\pm$ 0.001%. This kind of accuracy is invaluable in detecting postsynthetic modification of proteins.

SDS–polyacrylamide gel electrophoresis (SDS–PAGE)

This form of electrophoresis, described in Section 10.3.1, separates proteins on the basis of their shape (size), which in turn relates to their relative molecular masses. A series of proteins of known molecular mass (molecular weight markers) are run on a gel on a track adjacent to the protein of unknown molecular mass. The distance each marker protein moves through the gel is measured and a calibration curve of log M_r versus distance moved is plotted. The distance migrated by the protein of unknown M_r is also measured, and from the graph its log M_r and hence M_r is calculated. The method is suitable for proteins covering a large M_r range (10 000–300 000). The method is easy to perform and requires very little material. If silver staining (Section 10.3.7) is used, as little as 1 ng of protein is required. In practice SDS–PAGE is the most commonly used method for determining protein M_r values.

Molecular exclusion (gel filtration) chromatography

The elution volume of a protein from a molecular exclusion chromatography column having an appropriate fractionation range is determined largely by the size of the protein such that there is a logarithmic relationship between protein relative molecular mass and elution volume (Section 11.7.3). By calibrating the column with a range of proteins of known M_r, the M_r of a test protein can be calculated. The method is carried out on HPLC columns ($\sim 1 \times 30$ cm) packed with porous silica beads. Flow rates are about 1 cm^3 min^{-1}, giving a run time of about 12 min, producing sharp, well-resolved peaks. A linear calibration line is obtained by plotting a graph of log M_r versus K_d for the calibrating proteins. K_d is calculated from the following equation:

$$K_d = \frac{(V_e - V_o)}{(V_t - V_o)}$$

where V_o is the volume in which molecules that are wholly excluded from the column material emerge (the excluded volume), V_t is the volume in which small molecules that can enter all the pores emerge (the included volume) and V_e is the volume in which the marker protein elutes. This method gives values that are accurate to $\pm$ 10%.

Mass spectrometry

Using either electrospray ionisation (ESI) (Section 9.2.4) or matrix-assisted laser desorption ionisation (MALDI) (Section 9.3.7) intact molecular ions can be produced for proteins and hence their masses accurately measured by mass spectrometry. ESI produces molecular ions from molecules with molecular masses up to and in excess of 100 kDa, whereas MALDI produces ions from intact proteins up to and in excess of 200 kDa. In either case, only low picomole quantities of protein are needed. For example, $\alpha\beta_2$ crystallin gave a molecular mass value (20 200 $\pm$ 0.9), in excellent agreement with the deduced mass of 20 201. However, in addition about 10% of the analysed material produced an ion of mass 20 072.2. This showed that some of the purified protein molecules had lost their N-terminal amino acid (lysine). The deduced mass with the loss of N-terminal lysine was 20 072.8. Clearly mass spectrometry has the ability to provide highly accurate molecular mass measurements for proteins and peptides, which in turn can be used to deduce small changes made to the basic protein structure.

8.4.2 Amino acid analysis

The determination of which of the 20 possible amino acids are present in a particular protein, and in what relative amounts, is achieved by hydrolysing the protein to yield its component amino acids and identifying and quantifying them chromatographically. Hydrolysis is achieved by heating the protein with 6 M hydrochloride acid for 14 h at 110 °C *in vacuo*. Unfortunately, the hydrolysis procedure destroys or chemically modifies the asparagine, glutamine and tryptophan residues. Asparagine and glutamine are converted to their corresponding acids (Asp and Glu) and are quantified with them. Tryptophan is completely destroyed and is best determined spectrophotometrically on the unhydrolysed protein.

The amino acids in the protein hydrolysate may be separated chromatographically and quantified by postcolumn derivatisation with an appropriate reagent. In postcolumn derivatisation methods, the effluent stream from the chromatography column is mixed, in-line, with a reagent that reacts with the amino groups of amino acids to produce a coloured or fluorescent product. The effluent then continues to pass through an appropriate detector (colorimeter or fluorimeter) and the amount of colour/fluorescence recorded, on a chart recorder, where each amino acid is recorded as a separate peak, the area under the peak being proportional to the amount of that amino acid. The apparatus dedicated to the analysis of amino acids in mixtures by this technique is referred to as an amino acid analyser. In the original procedure, separation was achieved by ion-exchange chromatography on a sulphated polystyrene column and ninhydrin was used as the colour reagent and was sensitive down to about 50–100 pmol of the amino acid. Later, *o*-phthalaldehyde (Fig. 8.3) and fluorescamine, both of which give fluorescent products, became the reagents of choice, since they enabled as little as 10 pmol of an amino acid to be detected by fluorimetry.

In recent years, precolumn derivatisation of amino acids, followed by separation by reversed-phase HPLC has become attractive and has generally superseded the

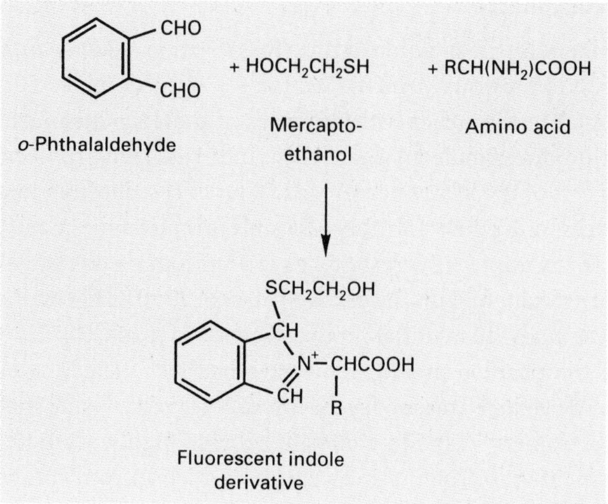

Fig. 8.3. The reaction of an amino acid with o-phthalaldehyde for pre- or postcolumn derivatisation.

original ion-exchange method for the quantification of amino acids in a protein hydrolysate. In this approach the amino acid hydrolysate is first treated with a molecule that (i) reacts with amino groups in amino acids, (ii) is hydrophobic, thus allowing separation of derivatised amino acids by reversed-phase HPLC and (iii) is easily detected by its ultraviolet absorbance of fluorescence. Reagents routinely used for precolumn derivatisation include o-phthalaldehyde (see Fig. 8.3) and 6-aminoquinolyl-N-hydroxysuccinimidyl carbamate (AQC), which both produce fluorescent derivatives, and phenylisothiocyanate, which produces a phenylthio-carbamyl derivative that is detected by its absorbance at 254 nm. Analysis times can be as little as 20 min, and sensitivity is down to 1 pmole or less of amino acid.

8.4.3 Primary structure determination

For many years the amino acid sequence of a protein was determined from studies made on the purified protein alone. This in turn meant that sequence data available were limited to those proteins that could be purified in sufficiently large amounts. Knowledge of the complete primary structure of the protein was (and still is) a pre-requisite for the determination of the three-dimensional structure of the protein, and hence an understanding of how that protein functions. However, nowadays the protein biochemist is normally satisfied with data from just a relatively short length of sequence either from the N terminus of the protein or from an internal sequence, obtained by sequencing peptides produced by cleavage of the native protein. The sequence data will then most likely be used for one of three purposes:

● To search sequence databases to see whether the protein of interest has already been isolated, and hence can therefore be identified. For this type of search extremely short lengths of sequence (three to five residues), known as sequence tags, need to be used. An example of this type of data search is given in Section 9.5.2.

- To search for sequence homology using computerised databases in order to identify the function of the protein. For example, the search may show significant sequence identity with the amino acid sequence of some known protein tyrosine kinases, strongly suggesting that the protein is also a tyrosine kinase.
- The sequence will be used to design an oligonucleotide probe for selecting appropriate clones from complementary DNA libraries. In this way the DNA coding for the protein can be isolated and the DNA sequence, and hence the protein sequence, determined. Obtaining a protein sequence in this way is far less laborious and time-consuming than having to determine the total protein sequence by analysis of the protein.

A further use of protein sequence data is in quality control in the biopharmaceutical industry. Many pharmaceutical companies produce products that are proteins, for example peptide hormones, antibodies, therapeutic enzymes, etc., and synthetic peptides also require analysis to confirm their identities. Sequence analysis, especially to determine sites and nature of postsynthetic modifications such as glycosylation, is necessary to confirm the structural integrity of these products.

Edman degradation

In 1950, Per Edman published a chemical method for the stepwise removal of amino acid residues from the N terminus of a peptide or protein. This series of reactions has come to be known as the Edman degradation, and the method remains, 50 years after its introduction, the most effective chemical means for removing amino acid residues in a stepwise fashion from a polypeptide chain. The reactions comprise three stages (see Fig. 8.4):

- *The coupling reaction:* In this step phenylisothiocyanate (PITC) reacts with the amino group to give the phenylthiocarbamyl (PTC) derivative of the peptide. The reaction is carried out in an inert atmosphere (argon) to avoid oxidation of the sulphur atom in PITC. Following the reaction, the PTC derivative is washed thoroughly with an organic solvent (e.g. benzene) to extract excess PITC and side products, and then dried under vacuum.
- *The cleavage reaction:* In this step, the dried PTC derivative is treated with an anhydrous acid (e.g. heptafluorobutyric acid). This results in the cleavage of the PTC-polypeptide at the peptide bond nearest to the PTC substituent thus releasing the original N-terminal amino acid residue as the 2-anilino-5-thiazolinone derivative, leaving the original polypeptide chain less its N-terminal amino acid residue. Following the cleavage reaction, the anhydrous acid is removed under vacuum and the thiazolinone derivative extracted from the remaining peptide with an organic solvent and recovered by evaporation of the organic solvent.

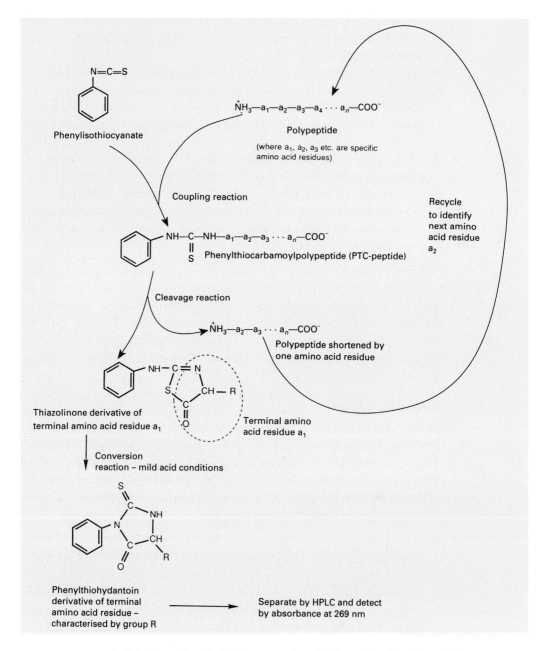

Fig. 8.4. Edman degradation for sequencing of amino acid residues (a, to a_n) in a polypeptide. Each cycle releases the N-terminal amino acid residue as a phenylthiohydantoin derivative, which is then identified chromatographically against reference compounds.

- *The conversion reaction:* Since the thiazolinone is a derivative of the N-terminal amino acid, it could, in principle, be used for identification of that amino acid. However, in practice this is not done, since thiazolinones are relatively unstable. A more stable derivative is obtained by heating the thiazolinone in 1 M HCl at 80 °C for 10 min to convert it to the more stable, isomeric 3-phenyl-2-thiohydantoin (PTH) derivative. This PTH-amino acid is therefore the end-product of one cycle of the Edman degradation and can be easily identified by reversed-phase (RP) HPLC. Thus, if PTH-alanine is identified, we know that the first amino acid residue in the protein was alanine. The remaining polypeptide chain may now be subjected to further cycles of Edman degradation. At the end of each cycle, a PTH-amino acid is recovered and identified. In this way the amino acid sequence of a polypeptide chain may be determined. Theoretically one should be able to apply a series of Edman degradation reactions to a protein and obtain a complete sequence. In practice this is not possible, since the Edman degradation gives only a 96–98% repetitive yield at each step. Thus, after a number of cycles, the yield of PTH-amino acid drops and the background level of PTH-amino acids increases. However, sequences of 20–40 amino acid residues are not uncommon and are frequently sufficient for the purposes outlined above.

The Edman degradation is invariably carried out in an automated analyser, where all steps, including injection onto the reversed-phase HPLC column and identification of the PTH derivative, are carried out automatically. Analysers can therefore be loaded and run overnight and data obtained first thing the following morning. Protein samples in solution are dried onto a small glass fibre disc that is inserted into the reaction chamber of the machine. This ensures that the protein is spread over a very large surface area (i.e. over every glass thread that goes to make up the glass fibre disc). Therefore, even though the protein is denatured by the rigorous chemical treatments of the Edman degradation, the insoluble protein is precipitated as an extremely thin film, thus allowing high reactivity at each step of the Edman cycle. Even proteins that have been blotted onto membranes from gels can be sequenced in the machine. Following blotting (e.g. from a two-dimensional gel), the protein spot of interest can be cut out and placed in the reaction cartridge. In this case it is necessary to use a particulary resistant form of membrane, poly(vinylidene difluoride) (PVDF), since normal nitrocellular membranes are unstable to many of the reagents involved in the Edman degradation. Nowadays sequence data can be obtained from as little as 10–100 ng of protein, the sensitivity of this method being limited only by the sensitivity of detection of the PTH derivatives by ultraviolet absorbance during HPLC.

Protein cleavage and peptide production

Clearly the Edman method determines the amino acid sequence from the N terminus of the protein and requires a free amino group at the N terminus for reaction with PITC. However, it is estimated that 50–70% of all proteins have their N-terminal amino group blocked (e.g. by a formyl, acetyl or acyl group). For such

Table 8.5	Specific cleavage of polypeptide
Reagent	Specificity
Enzymic cleavage	
Chymotrypsin	C-terminal side of hydrophobic amino acid residues, e.g. Phe, Try, Tyr, Leu
Endoproteinase Arg-C	C-terminal side of arginine
Endoproteinase Asp-N	Peptide bonds N-terminal to aspartate or cysteine residues
Trypsin	C-terminal side of arginine and lysine residues but Arg-Pro and Lys-Pro poorly cleaved
Endoproteinase Glu-C	C-terminal side of glutamate residues and some aspartate residues
Endoproteinase Lys-C	C-terminal side of lysine
Thermolysin	N-terminal side of hydrophobic amino acid residues excluding Trp
Chemical cleavage	
BNPS skatole N-Bromosuccinimide o-Iodosobenzoate	C-terminal side of tryptophan residues
Cyanogen bromide	C-terminal side of methionine residues
Hydroxylamine	Asparagine–glycine bonds
2-Nitro-5-thiocyanobenzoate	N-terminal side of cysteine residues

proteins determining an N-terminal amino acid sequence is not possible, so they have to be cleaved to produce peptides, one or more of which can be purified and sequenced to give details of a region from within the protein. (For the reasons described above for requiring protein sequence data, it is usually immaterial whether the sequence comes from the N terminus or from within the protein.) Peptides can be produced by either chemical or enzymatic cleavage of the native protein (see Table 8.5). Chemical methods include the use of cyanogen bromide, which cleaves at methionine residues, and N-bromosuccinimide, which cleaves at tryptophan residues. Methione is a relatively rare amino acid in proteins, and tryptophan even rarer, so these methods tend to produce large peptides. Enzymatic methods include the use of trypsin, which cleaves C-terminal to arginine and lysine residues, endoproteinase Arg-C, which cleaves C-terminal to arginine only, and endoproteinase Glu-C, which cleaves C-terminal to glutamate and some aspartate residues. Clearly it is useful to have the amino acid composition of the protein (Section 8.4.2) to help to decide which method to use; obviously it is better to cleave at an amino acid that is present at relatively low amounts, thus producing a small number of large peptides rather than a more complex mixture of smaller peptides. The peptide hydrolysate thus produced is then fractionated using RP-HPLC. It may seem a little odd to be separating peptides that invariably contain a large proportion of charged and polar groups using a method based on hydrophobicity. However, the standard conditions used to separate peptides mask the polar groups of peptides and give the peptides an overall hydrophobic characteristic. Peptides are frequently dissolved in 1% (v/v) trifluoroacetic acid prior to RP-HPLC. Under these acid conditions, carboxyl groups (-COO⁻) in the peptide (from the C terminus and the side-chains of any Asp or Glu residues present) are protonated (-COOH) thus masking the charged nature of this group. Any positively charged groups (form the N-terminal amino group and the side-chains of Lys, His and Arg residues) can pair with the trifluoroacetyl group (CF₃COO⁻), masking the positive charge and indeed now giving these groups hydrophobic character due to the hydrophobic trifluoroacetyl group. The overall appearance of the peptide under these conditions is therefore of a non-charged, hydrophobic molecule, with of course the side-chains of any hydrophobic residues present in the peptide (Leu, Tyr, Phe, etc.) also contributing to the peptide's hydrophobicity. All peptides then bind to a RP-HPLC column and can be sequentially eluted, in order of increasing hydrophobicity, by the application of a linear gradient of acetonitrile (methyl cyanide), which competes for the hydrophobic interaction between the peptide and the column material.

Mass spectrometry

Because of the absolute requirement to produce ions in the gas phase for the analysis of any sample by mass spectrometry (MS), for many years MS analysis was applicable only to small, non-polar molecules (< 500 M_r). However, recent developments in ionisation technology such as the introduction of fast atom bombardment (FAB), ESI and MALDI methods (see Chapter 9), now means that the analysis of large, charged molecules such as proteins and peptides are routinely achieved. Indeed, the analysis of proteins and peptides by MS is now becoming routine, particularly with the introduction of smaller (and cheaper) bench-top mass spectrometers. Although the Edman degradation still has applications in protein structure analysis, mass spectrometry is now used more routinely to determine amino acid sequence data. Also, of course, proteins with blocked N-terminal residues can be sequenced directly by MS. When peptides are fragmented it is fortunate that the break occurs predominantly at the peptide bond (although it must be noted that other fragmentations, such as internal cleavages, secondary fragmentations, etc. do occur, thus complicating the mass spectrum). This means that the peptide fragments produced each differ sequentially by the mass of one amino acid residue. The amino acid sequence can thus be readily deduced. In particular, if side-chain modifications occur, these can also be observed due to the corresponding increase in mass difference. The use of mass spectrometry to obtain sequence data from proteins and peptides is described more fully in Section 9.3. Tandem mass spectrometry (MS/MS or MS²) is also increasingly being used to obtain sequence data. A digest of the protein (e.g. with trypsin) is separated by MS. The ion corresponding to one peptide is selected in the first analyser and collided with argon gas in a collision cell to generate fragment ions. The fragment ions thus generated are then separated, according to mass, in a second analyser, identified, and the sequence determined as described in Section 9.3.

A further method, ladder sequencing (Section 9.5.5), has been developed, and combines the Edman chemistry with MS. Edman sequencing is carried out using a mixture of PITC and phenylisocyanate (PIC) (at about 5% of the concentration of PITC). N-terminal amino groups that react with PIC are effectively blocked as they are not cleaved at the acid cleavage step. Consequently, at each cycle, approximately 5% of the protein molecules are blocked. Thus, after 20 to 30 cycles of Edman degradation, a nested set of peptides is produced, each differing by the loss of one amino acid. Analysis of the mass of each of these polypeptides using ESI or MALDI allows the determination of the molecular mass of each polypeptide and the difference in mass between each molecule identifies the lost amino acid residue.

Detection of disulphide linkages

For proteins that contain more than one cysteine residue it is important to determine whether, and if so how many, cysteine residues are joined by disulphide bridges. The most commonly used method involves the use of MS (Section 9.5.6). The native protein (i.e. with disulphide bridges intact) is cleaved with a proteolytic enzyme (e.g. trypsin) to produce a number of small peptides. The same experiment is also carried out on proteins treated with dithiothreitol (DTT) which reduces (cleaves) the disulphide bridges. MALDI spectra of the tryptic digest before and after reduction with DTT allows identification of disulphide-linked peptides. Linked peptides from the native protein will disappear from the spectrum of the reduced protein and reappear as *two* peptides of lower mass. Knowledge of the exact mass of each of the two peptides, and knowledge of the cleavage site of the enzyme used, will allow easy identification of the two peptides from the known protein sequence. Thus, if the mass of two disulphide-linked peptides is M, and this is reduced to two separate chains of masses A and B, respectively, then $A + B = M + 2$. The extra two mass units derive from the fact that reduction of the disulphide bond results in an increase of mass of $+1$ for both cysteine residues.

$$-S - S- \xrightarrow{2H} -SH + HS-$$

Hydrophobicity profile

Having determined the amino acid sequence of a protein, analysis of the distribution of hydrophobic groups along the linear sequence can be used in a predictive manner. This requires the products of a hydrophobicity profile for the protein, which graphs the average hydrophobicity per residue against the sequence number. Averaging is achieved by evaluating, using a predictive algorithm, the mean hydrophobicity within a moving window that is stepped along the sequence from each residue to the next. In this way, a graph comprising a series of curves is produced and reveals areas of minima and maxima in hydrophobicity along the linear polypeptide chain. For membrane proteins, such profiles allow the identification of potential membrane-spanning segments. For example, an analysis of a thylakoid membrane protein revealed seven general regions of the protein sequence that contained spans of 20–28 amino acid residues, each of which contained predominantly hydrophobic residues flanked on either side by hydrophilic residues. These regions represent the seven membrane-spanning helical regions of the protein.

For membrane proteins defining aqueous channels, hydrophilic residues are also present in the transmembrane section. Pores comprise amphipathic α-helices, the polar sides of which line the channel, whereas the hydrophobic sides interact with the membrane lipids. More advanced algorithms are used to detect these sequences, since such helices would not necessarily be revealed by simple hydrophobicity analysis.

8.4.4 Glycoproteins

Glycoproteins result from the covalent attachment of carbohydrate chains (glycans), both linear and branched in structure, to various sites on the polypeptide backbone of a protein. These post-translational modifications are carried out by cytoplasmic enzymes within the endoplasmic reticulum and Golgi apparatus. The amount of polysaccharide attached to a given glycoprotein can vary enormously, from as little as a few per cent to more than 60% by weight. Glycoproteins tend to be found in the serum and in cell membranes. The precise role played by the carbohydrate moiety of glycoproteins includes stabilisation of the protein structure, protection of the protein from degradation by proteases, control of protein half-life in blood, the physical maintenance of tissue structure and integrity, a role in cellular adhesion and cell–cell interaction, and as an important determinant in receptor–ligand binding.

The major types of protein glycoconjugates are:

- N-linked;
- O-linked;
- glycosylphosphatidylinositol (GPI)-linked.

N-linked glycans are always linked to an asparagine residue side-chain (Fig. 8.5) at a consensus sequence Asn-X-Ser/Thr where X is any amino acid except proline. O-linked glycosylation occurs where carbohydrate is attached to the hydroxyl group of a serine or threonine residue (Fig. 8.5). However, there is no consensus sequence similar to that found for N-linked oligosaccharides. GPI membrane anchors are a more recently discovered modification of proteins. They are complex glycophospholipids that are covalently attached to a variety of externally expressed plasma membrane proteins. The role of this anchor is to provide a stable association of protein with the membrane lipid bilayer, and will not be discussed further here.

There is considerable interest in the determination of the structure of O- and N-linked oligosaccharides, since glycosylation can affect both the half-life and function of a protein. This is particularly important of course when producing therapeutic glycoproteins by recombinant methods as it is necessary to ensure that the correct carbohydrate structure is produced. It should be noted that prokaryotic cells do not produce glycoproteins, so cloned genes for glycoproteins need to be expressed in eukaryotic cells. The glycosylation of proteins is a complex

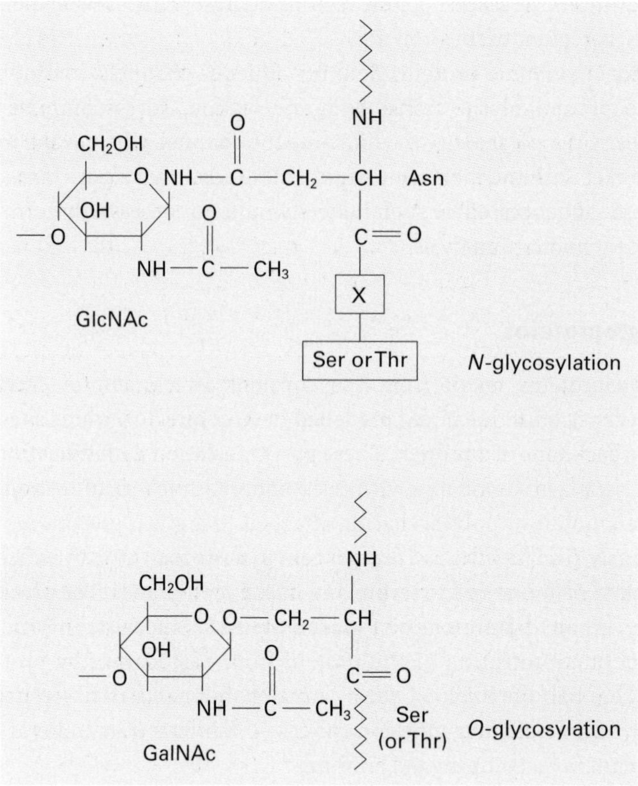

Fig. 8.5. The two types of oligosaccharide linkages found in glycoproteins.

subject. From one glycoprotein to another there are variations in the sites of glycosylation (e.g. only about 30% of consensus sequences for N-linked attachments are occupied by polysaccharide; the nature of the secondary structure at this position also seems to play a role in deciding whether glycosylation takes place), variations in the type of amino acid–carbohydrate bond, variations in the composition of the sugar chains, and variations in the particular carbohydrate sequences and linkages in each chain. There are eight monosaccharide units commonly found in mammalian glycoproteins, although other less common units are also known to occur. These eight are N-acetyl neuraminic acid (NeuNAc), N-glycolyl neuraminic acid (NeuGc), D-galactose (Gal), N-acetyl-D-glucosamine (GlcNac), N-acetyl-D-galactosamine (GalNAc), D-mannose (Man), L-fucose (Fuc) and D-xylose (Xyl). To further complicate the issue, within any population of molecules in a purified glycoprotein there can be considerable heterogeneity in the carbohydrate structure (glycoforms). This can include some molecules showing increased branching of sugar side-chains, reduced chain length and further addition of single carbohydrate units to the same polypeptide chain. The complete determination of the glycosylation status of a molecule clearly requires considerable effort. However, the steps involved are fairly straightforward and the following therefore provides a generalised (and idealised) description of the overall procedures used.

The first question to be asked about a purified protein is 'Is it a glycoprotein?' Glycoprotein bands in gels (e.g. on SDS-polyacrylamide gels) can be stained with cationic dyes such as Alcian Blue, which bind to negatively charged glycosaminoglycan side-chains, or by the periodic acid–Schiff reagent (PAS), where carbohydrate is initially oxidised by periodic acid then subsequently stained with Schiff's reagent. However, although they are both carbohydrate specific (i.e. non-glycosylated proteins are not stained) both methods suffer from low sensitivity. A more sensitive, and informative, approach is to use the specific carbohydrate-binding proteins known as lectins. Blots from SDS–PAGE, dot blots of the glycoprotein sample, or the glycoprotein sample adsorbed onto the walls of a microtitre plates can be challenged with enzyme-linked lectins. Lectins that bind to the glycoprotein can be identified by the associated enzymic activity. By repeating the experiment with a range of different lectins, one can not only confirm the presence of a glycoprotein but also identify which sugar residues are, or are not, present. Having confirmed the presence of glycoprotein the following procedures would normally be carried out.

- *Identification of the type and amount of each monosaccharide:*   Release of monosaccharides is achieved by hydrolysis in methanolic HCl at 80 °C for 18 h. The released monosaccharide can be separated and quantified by gas chromatography.
- *Protease digestion to release glycopeptide:*   A protease is chosen that cleaves the glycoprotein into peptides and glycopeptides of ideally 5–15 amino acid residues. Glycopeptides are then fractionated by HPLC and purified glycopeptides subjected to N-terminal sequence analysis to allow identification of the site of glycosylation.
- *Oligosaccharide profiling:*   Oligosaccharide chains are released from the polypeptide backbone either chemically, for example by hydrazinolysis to release N-linked oligosaccharide, or enzymatically using peptide-*N*-glucosidase F (PNGase F), which cleaves sugars at the asparagine link, or using endo-α-*N*-acetylgalactosaminidase (*O*-glycanase), which cleaves O-linked glycans. These released oligosaccharides can then be separated either by HPLC or by high performance anion exchange chromatography (HPAEC).
- *Structure analysis of each purified oligosaccharide:*   This requires the determination of the composition, sequence and nature of the linkages in each purified oligosaccharide. A detailed description is beyond the scope of this book, but would involve a mixture of complementary approaches including analysis by FAB–MS, gas chromatography–MS, lectin analysis following partial release of sugars and nuclear magnetic resonance (NMR) analysis.

8.4.5 Tertiary structure

The most commonly used method for determining protein three-dimensional structure is X-ray crystallography. A detailed description of the theory and methodology is beyond the scope of this book, requiring a detailed mathematical understanding of the process and computer analysis of the extensive data that are generated. The following is therefore a brief and idealised description of the overall process, and ignores the multitude of pitfalls and problems inherent in determining three-dimensional structures.

- Clearly the first step must be to produce a crystal of the protein (a crystal should be thought of as a three-dimensional lattice of molecules). Protein crystallisation is attempted using as homogeneous a preparation as possible, such preparations having a greater chance of yielding crystals than material that contains impurities. Because of our inadequate understanding of the physical processes involved in crystallisation, methods for growing protein crystals are generally empirical, but basically all involve varying the physical parameters that affect solubility of the protein – for example pH, ionic strength, temperature, presence of precipitating agents – to produce a state of supersaturation. The process involves extensive trial and error to find a procedure that results in crystals for a particular protein. Initially this involves a systematic screen of methods to identify those conditions that indicate crystallinity, followed by subsequent experiments that involve fine-tuning of these conditions. Basically, nucleation sites of crystal growth are formed by chance collisions of molecules forming molecular aggregates, and the probability that these aggregates will occur will be greater in a saturated solution. Clearly, to produce saturated solutions, tens of milligrams of proteins are required. This used to represent a considerable challenge for other than the most abundant proteins, but nowadays genetic engineering methodology allows the overproduction of most proteins from cloned genes almost on demand. The following are some of the methods that have proved successful.

    (a) *Dialysis.*   A state of supersaturation is achieved by dialysis of the protein solution against a solution containing a precipitant, or by a gradual change in pH or ionic strength. Because of frequent limitations on the amount of protein available, this approach often uses small volumes ($< 50\,mm^3$) for which a number of microdialysis techniques exist.

    (b) *Vapour diffusion.*   This process relies on controlled equilibration through the vapour phase to produce supersaturation in the sample. For example, in the hanging-drop method, a microdroplet (2–$20\,mm^3$) of protein is deposited on a glass coverslip; then the coverslip is inverted and placed over a sealed reservoir containing a precipitant solution, with the droplet initially having a precipitant concentration lower than that in the reservoir. Vapour diffusion will then gradually increase the concentration of the protein solution. Because of the small volumes involved this method readily lends itself to screening large numbers of different conditions.

      When produced, crystals may not be of sufficient size for analysis. In this case larger crystals can be obtained by using a small crystal to seed a supersaturated protein solution, which will result in a larger crystal.

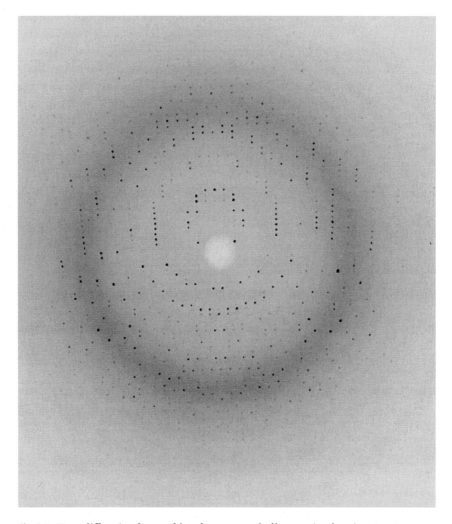

Fig. 8.6. X-ray diffraction frame of data from a crystal of herpes simplex virus type 1 thymidine kinase, complexed with substrate deoxythymidine, at 2 Å resolution. (Picture provided by John N. Champness, Matthew S. Bennett and Mark R. Sanderson of King's College London.)

- Once prepared, the crystal (which is extremely fragile) is mounted inside a quartz or glass capillary tube, with a drop of either mother liquor (the solution from which it was crystallised) or a stabilising solution drawn into one end of the capillary tube to prevent the crystal from drying out. The tube is then sealed and the crystal exposed to a beam of X-rays. Since the wavelength of X-rays is comparable to the planar separation of atoms in a crystal lattice, the crystal can be considered to act as a three-dimensional grating. The X-rays are therefore diffracted, interfering both in phase and out of phase to produce a diffraction pattern as shown in Fig. 8.6. Data collection technology necessary for recording the diffraction pattern is now highly sophisticated. Originally, conventional diffractometers and photographic film were used to detect diffracted X-rays. This involved wet developing of the film and subsequent digital scanning of the negative. Data collection by this method took many weeks. By contrast, modern area-detectors can collect data in under 24 h.

- Unfortunately the diffraction pattern alone is insufficient to determine the crystal structure. Each diffraction maximum has both an amplitude and a phase associated with it, and both need to be determined. But the phases are not directly measurable in a diffraction experiment and must be estimated from further experiments. This is usually done by the method of isomorphous replacement (MIR). The MIR method requires at least two further crystals of the protein (derivatives), each being crystallised in the presence of a different heavy-metal ion (e.g. Hg^{2+}, Cu^{2+}, Mn^{2+}). Comparison of the diffraction patterns from the crystalline protein and the crystalline heavy-metal atom derivative allows phases to be estimated. A more recent approach to producing a heavy-metal derivative is to clone the protein of interest into a methionine auxotroph, and then grow this strain in the presence of selenomethionine (a selenium-containing analogue of methionine). Selenomethionine is therefore incorporated into the protein in the place of methionine, and the final purified and crystallised protein has the selenium heavy metal conveniently included in its structure.

- Diffraction data and phase information having been collected, these data are processed by computer to construct an electron density map. The known sequence of the protein is then fitted into the electron density map using computer graphics, to produce a three-dimensional model of the protein (Fig. 8.7.). In the past there had been concern that the three-dimensional structure determined from the rigid molecules found in a crystal may differ from the true, more flexible, structure found in free solution. These concerns have been effectively resolved by, for example, diffusing substrate into an enzyme crystal and showing that the substrate is converted into product by the crystalline enzyme (there is sufficient mother liquor within the crystal to maintain the substrate in solution). In a more recent development, it is now becoming possible to determine the solution structure of protein using NMR. At present the method is capable of determining the structure of a protein up to about 20 000 kDa but will no doubt be developed to study larger proteins. Although the time-consuming step of producing a crystal is obviated, the methodology and data analysis involved are at present no less time-consuming and complex than that for X-ray crystallography.

8.5 PROTEOMICS AND PROTEIN FUNCTION

In order to completely understand how a cell works, it is necessary to understand the function (role) of every single protein in that cell. The analysis of any specific disease (e.g. cancer) will also require us to understand what changes have taken place in the protein component of the cell, so that we can use this information to understand the molecular basis of the disease, and thus design appropriate drug

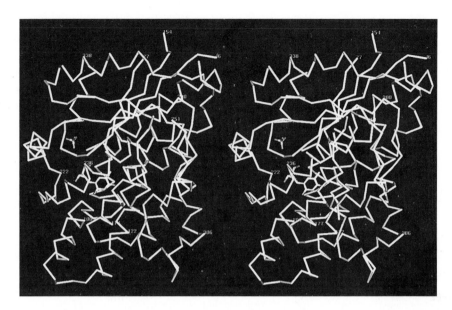

Fig. 8.7. (*Relaxed-eye stereo pair*): A Cα-trace of herpes simplex virus type 1 thymidine kinase from a crystallographic study of a complex of the enzyme with one of its substrates, deoxythymidine. The enzyme is an α–β protein, having a five-stranded parallel β-sheet surrounded by 14 α-helices. The active site, occupied by deoxythymidine, is a volume surrounded by four of the helices, the C-terminal edge of the β-sheet and a short 'flap' segment; a sulphate ion occupies the site of the β-phosphate of the absent co-substrate ATP. (Short missing regions of chain indicate where electron density calculated from the X-ray data could not be interpreted.) (Picture provided by John N. Champness, Matthew S. Bennett and Mark R. Sanderson of King's College London.)

therapies and develop diagnostic methods. (Just about every therapeutic drug that is currently in use has a protein as its target.) The completion of the Human Genome Project might suggest that it is not now necessary to study proteins directly, since the amino acid sequence of each protein can be deduced from the DNA sequence. This is not true for the following reasons:

- First, although the DNA in each cell type in the body is the same, different sets of genes are expressed in different tissues, and hence the protein component of a cell varies from cell type to cell type. For example, some proteins are found in nearly all cells (the so-called house-keeping genes) such as those involved in glycolysis, whereas specific cell types such as kidney, liver, brain, etc. contain specific proteins unique to that tissue and necessary for the functioning of that particular tissue/organ. It is therefore only by studying the protein component of a cell directly that we can identify which proteins are actually present.
- Secondly, it is now appreciated that a single DNA sequence (gene) can encode multiple proteins. This can occur in a number of ways:
    (i) Alternative splicing of the mRNA transcript.
    (ii) Variation in the translation 'stop' or 'start' sites.
    (iii) Frameshifting, where a different set of triplet codons is translated, to give a totally different amino acid sequence.

(iv) Post-translational modifications. The genome sequence defines the amino acid sequence of a protein, but tells us nothing of any post-translational modifications (Sections 8.2.1 and 9.5.3) that can occur once the polypeptide chain is synthesised at the ribosome. Up to 10 different forms (variants) of a single polypeptide chain can be produced by phosphorylation, glycosylation, etc.

The consequence of the above is that the total protein content of the human body is an order of magnitude more complex than the genome. The human genome sequence suggests there may be 30 000–40 000 genes (and hence proteins) whereas estimates of the actual number of proteins in human cells suggests possibly as many as 200 000 or even more. The dogma that one gene codes for one protein has been truly demolished!

From the above, I hope it is easy to appreciate the need to directly analyse the protein component of the cell, and the need for an understanding of the function of each individual protein in the cell. In recent years, development of new techniques (discussed below) has enhanced our ability to study the protein component of the cell and has led to the introduction of the terms proteome and proteomics. The total DNA composition of a cell is referred to as the genome, and the study of the structure and function of this DNA is called genomics. By analogy, the proteome is defined as the total protein component of a cell, and the study of the structure and function of these proteins is called proteomics. The ultimate aim of proteomics is to catalogue the identity and amount of every protein in a cell, and determine the function of each protein.

Earlier sections of this chapter and Chapter 11 describe the traditional, but still very valid approach to studying proteins, where individual proteins are extracted from tissue and purified so that studies can be made of the structure and function of the purified proteins. The subject of proteomics has developed from a different approach, where modern techniques allow us to view and analyse much of the total protein content of the cell in a single step. The development of these newer techniques has gone hand-in-hand with the development of techniques for the analysis of proteins by mass spectrometry, which has revolutionised the subject of protein chemistry. The cornerstone of proteomics has been two-dimensional (2-D) PAGE (described in Section 10.3) and the applications of this technique in proteomics are described below. However, although 2-D PAGE remains central to proteomics, the study of proteomics has stimulated the development of further methods for studying proteins and these will also be described below.

8.5.1 2-D PAGE

2-D PAGE has found extensive use in detecting changes in gene expressions between two different biological states, for example comparing normal and diseased tissue. In this case, a 2-D gel pattern would be produced of an extract from a diseased tissue such as a liver tumour and compared with the 2-D gel patterns of an extract from normal liver tissue. The two gel patterns are then compared to see whether there are any differences in the two patterns. If it is found that a protein is present (or is absent) only in the liver tumour sample, then by identifying this protein we are directed to the gene for this protein and can thus try to understand why this gene is expressed (or not) in the diseased state. In this way it is possible to obtain an understanding of the molecular basis of diseases. This approach can be taken to study *any* disease process where normal and diseased tissue can be compared, for example arthritis, kidney disease, or heart valve disease.

Under favourable circumstances up to 5000 protein spots can be identified on a large format 2-D gel. Thus with 2-D PAGE we now have the ability to follow changes in the expression of a significant proportion of the proteins in a cell or tissue type, rather than just one or two, which has been the situation in the past. The potential applications of proteome analysis are vast. Initially one must produce a 2-D map of the proteins expressed by an organism, tissue or cell under 'normal' conditions. This 2-D reference map and database can then be used to compare similar information from 'abnormal' or treated organisms, tissues or cells. For example, as well as comparing normal tissue with diseased tissue (as described above), we can:

- analyse the effects of drug treatment or toxins on cells;
- observe the changing protein component of the cell at different stages of tissue development;
- observe the response to extracellular stimuli such as hormones or cytokines;
- compare pathogenic and non-pathogenic bacterial strains;
- compare serum protein profiles from healthy individuals and Alzheimer or cancer patients to detect proteins, produced in the serum of patients, which can then be developed as diagnostic markers for diseases (e.g. by setting up an enzyme-linked immunosorbent assay (ELISA) to measure the specific protein).

As a typical example, a research group studying the toxic effect of drugs on the liver can compare the 2-D gel patterns from their 'damaged' livers with the normal liver 2-D reference map, thus identifying protein changes that occur as a result of drug treatment.

The sheer complexity and amount of data available from 2-D gel patterns is daunting, but fortunately there is a range of commercial 2-D gel analysis software, compatible with personal computer workstations, which can provide both qualitative and quantitative information from gel patterns, and can also compare patterns between two different 2-D gels (see below). This has allowed the construction of a range of databases of quantitative protein expression in a range of tissue and cell types. For example, an extensive series of 2-DE databases, known as SWISS-2D PAGE is maintained at Geneva University Hospital and is accessible via the World Wide Web at <http://au.expasy.org/ch2d/>. This facility therefore allows an individual laboratory to compare their own 2-D protein database with that in another laboratory.

The comparison of two gel patterns is made by using any one of a number of software packages designed for this purpose. One of the more interesting approaches to comparing gel patterns is the use of the Flicker program, which is available on the Web at <http://open2dprot.sourceforge.net/Flicker>. This program superimposes the two 2-D patterns to be compared and then alternately, and rapidly, displays one pattern and then the other. Spots that appear on both gel patterns (the majority) will be seen as fixed spots, but a spot that appears on one gel and not the other will seen to be flashing (hence 'flicker'). When one has compared two 2-DE patterns and identified any proteins spot(s) of interest, it is then necessary to identify each specific protein. In the majority of cases this is done by peptide mass-fingerprinting. The spot of interest is cut out of the gel and incubated in a solution of the proteolytic enzyme trypsin, which cleaves the protein C-terminal to each arginine and lysine residue. In this way the protein is reduced to a set of peptides. This collection of peptides is then analysed by MALDI–MS (see Section 9.3.7) to give an accurate mass measurement for each of the peptides in the sample. This set of masses, derived from the tryptic digestion of the protein, is highly diagnostic for this protein, as no other protein would give the same set of peptide masses (fingerprint). Using Web-based programs, such as Mascot or Protein Prospector (Section 9.7.2) this experimentally derived peptide mass-fingerprint is compared with databases of tryptic peptide mass-fingerprints generated from sequences of known proteins (or predicted sequences deduced from nucleotide sequences). If a match is found with a fingerprint from the database then the protein will be identified.

However, sometimes results from peptide mass-fingerprinting can be ambiguous. In this case it is necessary to obtain some partial amino acid sequence data from one of the peptides. This is done by tandem mass spectrometry (MS/MS; Section 9.3.3), where one of the peptides separated for mass-fingerprinting is further fragmented in a second analyser, and from the fragmentation pattern sequence data can be deduced (mass spectrometry conveniently fragments peptides at the peptide bond, such that the difference in the mass of fragments produced can be related to the loss of specific amino acids; Section 9.5.5). This partial sequence data is then used to search the protein sequence databases for sequence identity. Universal databases are available that store information on all types of protein from all biological species. These databases can be divided into two categories: (i) databases that are a simple repository of sequence data, mostly deduced directly from DNA sequences, for example the Tr EMBL database; and (ii) annotated databases where information in addition to the sequence is extracted by the biologist (the annotator) from the literature, review article, etc., for example the SWISS-PROT database.

An example of how sequence data can be produced is shown in Fig. 8.8. A lysate of 2×10^6 rat basophil leukaemic (RBL) cells were separated by 2-D electrophoresis and spot 2 chosen for analysis. This spot was digested *in situ* using trypsin and the resultant peptides extracted. This sample was then analysed by tandem MS using a triple quadrupole instrument (ESI–MS^2). MS of the peptide mixture showed a number of molecular ions relating to peptides. One of these (*m/z* 890) was selected for further analysis, being further fragmented in a quadrupole mass spectrometer to give fragment ions ranging from *m/z* 595.8 to 1553.6 (Fig. 8.8). The ions at *m/z* 1002.0, 1116.8, 1280.0, 1466.2 and 1553.6 are likely to be part of a Y ion series

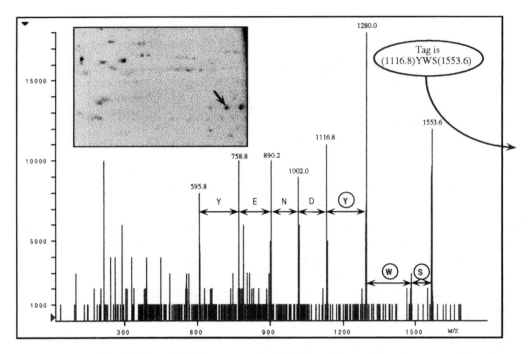

Fig. 8.8. Nano-ESI MS² spectrum of *m/z* 890 from RBL spot 2 showing construction of a sequence tag. The *y*-axis shows relative intensity. (Courtesy of Glaxo SmithKline, Stevenage, UK.)

(see Fig. 8.8) as they appear at higher *m/z* than the precursor at *m/z* 890. The gap between adjacent Y ions is related directly to an amino acid residue because the two flanking Y ions result from cleavage of two adjacent amide bonds. Therefore, with a knowledge of the relative molecular masses of each of the 20 naturally occurring amino acids, it is possible to determine the presence of a particular residue at any point within the peptide. The position of the assigned amino acid is deduced by virtue of the *m/z* ratio of the two ions. By reading several amino acids it was possible to assemble a sequence of amino acids, in this case (using the one-letter code) YWS. Database searching was then possible using the peptide 1778 Da, the position of the lower *m/z* Y ion (1116.8), the proposed amino acid sequence (YWS) and the higher Y ion at *m/z* 1553.6. This provides a sequence tag, which is written as (1116.8) YWS (1553.6).

A search of the SWISS-PROT database (Fig. 8.9), showed just two 'hits' from 40 000 entries, suggesting the protein is glyceraldehyde-3-phosphate dehydrogen-ase. The full sequence of this peptide is LISWYDNEYGYSNR and the MS/MS frag-mentation data give a perfect match. Other peptides in the sample can also be analysed in the same manner, confirming the identity of the protein.

A further development of 2-D PAGE has been the introduction of difference gel electrophoresis (DIGE). This again allows the comparison of protein components of similar mixtures, but has the advantage that only one 2-D gel has to be run

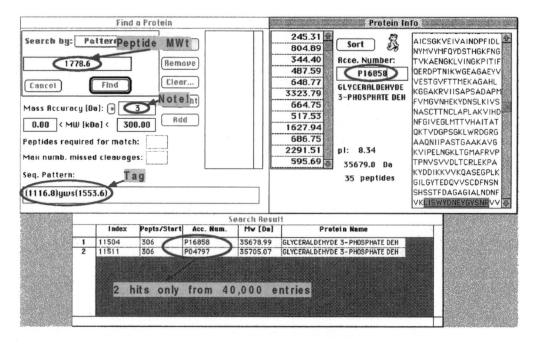

Fig. 8.9. The PeptideSearch™ input form and search result based on data obtained from nano-ESI MS2 of m/s 890 from RBL Spot 2. (Courtesy of Glaxo SmithKline, Stevenage, UK.)

rather than two. In this method the two samples to be compared are each treated with one of two different, yet structurally very similar, fluorescent dyes (cy3 and cy5). Each dye reacts with amino groups, so that each protein is fluorescently labelled by the dye binding to lysine residues and the N-terminal amino groups. The two protein solutions to be compared are then mixed and run on a *single* 2-D gel. Thus every protein in one sample superimposes with its differentially labelled identical counterpart in the other sample. Scanning of the gel at two different wavelengths that excite the two dye molecules reveals whether any individual spot is associated with only one dye molecule rather than two. Most spots will, of course, fluoresce at both wavelengths, but if a spot is associated with only one dye molecule then this tells us that that protein can have been present in only one of the extracts, and the wavelength at which it fluoresces tells you which extract it was originally in.

8.5.2 Isotope-coded affinity tags (ICAT)

Isotope-coded affinity tags (ICAT) uses mass spectrometry (rather than 2-D gels) to identify differences in the protein content of two complex mixtures. For example, the method can be used to identify protein differences between tumour and normal tissue, in the same way that 2-D PAGE can be used to address the same question (Section 8.5.1). This method uses two protein 'tags' that, whilst being in every other respect identical, differ slightly in molecular mass; hence one is 'heavy' and one is 'light'. Both contain (a) a chemical group that reacts with the amino acid cysteine, and (b) a biotin group. In both molecules these groups are joined by a linker region, but in one case the linker contains eight hydrogen atoms, in the other, eight deuterium atoms; one molecule (tag) is thus heavier than the other by 8 Da (see Fig. 9.26). One cell extract (e.g. from cancer cells) is thus treated with one tag (which binds to cysteine residues in all the proteins in the extract) and the second tag is used to treat the second extract (e.g. from normal cells). Both extracts are then treated with trypsin to produce mixtures of peptides, those peptides that contain cysteine having been 'tagged'. The two extracts are then combined and an avidin column used to affinity-purify the labelled peptides by binding to the biotin moiety. When released from the column this mixture of labelled peptides will contain pairs of identical peptides (derived from identical proteins) from the two cell extracts, each pair differing by a mass of 8 Da.

Analysis of this peptide mixture by liquid chromatography–MS will then reveal a series of peptide mass signals, each one existing as a 'pair' of signals separated by eight mass units. These data will reveal the relative abundance of each peptide in the pair. Since most proteins present in the two samples originally being compared will be present at much the same levels, most peptide pairs will have equal signal strengths. However, for proteins that exist in greater or lesser amounts in one of the extracts, different signal strengths will be observed for each of the peptides in the pair, reflecting the relative abundance of this protein in the two samples. Further analysis of either of these pairs via tandem mass spectrometry will provide some sequence data that should allow the protein to be identified. ICAT is discussed in more details in Section 9.6.2.

8.5.3 Determining the function of a protein

Successfully applied, the methods described in the preceding section will have provided the amino acid sequence (or partial sequence) of a protein of interest. The next step is to identify the function and role of this protein. The first step is invariably to search the databases of existing protein sequences to find a protein or proteins that have sequence homology with the protein of interest (the homology method). This is done using programs such as BLAST and PSI-BLAST. If sequence homology is found with a protein of known function, either from the same or different species, then this invariably identifies the function of the protein. However, this approach does not always work. For example, when the genome of the yeast *Saccharomyces cerevisiae* was completely sequenced in 1996, 6000 genes were identified. Of these, approximately 2000 coded for proteins that were already known to exist in yeast (i.e. had been purified and studied in previous years), 2000 had homology with known sequences and hence their function could be deduced by the homology method but 2000 could not be matched to any known genes, i.e. they were 'new', previously undiscovered genes. In these cases, there are a number of other computational methods that can be used to help to identify the protein's function. These include:

	A	B	C	D	E
P1	1	1	1	0	0
P2	0	0	1	1	1
P3	1	0	1	1	0
P4	0	1	1	0	1
P5	1	1	0	0	1
P6	0	1	1	0	1
P7	1	0	0	1	0
P8	1	0	1	1	0

Fig. 8.10. Phylogenic profile method. Five genomes, A–E, are shown (e.g. *E. coli*, *S. cerevisiae*, etc.). The presence (1) or absence (0) of eight proteins (P1–P8) in each of these genomes is shown. It can be seen that proteins P3 and P8 have the same phylogenic profile and therefore may have a functional linkage. P4 and P6 are similarly linked.

- *Phylogenic profile method:* This method aims to identify any other protein(s) that has the same phylogenic profile (i.e. the same pattern of presence or absence) as the unknown protein, in all known genomes. If such proteins are found it is inferred that the unknown protein is involved in the same cellular process as these other protein(s) (i.e. they are said to have a functional link) and will give a strong clue as to the function of the unknown protein. This method is based on the premise that two proteins would not always both be inherited into a new species (or neither inherited) unless the two proteins have a functional link. At the time of writing there are over 100 published genome sequences that can be surveyed with this method. Fig. 8.10 shows a simple, hypothetical example, where just five genomes are analysed.
- *Method of correlated gene neighbours:* If two genes are found to be neighbours in several different genomes, a functional linkage may be inferred between the two proteins. The central assumption of this approach is based on the observation that functionally related genes in prokaryotes tend to be linked to form operons (e.g. the *lac* operon). Although operons are rare in eukaryotic species, it does appear that proteins involved in the same biological process/pathway within the cell have their genes situated in close proximity (e.g. within 500 bp) in the genome. Thus, if two genes are found to be in close

proximity across a number of genomes, it can be inferred that the protein products of these genes have a functional linkage. This method is most robust for microbial genomics but works to some extent in human cells where operon-like clusters are also observed. As an example, this method correctly identified a functional link between eight enzymes in the biosynthetic pathway for the amino acid arginine in *Mycobacterium tuberculosis*.

- *Analysis of fusion:* This method is based on the observation that two genes may exist separately in one organism, whereas the genes are fused into a single multifunctional gene in another organism. The existence of the protein product of the fused gene, in which the two functions of the protein clearly interact (being part of the same protein molecule), suggests that in the first organism the two separate proteins also interact. It has been suggested that gene fusion events occur to reduce the regulational load of multiple interacting gene products.

- *Protein–protein interactions:* A further clue to identifying protein function can come from identifying protein–protein interactions, and methods to identify these are described in the next section.

8.5.4 Protein–protein interactions

Given the complex network of pathways that exist in the cell (signalling pathways, biosynthetic pathways, etc.), it is clear that all proteins must interact with other molecules to fulfil their role. Indeed, it is now apparent that proteins do not exist in isolation in the cell; proteins involved in a common pathway appear to exist in a loose interaction, sometimes referred to as a biomodule. Therefore, if one can identify an interaction between our unknown protein and a well-characterised protein, it can be inferred that the former has a function somehow related to the latter. For example, if the unknown protein is shown to interact with one or more proteins involved in the biosynthetic pathways for arginine, then this strongly suggests that the unknown protein is also involved in this pathway. Using this approach networks of interacting proteins are being identified in individual organisms. This has led to the development of the Database of Interacting Proteins (DIP), which can be found at <http://dip.doe-mbi.ucla.edu>. Given the current fad for inventing new words ending in 'ome', some refer to these maps of protein interactions as the interactome.

One of the most widely used, and successful, methods for investigating protein–protein interaction is the yeast two-hybrid (Y2H) system, which exploits the modular architecture of transcription factors. A transcription factor gene (GAL4) is split into the coding regions for two domains, a DNA-binding domain and a *trans*-activation domain. Both these domains are expressed, each linked to a different protein (one being the unknown protein, the other a protein with which it may interact), in separate yeast cells, which are then mated to produce diploid cells (the two proteins being studied are often referred to as the bait and prey). If, in this diploid cell, the bait and prey proteins bind to each other, they will bring together the two domains of the transcription factor, which will then be active and will bind to the promoter of a reporter gene (e.g. the *his* gene), inducing its expression. Identification of cells expressing the reporter gene product is evidence that the bait and prey proteins interact. In practice, following mating, diploids are selected on deficient medium (in this case, medium deficient in histidine), thus only yeast cells expressing interacting proteins survive (as they are capable of synthesising histidine). Once such a positive interaction is identified, the two interacting open reading frames (ORFs) are simply identified by sequencing a small part of the protein gene.

Using this approach, all 6000 ORFs from *S. cerevisiae* were individually cloned as both bait and prey. When the pool of 6000 prey clones was screened against each of the 6000 bait clones, 691 interactions were identified, only 88 of which were previously known. This therefore gave an indication of the function of over 600 proteins whose function was previously unknown. On a much larger scale, the same approach was used to identify protein–protein interactions in the fruit fly, *Drosophila melanogaster*. All 14 000 predicted *D. melanogaster* ORFs were amplified using the polymerase chain reaction (PCR) and each cloned into two-hybrid bait and prey vectors. A total of 45 417 two-hybrid positive colonies were obtained, from which 10 021 protein interactions involving 4500 proteins were obtained. The yeast 2-hybrid system is described in greater detail in Section 6.8.3.

8.5.5 Protein arrays

A newly developing area for studying protein–protein interactions is the use of protein arrays (chips). Although the basic principle for screening and identifying interacting molecules is much the same as for DNA arrays (Section 6.8.8), the production of protein arrays is more technically demanding owing mainly to the difficulty of binding proteins to a surface and ensuring that the protein is not denatured at any stage of the assay procedure.

In a protein array, proteins are immobilised as small spots (150–200 μm) onto a solid support (typically glass or a nitrocellulose membrane), using high precision contact printing (not unlike a dot-matrix printer) at a spot density of the order of 1500 spots cm^{-2}. A solution of the protein of unknown function is then incubated on the array surface for a period of time, then washed off, and the position(s) where the protein has bound, identified (see below). Since it is known which protein was immoblised in each position of the chip, each pair of interacting proteins can be identified.

Saccharomyces cerevisiae again provides a good example of the successful use of this technology where a protein array was used to identify yeast proteins that bind to the protein calmodulin (an important protein involved in calcium regulation). Five thousand eight hundred yeast ORFs were cloned into a yeast high copy expression vector, and each of the expressed proteins purified. Each protein was then spotted at high density onto nickel-coated glass microscope slides. Since each protein also contained a $(His)_6$-Tag (which binds to nickel; see Section 11.8.5) introduced at the C terminus, proteins were attached to the surface in an orientated manner, the C terminus being linked to the nickel-coated glass through the

(His)$_6$ sequence, while the rest of the molecule was therefore suitably orientated away from the surface of the array to be available for interaction with another protein. The array was then incubated in a solution of calmodulin that had been labelled with biotin. The calmodulin was then washed off and the positions where calmodulin had bound to the array were identified by incubating the array with a solution of fluorescently labelled avidin (the protein avidin binds strongly to the small molecular mass vitamin biotin: see Section 7.5.5). The use of ultraviolet light thus identified fluorescence where the screening molecules had bound. In total, 33 new proteins that bind calmodulin were discovered in this way.

Fig. 8.11 (see colour section) shows an interaction map of the yeast proteome. The authors constructed the map from published data on protein–protein interactions in yeast. The map contains 1584 proteins and 2358 interactions. Proteins are coloured according to their functional role, e.g. proteins involved in membrane fusion (blue), lipid metabolism (yellow), cell structure (green), etc. If one views the electronic version of this publication it is possible for the reader to zoom in and search for protein names and to read interactions more clearly.

Fig. 8.12 (see colour section) is a summary of Fig. 8.11 showing the number of interactions of proteins from each functional group with proteins of their own and other groups. The word function means the cellular role of the protein. Numbers in parentheses indicate, first, the number of interactions within a group and, secondly, the number of proteins within a group. Numbers on connecting lines indicate the numbers of interactions between proteins of the two connected groups. For example, in the upper left-hand corner, there are 77 interactions between the 21 proteins involved in membrane fusion and 141 proteins involved in vesicular transport. Looking at the bottom right of the diagram it can be seen that some proteins involved in RNA processing/modification not surprisingly also interact with proteins involved in RNA turnover, RNA splicing, RNA transcription and protein synthesis.

8.5.6 Systems biology

It can be seen from the section on proteomics that the study of proteins is moving away from methods that involve the purification and study of individual proteins. Nowadays proteins are more likely to be studied as a stained spot on a complex 2-D gel pattern, often present in as little as nanogram amounts, more often than not using analytical techniques such as mass spectrometry (see Chapter 9) and invariably requiring the interrogation of protein and genome sequence data on the Web (bioinformatics, Section 5.8). It is then necessary to determine which other proteins interact with the protein being studied. Proteomics is thus moving us away from studying proteins in isolation and encouraging us to consider the proteins in the cell as part of a dynamic interacting system. This has led to the development of the concept of systems biology, which can be defined as the study of living organisms in terms of their underlying network structure rather than just their individual molecular components. Since systems biology requires a study of all interacting components in the cell the new high throughput and quantitative techniques of proteomics are central to systems biology. Needless to say, the analysis of complex biological systems will generate massive volumes of data, which can be handled only by the computational methods that make up the subject of bioinformatics (see Section 5.8). The study of the cell is thus no longer the remit of the biologist alone. Systems biology has introduced cross-disciplinary studies involving biologists, computer scientists, chemists, engineers and mathematicians who can understand the language of each other's disciplines and who can integrate their work with the data acquisition, storage and analysis tools of bioinformatics.

8.6 SUGGESTIONS FOR FURTHER READING

CUTLER, P. (2004). *Protein Purification Protocols*. Humana Press, Totowa, NJ. (Detailed theory and practical procedures for a range of protein purification techniques.)

LIEBLER, D. C. (2002). *Introduction to Proteomics*. Humana Press, Totowa, NJ. (A good introduction to all aspects of proteomics, in particular the analysis of two-dimensional gels by mass spectrometry.)

SCOPES, R. K. (1996). *Protein Purification*, 3rd edn. Springer-Verlag, Berlin. (Principles and methods for a range of protein purification techniques.)

WALKER, J. M. (2005). *Proteomics Protocols*. Humana Press, Totowa, NJ, in press. (Theory and techniques of a spectrum of methods applied to proteomics.)

Chapter 9

Mass spectrometric techniques

9.1 INTRODUCTION

9.1.1 General

Mass spectrometry (MS) is an extremely valuable analytical technique in which the molecules in a test sample are converted to gaseous ions that are subsequently separated in a mass spectrometer according to their mass-to-charge ratio (m/z) and detected. The mass spectrum is a plot of the (relative) abundance of the ions at each m/z ratio. Note that it is the mass to charge ratios of ions (m/z) and not the actual mass that is measured. If, for example, a biomolecule is ionised by the addition of one or more protons (H^+) the instrument measures the m/z after addition of 1 Da for each proton if, the instrument is measuring positive ions or m/z minus 1 Da for each proton lost if it is measuring negative ions. The mass spectrum allows an accurate measure to be made of the relative molecular mass M_r (see Section 1.2.2 for details of this parameter) of each ionised molecule and in many cases details of its structure. The development of two ionisation techniques, electrospray ionisation (ESI) and matrix-assisted laser desorption/ionisation (MALDI) has enabled the accurate mass determination of high molecular mass compounds as well as low molecular mass molecules and has revolutionised the applicability of mass spectrometry to almost any biological molecule. Applications include the new science of proteomics (Section 8.5) as well as in drug discovery. The latter includes combinatorial chemistry, where a large number of similar molecules (combinatorial libraries) are produced and analysed to find the most effective compounds from a group of related organic chemicals. This chapter will cover the general principles of the technique and will concentrate on the applications of MS to protein structure.

The essential features of all mass spectrometers are therefore:

- production of ions in the gas phase;
- acceleration of the ions to a specific velocity in an electric field;
- separation of the ions in a mass analyser;
- detection of each species of a particular m/z ratio.

The instruments are calibrated with standard compounds of accurately known M_r values. In MS the carbon scale is used with mass of $^{12}C = 12.000000$. This level of

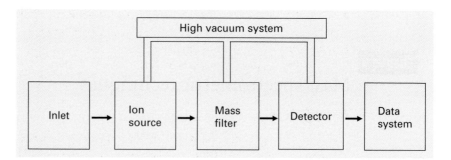

Fig. 9.1. Basic components of mass spectrometers.

accuracy is achievable in high resolution magnetic sector double-focusing and Fourier transform mass spectrometers (Section 9.7).

The mass analyser may separate ions by the use of either a magnetic or an electrical field. Alternatively the time taken for ions of different masses to travel a given distance in space is measured accurately in the time-of-flight (TOF) mass spectrometer (Section 9.3.7). Any material that can be ionised and whose ions can exist in the gas phase can be investigated by MS; remembering that very low pressures, i.e. high vacuum, in the region of 10^{-6} torr are required (1 torr is a measure of pressure that equals 1 mm of mercury (133.3 Pa)). The majority of biological MS investigations on proteins, oligosaccharides and nucleic acids is carried out with quadrupole, quadrupole–ion trap and TOF mass spectrometers. In the organic chemistry/biochemistry area of analysis of lower relative molecular mass compounds, the well-established magnetic sector mass spectrometers still find wide application and their main principles will also be described briefly.

The treatment of MS in this chapter will be strictly non-mathematical and non-technical. However, the intention is to give an overview of the types of instrumentation that are employed, the main uses of each, complementary techniques and the advantages/disadvantages of the different instruments and particular applications most suited to each type. Data analysis and sample preparation to obtain the best sensitivity for a particular type of compound will also be covered.

9.1.2 Components of a mass spectrometer

All mass spectrometers are basically similar (Fig. 9.1). They consist of the following:

- *A high vacuum system (10^{-6} torr or 1 μtorr):* These include turbomolecular pumps, diffusion pumps and rotary vane pumps.
- *A sample inlet:* This comprises a sample or a target plate; a high performance liquid chromatography (HPLC), gas chromatography (GC) or capillary electrophoresis system; solids probe; electron impact or direct chemical ionisation chamber.
- *An ion source (to convert molecules into gas-phase ions):* This can be MALDI, ESI, fast atom bombardment (FAB), electron impact or direct chemical ionisation.

- *A mass filter/analyser:* This can be: TOF; quadrupole–ion trap; magnetic sector or ion cyclotron Fourier transform (the last is also actually also a detector).
- *A detector:* This can be a conversion dynode; electron multiplier; microchannel plate or array detector.

9.1.3 Vacuum system

All mass analysers operate under vacuum in order to minimise collisions between ions and air molecules. Without a high vacuum, the ions produced in the source will not reach the detector. At atmospheric pressure, the mean free path of a typical ion is around 52 nm; at 1 mtorr, it is 40 mm; and at 1 μtorr, it is 40 m. In most instruments, two vacuum pump types are used, for example a rotary vane pump (to produce the main reduction in pressure) followed by a turbomolecular pump or diffusion pump to produce the high vacuum. The rotary vane pump can be an oil pump to provide initial vacuum (approximately 1 torr), while the turbomolecular pump provides a working high vacuum (1 mtorr to 1 ntorr). This is a high speed gas turbine with interspersed rotors (moving blades) and stators (i.e. fixed or stationary blades) whose rotation forces molecules through the blade system.

9.2 IONISATION

Ions may be produced from a neutral molecule by removing an electron to produce a positively charged cation, or by adding an electron to form an anion. Both positive- and negative-ion MS may be carried out but the methods of analysis in the following sections will be described mainly for positive-ion MS, since this is more common and the principles of separation and detection are essentially the same for both types of ion.

9.2.1 Electron impact ionisation

Electron impact ionisation (EI) is widely used for the analysis of metabolites, pollutants and pharmaceutical compounds, for example in drug testing programmes. EI has major applications as a mass detector for gas chromatography (GC/MS, Section 11.9.3). A stream of electrons from a heated metal filament is accelerated to 70 eV potential. (The electron volt, eV, is a measure of energy.) Sample ionisation occurs when the electrons stream across a high vacuum chamber into which molecules of the substance to be analysed (analyte) are allowed to diffuse (Fig. 9.2). Interaction with the analyte results in either loss of an electron from the substance (to produce a cation) or electron capture (to produce an anion). The analyte must be in the vapour state in the electron impact source, which limits the applicability to biological materials below approximately 400 Da. Before the advent of ESI and MALDI, the method did have some applicability to peptides, for example, whose volatility could be increased by chemical modification. A large amount of fragmentation of the analyte is common, which may or may not be desirable depending on the information required.

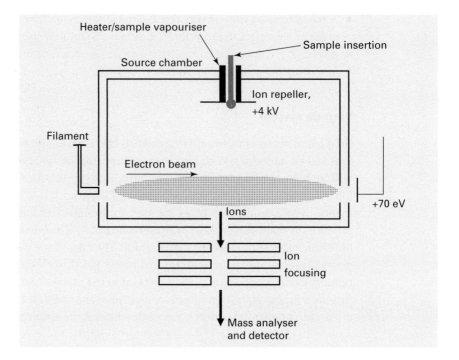

Fig. 9.2. Electron impact source. Electrons are produced by thermionic emission from a filament of tungsten or rhenium. The filament current is typically 0.1 mA. Electrons are accelerated towards the ion source chamber (held at a positive potential equal to the accelerating voltage) and acquire an energy equal to the voltage between the filament and the source chamber, typically 70 eV. The electron trap is held at a fixed positive potential with respect to the source chamber. Gaseous analyte molecules are introduced into the path of the electron beam where they are ionised. Owing to the positive ion repeller voltage and the negative excitation voltage that produce an electric field in the source chamber, the ions leave the source through the ion exit slit and are analysed.

Chemical bonds in organic molecules are formed by the pairing of electrons. Ionisation resulting in a cation requires the loss of an electron from one of these bonds (effectively knocked out by the bombarding electrons), but it leaves a bond with a single unpaired electron. This is a radical as well as being a cation and hence the representation as $M^{+\cdot}$, the (+) sign indicating the ionic state and the (·) a radical. Conversely, electron capture results both in an anion and also the addition of an unpaired electron and therefore a negatively charged radical, hence the symbol $M^{-\cdot}$. Such radical ions are termed molecular ions, parent ions or precursor ions and under the conditions of electron bombardment are relatively unstable. Their energy is in excess of that required for ionisation and has to be dissipated. This latter process results in the precursor ion disintegrating into a number of smaller fragment ions that may be relatively unstable and further fragmentation may occur. This gives rise to a series of daughter ions or product ions, which are recorded as the mass spectrum.

For the production of a radical cation, as it is not known where either the positive charge or the unpaired electron actually reside in the molecule, it is usual practice to place the dot signs outside the abbreviated bracket sign, '⁊'. When the precursor ion fragments, one of the products carries the charge and the other the unpaired electron, i.e. it splits into a radical and an ion. The product ions are therefore true ions and not radical ions. The radicals produced in the fragmentation process are neutral species and therefore do not take any further part in the MS but are pumped away by the vacuum system. Only the charged species are accelerated out of the source and into the mass analyser. It is also important to recognise that almost all possible bond breakages can occur and any given fragment will arise as both an ion and a radical. The distribution of charge and unpaired electron, however, is by no means equal. The distribution depends entirely on the thermodynamic stability of the products of fragmentation. Furthermore, any fragment ion may break down further (until single atoms are obtained) and hence not many ions of a particular type may survive, resulting in a low signal being recorded. A simple example is given by n-butane ($CH_3CH_2CH_2CH_3$) and some of the major fragmentations are shown Fig. 9.3a. The resultant EI spectrum is shown in Fig. 9.3b.

9.2.2 Chemical ionisation

Chemical ionisation (CI) is used for a range of samples similar to those for EI. It is particularly useful for the determination of molecular masses, as high intensity molecular ions are produced owing to less fragmentation. CI therefore gives rise to much cleaner spectra. The source is essentially the same as the EI source but it contains a suitable reagent gas such as methane (CH_4) or ammonia (NH_3) that is initially ionised by EI. The high gas pressure in the source results in ion–molecule reactions between reagent gas ions (such as NH_4^+ and CH_4^+) some of which react with the analyte to produce analyte ions. The mass differences from the neutral parent compounds therefore correspond to these adducts.

9.2.3 Fast atom bombardment

At the time of its development in the early 1980s, FAB revolutionised MS for the biologist. The important advance was that this soft ionisation technique, which led to the formation of ions with low internal energies and little consequent fragmentation, permitted analysis of biomolecules in solution without prior derivatisation. The sample is mixed with a relatively involatile, viscous matrix such as glycerol, thioglycerol or m-nitrobenzyl alcohol. The mixture, placed on a probe, is introduced into the source housing and bombarded with an ionising beam of neutral atoms (such as Ar, He, Xe) of high velocity. A later development was the use of a beam of caesium ions (Cs^+) and the term liquid secondary ion mass spectrometry (LSIMS) was introduced to distinguish this from FAB–MS. Pseudomolecular ion species arise as either protonated or deprotonated entities $(M + H)^+$ and $(M - H)^-$ respectively, which allows positive- and negative-ion mass spectra to be determined. The term pseudomolecular implies the mass of the ion formed from a substance of a given mass by the gain or loss of one or more protons. Other charged adducts can also be formed such as $(M + Na)^+$ and $(M + K)^+$.

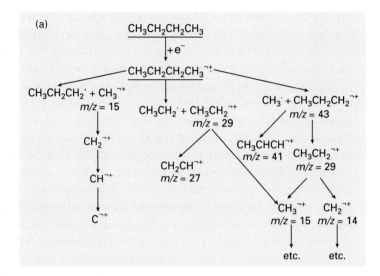

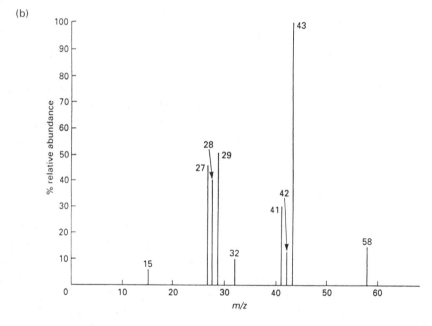

Fig. 9.3. Fragmentation pathways in *n*-butane and the electron impact ionisation spectrum. The pathway for fragmentation of *n*-butane is shown in (a) and the EI spectrum in (b). In the spectrum, the relative abundance is plotted from 0 to 100%, where the largest peak is set at 100% (base peak). Spectra represented in this way are said to be normalised.

9.2.4 Electrospray ionisation

This involves the production of ions by spraying a solution of the analyte into an electrical field. This is a soft ionisation technique and enables the analysis of large, intact (underivatised) biomolecules, such as proteins and DNA. The electrospray (ES) creates very small droplets of solvent-containing analyte. The essential principle in ES is that a spray of charged liquid droplets is produced by atomisation or nebulisation. Solvent (typically 50:50 water and organic solvent) is removed as the droplets enter the mass spectrometer. ESI is the result of the strong electric field (approximately 4 keV at the end of the capillary and 1 keV at the counter electrode) acting on the surface of the sample solution. As the solvent evaporates in the high vacuum region, the droplet size decreases and eventually charged analyte (free from solvent) remains. Ionisation can occur at atmospheric pressure and this method is also sometimes referred to as atmospheric pressure ionisation (API). The concentration of sample is usually around 1–10 pmol mm^{-3}. Typical solvents are 50:50 acetonitrile (or methanol):H_2O with 1% acetic acid or 0.1% formic acid. Ammonium hydroxide or trifluoroacetic acid (TFA, 0.02%) in 50:50 acetonitrile or methanol: H_2O can also be used. The organic acid (or the NH_4OH) aids ionisation of the analyte. At low pH, basic groups will be ionised. In the example of peptides these are the side groups of lysine, histidine and arginine and the N-terminal amino group. At alkaline pH the carboxylic acid side-chains as well as stronger anions such as phosphate and sulphate groups will be ionised. The presence of organic solvent assists in the formation of small droplets and facilitates evaporation. The flow rate into the source is normally around a few mm^3 min^{-1}, although higher flow rates can be tolerated (up to 1 cm^3 min^{-1}) if the solution is an eluant from on-line HPLC for example.

Smaller molecules usually produce singly charged ions but multiply charged ions are frequently formed from larger biomolecules, in contrast to MALDI, resulting in m/z ratios that are sufficiently small to be observed in the quadruple analyser. Thus masses of large intact proteins, DNA and organic polymers can also be accurately measured in electrospray MS although the m/z limit of measurement is normally 2000 or 3000 Da. For example, proteins are normally analysed in the positive ion mode, where charges are introduced by addition of protons. The number of basic amino acids in the protein (mainly lysine and arginine) determines the maximum number of charges carried by the molecule. The distribution of basic residues in most proteins is such that the multiple peaks (one for each $M + nH)^{n+}$ ion, are centred on an m/z of about 1000. In Fig. 9.6, a large protein with a mass of over 100 000 Da behaves as if it were multiple mass species around 1020 Da. For the species with 100 protons (H$^+$), i.e. with 100 charges, $z = 100$, $m/z = 1027.6$ therefore $(M + 100H)^{100+} = 1027.6$. When the computer processes the data for the multiple peaks, the average for each set of peaks gives a mass determination to a high accuracy. The peaks can be deconvoluted and presented as a single peak representing the M_r (in this example $M_r = 102\,658$). A diagrammatic representation of the ESI source is shown in Fig 9.4. A curtain or sheath gas (usually nitrogen) around the spray needle at a slow flow rate may be used to assist evaporation of the solvent at or below room temperature. This may be an advantage for thermally labile compounds.

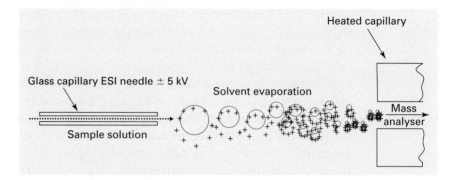

Fig. 9.4. Electrospray ionisation source. The ESI creates very small droplets of solvent-containing analyte by atomisation or nebulisation as the sample is introduced into the source through the fine glass (or other material) hollow needle capillary. The solvent evaporates in the high vacuum region as the spray of droplets enters the source. As the result of the strong electric field acting on the surface of the sample droplets, and electrostatic repulsion, their size decreases and eventually single species of charged analyte (free from solvent) remain. These may have multiple charges depending on the availability of ionisable groups.

Example 1 PROTEIN MASS DETERMINATION BY ESI

Question

A protein was isolated from human tissue and subjected to a variety of investigations. Relative molecular mass determinations gave values of approximately 12 000 by size exclusion chromatography and 13 000 by gel electrophoresis. After purification, a sample was subjected to electrospray ionisation mass spectrometry and the following data obtained.

m/z	773.9	825.5	884.3	952.3	1031.3
Abundance (%)	59	88	100	66	37

Given that $n_2 = (m_1 - 1)/(m_2 - m_1)$ and $M = n_2(m_2 - 1)$ and assuming that the only ions in the mixture arise by protonation, deduce an average molecular mass for the protein by this method.

Answer

M_r by exclusion chromatography = 12 000

M_r by gel electrophoresis = 13 000

Taking ESI peaks in pairs:

$m_1 - 1$	$m_2 - m_1$	n_2	$m_2 - 1$	M (Da)	z
951.3	79.0	12.041	1030.3	12 406.6	12
883.3	68.0	12.989	951.3	12 357.1	13
824.5	58.8	14.022	883.3	12 385.7	14
772.9	51.6	14.978	824.5	12 349.9	15

$\Sigma M = 49\,499.3$ Da

Mean $M = 12\,374.8$ Da

Note: Relative abundance values are not required for the determination of the mass.

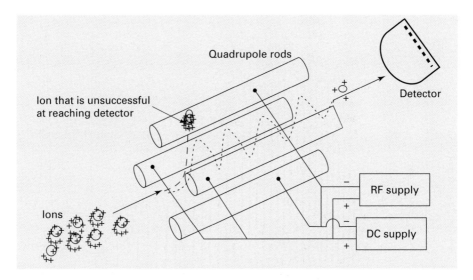

Fig. 9.5. Quadrupole analyser. The fixed (DC) and oscillating (RF) fields cause the ions to undergo complicated trajectories through the quadrupole filter. For a given set of fields, only certain trajectories are stable, which allows only ions of specific m/z to travel through to the detector. The efficiency of the quadrupole is impaired after a build up of ions that do not reach the detector. Therefore a set of pre-filters is added to the quadrupole to remove the ions that would otherwise affect the main quadrupole.

9.3 MASS ANALYSERS

9.3.1 Introduction

Once ions are created and leave the ion source, they pass into a mass analyser, the function of which is to separate the ions and to measure their masses. (Remember, what is really measured is the mass-to-charge ratio (m/z) for each ion.) At any given moment, ions of a particular mass are allowed to pass through the analyser, where they are counted by the detector. Subsequently, ions of a different mass are allowed to pass through the analyser and again the detector counts the number of ions. In this way, the analyser scans through a large range of masses. In the majority of instruments, a particular type of ionisation is coupled to a particular mass analyser that operates by a particular principle. That is, EI, CI and FAB are combined with magnetic sector instruments, ESI and its derivatives with quadrupole (or its variant ion trap) and MALDI is coupled to TOF detection.

9.3.2 Quadrupole mass spectrometry

The quadrupole analyser consists of four parallel cylindrical rods (Fig. 9.5). A direct current (DC) voltage and a superimposed radio frequency (RF) voltage are applied to each rod, creating a continuously varying electric field along the length of the analyser. Once in this field, ions are accelerated down the analyser towards the detector. The varying electric field is precisely controlled so that, during each stage of a scan, ions of one particular mass-to-charge ratio pass down the length of

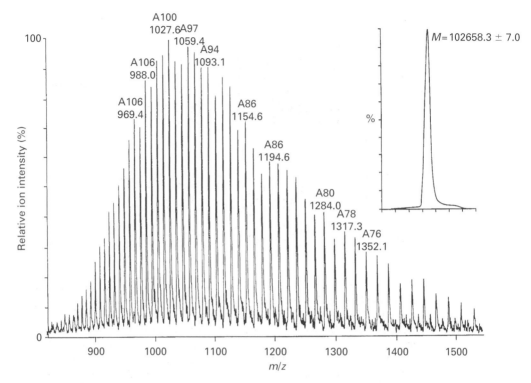

Fig. 9.6. Large intact protein mass accurately measured in electrospray MS. The species of ions are annotated by the charge state, for example with 99, 100, 101 charges, etc., and the associated m/z value. The inset shows the 'deconvoluted spectrum'.

the analyser. Ions with any other mass-to-charge value impact on the quadrupole rods and are not detected. By changing the electric field (scanning), the ions of different m/z successively arrive at the detector. Quadrupoles can routinely analyse up to m/z 3000, which is extremely useful for biological MS, since, as we have seen, proteins and other biomolecules normally give a charge distribution of m/z that is centred at a value below this (Fig. 9.6). Note that hexapole and octapole devices are also used to direct a beam into the next section of a triple quadrupole or into an ion trap, for example, but the principle is the same.

9.3.3 Ion trap mass spectrometry

Ion trap mass spectrometers use ESI to produce ions, all of which are transferred into, and subsequently measured almost simultaneously (within milliseconds), in a device called an ion trap (Fig. 9.7). The trap must then be refilled with the ions that are arriving from the source. Therefore, although the trap does not measure 100% of all ions produced (it depends on the cycle time to refill the trap then analyse the ions), this results nevertheless in a great improvement in sensitivity relative to quadrupole mass spectrometers, where at any given moment only ions of one particular m/z are detected. ESI–ion trap mass spectrometers have found

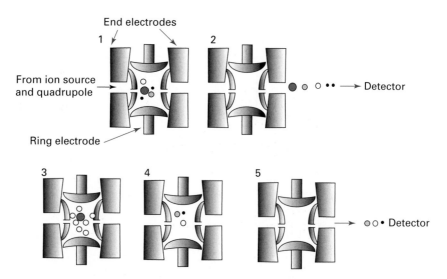

Fig. 9.7. Diagram of an ion trap.   The ion trap contains three hyperbolic electrodes which form a cavity in a cylindrical device of around 5 cm diameter, in which the ions are trapped (stored) and subsequently analysed. Each end-cap electrode has a small hole in the centre. Ions produced from the source enter the trap through the quadrupole and the entrance end-cap electrode. Potentials are applied to the electrodes to trap the ions (diagrams 1 and 2). The ring electrode has an alternating potential of constant radio frequency but variable amplitude. This results in a three-dimensional electrical field within the cavity. The ions are trapped in stable oscillating trajectories that depend on the potentials and the m/z of the ions. To detect these ions, the potentials are varied, resulting in the ion trajectories becoming unstable and the ions are ejected in the axial direction out of the trap in order of increasing m/z into the detector. A very low pressure of helium is maintained in the trap, which 'cools' the ions into the centre of the trap by low speed collisions that normally do not result in fragmentation. These collisions merely slow the ions down so that, during scanning, the ions leave quickly in a compact packet, producing narrower peaks with better resolution. In sequencing, all the ions are ejected except those of a particular m/z ratio that has been selected for fragmentation (see diagrams 3, 4 and 5). The steps are: (3) selection of precursor ion, (4) collision induced dissociation of this ion, and (5) ejection and detection of the fragment ions.

wide application for the analysis of peptides and small biomolecules such as in protein identification by tandem MS, liquid chromatography/mass spectrometry (LC/MS), combinatorial libraries and rapid analysis in drug discovery and drug development. Ion trap MS permits structural information to be readily obtained (and sequence information in the case of polypeptides). Not only can tandem MS analysis be carried out but also, owing to the high efficiency of each stage, further fragmentation of selected ions may be carried out to MS to the power n (MS^n) (Fig. 9.8). The instrument still allows accurate molecular mass determination to over 100 000 Da at greater than 0.01% mass accuracy.

The MS^n procedure in an ion trap involves ejecting all ions that are stored in the trap, except those corresponding to the selected m/z value. To perform tandem MS (MS^2) a collision gas is introduced (a low pressure of helium) and collision-induced dissociation (CID) occurs (Fig. 9.7). The fragment ions are then ejected in

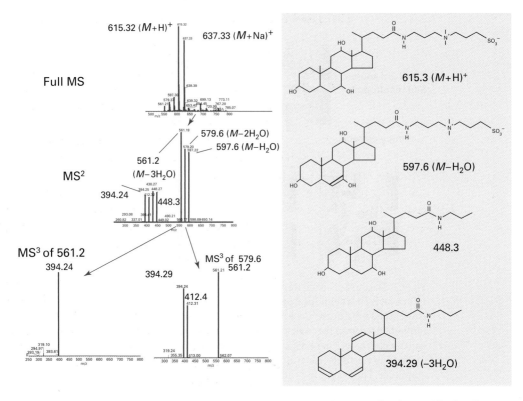

Fig. 9.8. Structural analysis, MS^n in an ion trap. In this example, of a steroid-related compound, the structure can be analysed when the $(M+H)^+$ at 615.3 are selected to be retained in the ion trap. These ions are subjected to collision-induced dissociation (CID) resulting in loss of the aliphatic sulphonate from the quaternary ammonium group and partial loss of some hydroxyl groups in the tandem MS experiment. The major fragment ions (561.2 and 579.6) are further selected for CID (MS^3), resulting in subsequent losses of more hydroxyl groups from specific parts of the steroid ring.

turn and the fragment spectrum determined. The process can be repeated successively where all the fragment ions stored in the trap except those fragment ions corresponding to another selected m/z value are ejected. This fragment ion can then be further fragmented to obtain more structural information, as illustrated for the example shown in Fig. 9.8. This technique has a big advantage, since no additional mass spectrometers or collision cells are required. The limitation is sensitivity, which decreases with each MS experiment, although the claimed record in an ion trap is currently MS^{14}.

9.3.4 Nanospray and on-line tandem mass spectrometry

The sensitivity with ESI can be greatly improved with a reduction in flow rate. Nanospray is therefore the technique of choice for ultimate sensitivity when sample amounts are limited. There are two ways of achieving this. Both static and dynamic nanospray techniques are widely used. Flow rates in both nanospray techniques are in the order of tens of nm^3 min^{-1}, which leads to low sample consumption and low signal-to-noise ratios.

First, in static nanospray, glass needles are used with a very finely drawn out capillary tip (coated with gold to allow the needle to be held at the correct kilovolt potential; see Fig. 9.4). The needles are filled with 1–2 mm^3 of sample and accurately positioned at the entrance to the source. Closed-circuit television (CCTV) is used to accurately determine the position of the capillary. The solution is drawn into the source by electrostatic pressure, although a low pressure may be applied with an air-filled syringe behind the other (open) end of the needle if necessary. In dynamic nanospray experiments, small diameter microbore HPLC or capillary columns are also used to achieve separation at low flow rates. This can be combined with a stream splitter device, which can further reduce flow rate (Section 11.3.2). The stream splitter can be used to divert a percentage of the solvent flow from the pump, say 99–99.9%, to waste and allow the remainder to pass through the column. This allows for much more accurate flow rates, since it is extremely difficult to directly and accurately pump at 0.5 mm^3 or even 50 nm^3 min^{-1} with a high pressure pump. Therefore one can use a pump that functions more efficiently at flow rates of 50–500 mm^3 min^{-1} to pass 0.5 nm^3 min^{-1} or less into the microcolumn.

Nanospray sources are used in triple quadrupole, ion trap and hybrid MALDI instruments. Computer programs can be set up to perform tandem MS, during the chromatographic separation, on each component as it elutes from the column, if it gives a signal above a threshold that is set by the operator.

9.3.5 Magnetic sector analyser

A magnetic sector analyser is shown diagrammatically in Fig. 9.9. The ions are accelerated by an electric field. The electric sector acts as a kinetic energy filter and allows only ions of a particular kinetic energy to pass, irrespective of the m/z. This greatly increases the resolution, since the ions emerge from the electrostatic analyser (ESA) with the whole range of masses but the same velocity. A given ion with the appropriate velocity then enters the magnetic sector analyser. It will travel in a curved trajectory in the magnetic field with a radius depending on the m/z and the velocity of the ion (the latter has already been selected). Thus only ions of a particular m/z will be detected at a particular magnetic field strength. The trajectory of the ions is through a sector of the circular poles of the magnet, hence the term magnetic sector. Fig. 9.9 shows several possible trajectories for a given ion in the magnetic field. Only one set of ions will be focused on the detector. If the field is changed, these ions will be defocused because they will not be deflected to the correct extent. A new set of ions will be deflected and collected at the detector. By starting at either end of the magnet range, the ions can be scanned from high to low mass or from low to high mass. This magnetic scanning is the most commonly used type of analysis in this instrument. Alternatively, the mass spectrum can be scanned electrically by varying the voltage, V, while holding the magnetic field B constant. This type of instrument is called a two-sector or double-focusing MS and resolving power to parts per million may be obtained.

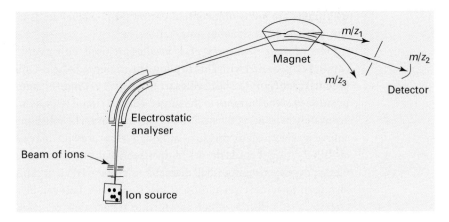

Fig. 9.9. Double-focusing magnetic sector mass spectrometer. The figure shows the 'forward geometry' arrangement where the electrostatic analyser is before the magnetic sector (known as EB; E for electric, B for magnetic). Similar results may be obtained if the reverse geometry (BE) type is used. The radial path followed by each ion is shown by scanning the magnetic field, B, and each ion of a particular m/z value can be brought into the detector slit in turn.

9.3.6 Plasma desorption ionisation

Plasma desorption ionisation mass spectrometry (PDMS) was the first mass spectrometer to be able to analyse proteins and other large biomolecules (although only those of relatively low M_r, less than 35 000). The technique and instruments developed are now obsolete and clearly overtaken by the much more powerful, sensitive and accurate instruments described elsewhere in this chapter. PDMS instruments are, however, still in use in some laboratories and research publications still appear with mass spectra obtained with this instrument. A basic understanding of the principle is therefore worth including. The source of the plasma (atomic nuclei stripped of electrons) is radioactive californium, ^{252}Cf, and two typical emission nuclei are the 100 MeV Ba^{20+} and Tc $^{18+}$, formed by the decay of the Cf, which are ejected in opposite directions, almost collinearly and with equal velocity. This is a pulsed technique, i.e. particles are emitted at discrete time intervals and require a TOF mass detector. The plasma particle emitted in the direction opposite to that passing through the sample triggers a time counter and the desorbed sample ions are accelerated electrically and detected as for other TOF analysers (Section 9.3.7).

9.3.7 MALDI, TOF mass spectrometry, MALDI–TOF

Matrix-assisted laser desorption ionisation (MALDI) produces gas phase protonated ions by excitation of the sample molecules from the energy of a laser transferred via an ultraviolet (UV) light-absorbing matrix. The matrix is a conjugated organic compound (normally a weak organic acid such as a derivative of cinnamic acid and dihydroxybenzoic acid) that is intimately mixed with the sample. Examples of MALDI matrix compounds and their application for particular

Table 9.1 Examples of MALDI matrix compounds

Compound	Structure	Application
α-Cyano-4-hydroxycinnamic acid (CHCA)		Peptides <10 kDa (glycopeptides)
Sinapinic acid (3,5-dimethoxy-4-hydoxycinnamic acid, SA)		Proteins > 10 kDa
'Super DHB', mixture of 10% 5-methoxysalycilic acid (2-hydroxy-5-methoxybenzoic acid) with DHB		Proteins, glycosylated proteins
2,5-Dihydroxybenzoic acid (DHB), (gentistic acid)		Neutral carbohydrates, synthetic polymers, (oligos)
3-Hydroxypicolinic acid		Oligonucleotides
2-(4-hydroxy-phenylazo)-benzoic acid (HABA)		Oligosaccharides, proteins

biomolecules are shown in Table 9.1. These are designed to maximally absorb light at the wavelength of the laser, typically a nitrogen laser of 337 nm or a neodymium/yttrium-aluminium-garnet (Nd-YAG) at 355 nm.

The sample (1–10 pmol mm^{-3}) is mixed with an excess of the matrix and dried onto the target plate, where sample and matrix co-crystallise on drying. Pulses of laser light of a few nanoseconds' duration cause rapid excitation and vaporisation of the crystalline matrix and the subsequent ejection of matrix and analyte ions into the gas phase (Fig. 9.10). This generates a plume of matrix and analyte ions that are analysed in a TOF mass analyser. The particular advantage of MALDI is the

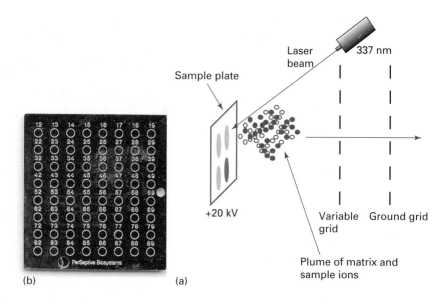

(b)   (a)

Fig. 9.10. MALDI ionisation mechanism and MALDI–TOF sample plate. (a) The sample
(A) is mixed, in solution, with a 'matrix' – the organic acid in excess of the analyte (in a
ratio between 1000:1 to10 000:1) and transferred to the MALDI plate. An ultraviolet laser
is directed to the sample (with a beam diameter of a few micrometres) for desorption.
The laser radiation of a few nanoseconds' duration is absorbed by the matrix molecules,
causing rapid heating of the region around the area of laser impact and electronic
excitation of the matrix. The immediate region of the sample explodes into the high
vacuum of the mass spectrometer, creating gas-phase protonated molecules of both the
acid and the analyte.

The laser flash ionises matrix molecules (neutral fragments (M) and matrix ions (MH)$^+$,
($M{-}H$)$^-$ and sample neutral fragments (A). Sample molecules are ionised by gas-phase
proton transfer from the matrix:

$$MH^+ + A \rightarrow M + AH^+$$

$$(M{-}H)^- + A \rightarrow (A{-}H)^- + M$$

The matrix serves as an absorbing medium for the ultraviolet light converting the
incident laser energy into molecular electronic energy, both for desorption and ionisation
and as a source of H$^+$ to transfer to, and ionise, the analyte molecule. (b) 100-spot MALDI
sample plate.

ability to produce large mass ions, with high sensitivity. MALDI is a very soft ionisation technique that does not produce abundant amounts of fragmentation like
some other ionisation methods. Since the molecular ions are produced with little
fragmentation, it is a valuable technique for examining mixtures (see Fig. 9.14 and
compare this to the more complex spectrum in Fig. 9.6).

TOF is the best type of mass analyser to couple to MALDI, as this technique has a
virtually unlimited mass range. Proteins and other macromolecules of M_r greater
than 400 000 have been accurately measured. The principle of TOF is illustrated
in Fig. 9.11 and the main components of the instrument are shown in Fig. 9.12.

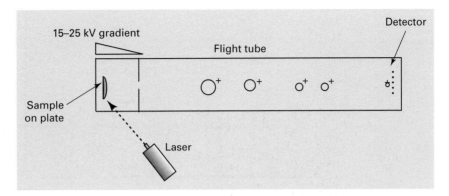

Fig. 9.11. Principle of time-of-flight (TOF). The ions enter the flight tube, where the lighter ions travel faster than the heavier ions to the detector. If the ions are accelerated with the same potential at a fixed point and a fixed initial time, the ions will separate according to their m/z ratios. This time-of-flight can be converted to mass. Typically a few hundred pulses of laser light are used, each of around a few nanoseconds' duration and the information is accumulated to build up a good spectrum. With the benefit of a camera that is used to follow the laser flashes one can move or 'track' the laser beam around the MALDI plate to find so-called sweet spots where the composition of co-crystallised matrix and sample is optimal for good sensitivity.

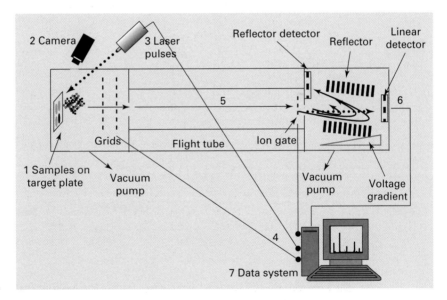

Fig. 9.12. MALDI–TOF instrument components. (1) Sample mixed with matrix is dried on the target plate, which is introduced into high vacuum chamber. (2) The camera allows viewing of the position of the laser beam, which can be tracked to optimise the signal. (3) The sample/matrix is irradiated with laser pulses. (4) The clock is started to measure time-of-flight. (5) Ions are accelerated by the electric field to the same kinetic energy and are separated according to mass as they fly through the flight tube. (6) Ions strike the detector either in linear (dotted arrow) or reflectron (full arrows) mode at different times, depending on their m/z ratio. (7) A data system controls instrument parameters, acquires signal versus time and processes the data.

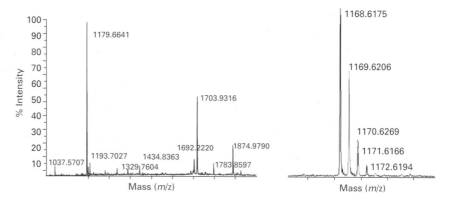

Fig. 9.13. Two examples of MALDI–TOF peptide spectra. The left-hand spectrum is from a protein digest mixture and the right-hand image is an expanded one of a small part of a spectrum showing ^{13}C-containing forms; see Section 9.5.4.

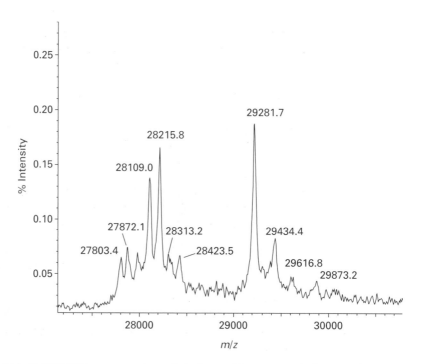

Fig. 9.14. MALDI–TOF spectrum of protein isoforms. The spectrum is almost exclusively singly charged ions representing the molecular ion species of the constitutent proteins. Compare this spectrum with the electrospray spectrum of another protein (Fig. 9.6) where the multiply charged ions result in multiple peaks that would make it harder to interpret masses of mixtures. (I acknowledge the assistance of Bruker Daltonics, who carried out the analysis.)

Sample concentration for MALDI

Maximum sensitivity is achieved in MALDI–TOF if samples are diluted to a particular concentration range. If the sample concentration is unknown a dilution series may be needed to produce a satisfactory sample/matrix spot of suitable concentration on the MALDI plate. Peptides and proteins seem to give best spectra at around 0.1–10 pmol mm^{-3} (Figs. 9.13 and 9.14). Some proteins, particularly glycoproteins, may yield better results at concentrations up to 10 pmol mm^{-3}. Oligonucleotides give better spectra at around 10–100 pmol mm^{-3}, whilst polymers require a concentration around 100 pmol nm^3. (Note: 1 pmol mm^{-3} = 10^{-6} mol dm^{-3}.)

Example 2 PEPTIDE MASS DETERMINATION(I)

Question

A peptide metabolite and an enzyme digest of it were analysed by a combination of mass spectrometric techniques giving the data listed below:

(i) The peptide showed two signals at 3841.5 and 1741 in the MALDI–TOF.

(ii) Five signals could be discerned when the peptide was introduced into a mass spectrometer via an electrospray ionization source:

m/z	498.2	581.1	697.1	871.2	1161.2

(iii) HPLC-MS of the digest indicated *four* components; the $[M + H]^+$ data for the components being $m/z = 176, 625, 1229$ and 1508. The ions corresponding to the MS of the '625' component appeared at $m/z = 521, 406,$ $293, 130$ and 113.

(iv) HPLC-MS–MS of the $m/z = 406$ ion of the '625' component identified two ions at $m/z = 378$ and 336 and of the $m/z = 113$ ion gave $m/z = 85$ and 57, in the product ion spectra.

Use the above data to compare and contrast the different ionisation methods, deduce a molecular mass for the peptide and determine a sequence for the '625' component.

Use the amino acid residue mass values in Table 9.2.

Answer

The data in (i) are $m/z = 3481.5$ and $m/z = 1741$. These data could represent either of the following possibilities:

(a) $m/z = 3481.5 \equiv (M + H)^+$
when $m/z = 1741 \equiv (M + H)^{2+}$, giving $M = 3480.5$

(b) $m/z = 3481.5 \equiv (2M + H)^+$
when $m/z = 1741 \equiv (M + H)^+$, giving $M = 1740$

Consideration of the data in (ii) allows a choice to be made between these two alternatives, using $n_2 = (m_1 - 1)/(m_2 - m_1)$ and $M = n_2(m_2 - 1)$.

Example 2 (Cont.)

$m_1 - 1$	$m_2 - m_1$	n_2	$m_2 - 1$	M(Da)	z
870.2	290	3.0006	1160.2	3481.2	3
696.1	174.1	3.9982	870.2	3479.3	4
580.1	116	5.0000	696.1	3481.1	5
497.2	82.9	5.9975	580.1	3479.2	6

$$\Sigma M = 13920.8 \, \text{Da}$$
$$\text{Mean } M = 3480.2 \, \text{Da}$$

The mean M result confirms set (a) of the conclusions above concerning the data obtained from the MALDI experiments.

The data in (iii) indicate that four products arise from the enzymatic digest of the original peptide. As these products arise directly from the original, the sum of these masses will be related to the M of the pepide.

Therefore

$$176 + 625 + 1229 + 1508 = 3538 \, \text{Da}$$

The difference between this mass and the M determined above is

$$3538 - 3480.2 = 57.8 \approx 58 \, \text{Da}$$

The difference of 58 mass units is explained as follows.

Each of the enzyme digest products is protonated (to be 'seen' in the mass spectrometer). Hence this accounts for 4 units. The remaining 54 unit increase arises from the enzymic hydrolysis. From a linear peptide, four products arise from three cleavage points (three cuts in a piece of string give four pieces). Each cleavage point requires the input of one water molecule (hydrolysis, $H_2O = 18$). Three cleavage points require $3 \times 18 = 54$.

The $m/z = 625$, $(M + H)^+$, peak was subjected to further mass spectrometry and sequence ions were observed.

m/z	624		521		406		293		130		113
Δ		103		115		113		163		17	
aa		Cys		Asp		Ile/Leu		Tyr		Ile/Leu	

The loss of 113 from the $m/z = 406$ ion indicates either Ile or Leu. MS^2 shows consecutive losses of 28 (CO) and 42 ($CH_2 = CH = CH_3$) which is indicative of Leu. The loss of 17 (not a sequence ion) from 130 confirms this as the C-terminal amino acid.

The predicted sequence, from the N-terminal end is

Cys-Asp-Leu-Tyr-Ile

Delayed extraction

In the first MALDI–TOF instruments, the ions in the plume of material generated by the laser pulse were continuously extracted by a high electrostatic field. Since this plume of material occupies a small but finite volume of space, ions arising at different places could have different energies. This energy spread (and

Example 3 PEPTIDE MASS DETERMINATION (II)

Consider the following mass spectrometric data obtained for a peptide metabolite.

(i) The MALDI spectrum showed two signals at $m/z = 1609$ and 805.

(ii) There were two significant signals in positive ion trap MS mass spectrum at $m/z = 805$ and 827, the latter signal being enhanced on addition of sodium chloride.

(iii) Signals at $m/z = 161.8, 202.0, 269.0$ and 403.0 were observed when the sample was introduced into the mass spectrometer via an electrospray ionization source.

Use these data to give an account of the ionisation methods used. Discuss the significance of the data and deduce a relative molecular mass for the metabolite. Use the amino acid residue mass values in Table 9.2.

Answer

(i) Signals in the MALDI spectrum were observed at $m/z = 1609$ and 805. These data could represent the following possibilities:

(a) $m/z = 1609 \equiv (M + H)^+$

when $m/z = 805 \equiv (M + 2H)^{2+}$
and $m/z = 403 \equiv (M + 4H)^{4+}$, giving $M = 1608$ Da

(b) $m/z = 1609 \equiv (2M + H)^+$

when $m/z = 805 \equiv (M + H)^+$
and $m/z = 403 \equiv (M + 2H)^{2+}$, giving $M = 804$ Da

(ii) The distinction between the above options can be made by considering the ion trap data. This mode of ionisation gave peaks at $m/z = 805$ and 827, the latter being enhanced on the addition of sodium chloride. This evidence suggests:

$m/z = 805 \equiv (M + H)^+$
$m/z = 827 \equiv (M + Na)^+$

giving $M = 804$ Da and supports option (b) from the MALDI data.

(iii) The multiply charged ions observed in the electrospray ionization method allow an average M to be calculated. Using the standard formula;

$m_1 - 1$	$m_2 - m_1$	n_2	$m_2 - 1$	M (Da)	z
268.0	134	2.0	402.0	804	2
201.0	67	3.0	268.0	804	3
160.8	40.2	4.0	201.0	804	4

The molecular mass is clearly 804 Da, confirming the above conclusions.

fragmentation occurring during this initial extraction period) usually broadens the peak corresponding to any particular ion, which leads to lower mass accuracy. However, if extraction is delayed until all ions have formed, this spread is minimised. The procedure is known as delayed extraction (DE), whereby the ions are formed in either a weak field or no field during a predetermined time

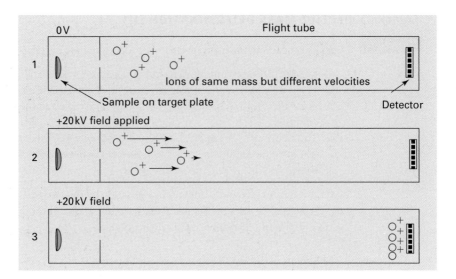

Fig. 9.15. Delayed extraction (DE). (1) No applied electric field. The ions spread out. (2) Field applied. The potential gradient accelerates slow ions more than fast ones. (3) Slow ions catch up with faster ones at the detector.

delay, and then extracted by the application of a high voltage pulse. The degree of fragmentation of ions (Section 9.3.8) can also be controlled, to some extent, by the length of the time delay. Delayed extraction is illustrated in Fig. 9.15.

9.3.8 Post-source decay

Post-source decay (PSD) is the process of fragmentation that may occur after an ion (the precursor ion) has been extracted from the source. Many biological molecules, particularly peptides, give rise to ions that dissociate over a time span of microseconds and most precursor ions will have been extracted before this dissociation is complete. The fragment ions generated will have the same velocity as the precursor and cause peak broadening and loss of resolution in a linear TOF analyser (Fig. 9.16). The problem is overcome by the use of a reflector.

The reflector

A reflector (or reflectron) is a type of ion mirror that provides higher resolution in MALDI–TOF. The reflector increases the overall path length for an ion and it corrects for minor variation in the energy spread of ions of the same mass. Both effects improve resolution. The device has a gradient electric field and the depth to which ions will penetrate this field, before reversal of direction of travel, depends upon their energy. Higher energy ions will travel further and lower energy ions a shorter distance. The flight times thus become focused, while neutral fragments are unaffected by the deflection. Fig. 9.16 shows a diagrammatic representation of a MALDI–TOF instrument that includes the facility for both linear and reflectron modes of ion collection. The reflectron improves resolution and mass accuracy and also allows structure and sequence information (in the case of peptides) to be obtained by PSD analysis.

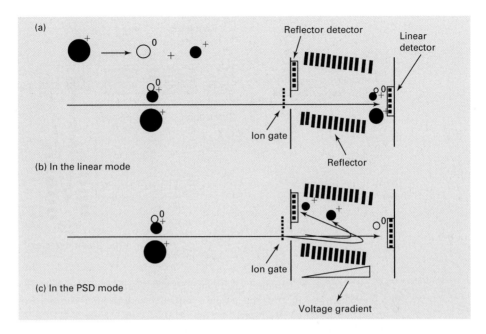

(a)

Reflector detector

Linear detector

Ion gate

Reflector

(b) In the linear mode

(c) In the PSD mode

Ion gate

Voltage gradient

Fig. 9.16. The MALDI–TOF reflector. Post-source decay (PSD) theory. (a) Fragment ions arising by PSD as well as the neutral fragments and the precursor ions have the same velocity and reach the detector simultaneously. This prevents a distinction between precursor and PSD fragment. (b) In the linear mode the charged fragments are not separated. (c) In the reflector mode, the fragment that does not retain the charge (neutral, denoted by $\bigcirc^0$) is not deflected in the reflector but the charged fragments ($\bullet^+$) are deflected according to their m/z ratios and a spectrum of the fragment (daughter) ions is recorded, albeit of a limited m/z range for each setting of the reflector voltages.

Sequencing peptides by PSD analysis in MALDI–TOF is less straightforward (and in a large percentage of experiments is unsuccessful) than tandem MS on a quadrupole ESI or ion trap instrument. At any given setting of the reflector/ion mirror, charged fragments of a particular range of m/z are focused in the reflector (Fig. 9.16). Fragment ions of m/z above and below this narrow range are poorly focused. Therefore, since only fragment ions of a limited mass range are focused for a given mirror ratio in the reflector, a number of spectra are run at different settings and stitched together to generate a composite spectrum.

Types of MALDI sample plates

MALDI sample plate types that are available include 100-well stainless steel flat plates. These are good for multiple sample analysis where close external calibration is used; that is, the use of a compound or compounds of known molecular mass placed on an adjacent spot to calibrate the instrument. It is also easier to see crystallisation of the matrix on this type of surface. Four-hundred-spot Teflon-coated plates have particular application for concentrating samples for increased sensitivity. Owing to the very small diameter of the spots, it is difficult to spot accurately manually but these plates are good for automated sample spotting. Only in the centre of each spot is the surface of the plate exposed, therefore the

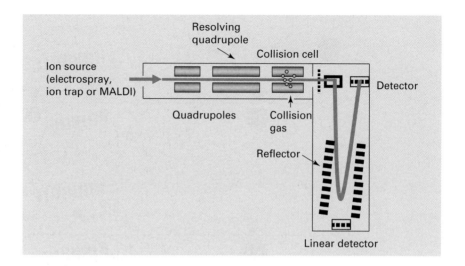

Fig. 9.17. Diagram of a hybrid quadrupole TOF MS. The diagram shown here does not represent any specific instrument from a particular manufacturer. The source may be an ion trap device, an electrospray or even a MALDI source (in the 'MALDI Q-TOF' from Micromass). Other hybrid instruments include the Bruker Daltonics 'BioTOF III, ESI-Q-q-TOF System' and the 'QSTAR' Hybrid LC-MS/MS from Applied Biosystems with an electrospray, nanospray or an optional MALDI source. The Shimadzu Biotech 'AXIMA MALDI QIT TOF' combines a MALDI source with an ion trap and reflectron TOF mass analyser.

sample does not 'wet' over the whole surface but concentrates itself into the centre of each spot as it dries. Gold-coated plates with wells (2 mm diameter, see Fig. 9.10b) are good surfaces on which to contain the spread of sample and matrix when used with high organic solvents, for example tetrahydrofuran preparations for polymers. They also allow on-plate reactions within the well with thiol-containing reagents that bind to the gold surface.

9.3.9 Novel hybrid instruments

There are a number of commercial developments of hybrid MS instruments that involve coupling an electrospray, ion trap or MALDI ion source with a hybrid quadrupole orthogonal acceleration TOF mass spectrometer (Fig. 9.17). This potentially leads to improved tandem MS performance from MALDI phase samples. The intention of the development of these instruments is to combine the best features of both types of ion source with the best features all types of analyser in order to improve tandem MS capability and increase sensitivity. Hybrid magnetic sector instruments are also manufactured where the first mass spectrometer is a two-sector device and the second mass spectrometer is a quadrupole.

9.3.10 Fourier transform ion cyclotron resonance mass spectrometry

The recent development of Fourier transform ion cyclotron resonance (FT-ICR) MS has great potential in analysis of a wide range of biomolecules. It is potentially the

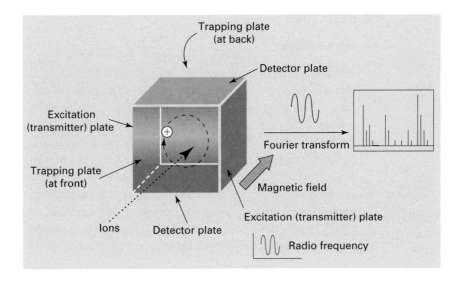

Fig. 9.18. Schematic diagram of the Fourier transform ion cyclotron resonance (FT-ICR) instrument. The technique involves trapping, excitation and detection of ions to produce a mass spectrum. The trapping plates to maintain the ions in orbit are at the front and back in the schematic. The excitation or transmitter plates, where the radio frequency pulse is given to the ions, are shown at each side and the detector plates that detect the image current, which is Fourier transformed, are shown at the top and bottom. The sample source is normally electrospray or MALDI. The ions are focused and transferred into the analyser cell under high vacuum. The analyser cell is a type of ion-trap in a spatially uniform static magnetic field which constrains the ions in a circular orbit, the frequency of which is determined by the mass, charge and velocity of the ion. Whilst the ions are in these stable orbits between the detector electrodes they will not give a measurable signal. In order to achieve this, ions of a given m/z ratio are excited to a wider orbital radius by applying a radio frequency signal of a few milliseconds' duration. One frequency excites ions of one particular m/z value, which results in the ions producing a detectable image current. This time-dependent image current is Fourier transformed to obtain the component frequencies, which correspond to the m/z ratios of the different ions. The angular frequency measurements produce values for m/z. Therefore the mass spectrum is determined to a very high mass resolution since frequency can be measured more accurately than any other physical property. After excitation, the ions relax back to their previous orbits and high sensitivity can be achieved by repeating this process many times.

most sensitive mass spectrometric technique and has almost unlimited mass resolution, $>10^6$ is observable with most instruments. The instrument also allows tandem MS to be carried out. The ions can be generated by a variety of techniques, such as an ESI or a MALDI source. FT-ICR MS is based on the principle of ions, which, whilst orbiting in a magnetic field, are excited by radio frequency signals. As a result, the ions produce a detectable image current on the cell in which they are trapped. The time-dependent image current is Fourier transformed to obtain the component frequencies of the different ions, which correspond to their m/z (Fig. 9.18).

9.4 **DETECTORS**

9.4.1 **Introduction**

The ions from the mass analyser impinge on a surface of a detector where the charge is neutralised, either by collection or donation of electrons. An electric current flows that is amplified and ultimately converted into a signal that is processed by a computer. The total ion current (TIC) is the sum of the current carried by all the ions being detected at any given moment and is a very useful parameter to measure during on-line MS. A plot of ion current versus time complements the ultraviolet trace that is also normally recorded during the chromatography run. Unlike the ultraviolet trace, which depends on the absorbance of each component at the particular wavelength(s) set on the ultraviolet detector, the TIC is of course independent of the light-absorbing properties of a substance and depends only upon its ionisability in the instrument.

9.4.2 **Electron multiplier and conversion dynode**

Electron multipliers are used as detectors for all types of mass spectrometers. These are frequently combined with a conversion dynode, which is a device to increase sensitivity. The ion beam from the mass analyser is focused onto the conversion dynode, which emits electrons in direct proportion to the number of bombarding ions. A positive ion or a negative ion hits the conversion dynode, causing the emission of secondary particle containing secondary ions, electrons and neutral particles (Fig. 9.19). These secondary particles are accelerated into the dynodes of the electron multiplier. They strike the dynodes with sufficient energy to dislodge electrons, which pass further into the electron multiplier, colliding with the dynodes, producing more and more electrons.

9.5 **STRUCTURAL INFORMATION BY TANDEM MASS SPECTROMETRY**

9.5.1 **Introduction**

As mentioned above, the newer ionisation techniques ESI and MALDI are soft ionisation techniques (as is FAB and its derivative techniques). In contrast to EI, they do not produce significant amounts of fragment ions. Therefore in order to obtain structural information on biomolecules and sequence information (in the case of proteins and peptides), tandem MS has been developed. The technique can also be applied to obtain sequence information on oligosaccharides (Section 9.5.6) and oligonucleotides (Fig. 9.20). Although it is unlikely that this method will ever replace DNA sequencing gels, it can be used to identify positions of modified or labelled bases that might not be picked up by the Sanger dideoxy sequencing method.

Structural information can be obtained on almost any type of organic molecule, on an instrument that is suitable for that type of sample. This includes

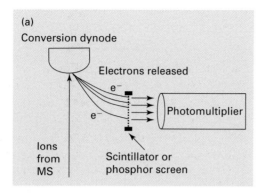

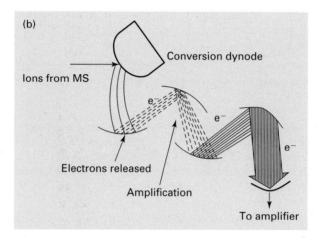

Fig. 9.19. Conversion dynode and electron multiplier. (a and b) Each ion strikes the conversion dynode (which converts ions to electrons), which emits a number of electrons that travel to the next, higher voltage dynode. The secondary electrons from the conversion dynode are accelerated and focused onto a second dynode, which itself emits secondary electrons. Each electron then produces several more electrons. Amplification is achieved through the 'cascading effect' of secondary electrons from dynode to dynode that finally results in a measurable current at the end of the electron multiplier. The cascade of electrons continues until a sufficiently large current for normal amplification is obtained. A series of up to 10–20 dynodes (set at different potentials) provides an amplification gain of 10^6 or 10^7.

investigation of organic compounds on a magnet sector MS where two double-focusing magnetic sector machines can be combined into a four-sector device coupled through a collision cell. The general procedure is that a mixture of ions is generated in the ion source of the mass spectrometer as normal and the ions are allowed to pass through the first mass analyser, where an ion of a particular m/z is selected (but not detected). This ion then enters the collision cell and collides with an inert collision gas such as helium or argon. The kinetic energy of this ion is converted to vibrational energy and the ion fragments. This is known as

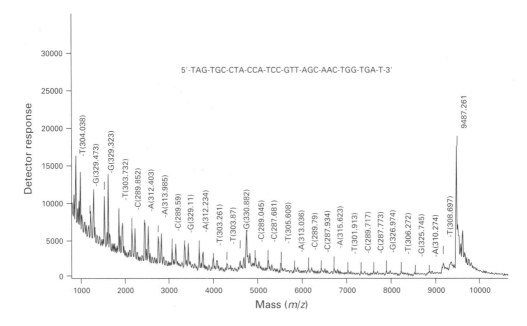

Fig. 9.20. DNA sequencing by MS. This shows an example of a 36-mer oligonucleotide sequenced by in-source decay on MALDI–TOF. The sequence is reconstructed from the mass differences between the peaks, which correspond to consecutive loss of a particular nucleotide at each fragmentation. (I acknowledge the use of the spectrum from Applied Biosystems.)

collision-induced dissociation (CID) or collision-activated dissociation (CAD). The m/z values of the fragment ions are then determined in a second mass spectrometer (see Fig. 9.21 for an illustration of the principle in a quadrupole mass spectrometer). Collision cells may be placed in any of the field-free regions, leading to a wide variety of experimental methodologies for many different applications. For example, as well as in the triple quadrupole MS this can be done in a hybrid instrument such as the Q-TOF (Section 9.3.9). Since the principles of tandem MS are similar for most instrument configurations, further discussion will focus on electrospray tandem MS. The procedure for obtaining structural and sequence information on polypeptides in ion trap MS has been described above (Section 9.3.3).

9.5.2 Sequencing of proteins and peptides

The structural identification of proteins involves protease cleavage, mostly by trypsin. Owing to the specificity of this protease, tryptic peptides usually have basic groups at the N and C termini. Trypsin cleaves after lysine and arginine residues, both of which have basic side-chains (an amino and a guanidino group, respectively). This results in a large proportion of high energy doubly charged positive ions that are more easily fragmented. The digestion of the protein into peptides is followed by identification of the peptides by (m/z), either as very accurate masses alone or by using a second fragmentation that gives ladders of

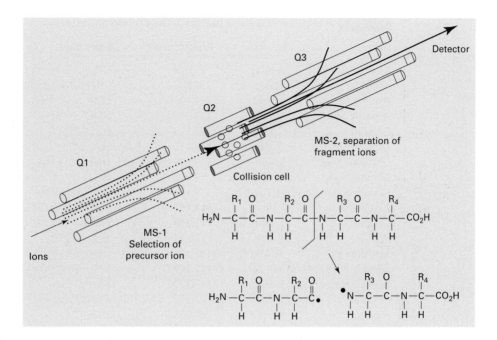

Fig. 9.21. Quadrupole MS sequencing. An ion of a particular m/z value is selected in the first quadrupole, Q1, as in Fig. 9.5, but instead of being detected, it passes through the second quadrupole, Q2, where it is subjected to collision with the collision gas. The Q3 acts like a second quadrupole mass spectrometer, MS-2, to scan m/z to obtain a spectrum of the fragment ions. The collision cell, Q2, is frequently a radio frequency (RF)-only quadrupole containing the appropriate collision gas. No mass filtering occurs here, the RF merely constrains the ions to allow a greater number of collisions to occur. The fragmentation depicted here is at the peptide bond and one of the fragments will retain the charge, resulting in either a y-series or a b-series ion, see Fig. 9.22.

fragments cleaved at the peptide bonds. Although a wide variety of fragmentations may occur, there is a predominance of peptide bond cleavage, which gives rise to peaks in the spectrum that differ sequentially by the residue mass. The mass differences are thus used to reconstruct the amino acid sequence (primary structure) of the peptide (Table 9.2).

Different series of ions, a, b, c and x, y, z, may be recognised, depending on which fragment carries the charge. Ions x, y and z arise by retention of charge on the C-terminal fragment of the peptide. For example, the z_1 ion is the first C-terminal residue; y_1 also contains the NH group (15 atomic mass units greater) and x_1 includes the carbonyl group; y_2 comprises the first two C-terminal residues, and so on. The a, b, and c ion series arise from the N-terminal end of the peptide, when the fragmentation results in retention of charge on these fragments. Fig. 9.22a shows an idealised peptide subjected to fragmentation. Particular series will generally predominate so that the peptide may be sequenced from both ends by obtaining complementary data (Fig. 9.22b). In addition, ions can arise from side-chain fragmentation, which enables a distinction to be made between isomeric amino

Table 9.2 Symbols and residue masses of the protein amino acids

Name	Symbol	Residue mass[a]	Side-chain
Alanine	A, Ala	71.079	CH_3-
Arginine	R, Arg	156.188	$HN=C(NH_2)-NH-(CH_2)_3$-
Asparagine	N, Asn	114.104	$H_2N-CO-CH_2$-
Aspartic acid	D, Asp	115.089	$HOOC-CH_2$-
Cysteine	C, Cys	103.145	$HS-CH_2$-
Glutamine	Q, Gln	**128.131**	$H_2N-CO-(CH_2)_2$-
Glutamic acid	E, Glu	129.116	$HOOC-(CH_2)_2$-
Glycine	G, Gly	57.052	H-
Histidine	H, His	137.141	Imidazole-CH_2-
Isoleucine	I, Ile	**113.160**	$CH_3-CH_2-CH(CH_3)$-
Leucine	L, Leu	**113.160**	$(CH_3)_2-CH-CH_2$-
Lysine	K, Lys	**128.17**	$H_2N-(CH_2)_4$-
Methionine	M, Met	131.199	$CH_3-S-(CH_2)_2$-
Metsulphoxide	Met.SO	**147.199**	$CH_3-S(O)-(CD_2)_2$-
Phenylalanine	F, Phe	**147.177**	Phenyl-CH_2-
Proline	P, Pro	97.117	Pyrrolidone-CH-
Serine	S, Ser	87.078	$HO-CH_2$-
Threonine	T, Thr	101.105	$CH_3-CH(OH)$-
Tryptophan	W, Trp	186.213	Indole-$NH-CH=C-CH_2$-
Tyrosine	Y, Tyr	163.176	4-OH-Phenyl-CH_2-
Valine	V, Val	99.133	$CH_3-CH(CH_2)$-

[a]Residue mass is the mass in a peptide bond, i.e. after loss of H_2O when the peptide bond is formed. The numbers in bold in the residue mass column indicate amino acids that may be ambiguous in a sequence determined by tandem MS due to close similarity or identity in mass.

acids such as leucine and isoleucine. The protein is identified by searching databases of expected masses from all known peptides from every protein (or translations from DNA) and theoretical masses from fragmented peptides. The sensitivity of tandem MS has been claimed down to zeptomole level (see Table 9.3).

9.5.3 Comparison of mass spectrometry and Edman sequencing

Edman degradation to obtain the complete sequence of a protein is uncommon nowadays, since genomes are available to search with fragmentary sequences. Most intact proteins, if they are not processed from a secretory or pro-peptide form, are blocked at the N terminus, most commonly with an acetyl group. Other N-terminal blocking includes fatty acylation, most commonly with a myristoyl, C_{12} fatty acid, attached through a glycine residue, but the presence of many shorter chain fatty acids is known to occur. Cyclisation of glutamine to a pyroglutamyl residue and post-translational modification to N-terminal trimethylalanine and dimethylproline also occur. In the case of recombinant proteins overexpressed in *Escherichia coli*, the initiator residue *N*-formylmethionine is often incompletely removed. All these modifications leave the N-terminal residue without a free

(a)

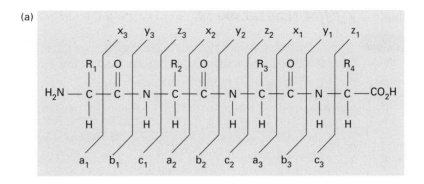

(b)

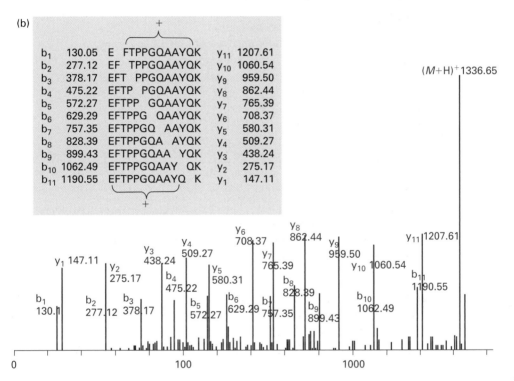

b_1	130.05	E FTPPGQAAYQK	y_{11}	1207.61
b_2	277.12	EF TPPGQAAYQK	y_{10}	1060.54
b_3	378.17	EFT PPGQAAYQK	y_9	959.50
b_4	475.22	EFTP PGQAAYQK	y_8	862.44
b_5	572.27	EFTPP GQAAYQK	y_7	765.39
b_6	629.29	EFTPPG QAAYQK	y_6	708.37
b_7	757.35	EFTPPGQ AAYQK	y_5	580.31
b_8	828.39	EFTPPGQA AYQK	y_4	509.27
b_9	899.43	EFTPPGQAA YQK	y_3	438.24
b_{10}	1062.49	EFTPPGQAAY QK	y_2	275.17
b_{11}	1190.55	EFTPPGQAAYQ K	y_1	147.11

$(M+H)^+$ 1336.65

Fig. 9.22. Peptide fragment ion nomenclature and tandem MS spectrum of a peptide. (a) Charge may be retained by either the N- or C-terminal fragment, resulting in the a, b and c series of ions or x, y and z series, respectively. b- and y-series ions frequently predominate. Corresponding neutral fragments are of course not detected. The sequence of the peptide, from a mutant haemoglobin, is EFTPPGQAAYQK. The figure shows the tandem mass spectrum from collision-induced dissociation of the doubly charged $(M + 2H)^{2+}$ precursor, $m/z = 668.3$. Cleavage at each peptide bond results in the b or y ions when the positive charge is retained by the fragment containing the N or C terminus of the peptide, respectively (see inset).

proton on the alpha nitrogen and Edman chemistry cannot proceed. Mass spectrometry has therefore been essential for their correct structural identification. The protein-sequencing instruments are still important for solid-phase sequencing to identify post-translational modifications; in particular, sites of phosphorylation

Example 4 PEPTIDE SEQUENCING (I)

Question

An oligopeptide obtained by tryptic digestion was investigated by ESI–MS and ion trap MS–MS both in positive mode, and gave the following m/z data:

ESI	223.2	297.3							
Ion trap	146	203	260	357	444	591	648	705	802	890

(i) Predict the sequence of the oligopeptide. Use the amino acid residual mass values in the table below.

(ii) Determine the average molecular mass.

(iii) Identify the peaks in the ESI spectrum.

(See table 9.2 for amino acid residue mass.)

Note: Trypsin cleaves on the C-terminal side of arginine and lysine.

Answer

(i) The highest mass peak in the ion trap MS spectrum is $m/z = 890$, which represents $(M + H)^+$.

Hence $M = 889$ Da.

m/z	146	203	260	357	444	591	648	705	802	889
Δ		57	57	97	87	147	57	57	97	87
aa		Gly	Gly	Pro	Ser	Phe	Gly	Gly	Pro	Ser

The mass differences (Δ), between sequence ions, represent the amino acid(aa) residue masses. The lowest mass sequence ion, $m/z = 146$, is too low for arginine and must therefore represent Lys + OH. The sequence in conventional order from the N-terminal end would be:

Ser-Pro-Gly-Gly-Phe-Ser-Pro-Gly-Gly-Lys

(ii) The summation of the residues = 889 Da, which is a check on the mass spectrometry value for M.

(iii) The m/z values in the ESI spectrum represent multiply charged species and may be identified as follows:

$m/z = 223.2 \equiv (M + 4H)^{4+}$ from $889/223.2 = 3.98$

$m/z = 297.3 \equiv (M + 3H)^{3+}$ from $889/297.3 = 2.99$

Remember that z must be an integer and hence values need to be rounded to the nearest whole number.

and a combination of microsequencing and MS techniques are now commonly employed for complete covalent structure determination of proteins.

9.5.4 Carbon isotopes and finding the charge state of a peptide

Since the mass detector operates on the basis of m/z, mass assignment is normally made assuming a single charge per ion (i.e. $m/z = m + 1$ in positive ion mode).

Example 5 PEPTIDE SEQUENCING (II)

Question Determine the primary structure of the oligopeptide that gave the following, positive mode, MS–MS data:

m/z	149	305	442	529	617

Use the amino acid residual mass values in Table 9.2.

Answer $m/z = 617 \equiv (M + H)^+$

m/z	149	305	442	529	616
Δ		156	137	87	87
aa		Arg	His	Ser	Ser

Conventional order for the sequence would be:
Ser-Ser-His-Arg-?
It is important to note that no assignment has been given for the remaining $m/z =$ 149. It may not in fact be a sequence ion and more information would be required, such as an accurate molecular mass of the oligopeptide, in order to proceed further. It is, however, possible to speculate as to the nature of this ion. If the $m/z = 149$ ion is the C-terminal amino acid then it would end in-OH and be 17 mass units greater than the corresponding residue mass. The difference between 149 and 17 is 132, which is extremely close to methionine, so this amino acid remains a possibility to end the chain.

However, since there is around 1.1% ^{13}C natural abundance, with increasing size, peptides will have a greater chance of containing at least one ^{13}C and two ^{13}C, etc. A peptide of 20 residues has approximately equal peak heights of the 'all ^{12}C peptide' and of the peptide with one ^{13}C. A singly charged peptide will show adjacent peaks differing in one mass unit; a doubly charged peptide will show adjacent peaks differing in half a mass unit and so on (Fig. 9.23 and Table 9.3). In the example illustrated (Fig. 9.23), angiotensin has an M_r calculated from its sequence as 1295.69. The experimentally derived values are, for the singly charged ion, $[(M + H)/1] = 1296.65$ and for the doubly charged ion, $[(M + 2H)/2] = 648.82$. For elements such as chlorine, the isotopic abundance ^{35}Cl: ^{37}Cl is approximately 3:1. If a compound contains a single chlorine atom, two ion species will be observed, with peak intensities in an approximate ratio of 3:1. If a compound contains two chlorine atoms then three peaks will be seen. The technique is particularly useful for determining which are the high energy doubly charged tryptic peptides, for tandem MS.

9.5.5 Ladder sequencing

This technique is an alternative to tandem MS and involves the generation of a set of fragments of a polypeptide chain followed by analysis of the mass of each component. Each component in the polypeptide mixture differs from the next by

Example 6 PEPTIDE MASS DETERMINATION (III)

Question

An unknown peptide and an enzymatic digest of it were analysed by mass spectrometric and chromatographic methods as follows:

   (i) MALDI–TOF mass spectrometry of the peptide gave two signals at $m/z =$ 3569 and 1785;

  (ii) MALDI–TOF of the hydrolysate showed signals at $m/z =$ 766, 891, 953 and 1016;

 (iii) the data obtained from analysis of the peptide using coupled HPLC–MS operating through an electrospray ionisation source were $m/z =$ 510.7, 595.7, 714.6, 893.0 and 1190.3;

 (iv) when the hydrolysate was analysed by HPLC, four distinct components could be discerned.

Explain what information is available from these observations and determine a molecular mass, using the amino acid residue mass values in Table 9.2, for the unknown peptide.

Answer

  (i) Signals from MALDI–TOF were observed at $m/z =$ 3569 and 1785. These data could represent either of the following possibilities:

    (a) $m/z = 3569 \equiv (M + H)^+$
       when $m/z = 1785 \equiv (M + 2H)^{2+}$, giving $M = 3568$

    (b) $m/z = 3569 \equiv (2M + H)^+$,
       when $m/z = 1785 \equiv (M + H)^+$, giving $M = 1784$

  (ii) It is possible to distinguish between these two options by considering the MALDI–TOF of the products of hydrolysis. Four m/z values were obtained: 766, 891, 953 and 1016.
     Each is a protonated species and the sum of these masses, 3626, will be of the order of the M of the original peptide. The value of this sum supports option (a) in (i) above.

 (iii) Electrospray ionisation data represent multiply charged ions. Using the standard formula the mean M may be obtained.

$m_1 - 1$	$m_2 - m_1$	n_2	$m_2 - 1$	$M\,(Da)$	z
892.0	297.3	3.0003	1189.3	3568.3	3
713.6	178.4	4.0000	892.0	3568.0	4
594.7	118.9	5.0016	713.6	3569.2	5
509.7	85	5.9964	594.7	3566.1	6

        $\Sigma M = 14271.6$ Da
      Mean $M = 3567.9$ Da

This more precise value confirms the conclusions found above. For an explanation of the mass difference between M_r and the sum of the hydrolysate products, refer to the answer to Example 2.

   The data in (iv) are confirmatory chromatographic evidence that only four hydrolysis products were obtained.

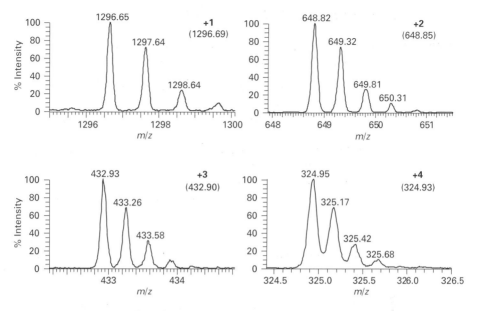

Fig. 9.23. Spectra of a multiply charged peptide. Finding the charge state of a peptide involves zooming in on a particular part of the mass spectrum to obtain a detailed image of the mass differences between different peaks that arise from the same biomolecule, due to isotopic abundance. This is due mainly to ^{12}C and its ^{13}C isotope, as described in the text.

Table 9.3 **Mass differences due to isotopes in multiply charged peptides**

Charge on peptide	Apparent mass	Mass difference between isotope peaks
Single charge	$[(M+H)/1]$	1 Da
Double charge	$[(M+2H)/2]$	0.5 Da
Triple charge	$[(M+3H)/3]$	0.33 Da
n charges	$[(M+nH)/n]$	$1/n$ Da

loss of a mass that is characteristic of the residue weight (which may involve a modified side-chain) thus enabling the sequence of the polypeptide to be read. The ladder of degraded peptides can be generated by Edman chemistry (Section 8.4.3) or by exopeptidase digestion from the N or the C terminus. The Edman chemistry is modified to carry out the coupling step with phenylisothiocyanate (PITC) in the presence of a small amount of phenylisocyanate, which acts as a chain-terminating agent. This has some analogy to the dideoxy Sanger DNA sequencing methodology. This is essentially a subtractive technique (one looks at the mass of the remaining fragment after each cycle). For example when a phosphoserine residue is encountered, a loss of 167.1 Da is observed in place of 87.1 for loss of a serine residue. This technique therefore avoids one of the major problems of analysing post-translational modifications, since the majority of modifications are stable during the Edman chemistry. The technique of ladder sequencing has particular application in MALDI–TOF MS, which has high sensitivity and greater ability to analyse mixtures.

9.5.6 **Post-translational modification of proteins**

Many chemically distinct types of post-translational modification of proteins are known to occur. These include the wide variety of acylations at the N terminus of proteins (mentioned above) as well as acylations at the C terminus and at internal sites. In this section, examples of the application of MS techniques employed for analysis of glycosylation, phosphorylation and disulphide bonds are given. An up-to-date list of the broad chemical diversity of known modifications and the side-chains of the amino acids to which they are attached is in the website 'Delta Mass', which is a database of protein post-translational modifications that can be found at <http://www.abrf.org/index.cfm/dm.home>. There are hyperlinks to references to the modifications.

Protein phosphorylation and identification of phosphopeptides

The reversible covalent phosphorylation of eukaryotic proteins is a common regulatory mechanism for protein activity (Sections 15.5.4 and 16.5.3). The modified residues are O-phosphoserine, O-phosphothreonine and O-phosphotyrosine but many other amino acids in proteins can be phosphorylated: O-phospho-Asp; S-phospho-Cys; N-phospho-Arg; N-phospho-His and N-phospho-Lys. Analysis of modified peptides by MS is essential to confirm the exact location and number of phosphorylated residues, especially if no ^{32}P or other radiolabel is present. The identification of either positive or negative ions may yield more information, depending on the mode of ionisation and fragmentation of an individual peptide. Phosphopeptides may give better spectra in the negative-ion mode, since they have a strong negative charge due to the phosphate group. Phosphopeptides may not run well on MALDI–TOF and methods have been successfully developed for this type of instrument that employ examination of spectra before and after dephosphorylation of the peptide mixture with phosphatases.

Mass spectrometry of glycosylation sites and structures of the sugars

The attachment points of N-linked (through asparagine) and O-linked (through serine) glycosylation sites and the structures of the complex carbohydrates can be determined by MS. The loss of each monosaccharide unit of distinct mass can be interpreted to reconstruct the glycosylation pattern (Fig. 9.24).

The 'GlycoMod' website, part of the 'ExPASy' suite, provides valuable assistance in interpretation of the spectra. GlycoMod is a tool that can predict the possible oligosaccharide structures that occur on proteins from their experimentally determined masses. The program can be used for free or derivatised oligosaccharides and for glycopeptides. Another algorithm 'GlycanMass', also part of the ExPASy suite, can be used to calculate the mass of an oligosaccharide structure from its oligosaccharide composition. GlyocoMod and GlycanMass may be found at <http://us.expasy. org/tools/glycomod/> and <http://us.expasy.org/tools/glycomod/glycanmass.html>, respectively.

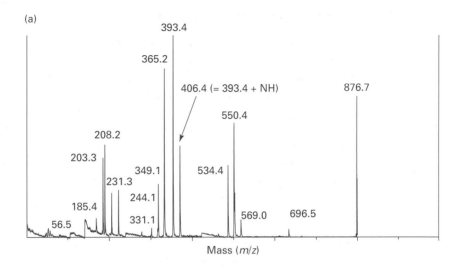

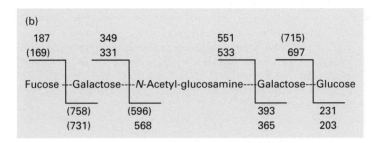

Fig. 9.24. MALDI–TOF PSD MS of carbohydrates. (a) PSD MS spectrum of the carbohydrate Fuc1–2Gal1–3GlucNAc1–3Gal1–4Glc using 2,5-dihydroxybenzoic acid as matrix. On careful inspection of the spectrum one can observe a number of abrupt changes in baseline corresponding to where the PSD spectra have been 'stitched' together. The peak at 876.7 Da is due to the mass of the intact molecule as a sodium adduct, i.e. the parent ion at 876.7 = $[M + Na]^+$. (b) Interpretation of the spectrum. Experimentally derived fragment masses are mainly within 1 Da of the theoretical. The masses in parentheses were not seen in this experiment.

Identification of disulphide linkages by mass spectrometry

MS is also used in the location of disulphide bonds in a protein. The identification of the position of the disulphide linkages involves the fragmentation of proteins into peptides under low pH conditions to minimise disulphide exchange. Proteases with active site thiols should be avoided (e.g. papain, bromelain). Pepsin and cyanogen bromide are particularly useful. The disulphide-linked peptide fragments are separated and identified under mild oxidising conditions by HPLC–MS. The separation is repeated after reduction with reagents such as mercaptoethanol and dithiothreitol (DTT) to cleave -S–S- bonds and the products reanalysed as before. Peptides that were disulphide linked disappear from the spectrum and reappear at the appropriate positions for the individual components.

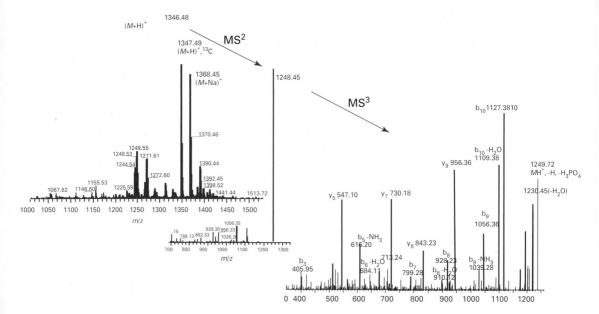

Fig. 9.25. MS identification of phosphopeptides. Sequence is YEILNS^{P}EKAC where S^P is phosphoserine. The MS^2 and MS^3 spectra are shown. The first tandem MS experiment results mainly in loss of H_3PO_4, 98 Da. Particular problems may also be associated with electrospray mass spectrometry of phosphopeptides, where a high level of Na$^+$ and K$^+$ adducts is seen regularly.

9.5.7 Selected ion monitoring

Selected ion monitoring (SIM) is typically used to look for ions that are characteristic of a target compound or family of compounds. This technique has particular application for on-line chromatography–MS, where the instruments can be set up to monitor selected ion masses as the components elute successively from the capillary LC or reverse-phase HPLC column for example (Sections 11.3.3 and 11.9.3). Detection programs or algorithms that are set up to carry out tandem MS on each component as it elutes from a chromatography column can be adapted to enable selective detection of many types of post-translationally modified peptides. This technique can selectively detect low mass fragment ions that are characteristic markers and identify the presence of post-translational modifications such as phosphorylation, glycosylation, sulphation and acylation in any particular peptide. For example, phosphopeptides can be identified by production of phosphate-specific fragment ions of 63 Da (PO_2^-) and 79 Da (PO_3^-) by collision-induced dissociation during negative ion HPLC-ES–MS. Glycopeptides can be identified by characteristic fragment ions including hexose$^+$ (163 Da) and N-acetylhexosamine$^+$ (204 Da). Phosphoserine- and phosphothreonine-containing peptides can also be identified by a process known as neutral loss scanning, where these peptides show loss of 98 Da by β-elimination of H_3PO_4 (Fig. 9. 25).

9.6 ANALYSING PROTEIN COMPLEXES

MS is frequently used to identify partner proteins that interact with a particular protein of interest. Interacting proteins can be isolated by a number of methods including immunoprecipitation of tagged proteins from cell transfection, affinity chromatography and surface plasmon resonance. Surface plasmon resonance (SPR; Section 16.3.2) technology has widespread application for biomolecular interaction analysis and, during characterization of protein–ligand and protein–protein interactions, direct analysis by MALDI–TOF MS of samples bound to the Biacore chips is now possible (where interaction kinetic data are also obtained; Section 16.3.2). Direct analysis of protein complexes by MS is also possible. As well as accurate molecular mass of large biopolymers such as proteins of mass greater than 400 kDa, intact virus particles of 40×10^6 Da (40 MDa) have been analysed using ESI–TOF. An icosahedral virus consisting of a single-stranded RNA surrounded by a homogeneous protein shell with a total mass of 6.5×10^6 Da and a rod-shaped RNA virus with a total mass of 40.5×10^6 Da were studied on this ESI–TOF hybrid mass spectrometer.

9.6.1 Sample preparation and handling

Mass analysis by ES–MS and MALDI–TOF is affected, seriously in some cases, by the presence of particular salts, buffers and detergents. Keratin contamination from flakes of skin and hair can be a major problem particularly when gels and slices are involved; therefore gloves and laboratory coats must be worn. Work on a clean surface in a hood with air filter if possible and use a dedicated box of clean polypropylene microcentrifuge tubes tested to confirm that it does not leach out polymers, mould-release agents, plasticisers, etc. Sample clean-up to remove or reduce levels of buffer salts, EDTA, DMSO, non-ionic and ionic detergents (e.g. SDS), etc. can be achieved by dilution, washing, drop dialysis, and ion-exchange resins. If one is analysing samples by MALDI–TOF, on-plate washing can remove buffers and salts. Sample clean-up can also be achieved by pipette tip chromatography (Section 11.2.5). This consists of a miniature C_{18} reverse-phase chromatography column, packed in a 10 nm^3 pipette tip. The sample, in low or zero organic solvent-containing buffer, is loaded into the tip with a few up and down movements of the pipette piston to ensure complete binding of the sample. Since most contaminants described above will not bind, the sample is trapped on the reverse-phase material and eluted with a solvent containing high organic solvent (typically 50–75% acetonitrile). This is particularly applicable for clean-up of samples after in-gel digestion of protein bands separated on SDS–PAGE. Coomassie Brilliant Blue dye is also removed by this procedure. The technique can be used to concentrate samples and fractionate a mixture. Purification can also be carried out to specifically bind one particular component in a mixture. Immobilised metal ion affinity columns are used to enrich phosphopeptides.

9.6.2 **Quantitative analysis of complex protein mixtures by mass spectrometry**

Proteome analysis (described in Section 8.5) involves the following basic steps:

- run a gel (one-dimensional (1-D) or two-dimensional (2-D)),
- stain,
- scan to identify spots of interest,
- excise gel spots,
- extract and digest proteins,
- mass analyse the resulting peptides,
- search database.

The initial separation of proteins currently relies on gel electrophoresis, which has a number of limitations including the difficulty in analysing all the proteins expressed owing to huge differences in expression levels. Although thousands of proteins can be reproducibly separated on one 2-D gel from approximately 1 mg of tissue/biopsy or biological fluid, the dynamic range of protein expression can be as high as nine orders of magnitude. One development that has helped to over-come some of the problems is the isotope-coded affinity tag (ICAT) strategy for quantifying differential protein expression. The heavy and light forms of the sulphydryl (thiol-)-specific ICAT reagent (whose structure is illustrated in Fig. 9.26) are used to derivatise proteins in respective samples isolated from cells or tissues in different states. The two samples are combined and proteolysed, nor-mally with trypsin, for reasons explained above. The labelled peptides are purified by affinity chromatography utilising the biotin group on the ICAT reagent then analysed by MS on either LC–MS–MS (including ion trap) or MALDI–TOF instru-ments. The relative intensities of the ion from the two isotopically tagged forms of each specific peptide indicate their relative abundance. These pairs of peptides are easily detected because they coelute from reverse-phase microcapillary liquid chromatography (RP-μLC) and contain eight mass units of difference owing to the two forms of the ICAT tag. An initial MS scan identifies the peptides from proteins that show differential expression by measuring relative signal intensities of each ICAT-labelled peptide pair. Peptides of interest are then selected for sequencing by tandem MS and the particular protein from which a peptide originated can be identified by database searching the tandem MS spectral data.

Sequence tag methodology can permit the identification of a protein with only one peptide from that particular protein. This is especially useful if the protein is in a mixture. The data that are used in the search comprise the mass (or m/z) of the intact peptide and a small number of fragment ion masses. An example is illus-trated in Fig. 9.27.

9.7 **COMPUTING AND DATABASE ANALYSIS**

9.7.1 **Organic compound databases**

MS organic compound databases are available to identify the compound(s) in the analyte. The spectra in the databases are obtained by electron impact ionisation.

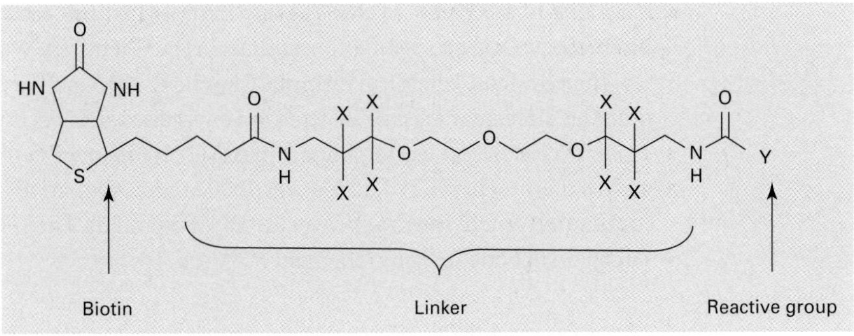

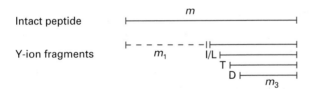

Fig. 9.26. Structure of the ICAT reagent. The ICAT reagent is in two forms, heavy (8 deuterium atoms) and light (no deuterium). The reagent has three elements: an affinity tag (biotin), to isolate ICAT-labelled peptides: a linker in two forms that has stable isotopes incorporated and a reactive group (Y) with specificity towards thiol groups (or other functional groups in proteins (e.g. SH, NH_2, COOH) (cysteines). The heavy reagent is D8-ICAT (where X is deuterium) and light reagent is D8-ICAT (where X is hydrogen). Two protein mixtures representing two different cell states are treated with the isotopically light and heavy ICAT reagents; an ICAT reagent is covalently attached to each cysteine residue in every protein. The protein mixtures are combined, proteolysed and ICAT-labelled peptides are isolated on an avidin column utilising the biotin tag. Peptides are separated by microbore HPLC. Since each pair of ICAT-labelled peptides is chemically identical they are easily visualised because they coelute, with an 8 Da mass difference. The ratios of the original amounts of proteins from the two cell states are strictly maintained in the peptide fragments. The relative quantification is determined by the ratio of the peptide pairs. The protein is identified by database searching with the sequence information from tandem MS analysis by selecting peptides that show differential expression between samples.

Intact peptide ⊢————————— m —————————⊣

Y-ion fragments ⊢– – – – – – –⊣⊢————————⊣
                         m_1 I/L ⊢————————⊣
                                      T ⊢————————⊣
                                      D ⊢————————⊣
                                            m_3

Sequence tag: peptide mass, m + mass, m_1 + sequence (-I/L-T-D-) + mass m_3

Fig. 9.27. Example of protein identification by sequence tag. In this example, the search data are based on the molecular mass of the intact peptide (m) and five fragmention masses. This defines the sequence tag of three residues positioned with respect to the N and C termini between masses m_1 and m_3.

Two such databases are:

● Integrated Spectral Data Base System for Organic Compounds (SDBS) from the National Institute of Advanced Industrial Science and Technology NIMC Spectral Database System. Data on specific compounds can be searched with compound name, molecular formula, number of atoms (CHNO) and molecular mass. The database contains 19 000 electron impact mass spectra and also includes 47 000 Fourier transform infrared (FT-IR) spectra; 11 500 ^{1}H-NMR spectra and 10 200 ^{13}C-NMR spectra. The URL is <http://www.aist.go.jp/RIODB/SDBS/menu-e.html>.

- NIST Chemistry WebBook. NIST is the National Institute for Standards and Technology. Data on specific compounds in the Chemistry WebBook can be searched by name, chemical formula, Chemical Abstracts Service registry number, molecular mass or selected ion energetics and spectral properties. This site comprises electron impact mass spectra for over 15 000 compounds as well as thermochemical data for over 7000 organic and small inorganic compounds and IR spectra for over 16 000 compounds. The URL is <http://webbook.nist.gov./chemistry/>.

9.7.2 Identification of proteins

Database searches to identify a particular protein that has been analysed by MS is particularly important. This section gives an overview of websites for proteomic identification.

The identification of proteins can be carried out by using many websites, for example 'Mascot' from Matrix Science <http://www.matrixscience.com/cgi/index.pl?page=/search_form_select.html> and 'Protein prospector' <http://128.40.158.151/mshome3.4.htm>. The search can be limited by searching particular species or genera e.g. 'mammalia' only, thus increasing the speed. However, when looking for a homologous sequence the species should not be defined. The modification of cysteine residues, if any, should be included otherwise the number of peptides matched to the theoretical list will be decreased, producing a worse hit. If no cysteine modification has been carried out, and if the protein originates from a gel sample, then much of this residue will have been converted to acrylamide-modified cysteine. Unmatched masses should be re-searched, since sometimes two or more proteins run together on electrophoresis. Note the delta p.p.m. (the difference between the theoretical and the experimental mass of a particular peptide), which should be low and consistent. This gives an indication of whether the result is genuine. If an internal calibration has been performed the mass accuracy parameter can be set to 20 p.p.m. For a close external calibration this should be set to 50 p.p.m. If a hit is not found with the first search, this parameter can be increased.

Different databases can be searched. NCBInr is the largest database whilst Swiss Prot is smaller. However Swiss Prot provides the most information with the protein hits. If it is known that the protein is not larger than, for example 100 kDa then the mass range should be limited to prevent false hits. Although the search will be refined by limiting to a particular mass range of the intact protein, the possibility of subunits or fragments must be considered. Some information on the isoelectric point of a protein will also be known for a 2-D gel sample but this should also be treated with caution. If a number of larger size peptides are seen in the digest then the missed cleavages parameter should be increased. Typically this is set to 1 or 2. If the possibility of post-translational or other modification is uncertain, then the top three options should be selected, i.e. acetylation of the N terminus, oxidation of Met, and conversion of Glu to pyro-Glu. If phosphorylation of S, T or Y is selected when not suspected this may lead to false hits. More than one amino acid can usually be listed in the box (e.g. 'STY 80' to select any phosphorylation). The list of peptide masses should be input to four decimal places if possible. In the initial search, use masses from the higher signal intensity peaks and set the minimum number of peptides low as compared with the number of masses in the peptide list. To increase the specificity of the search this number can be increased. If no hits are found then this number can be decreased in subsequent passes. Be sure to select whether the fragment and precursor ions have been calculated from monoisotopic or average masses.

De-isotoping software is available to artificially remove the ^{13}C peaks arising from the presence of the ^{13}C isotopic form of carbon in otherwise chemically identical peptides. This simplifies the spectrum but more importantly this will ensure that the search algorithm will not be not confused and will attempt to find two or more distinct peptides that each differ by 1 Da. This is particularly valuable when one is analysing peptide mixtures, since overlapping isotope clusters are thus identified correctly and only the genuine ^{12}C peaks are reported. If the resolution of the mass spectrum is not sufficient to resolve individual isotope peaks then the average mass is often reported. This is still the case with larger polypeptides and proteins (see Fig. 9.14) but, in modern instruments, the all ^{12}C, one ^{13}C, two ^{13}C, etc. peptide forms can be resolved (see Fig. 9.13).

Various software packages (including commercial software packages such as *SEQUEST*) are available to use the information on the fragment ions obtained from a tandem MS experiment to search protein (and DNA translation) databases to identify the sequence and the protein from which it is derived. Once the protein has been identified, one can view the full protein summary and link to protein structure, Swiss 2-D PAGE, nucleic acid databases, etc.

9.8 **SUGGESTIONS FOR FURTHER READING**

AEBERSOLD, R. and MANN, M. (2003). Mass spectrometry-based proteomics. *Nature*, **422**, 198–207. (There are also a number of other, very informative proteomics reviews in this issue between pp. 193 and 225.)

HERNANDEZ, H. and ROBINSON, C. V. (2001). Dynamic protein complexes: insights from mass spectrometry. *Journal of Biological Chemistry*, **276**, 46685–46688.

LARSEN, M. R., SØRENSEN, G. L., FEY, S. J., LARSEN, P. M. and PROEPSTORFF, P. (2001). Phospho-proteomics: evaluation of the use of enzymatic de-phosphorylation and differential mass spectrometric peptide mass mapping for site specific phosphorylation assignment in proteins separated by gel electrophoresis. *Proteomics*, **1**, 223–238. (The paper reviews methods for identification of this important and widespread post-translational modification.)

MOSELEY, M. A. (2001). Current trends in differential expression proteomics: isotopically coded tags. *Trends in Biotechnology*, **19** (Suppl.), S10–S16. (A review of developments in isotopically coded tags, an innovation that allows quantitative analysis of differences in expression levels of protein between cells and tissues in different states, e.g. between diseased and normal.)

NELSON, R. W., NEDELKOV, D. and TABBS, K. A. (2000). Biosensor chip mass spectrometry: a chip-based proteomics approach. *Electrophoresis*, **21**, 1155–1163. (This is a review of biomolecular interaction analysis–mass spectrometry for the detailed characterization of proteins and protein–protein interactions and the development of biosensor chip mass spectrometry as a new chip-based proteomics approach.)

SIMPSON, R. J. (2003). *Proteins and Proteomics.* Cold Spring Harbor Laboratory Press, Cold Spring Harbor, NY. (This volume includes extensive coverage of protein mass spectrometry techniques).

Websites

The ExPASy (*E*xpert *P*rotein *A*nalysis *Sy*stem) server of the Swiss Institute of Bioinformatics (SIB) contains a large suite of programs for the analysis of protein sequences, structures and proteomics as well as 2-D PAGE analysis (2-D gel documentation and 2-D gel image analysis programs). The ExPASy suite of programmes is at <http://www.expasy.ch/> and <http://us.expasy.org/tools/>. Glyocomod and GlycanMass are found at <http://us.expasy.org/tools/glycomod/> and <http://us.expasy.org/tools/glycomod/glycanmass.html>, respectively.

Also, Deltamass is a database of protein post-translational modifications at <http://www.abrf.org/index.cfm/dm.home>, which can be accessed to determine whether post-translational modifications are present. There are hyperlinks to references to the modifications.

There is also a prediction program 'findmod' for finding potential protein post-translational modifications in the ExPASy suite at <http://expasy.org/tools/findmod/>.

Information and protocols for sample clean-up are found at the URLs <www.millipore.com/ziptip> and <http://www.nestgrp.com/protocols/protocols.shtml#massspec>'Stylus™ Pipette Tips for Protein Sample Preparation'.

Products for Phosphorylated Peptide and Protein Enrichment and Detection IMAC columns and chromatography may be found at <http:// www.piercenet. com/files/phosphor.pdf> and GelCode Phosphoprotein Staining Kit at <http:// www. piercenet.com/>.

Chapter 10

Electrophoretic techniques

10.1 **GENERAL PRINCIPLES**

The term electrophoresis describes the migration of a charged particle under the influence of an electric field. Many important biological molecules, such as amino acids, peptides, proteins, nucleotides and nucleic acids, possess ionisable groups and, therefore, at any given pH, exist in solution as electrically charged species either as cations (+) or anions (−). Under the influence of an electric field these charged particles will migrate either to the cathode or to the anode, depending on the nature of their net charge.

The equipment required for electrophoresis consists basically of two items, a power pack and an electrophoresis unit. Electrophoresis units are available for running either vertical or horizontal gel systems. Vertical slab gel units are commercially available and routinely used to separate proteins in acrylamide gels (Section 10.2). The gel is formed between two glass plates that are clamped together but held apart by plastic spacers. The most commonly used units are the so-called minigel apparatus (Fig. 10.1). Gel dimensions are typically 8.5 cm wide × 5 cm high, with a thickness of 0.5–1 mm. A plastic comb is placed in the gel solution and is removed after polymerisation to provide loading wells for up to 10 samples. When the apparatus is assembled, the lower electrophoresis tank buffer surrounds the gel plates and affords some cooling of the gel plates. A typical horizontal gel system is shown in Fig. 10.2. The gel is cast on a glass or plastic sheet and placed on a cooling plate (an insulated surface through which cooling water is passed to conduct away generated heat). Connection between the gel and electrode buffer is made using a thick wad of wetted filter paper (Fig. 10.2: note, however, that agarose gels for DNA electrophoresis are run submerged in the buffer (Section 10.4.1). The power pack supplies a direct current between the electrodes in the electrophoresis unit. All electrophoresis is carried out in an appropriate buffer, which is essential to maintain a constant state of ionisation of the molecules being separated. Any variation in pH would alter the overall charge and hence the mobilities (rate of migration in the applied field) of the molecules being separated.

In order to understand fully how charged species separate it is necessary to look at some simple equations relating to electrophoresis. When a potential difference (voltage) is applied across the electrodes, it generates a potential

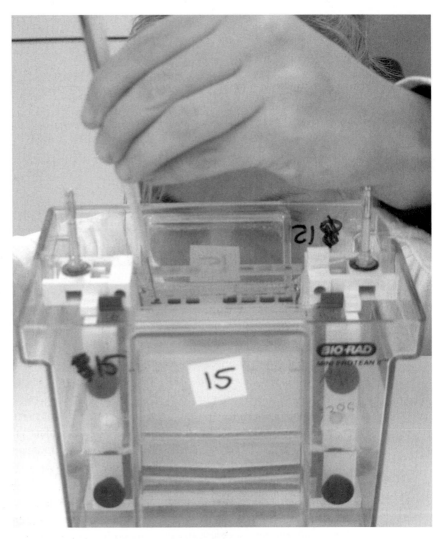

Fig. 10.1. Photograph showing samples being loaded into the wells of an SDS–PAGE minigel. Six wells that have been loaded can be identified by the blue dye (bromophenol blue) that is incorporated into the loading buffer.

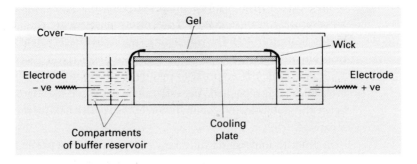

Fig. 10.2. A typical horizontal apparatus, such as that used for immunoelectrophoresis, isoelectric focusing and the electrophoresis of DNA and RNA in agarose gels.

gradient, E, which is the applied voltage, V, divided by the distance, d, between the electrodes. When this potential gradient E is applied, the force on a molecule bearing a charge of q coulombs is Eq newtons. It is this force that drives a charged molecule towards an electrode. However, there is also a frictional resistance that retards the movement of this charged molecule. This frictional force is a measure of the hydrodynamic size of the molecule, the shape of the molecule, the pore size of the medium in which electrophoresis is taking place and the viscosity of the buffer. The velocity, v, of a charged molecule in an electric field is therefore given by the equation:

$$v = \frac{Eq}{f}$$
(10.1)

where f is the frictional coefficient.

More commonly the term electrophoretic mobility (μ), of an ion is used, which is the ratio of the velocity of the ion to field strength (v/E). When a potential difference is applied, therefore, molecules with different overall charges will begin to separate owing to their different electrophoretic mobilities. Even molecules with similar charges will begin to separate if they have different molecular sizes, since they will experience different frictional forces. As will be seen below, some forms of electrophoresis rely almost totally on the different charges on molecules to effect separation, whilst other methods exploit differences in molecular size and therefore encourage frictional effects to bring about separation.

Provided the electric field is removed before the molecules in the sample reach the electrodes, the components will have been separated according to their electrophoretic mobility. Electrophoresis is thus an incomplete form of electrolysis. The separated samples are then located by staining with an appropriate dye or by autoradiography (Section 14.2.3) if the sample is radiolabelled.

The current in the solution between the electrodes is conducted mainly by the buffer ions, a small proportion being conducted by the sample ions. Ohm's law expresses the relationship between current (I), voltage (V) and resistance (R):

$$\frac{V}{I} = R$$
(10.2)

It therefore appears that it is possible to accelerate an electrophoretic separation by increasing the applied voltage, which would result in a corresponding increase in the current flowing. The distance migrated by the ions will be proportional to both current and time. However, this would ignore one of the major problems for most forms of electrophoresis, namely the generation of heat.

During electrophoresis the power (W, watts) generated in the supporting medium is given by

$$W = I^2 R$$
(10.3)

Most of this power generated is dissipated as heat. Heating of the electrophoretic medium has the following effects:

- An increased rate of diffusion of sample and buffer ions leading to broadening of the separated samples.
- The formation of convection currents, which leads to mixing of separated samples.
- Thermal instability of samples that are rather sensitive to heat. This may include denaturation of proteins (e.g. thus the loss of enzyme activity).
- A decrease of buffer viscosity, and hence a reduction in the resistance of the medium.

If a constant voltage is applied, the current increases during electrophoresis owing to the decrease in resistance (see Ohm's law, equation 10.2) and the rise in current increases the heat output still further. For this reason, workers often use a stabilised power supply, which provides constant power and thus eliminates fluctuations in heating.

Constant heat generation is, however, a problem. The answer might appear to be to run the electrophoresis at very low power (low current) to overcome any heating problem, but this can lead to poor separations as a result of the increased amount of diffusion resulting from long separation times. Compromise conditions, therefore, have to be found with reasonable power settings, to give acceptable separation times, and an appropriate cooling system, to remove liberated heat. While such systems work fairly well, the effects of heating are not always totally eliminated. For example, for electrophoresis carried out in cylindrical tubes or in slab gels, although heat is generated uniformly through the medium, heat is removed only from the edges, resulting in a temperature gradient within the gel, the temperature at the centre of the gel being higher than that at the edges. Since the warmer fluid at the centre is less viscous, electrophoretic mobilities are therefore greater in the central region (electrophoretic mobilities increase by about 2% for each 1 °C rise in temperature), and electrophoretic zones develop a bowed shape, with the zone centre migrating faster than the edges.

A final factor that can effect electrophoretic separation is the phenomenon of electroendosmosis (also known as electroosmotic flow), which is due to the presence of charged groups on the surface of the support of the support medium. For example, paper has some carboxyl groups present, agarose (depending on the purity grade) contains sulphate groups and the surface of glass walls used in capillary electrophoresis (Section 10.5) contains silanol (Si—OH) groups. Figure 10.3 demonstrates how electroendosmosis occurs in a capillary tube, although the principle is the same for any support medium that has charged groups on it. In a fused-silica capillary tube, above a pH value of about 3, silanol groups on the silica capillary wall will ionise, generating negatively charged sites. It is these charges that generate electroendosmosis. The ionised silanol groups create an electrical double layer, or region of charge separation, at the capillary wall/electrolyte interface. When a voltage is applied, cations in the electrolyte near the capillary wall migrate towards the cathode, pulling electrolyte solution with them. This creates a net electroosmotic flow towards the cathode.

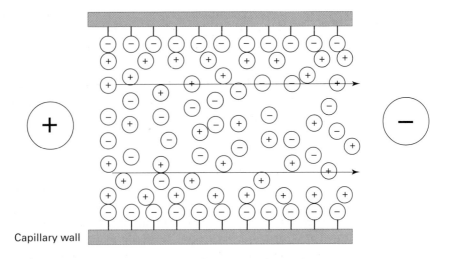

Capillary wall

• Acidic silanol groups impart negative charge on wall
• Counter ions migrate toward cathode, dragging solvent along

Fig. 10.3. Electroosmotic flow through a glass capillary. Electrolyte cations are attracted to the capillary walls, forming an electrical double layer. When a voltage is applied, the net movement of electrolyte solution towards the cathode is known as electro-endosmotic flow.

10.2 SUPPORT MEDIA

The pioneering work on electrophoresis by A. Tiselius and co-workers was performed in free solution. However, it was soon realised that many of the problems associated with this approach, particularly the adverse effects of diffusion and convection currents, could be minimised by stabilising the medium. This was achieved by carrying out electrophoresis on a porous mechanical support, which was wetted in electrophoresis buffer and in which electrophoresis of buffer ions and samples could occur. The support medium cuts down convection currents and diffusion so that the separated components remain as sharp zones. The earliest supports used were filter paper or cellulose acetate strips, wetted in electrophoresis buffer. Nowadays these media are infrequently used, although cellulose acetate still has its uses (see Section 10.3.6). In particular, for many years small molecules such as amino acids, peptides and carbohydrates were routinely separated and analysed by electrophoresis on supports such as paper or thin-layer plates of cellulose, silica or alumina. Although occasionally still used nowadays, such molecules are now more likely to be analysed by more modern and sensitive techniques such as high performance liquid chromatography (Section 11.3.2). While paper or thin-layer supports are fine for resolving small molecules, the separation of macromolecules such as proteins and nucleic acids on such supports is poor.

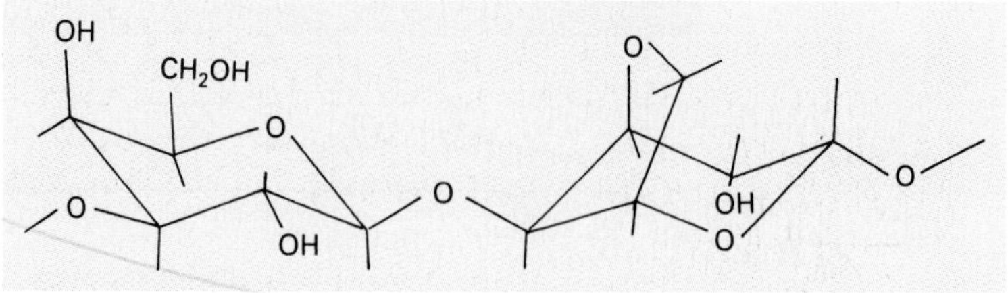

Fig. 10.4. Agarobiose, the repeating unit of agarose.

However, the introduction of the use of gels as a support medium led to a rapid improvement in methods for analysing macromolecules. The earliest gel system to be used was the starch gel and, although this still has some uses, the vast majority of electrophoretic techniques used nowadays involve either agarose gels or polyacrylamide gels.

10.2.1 Agarose gels

Agarose is a linear polysaccharide (average relative molecular mass about 12 000) made up of the basic repeat unit agarobiose, which comprises alternating units of galactose and 3,6-anhydrogalactose (Fig. 10.4). Agarose is one of the components of agar that is a mixture of polysaccharides isolated from certain seaweeds. Agarose is usually used at concentrations of between 1% and 3%. Agarose gels are formed by suspending dry agarose in aqueous buffer, then boiling the mixture until a clear solution forms. This is poured and allowed to cool to room temperature to form a rigid gel. The gelling properties are attributed to both inter- and intramolecular hydrogen bonding within and between the long agarose chains. This cross-linked structure gives the gel good anticonvectional properties. The pore size in the gel is controlled by the initial concentration of agarose; large pore sizes are formed from low concentrations and smaller pore sizes are formed from the higher concentrations. Although essentially free from charge, substitution of the alternating sugar residues with carboxyl, methyoxyl, pyruvate and especially sulphate groups occurs to varying degrees. This substitution can result in electroendosmosis during electrophoresis and ionic interactions between the gel and sample in all uses, both unwanted effects. Agarose is therefore sold in different purity grades, based on the sulphate concentration – the lower the sulphate content, the higher the purity.

Agarose gels are used for the electrophoresis of both proteins and nucleic acids. For proteins, the pore sizes of a 1% agarose gel are large relative to the sizes of proteins. Agarose gels are therefore used in techniques such as immunoelectrophoresis (Section 7.4.1) or flat-bed isoelectric focusing (Section 10.3.4), where the proteins are required to move unhindered in the gel matrix according to their native charge. Such large pore gels are also used to separate much larger molecules such as DNA or RNA, because the pore sizes in the gel are still large enough for DNA or RNA molecules to pass through the gel. Now, however, the pore size and molecule size are more comparable and frictional effects begin to play a role in the separation of these molecules (Section 10.4). A further advantage of using agarose is the availability of low melting temperature agarose (62–65 °C). As the name suggests, these gels can be reliquified by heating to 65 °C and thus, for example, DNA samples separated in a gel can be cut out of the gel, returned to solution and recovered.

Owing to the poor elasticity of agarose gels and the consequent problems of removing them from small tubes, the gel rod system sometimes used for acrylamide gels is not used. Horizontal slab gels are invariably used for isoelectric focusing or immunoelectrophoresis in agarose. Horizontal gels are also used routinely for DNA and RNA gels (Section 10.4), although vertical systems have been used by some workers.

10.2.2 Polyacrylamide gels

Electrophoresis in acrylamide gels is frequently referred to as PAGE, being an abbreviation for polyacrylamide gel electrophoresis.

Cross-linked polyacrylamide gels are formed from the polymerisation of acrylamide monomer in the presence of smaller amounts of N,N'-methylene-bisacrylamide (normally referred to as 'bis'-acrylamide) (Fig. 10.5). Note that bis-acrylamide is essentially two acrylamide molecules linked by a methylene group, and is used as a cross-linking agent. Acrylamide monomer is polymerised in a head-to-tail fashion into long chains and occasionally a bis-acrylamide molecule is built into the growing chain, thus introducing a second site for chain extension. Proceeding in this way a cross-linked matrix of fairly well-defined structure is formed (Fig. 10.5). The polymerisation of acrylamide is an example of free-radical catalysis, and is initiated by the addition of ammonium persulphate and the base N,N,N',N'-tetramethylenediamine (TEMED). TEMED catalyses the decomposition of the persulphate ion to give a free radical (i.e. a molecule with an unpaired electron):

$$S_2O_8^{2-} + e^- \rightarrow SO_4^{2-} + SO_4^-{}^{\bullet}$$

If this free radical is represented as R$^{\bullet}$ (where the dot represents an unpaired electron) and M as an acrylamide monomer molecule, then the polymerisation can be represented as follows:

R$^{\bullet}$ + M → RM$^{\bullet}$

RM$^{\bullet}$ + M → RMM$^{\bullet}$

RMM$^{\bullet}$ + M → RMMM$^{\bullet}$ etc.

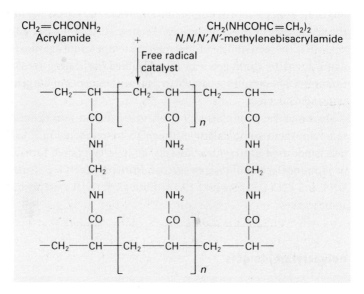

Fig. 10.5. The formation of a polyacrylamide gel from acrylamide and bis-acrylamide.

Free radicals are highly reactive species due to the presence of an unpaired elec-tron that needs to be paired with another electron to stabilise the molecule. R·therefore reacts with M, forming a single bond by sharing its unpaired electron with one from the outer shell of the monomer molecule. This therefore produces a new free radical molecule $R-M'$, which is equally reactive and will attack a further monomer molecule. In this way long chains of acrylamide are built up, being cross-linked by the introduction of the occasional bis-acrylamide molecule into the growing chain. Oxygen mops up free radicals and therefore all gel solutions are normally degassed (the solutions are briefly placed under vacuum to remove loosely dissolved air) prior to use. The degassing of the gel solution also serves a second purpose. The polymerisation of acrylamide is an exothermic reac-tion (i.e. heat is liberated) and the warming up of the gel solution as it sets can liberate air bubbles that become trapped in the polymerised gel. The degassing step prevents this possibility.

Photopolymerisation is an alternative method that can be used to polymer-ise acrylamide gels. The ammonium persulphate and TEMED are replaced by riboflavin and when the gel is poured it is placed in front of a bright light for 2–3 h. Photodecomposition of riboflavin generates a free radical that initiates polymerisation.

Acrylamide gels are defined in terms of the total percentage of acrylamide present, and the pore size in the gel can be varied by changing the concentrations of both the acrylamide and bis-acrylamide. Acrylamide gels can be made with a content of between 3% and 30% acrylamide. Thus low percentage gels (e.g. 4%) have large pore sizes and are used, for example, in the electrophoresis of proteins, where free movement of the proteins by electrophoresis is required without any noticeable frictional effect, for example in flat-bed isoelectric focusing (Section 10.3.4) or the stacking gel system of an SDS–polyacrylamide gel (Section 10.3.1).

Low percentage acrylamide gels are also used to separate DNA (Section 10.4). Gels of between 10% and 20% acrylamide are used in techniques such as SDS–gel electrophoresis, where the smaller pore size now introduces a sieving effect that contributes to the separation of proteins according to their size (Section 10.3.1).

Proteins were originally separated on polyacrylamide gels that were polymerised in glass tubes, approximately 7 mm in diameter and about 10 cm in length. The tubes were easy to load and run, with minimum apparatus requirements. However, only one sample could be run per tube and, because conditions of separation could vary from tube to tube, comparison between different samples was not always accurate. The later introduction of vertical gel slabs allowed running of up to 20 samples under identical conditions in a single run. Vertical slabs are now used routinely both for the analysis of proteins (Section 10.3) and for the separation of DNA fragments during DNA sequence analysis (Section 10.4). Although some workers prepare their own acrylamide gels, others purchase commercially available ready-made gels for techniques such as SDS–PAGE, native gels and isoelectric focusing (IEF) (see below).

10.3 ELECTROPHORESIS OF PROTEINS

10.3.1 Sodium dodecyl sulphate–polyacrylamide gel electrophoresis

SDS–polyacrylamide gel electrophoresis (SDS–PAGE) is the most widely used method for analysing protein mixtures qualitatively. It is particularly useful for monitoring protein purification and, because the method is based on the separation of proteins according to size, it can also be used to determine the relative molecular mass of proteins. SDS ($CH_3-(CH_2)_{10}-CH_2OSO_3^-Na^+$) is an anionic detergent. Samples to be run on SDS–PAGE are firstly boiled for 5 min in sample buffer containing β-mercaptoethanol and SDS. The mercaptoethanol reduces any disulphide bridges present that are holding together the protein tertiary structure, and the SDS binds strongly to, and denatures, the protein. Each protein in the mixture is therefore fully denatured by this treatment and opens up into a rod-shaped structure with a series of negatively charged SDS molecules along the polypeptide chain. On average, one SDS molecule binds for every two amino acid residues. The original native charge on the molecule is therefore completely swamped by the negatively charged SDS molecules. The rod-like structure remains, as any rotation that tends to fold up the protein chain would result in repulsion between negative charges on different parts of the protein chain, returning the conformation back to the rod shape. The sample buffer also contains an ionisable tracking dye, usually bromophenol blue, that allows the electrophoretic run to be monitored, and sucrose or glycerol, which gives the sample solution density thus allowing the sample to settle easily through the electrophoresis buffer to the bottom when injected into the loading well (see Fig. 10.1). Once the samples are all loaded, a current is passed through the gel. The samples to be separated are not in fact loaded directly into the main separating gel. When the main separating gel (normally about 5 cm long) has been poured between the glass plates and allowed to set, a shorter (approximately 0.8 cm) stacking gel is poured on top of the separating gel and it is into this gel that the wells are formed and the proteins loaded. The purpose of this stacking gel is to concentrate the protein sample into a sharp band before it enters the main separating gel. This is achieved by utilising differences in ionic strength and pH between the electrophoresis buffer and the stacking gel buffer and involves a phenomenon known as isotacho-phoresis. The stacking gel has a very large pore size (4% acrylamide), which allows the proteins to move freely and concentrate, or stack, under the effect of the electric field. The band-sharpening effect relies on the fact that negatively charged glycinate ions (in the electrophoresis buffer) have a lower electrophoretic mobility than do the protein–SDS complexes, which, in turn, have lower mobility than the chloride ions (Cl$^-$) of the loading buffer and the stacking gel buffer. When the current is switched on, all the ionic species have to migrate at the same speed otherwise there would be a break in the electrical circuit. The glycinate ions can move at the same speed as Cl$^-$ only if they are in a region of higher field strength. Field strength is inversely proportional to conductivity, which is proportional to concentration. The result is that the three species of interest adjust their concentrations so that [Cl$^-$] > [protein–SDS] > [glycinate]. There is only a small quantity of protein–SDS complexes, so they concentrate in a very tight band between glycinate and Cl$^-$ boundaries. Once the glycinate reaches the separating gel it becomes more fully ionised in the higher pH environment and its mobility increases. (The pH of the stacking gel is 6.8, that of the separating gel is 8.8.) Thus, the interface between glycinate and Cl$^-$ leaves behind the protein–SDS complexes, which are left to electrophorese at their own rates. The negatively charged protein–SDS complexes now continue to move towards the anode, and, because they have the same charge per unit length, they travel into the separating gel under the applied electric field with the same mobility. However, as they pass through the separating gel the proteins separate, owing to the molecular sieving properties of the gel. Quite simply, the smaller the protein the more easily it can pass through the pores of the gel, whereas large proteins are successively retarded by frictional resistance due to the sieving effect of the gels. Being a small molecule, the bromophenol blue dye is totally unretarded and therefore indicates the electrophoresis front. When the dye reaches the bottom of the gel, the current is turned off, and the gel is removed from between the glass plates and shaken in an appropriate stain solution (usually Coomassie Brilliant Blue, see Section 10.3.7) and then washed in destain solution. The destain solution removes unbound background dye from the gel, leaving stained proteins visible as blue bands on a clear background. A typical minigel would take about 1 h to prepare and set, 40 min to run at 200 V and have a 1 h staining time with Coomassie Brilliant Blue. Upon destaining, strong protein bands would be seen in the gel within 10–20 min, but overnight destaining is needed to completely remove all background stain. Vertical slab gels are invariably run, since this allows up to 10 different samples to be loaded onto a single gel. A typical SDS–polyacrylamide gel is shown in Fig. 10.6.

Typically, the separating gel used is a 15% polyacrylamide gel. This gives a gel of a certain pore size in which proteins of relative molecular mass (M_r) 10 000 move through the gel relatively unhindered, whereas proteins of M_r 100 000 can only

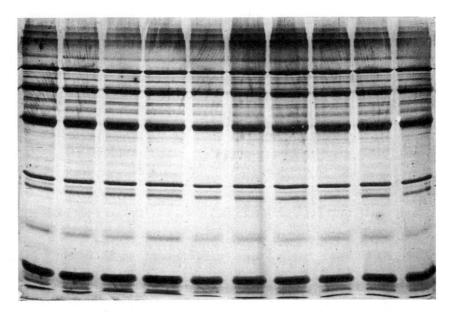

Fig. 10.6. A typical SDS–polyacrylamide gel. All 10 wells in the gel have been loaded with the same complex mixture of proteins. (Courtesy of Bio-Rad Laboratories.)

just enter the pores of this gel. Gels of 15% polyacrylamide are therefore useful for separating proteins in the range M_r 100 000 to 10 000. However, a protein of M_r 150 000, for example, would be unable to enter a 15% gel. In this case a larger-pored gel (e.g. a 10% or even 7.5% gel) would be used so that the protein could now enter the gel and be stained and identified. It is obvious, therefore, that the choice of gel to be used depends on the size of the protein being studied. The fractionation range of different percentage acrylamide gels is shown in Table 10.1. This shows, for example, that in a 10% polyacrylamide gel proteins greater than 200 kDa in mass cannot enter the gel, whereas proteins with relative molecular mass (M_r) in the range 200 000 to 15 000 will separate. Proteins of M_r 15 000 or less are too small to experience the sieving effect of the gel matrix, and all run together as a single band at the electrophoresis front.

The M_r of a protein can be determined by comparing its mobility with those of a number of standard proteins of known M_r that are run on the same gel. By plotting a graph of distance moved against log M_r for each of the standard proteins, a calibration curve can be constructed. The distance moved by the protein of unknown M_r is then measured, and then its log M_r and hence M_r can be determined from the calibration curve.

SDS–gel electrophoresis is often used after each step of a purification protocol to assess the purity or otherwise of the sample. A pure protein should give a single band on an SDS–polyacrylamide gel, unless the molecule is made up of two unequal subunits. In the latter case two bands, corresponding to the two subunits, will be seen. Since only submicrogram amounts of protein are needed for the gel, very little material is used in this form of purity assessment and at the same time a

Table 10.1 The relationship between acrylamide gel concentration and protein fractionation range

Acrylamide concentration (%)	Protein fractionation range ($M_r \times 10^{-3}$)
5	60–350
10	15–200
15	10–100

value for the relative molecular mass of the protein can be determined on the same gel run (as described above), with no more material being used.

Example 1   MOLECULAR MASS DETERMINATION BY ELECTROPHORESIS

Question

The following table shows the distance moved in an SDS–polyacrylamide gel by a series of marker proteins of known relative molecular mass (M_r). A newly purified protein (X) run on the same gel showed a single band that had moved a distance of 45 mm. What was the M_r of protein X?

Protein	M_r	Distance moved (mm)
Transferrin	78 000	6.0
Bovine serum albumin	66 000	12.5
Ovalbumin (egg albumin)	45 000	32.0
Glyceraldehyde-3-phosphate dehydrogenase	36 000	38.0
Carbonic anhydrase	29 000	50.0
Trypsinogen	24 000	54.0
Soyabean trypsin inhibitor	20 100	61.0
β-Lactoglobulin	18 400[a]	69.0
Myoglobin	17 800	69.0
Lysozyme	14 300	79.0
Cytochrome c	12 400	86.5

[a] Note: β-lactoglobulin has a relative molecular mass of 36 800 but is a dimer of two identical subunits of 18 400 relative molecular mass. Under the reducing conditions of the sample buffer the disulphide bridges linking the subunits are reduced and thus the monomer chains are seen on the gel.

Answer

Construct a calibration graph by plotting log M_r versus distance moved for each of the marker proteins. From a graph of log M_r versus the distance moved by each protein you can determine a relative molecular mass for protein X of approximately 31 000. Note that this method is accurate to ± 10%, so your answer is 31 000 ± 3100.

10.3.2 Native (buffer) gels

While SDS–PAGE is the most frequently used gel system for studying proteins, the method is of no use if one is aiming to detect a particular protein (often an enzyme) on the basis of its biological activity, because the protein (enzyme) is denatured by the SDS–PAGE procedure. In this case it is necessary to use non-denaturing conditions. In native or buffer gels, polyacrylamide gels are again used (normally a 7.5% gel) but the SDS is absent and the proteins are *not* denatured prior to loading. Since all the proteins in the sample being analysed carry their native charge at the pH of the gel (normally pH 8.7), proteins separate according to their different electrophoretic mobilities *and* the sieving effects of the gel. It is therefore not possible to predict the behaviour of a given protein in a buffer gel but, because of the range of different charges and sizes of proteins in a given protein mixture, good resolution is achieved. The enzyme of interest can be identified by incubating the gel in an appropriate substrate solution such that a coloured product is produced at the site of the enzyme. An alternative method for enzyme detection is to include the substrate in an agarose gel that is poured over the acrylamide gel and allowed to set. Diffusion and interaction of enzyme and substrate between the two gels results in colour formation at the site of the enzyme. Often, duplicate samples will be run on a gel, the gel cut in half and one half stained for activity, the other for total protein. In this way the total protein content of the sample can be analysed and the particular band corresponding to the enzyme identified by reference to the activity stain gel.

10.3.3 Gradient gels

This is again a polyacrylamide gel system, but instead of running a slab gel of uniform pore size throughout (e.g. a 15% gel) a gradient gel is formed, where the acrylamide concentration varies uniformly from, typically, 5% at the top of the gel to 25% acrylamide at the bottom of the gel. The gradient is formed via a gradient mixer (Section 11.3.1) and run down between the glass plates of a slab gel. The higher percentage acrylamide (e.g. 25%) is poured between the glass plates first and a continuous gradient of decreasing acrylamide concentration follows. Therefore at the top of the gel there is a large pore size (5% acrylamide) but as the sample moves down through the gel the acrylamide concentration slowly increases and the pore size correspondingly decreases. Gradient gels are normally run as SDS gels with a stacking gel. There are two advantages to running gradient gels. First, a much greater range of protein M_r values can be separated than on a fixed-percentage gel. In a complex mixture, very low molecular weight proteins travel freely through the gel to begin with, and start to resolve when they reach the smaller pore sizes towards the lower part of the gel. Much larger proteins, on the other hand, can still enter the gel but start to separate immediately due to the sieving effect of the gel. The second advantage of gradient gels is that proteins with very similar M_r values may be resolved, although they cannot otherwise be resolved in fixed percentage gels. As each protein moves through the gel the pore sizes become smaller until the protein reaches its pore size limit. The pore size in the gel is now too small to allow passage of the protein, and the protein sample stacks up at this point as a sharp band. A similar-sized protein, but with slightly lower M_r will be able to travel a little further through the gel before reaching its

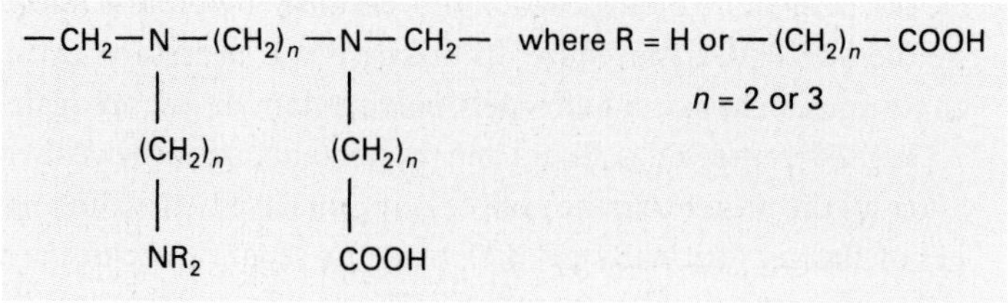

$$-CH_2-N-(CH_2)_n-N-CH_2- \quad \text{where } R = H \text{ or } -(CH_2)_n-COOH$$

$$n = 2 \text{ or } 3$$

$$(CH_2)_n \qquad (CH_2)_n$$

$$NR_2 \qquad COOH$$

Fig. 10.7. The general formula for ampholytes.

pore size limit, at which point it will form a sharp band. These two proteins, of slightly different M_r values, therefore separate as two, close, sharp bands.

10.3.4 Isoelectric focusing gels

This method is ideal for the separation of amphoteric substances such as proteins because it is based on the separation of molecules according to their different isoelectric points (Section 8.1). The method has high resolution, being able to separate proteins that differ in their isoelectric points by as little as 0.01 of a pH unit. The most widely used system for IEF utilises horizontal gels on glass plates or plastic sheets. Separation is achieved by applying a potential difference across a gel that contains a pH gradient. The pH gradient is formed by the introduction into the gel of compounds known as ampholytes, which are complex mixtures of synthetic polyamino-polycarboxylic acids (Fig. 10.7). Ampholytes can be purchased in different pH ranges covering either a wide band (e.g. pH 3–10) or various narrow bands (e.g. pH 7–8), and a pH range is chosen such that the samples being separated will have their isoelectric points (pI values) within this range. Commercially available ampholytes include Bio-Lyte and Pharmalyte.

Traditionally 1–2 mm thick IEF gels have been used by research workers, but the relatively high cost of ampholytes makes this a fairly expensive procedure if a number of gels are to be run. However, the introduction of thin-layer IEF gels, which are only 0.15 mm thick and which are prepared using a layer of electrical insulation tape as the spacer between the gel plates, has considerably reduced the cost of preparing IEF gels, and such gels are now commonly used. Since this method requires the proteins to move freely according to their charge under the electric field, IEF is carried out in low percentage gels to avoid any sieving effect within the gel. Polyacrylamide gels (4%) are commonly used, but agarose is also used, especially for the study of high M_r proteins that may undergo some sieving even in a low percentage acrylamide gel.

To prepare a thin-layer IEF gel, carrier ampholytes, covering a suitable pH range, and riboflavin are mixed with the acrylamide solution, and the mixture is then poured over a glass plate (typically 25 cm × 10 cm), which contains the spacer. The second glass plate is then placed on top of the first to form the gel cassette, and the gel polymerised by photopolymerisation by placing the gel in front of a bright light. The photodecomposition of the riboflavin generates a free radical, which initiates polymerisation (Section 10.2.2). This takes 2–3 h. Once the gel has set, the glass plates are prised apart to reveal the gel stuck to one of the glass sheets. Electrode wicks, which are thick (3 mm) strips of wetted filter paper (the anode is phosphoric acid, the cathode sodium hydroxide) are laid along the long length of each side of the gel and a potential difference applied. Under the effect of this potential difference, the ampholytes form a pH gradient between the anode and cathode. The power is then turned off and samples applied by laying on the gel small squares of filter paper soaked in the sample. A voltage is again applied for about 30 min to allow the sample to electrophorese off the paper and into the gel, at which time the paper squares can be removed from the gel. Depending on which point on the pH gradient the sample has been loaded, proteins that are initially at a pH region below their isoelectric point will be positively charged and will initially migrate towards the cathode. As they proceed, however, the surrounding pH will be steadily increasing, and therefore the positive charge on the protein will decrease correspondingly until eventually the protein arrives at a point where the pH is equal to its isoelectric point. The protein will now be in the zwitterion form with no net charge, so further movement will cease. Likewise, substances that are initially at pH regions above their isoelectric points will be negatively charged and will migrate towards the anode until they reach their isoelectric points and become stationary. It can be seen that as the samples will always move towards their isoelectric points it is not critical where on the gel they are applied. To achieve rapid separations (2–3 h) relatively high voltages (up to 2500 V) are used. As considerable heat is produced, gels are run on cooling plates (10 °C) and power packs used to stabilise the power output and thus to minimise thermal fluctuations. Following electrophoresis, the gel must be stained to detect the proteins. However, this cannot be done directly, because the ampholytes will stain too, giving a totally blue gel. The gel is therefore first washed with fixing solution (e.g. 10% (v/v) trichloroacetic acid). This precipitates the proteins in the gel and allows the much smaller ampholytes to be washed out. The gel is stained with Coomassie Brilliant Blue and then destained (Section 10.3.7). A typical IEF gel is shown in Fig. 10.8. The technique is very similar to the technique of chromatofocusing (Section 11.6.3).

The pI of a particular protein may be determined conveniently by running a mixture of proteins of known isoelectric point on the same gel. A number of mixtures of proteins with differing pI values are commercially available, covering the pH range 3.5–10. After staining, the distance of each band from one electrode is measured and a graph of distance for each protein against its pI (effectively the pH at that point) plotted. By means of this calibration line, the pI of an unknown protein can be determined from its position on the gel.

IEF is a highly sensitive analytical technique and is particularly useful for studying microheterogeneity in a protein. For example, a protein may show a single band on an SDS gel, but may show three bands on an IEF gel. This may occur, for example, when a protein exists in mono-, di- and tri-phosphorylated forms. The difference of a couple of phosphate groups has no significant effect on the overall relative molecular mass of the protein, hence a single band on SDS gels, but the small charge difference introduced on each molecule can be detected by IEF.

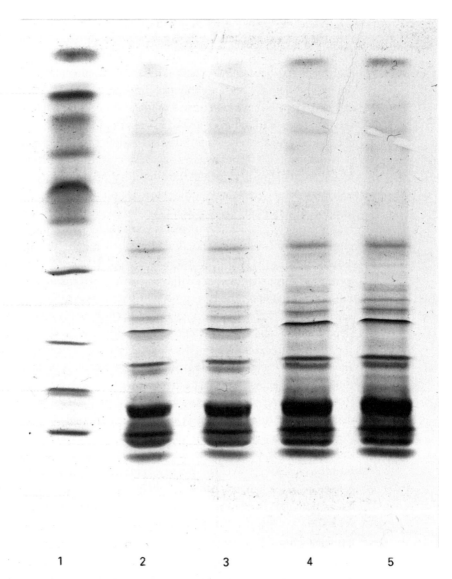

Fig. 10.8. A typical isoelectric focusing gel. Track 1 contains a mixture of standard proteins of known isoelectric points. Tracks 2–5 show increasing loadings of venom from the Japanese water moccasin snake. (Courtesy of Bio-Rad Laboratories Ltd.)

The method is particularly useful for separating isoenzymes (Section 8.2), which are different forms of the same enzyme often differing by only one or two amino acid residues. Since the proteins are in their native form, enzymes can be detected in the gel either by washing the unfixed and unstained gel in an appropriate substrate or by overlayering with agarose containing the substrate. The approach has found particular use in forensic science, where traces of blood or other biological fluids can be analysed and compared according to the composition of certain isoenzymes.

Although IEF is used mainly for analytical separations, it can also be used for preparative purposes. In vertical column IEF, a water-cooled vertical glass column is used, filled with a mixture of ampholytes dissolved in a sucrose solution containing a density gradient to prevent diffusion. When the separation is complete, the current is switched off and the sample components run out through a valve in the base of the column. Alternatively, preparative IEF can be carried out in beds of granulated gel, such as Sephadex G-75 (Section 11.8.2).

10.3.5 Two-dimensional polyacrylamide gel electrophoresis

This technique combines the technique of IEF (first dimension), which separates proteins in a mixture according to charge (pI), with the size separation technique of SDS–PAGE (second dimension). The combination of these two techniques to give two-dimensional (2-D) PAGE provides a highly sophisticated analytical method for analysing protein mixtures. To maximise separation, most workers use large format 2-D gels (20 cm × 20 cm), although the minigel system can be used to provide useful separation in some cases. For large-format gels, the first dimension (isoelectric focusing) is carried out in an acrylamide gel that has been cast on a plastic strip (18 cm × 3 mm wide). The gel contains ampholytes (for forming the pH gradient) together with 8 M urea and a non-ionic detergent, both of which denature and maintain the solubility of the proteins being analysed. The denatured proteins therefore separate in this gel according to their isoelectric points. The IEF strip is then incubated in a sample buffer containing SDS (thus binding SDS to the denatured proteins) and then placed between the glass plates of, and on top of, a previously prepared 10% SDS–PAGE gel. Electrophoresis is commenced and the SDS-bound proteins run into the gel and separate according to size, as described in Section 10.3.1. The IEF gels are provided as dried strips and need rehydrating overnight. The first dimension IEF run then takes 6–8 h, the equilibration step with SDS sample buffer takes about 15 min, and then the SDS–PAGE step takes about 5 h. A typical 2-D gel is shown in Fig. 10.9. Using this method one can routinely resolve between 1000 and 3000 proteins from a cell or tissue extract and in some cases workers have reported the separation of between 5000 and 10 000 proteins. The applications of 2-D PAGE, and a description of the method's central role in proteomics is described in Section 8.5.1.

10.3.6 Cellulose acetate electrophoresis

Although one of the older methods, cellulose acetate electrophoresis still has a number of applications. In particular it has retained a use in the clinical analysis of serum samples. Cellulose acetate has the advantage over paper in that it is a much more homogeneous medium, with uniform pore size, and does not adsorb proteins in the way that paper does. There is therefore much less trailing of protein bands and resolution is better, although nothing like as good as that achieved with polyacrylamide gels. The method is, however, far simpler to set up and run. Single

pl

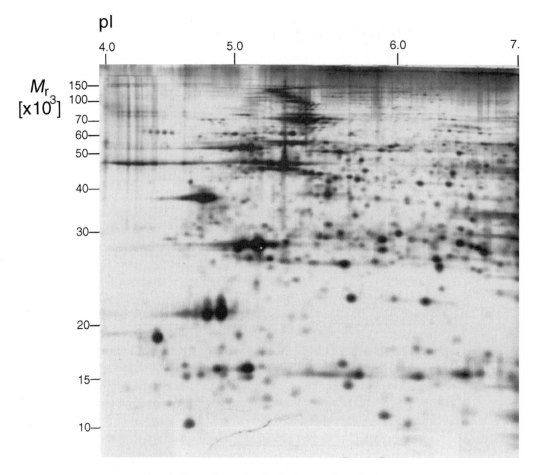

Fig. 10.9. A typical two-dimensional gel. The sample applied was 100 μg of total protein extracted from a normal dog heart ventricle. The first dimension was carried out using a pH 4–7 isoelectric-focusing gel. The second dimension was a 12% SDS–PAGE vertical slab gel. The pattern was visualised by silver staining. (Courtesy of Monique Heinke and Dr Mike Dunn, Division of Cardiothoracic Surgery, Imperial College School of Medicine, Heart Science Centre, Harefield, UK.)

samples are normally run on cellulose acetate strips (2.5 cm × 12 cm), although multiple samples are frequently run on wider sheets. The cellulose acetate is first wetted in electrophoresis buffer (pH 8.6 for serum samples) and the sample (1–2 mm³) loaded as a 1 cm wide strip about one-third of the way along the strip. The ends of the strip make contact with the electrophoresis buffer tanks via a filter paper wick that overlaps the end of the cellulose acetate strip, and electrophoresis conducted at 6–8 V cm⁻¹ for about 3 h. Following electrophoresis, the strip is stained for protein (see Section 10.3.7), destained, and the bands visualised. A typical serum protein separation shows about six major bands. However, in many disease states, this serum protein profile changes and a clinician can obtain information concerning the disease state of a patient from the altered pattern. Although

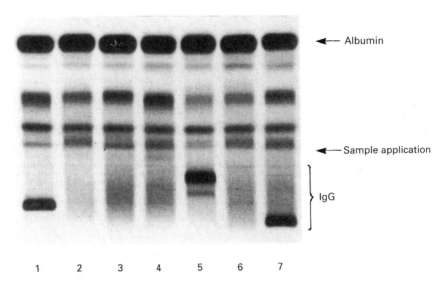

Fig. 10.10. Electrophoresis of human serum samples on an agarose gel. Tracks 2, 3, 4 and 6 show normal serum protein profiles. Tracks 1, 5 and 7 show myeloma patients, who are identified by the excessive production of a particular monoclonal antibody seen in the IgG fraction. (Courtesy of Charles Andrews and Nicholas Cundy, Edgware General Hospital, London.)

still frequently used for serum analysis, electrophoresis on cellulose acetate is being replaced by the use of agarose gels, which give similar but somewhat better resolution. A typical example of the analysis of serum on an agarose gel is shown in Fig. 10.10. Similar patterns are obtained when cellulose acetate is used.

Enzymes can easily be detected, in samples electrophoresed on cellulose acetate, by using the zymogram technique. The cellulose strip is laid on a strip of filter paper soaked in buffer and substrate. After an appropriate incubation period, the strips are peeled apart and the paper zymogram treated accordingly to detect enzyme product; hence, it is possible to identify the position of the enzyme activity on the original strip. An alternative approach to detecting and semiquantifying *any* particular protein on a strip is to treat the strip as the equivalent of a protein blot and to probe for the given protein using primary antibody and then enzyme-linked secondary antibody (Section 10.3.8). Substrate colour development indicates the presence of the particular protein and the amount of colour developed in a given time is a semiquantitative measure of the amount of protein. Thus, for example, large numbers of serum samples can be run on a wide sheet, the sheet probed using antibodies, and elevated levels of a particular protein identified in certain samples by increased levels of colour development in these samples.

10.3.7 Detection, estimation and recovery of proteins in gels

The most commonly used general protein stain for detecting protein on gels is the sulphated trimethylamine dye Coomassie Brilliant Blue R-250 (CBB). Staining is usually carried out using 0.1% (w/v) CBB in methanol:water:glacial acetic acid (45:45:10, by vol.). This acid–methanol mixture acts as a denaturant to precipitate or fix the protein in the gel, which prevents the protein from being washed out whilst it is being stained. Staining of most gels is accomplished in about 2 h and destaining, usually overnight, is achieved by gentle agitation in the same acid–methanol solution but in the absence of the dye. The Coomassie stain is highly sensitive; a very weakly staining band on a polyacrylamide gel would correspond to about 0.1 μg (100 ng) of protein. The CBB stain is not used for staining cellulose acetate (or indeed protein blots) because it binds quite strongly to the paper. In this case, proteins are first denatured by brief immersion of the strip in 10% (v/v) trichloroacetic acid, and then immersed in a solution of a dye that does not stain the support material, for example Procion blue, Amido black or Procion S.

Although the Coomassie stain is highly sensitive, many workers require greater sensitivity such as that provided by silver staining. Silver stains are based either on techniques developed for histology or on methods based on the photographic process. In either case, silver ions (Ag^+) are reduced to metallic silver on the protein, where the silver is deposited to give a black or brown band. Silver stains can be used immediately after electrophoresis, or, alternatively, after staining with CBB. With the latter approach, the major bands on the gel can be identified with CBB and then minor bands, not detected with CBB, resolved using the silver stain. The silver stain is at least 100 times more sensitive than CBB, detecting proteins down to 1 ng amounts. Other stains with similar sensitivity include the fluorescent stains Sypro Orange (30 ng) and Sypro Ruby (10 ng).

Glycoproteins have traditionally been detected on protein gels by use of the periodic acid–Schiff (PAS) stain. This allows components of a mixture of glycoproteins to be distinguished. However, the PAS stain is not very sensitive and often gives very weak, red-pink bands, difficult to observe on a gel. A far more sensitive method used nowadays is to blot the gel (Section 10.3.8) and use lectins to detect the glycoproteins. Lectins are protein molecules that bind carbohydrates, and different lectins have been found that have different specificities for different types of carbohydrate. For example, certain lectins recognise mannose, fucose, or terminal glucosamine of the carbohydrate side-chains of glycoproteins. The sample to be analysed is run on a number of tracks of an SDS–polyacrylamide gel. Coloured bands appear at the point where the lectins bind if each blotted track is incubated with a different lectin, washed, incubated with a horseradish peroxidase-linked antibody to the lectin, and then peroxidase substrate added. In this way, by testing a protein sample against a series of lectins, it is possible to determine not only that a protein is a *glyco*protein, but to obtain information about the type of glycosylation.

Quantitative analysis (i.e. measurements of the relative amounts of different proteins in a sample) can be achieved by scanning densitometry. A number of commercial scanning densitometers are available, and work by passing the stained gel track over a beam of light (laser) and measuring the transmitted light. A graphic presentation of protein zones (peaks of absorbance) against migration distance is produced, and peak areas can be calculated to obtain quantitative data. However, such data must be interpreted with caution because there is only a limited range of protein concentrations over which there is a linear relationship between absorbance and concentration. Also, equal amounts of different proteins do not always stain equally with a given stain, so any data comparing the relative amounts of protein can only be semiquantitative. An alternative and much cheaper way of obtaining such data is to cut out the stained bands of interest, elute the dye by shaking overnight in a known volume of 50% pyridine, and then to measure spectrophotometrically the amount of colour released. More recently gel documentation systems have been developed, which are replacing scanning densitometers. Such benchtop systems comprise a video imaging unit (computer linked) attached to a small 'darkroom' unit that is fitted with a choice of white or ultraviolet light (transilluminator). Gel images can be stored on the computer, enhanced accordingly and printed as required on a thermal printer, thus eliminating the need for wet developing in a purpose built darkroom, as is the case for traditional photography.

Although gel electrophoresis is used generally as an analytical tool, it can be utilised to separate proteins in a gel to achieve protein purification. Protein bands can be cut out of protein blots and sequence data obtained by placing the blot in a protein sequencer (see Section 8.4.3). Stained protein bands can be cut out of protein gels and the protein recovered by electrophoresis of the protein out of the gel piece (electroelution). A number of different designs of electroelution cells are commercially available, but perhaps the easiest method is to seal the gel piece in buffer in a dialysis sac and place the sac in buffer between two electrodes. Protein will electrophorese out of the gel piece towards the appropriate electrode but will be retained by the dialysis sac. After electroelution, the current is reversed for a few seconds to drive off any protein that has adsorbed to the wall of the dialysis sac and then the protein solution within the sac is recovered.

10.3.8 Protein (western) blotting

Although essentially an analytical technique, PAGE does of course achieve fractionation of a protein mixture during the electrophoresis process. It is possible to make use of this fractionation to examine further individual separated proteins. The first step is to transfer or blot the pattern of separated proteins from the gel onto a sheet of nitrocellulose paper. The method is known as protein blotting, or western blotting by analogy with Southern blotting (Section 5.9.2), the equivalent method used to recover DNA samples from an agarose gel. Transfer of the proteins from the gel to nitrocellulose is achieved by a technique known as electroblotting. In this method a sandwich of gel and nitrocellulose is compressed in a cassette and immersed, in buffer, between two parallel electrodes (Fig. 10.11). A current is passed at right angles to the gel, which causes the separated proteins to electrophorese out of the gel and into the nitrocellulose sheet. The nitrocellulose with its transferred protein is referred to as a blot. Once transferred onto nitrocellulose, the separated proteins can be examined further. This

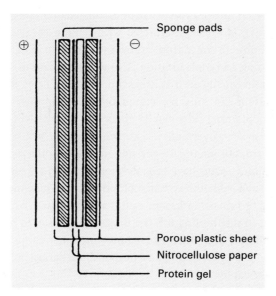

Fig. 10.11. Diagrammatic representation of electroblotting. The gel to be blotted is placed on top of a sponge pad saturated in buffer. The nitrocellulose sheet is then placed on top of the gel, followed by a second sponge pad. This sandwich is supported between two rigid porous plastic sheets and held together with two elastic bands. The sandwich is then placed between parallel electrodes in a buffer reservoir and an electric current passed. The sandwich must be placed such that the immobilising medium is between the gel and the anode for SDS–polyacrylamide gels, because all the proteins carry a negative charge.

involves probing the blot, usually using an antibody to detect a specific protein. The blot is first incubated in a protein solution, for example 10% (w/v) bovine serum albumin, or 5% (w/v) non-fat dried milk (the so-called blotto technique), which will block all remaining hydrophobic binding sites on the nitrocellulose sheet. The blot is then incubated in a dilution of an antiserum (primary antibody) directed against the protein of interest. This IgG molecule will bind to the blot if it detects its antigen, thus identifying the protein of interest. In order to visualise this interaction the blot is incubated further in a solution of a secondary antibody, which is directed against the IgG of the species that provided the primary antibody. For example, if the primary antibody was raised in a rabbit then the secondary antibody would be anti-rabbit IgG. This secondary antibody is appropriately labelled so that the interaction of the secondary antibody with the primary antibody can be visualised on the blot. Anti-species IgG molecules are readily available commercially, with a choice of a different labels attached. One of the most common detection methods is to use an enzyme-linked secondary antibody (Fig. 10.12). In this case, following treatment with enzyme-labelled secondary antibody, the blot is incubated in enzyme–substrate solution, when the enzyme converts the substrate into an insoluble coloured product that is precipitated onto the nitrocellulose. The presence of a coloured band therefore indicates the position of the protein of interest. By careful comparisons of the blot with a

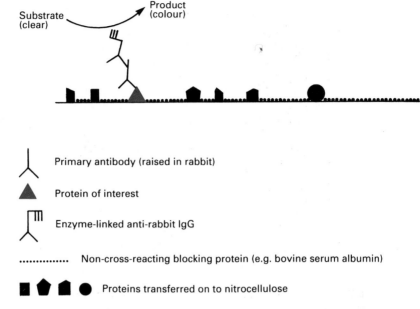

Primary antibody (raised in rabbit)

Protein of interest

Enzyme-linked anti-rabbit IgG

.... Non-cross-reacting blocking protein (e.g. bovine serum albumin)

■⬠▲● Proteins transferred on to nitrocellulose

Fig. 10.12. The use of enzyme-linked second antibodies in immunodetection of protein blots. First, the primary antibody (e.g. raised in a rabbit) detects the protein of interest on the blot. Secondly, enzyme-linked anti-rabbit IgG detects the primary antibody. Thirdly, addition of enzyme substrate results in coloured product deposited at the site of protein of interest on the blot.

stained gel of the same sample, the protein of interest can be identified. The enzyme used in enzyme-linked antibodies is usually either alkaline phosphatase, which converts colourless 5-bromo-4-chloro-indolylphosphate (BCIP) substrate into a blue product, or horseradish peroxidase, which, with H_2O_2 as a substrate, oxidises either 3-amino-9-ethylcarbazole into an insoluble brown product, or 4-chloro-1-naphthol into an insoluble blue product. An alternative approach to the detection of horseradish peroxidase is to use the method of enhanced chemiluminescence (ECL). In the presence of hydrogen peroxide and the chemiluminescent substrate luminol (Fig. 10.13) horseradish peroxidase oxidises the luminol with concomitant production of light, the intensity of which is increased 1000-fold by the presence of a chemical enhancer. The light emission can be detected by exposing the blot to a photographic film. Corresponding ECL substrates are available for use with alkaline-phosphatase-labelled antibodies. The principle behind the use of enzyme-linked antibodies to detect antigens in blots is highly analogous to that used in enzyme-linked immunosorbent assays (Section 7.7.3).

Although enzymes are commonly used as markers for second antibodies, other markers can also be used. These include:

● ^{125}I-labelled secondary antibody: Binding to the blot is detected by autoradiography (Section 14.2.3).

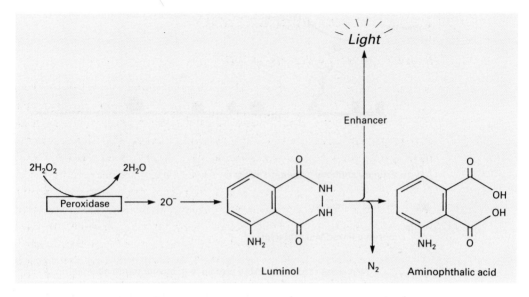

Fig. 10.13. The use of enhanced chemiluminescence to detect horseradish peroxidase.

- *Fluorescein isothiocyanate-labelled secondary antibody:* This fluorescent label is detected by exposing the blot to ultraviolet light.
- *^{125}I-labelled protein A:* Protein A is purified from *Staphylococcus aureus* and specifically binds to the Fc region of IgG molecules. ^{125}I-labelled protein A is therefore used instead of a second antibody, and binding to the blot is detected by autoradiography.
- *Gold-labelled secondary antibodies:* Second antibodies (anti-species IgG) coated with minute gold particles are commercially available. These are directly visible as a red colour when they bind to the primary antibody on the blot.
- *Biotinylated secondary antibodies:* Biotin is a small molecular weight vitamin that binds strongly to the egg protein avidin ($K_d = 10^{-15}$ M). The blot is incubated with biotinylated second antibody, then incubated further with enzyme-conjugated avidin. Since multiple biotin molecules can be linked to a single antibody molecule, many enzyme-linked avidin molecules can bind to a single biotinylated antibody molecule, thus providing an enhancement of the signal. The enzyme used is usually alkaline phosphatase or horseradish peroxidase.

In addition to the use of labelled antibodies or proteins, other probes are sometimes used. For example, radioactively labelled DNA can be used to detect DNA-binding proteins on a blot. The blot is first incubated in a solution of radiolabelled DNA, then washed, and an autoradiograph of the blot made. The presence of radioactive bands, detected on the autoradiograph, identifies the positions of the DNA-binding proteins on the blot.

10.4 ELECTROPHORESIS OF NUCLEIC ACIDS

10.4.1 Agarose gel electrophoresis of DNA

For the majority of DNA samples, electrophoretic separation is carried out in agarose gels. This is because most DNA molecules and their fragments that are analysed routinely are considerably larger than proteins and therefore, because most DNA fragments would be unable to enter a polyacrylamide gel, the larger pore size of an agarose gel is required. For example, the commonly used plasmid pBR322 has an M_r of 2.4×10^6. However, rather than use such large numbers it is more convenient to refer to DNA size in terms of the number of base-pairs. Although, originally, DNA size was referred to in terms of base-pairs (bp) or kilobase-pairs (kbp), it has now become the accepted nomenclature to abbreviate kbp to simply kb when referring to double-stranded DNA. pBR322 is therefore 4.36 kb. Even a small restriction fragment of 1 kb has an M_r of 620,000. When talking about single-stranded DNA it is common to refer to size in terms of nucleotides (nt). Since the charge per unit length (owing to the phosphate groups) in any given fragment of DNA is the same, all DNA samples should move towards the anode with the same mobility under an applied electrical field. However, separation in agarose gels is achieved because of resistance to their movement caused by the gel matrix. The largest molecules will have the most difficulty passing through the gel pores (very large molecules may even be blocked completely), whereas the smallest molecules will be relatively unhindered. Consequently the mobility of DNA molecules during gel electrophoresis will depend on size, the smallest molecules moving fastest. This is analogous to the separation of proteins in SDS–polyacrylamide gels (Section 10.3.1), although the analogy is not perfect, as double-stranded DNA molecules form relatively stiff rods and it is not completely understood how they pass through the gel, it is probable that long DNA molecules pass through the gel pores end-on. While passing through the pores, a DNA molecule will experience drag; so the longer the molecule, the more it will be retarded by each pore. Sideways movement may become more important for very small double-stranded DNA and for the more flexible single-stranded DNA. It will be obvious from the above that gel concentrations must be chosen to suit the size range of the molecules to be separated. Gels containing 0.3% agarose will separate double-stranded DNA molecules of between 5 and 60 kb size, whereas 2% gels are used for samples of between 0.1 and 3 kb. Many laboratories routinely use 0.8% gels, which are suitable for separating DNA molecules in the range 0.5–10 kb. Since agarose gels separate DNA according to size, the M_r of a DNA fragment may be determined from its electrophoretic mobility by running a number of standard DNA markers of known M_r on the same gel. This is most conveniently achieved by running a sample of bacteriophage λ DNA (49 kb) that has been cleaved with a restriction enzyme such as EcoRI. Since the base sequence of λ DNA is known, and the cleavage sites for EcoRI are known, this generates fragments of accurately known size (Fig. 10.14).

DNA gels are invariably run as horizontal, submarine or submerged gels; so named because such a gel is totally immersed in buffer. Agarose, dissolved in gel

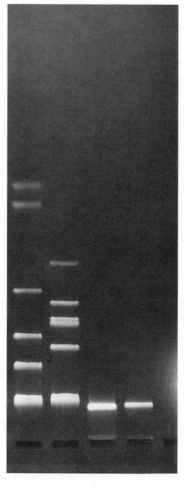

Fig. 10.14. Photograph showing four tracks from a 0.8% agarose submarine gel. The gel was run at 40 V in Tris/borate/EDTA buffer for 16 h, stained with ethidium bromide and viewed under ultraviolet light. Sample loadings were about 0.5 μg of DNA per track. Tracks 1 and 2, λ DNA (49 kb). Track 3, λ DNA cleaved with the enzyme *Eco*RI to generate fragments of the following size (in order from the origin): 21.80 kb, 7.52 kb, 5.93 kb, 5.54 kb, 4.80 kb, 3.41 kb. Track 4, λ DNA cleaved with the enzyme *Hind*III to generate fragments of the following size (in order from the origin): 23.70 kb, 9.46 kb, 6.75 kb, 4.26 kb, 2.26 kb, 1.98 kb. (Courtesy of Stephen Boffey, University of Hertfordshire.)

buffer by boiling, is poured onto a glass or plastic plate, surrounded by a wall of adhesive tape or a plastic frame to provide a gel about 3 mm in depth. Loading wells are formed by placing a plastic well-forming template or comb in the poured gel solution, and removing this comb once the gel has set. The gel is placed in the electrophoresis tank, covered with buffer, and samples loaded by directly injecting the sample into the wells. Samples are prepared by dissolving them in a buffer solution that contains sucrose, glycerol or Ficoll, which makes the solution dense and allows it to sink to the bottom of the well. A dye such as bromophenol blue is also included in the sample solvent; it makes it easier to see the sample that is being loaded and also acts as a marker of the electrophoresis front. No stacking gel (Section 10.3.1) is needed for the electrophoresis of DNA because the mobilities of DNA molecules are much greater in the well than in the gel, and therefore all the molecules in the well pile up against the gel within a few minutes of the current being turned on, forming a tight band at the start of the run. General purpose gels are approximately 25 cm long and 12 cm wide, and are run at a voltage gradient of about $1.5\ V\,cm^{-1}$ overnight. A higher voltage would cause excessive heating. For rapid analyses that do not need extensive separation of DNA molecules, it is common to use mini-gels that are less than 10 cm long. In this way information can be obtained in 2–3 h.

Once the system has been run, the DNA in the gel needs to be stained and visualised. The reagent most widely used is the fluorescent dye ethidium bromide. The gel is rinsed gently in a solution of ethidium bromide ($0.5\ \mu g\,cm^{-3}$) and then viewed under ultraviolet light (300 nm wavelength). Ethidium bromide is a cyclic planar molecule that binds between the stacked base-pairs of DNA (i.e. it intercalates) (Section 5.7.4). The ethidium bromide concentration therefore builds up at the site of the DNA bands and under ultraviolet light the DNA bands fluoresce orange-red. As little as 10 ng of DNA can be visualised as a 1 cm wide band. It should be noted that extensive viewing of the DNA with ultraviolet light can result in damage of the DNA by nicking and base-pair dimerisation. This is of no consequence if a gel is only to be viewed, but obviously viewing of the gel should be kept to a minimum if the DNA is to be recovered (see below). It is essential to protect one's eyes by wearing goggles when ultraviolet light is used. If viewing of gels under ultraviolet is carried out for long periods, a plastic mask that covers the whole face should be used to avoid 'sunburn'.

10.4.2 DNA sequencing gels

Although agarose gel electrophoresis of DNA is a 'workhorse' technique for the molecular biologist, a different form of electrophoresis has to be used when DNA sequences are to be determined. Whichever DNA sequencing method is used (Section 5.11), the final analysis usually involves separating single-stranded DNA molecules shorter than about 1000 nt and differing in size by only 1 nt. To achieve this it is necessary to have a small-pored gel and so acrylamide gels are used instead of agarose. For example, 3.5% polyacrylamide gels are used to separate DNA in the range 80–1000 nt and 12% gels to resolve fragments of between 20 and 100 nt. If a wide range of sizes is being analysed it is often convenient to run a gradient gel, for example from 3.5% to 7.5%. Sequencing gels are run in the presence of denaturing agents, urea and formamide. Since it is necessary to separate DNA molecules that are very similar in size, DNA sequencing gels tend to be very long (100 cm) to maximise the separation achieved. A typical DNA sequencing gel is shown in Fig. 5.38.

As mentioned above, electrophoresis in agarose can be used as a preparative method for DNA. The DNA bands of interest can be cut out of the gel and the DNA recovered by: (a) electroelution, (b) macerating the gel piece in buffer, centrifuging and collecting the supernatant; or (c), if low melting point agarose is used, melting the gel piece and diluting with buffer. In each case, the DNA is finally recovered by precipitation of the supernatant with ethanol.

10.4.3 Pulsed-field gel electrophoresis

The agarose gel methods for DNA described above can fractionate DNA of 60 kb or less. The introduction of pulsed-field gel electrophoresis (PFGE) and the further development of variations on the basic technique now means that DNA fragments up to 2×10^3 kb can be separated. This therefore allows the separation of whole chromosomes by electrophoresis. The method basically involves electrophoresis in agarose where two electric fields are applied alternately at different angles for defined time periods (e.g. 60 s). Activation of the first electric field causes the coiled molecules to be stretched in the horizontal plane and start to move through the gel. Interruption of this field and application of the second field force the molecule to move in the new direction. Since there is a length-dependent relaxation behaviour when a long-chain molecule undergoes conformational change in an electric field, the smaller a molecule, the quicker it realigns itself with the new field and is able to continue moving through the gel. Larger molecules take longer to realign. In this way, with continual reversing of the field, smaller molecules draw ahead of larger molecules and separate according to size. Fig. 10.15 shows the separation of yeast chromosomes that vary in size from 260 to 850 kb. Needless to say the physics of designing a PFGE system is complex and in recent years a number of different developments on the same basic theme have resulted in a bewildering array of related techniques. Detailed description of these techniques is beyond the scope of this chapter but the names of a few of these techniques indicate the principles involved, for example orthogonal field alternating gel electrophoresis (OFAGE), field inversion gel electrophoresis (FIGE), transverse alternating field gel electrophoresis (TAFE), contour-clamped homogeneous electric field electrophoresis (CHEF), and rotating field electrophoresis (RFE).

10.4.4 Electrophoresis of RNA

Like that of DNA, electrophoresis of RNA is usually carried out in agarose gels, and the principle of the separation, based on size, is the same. Often one requires a rapid method for checking the integrity of RNA immediately following extraction but before deciding whether to process it further. This can be achieved easily by electrophoresis in a 2% agarose gel in about 1 h. Ribosomal RNAs (18 S and 28 S) are clearly resolved and any degradation (seen as a smear) or DNA contamination is seen easily. However, if greater resolution is required, a smaller-pored acrylamide gel is used to enhance resolution, for example to resolve transfer RNAs (4 S) from 5 S ribosomal RNA. This can be achieved on a 2.5–5% acrylamide

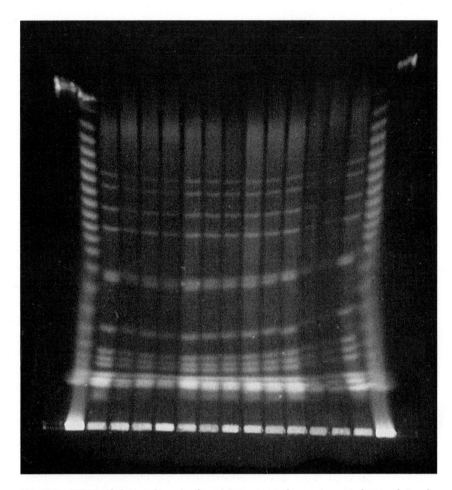

Fig. 10.15. CHEF gel electrophoresis of yeast (repeat samples run in central 13 tracks) and bacteriophage λ multimers (the 'ladders' on the two outside lanes). Every step of the ladder in the two outer lanes is about 43.5 kb and 20 steps are resolved up to 850 kb. The yeast chromosomes are of sizes 260, 290, 370, 460, 580/600, 700, 780, 820 and 850 kb. (Courtesy of Margit Burmeister, University of Michigan.)

gradient gel with an overnight run. Both these methods involve running native RNA. There will almost certainly be some secondary structure within the RNA molecule owing to intramolecular hydrogen bonding (see e.g. the clover leaf structure of tRNA, Fig. 5.6). For this reason native RNA run on gels can be stained and visualised with ethidium bromide. However, if the study objective is to determine RNA size by gel electrophoresis, then full denaturation of the RNA is needed to prevent hydrogen bond formation within or even between polynucleotides that will otherwise affect the electrophoretic mobility. There are three denaturing agents (formaldehyde, glyoxal and methylmercuric hydroxide) that are compatible with both RNA and agarose. Either one of these may be incorporated into the agarose gel and electrophoresis buffer, and the sample is heat denatured in the presence of the denaturant prior to electrophoresis. After heat denaturation, each of these agents forms adducts with the amino groups of guanine and uracil, thereby preventing hydrogen bond reformation at room temperature during electrophoresis. It is also necessary to run denaturing gels if the RNA is to be blotted (northern blots, Section 5.9.2) and probed, to ensure that the base sequence is available to the probe. Denatured RNA stains only very weakly with ethidium bromide, so acridine orange is commonly used to visualise RNA on denaturing gels. However, it should be noted that many workers will be using radiolabelled RNA and will therefore identify bands by autoradiography. An example of the electrophoresis of RNA is shown in Fig. 10.16.

10.5 CAPILLARY ELECTROPHORESIS

The technique has variously been referred to as high performance capillary electrophoresis (HPCE), capillary zone electrophoresis (CZE), free solution capillary electrophoresis (FSCE) and capillary electrophoresis (CE), but the term CE is the one most common nowadays. The microscale nature of the capillary used, where only microlitres of reagent are consumed by analysis and only nanolitres of sample needed for analysis, together with the ability for on-line detection down to femtomole (10^{-15} moles) sensitivity in some cases has for many years made capillary electrophoresis the method of choice for many biomedical and clinical analyses. Capillary electrophoresis can be used to separate a wide spectrum of biological molecules including amino acids, peptides, proteins, DNA fragments (e.g. synthetic oligonucleotides) and nucleic acids, as well as any number of small organic molecules such as drugs or even metal ions (see below). The method has also been applied successfully to the problem of chiral separations (Section 11.5.5).

As the name suggests, capillary electrophoresis involves electrophoresis of samples in very narrow-bore tubes (typically 50 μm internal diameter, 300 μm external diameter). One advantage of using capillaries is that they reduce problems resulting from heating effects. Because of the small diameter of the tubing there is a large surface-to-volume ratio, which gives enhanced heat dissipation. This helps to eliminate both convection currents and zone broadening owing to increased diffusion caused by heating. It is therefore not necessary to include a stabilising medium in the tube and allows free-flow electrophoresis.

Theoretical considerations of CE generate two important equations:

$$t = \frac{L^2}{\mu V} \tag{10.4}$$

where t is the migration time for a solute, L is the tube length, μ is the electrophoretic mobility of the solute, and V is the applied voltage.

The separation efficiency, in terms of the total number of theoretical plates, N, is given by

$$N = \frac{\mu V}{2D} \tag{10.5}$$

where D is the solute's diffusion coefficient.

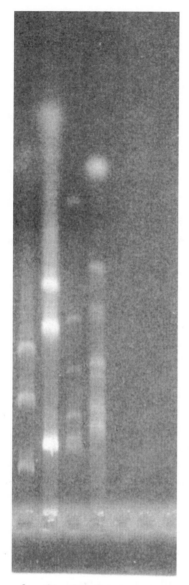

1   2   3   4

Fig. 10.16. Gel electrophoresis of RNA in a 1.4% agarose gel. Track 1 is total RNA from the tobacco plant denatured with glyoxal prior to running. Track 2 is the same sample, *not* denatured. The two faster-running major bands are 18 S and 25 S ribosomal RNA. The slower running major band is nuclear DNA. Tracks 3 and 4 show a mixture of RNA marker fragments, with (track 3) and without (track 4) glyoxal treatment. The sizes of the marker RNA fragments are 0.24, 1.4, 2.4, 4.4, 7.5 and 9.5 kb. Note that, with each sample, denaturation results in lower mobilities for the components of each sample. (Courtesy of Debbie Cook and Robert Slater, Department of Life Sciences, University of Hertfordshire.)

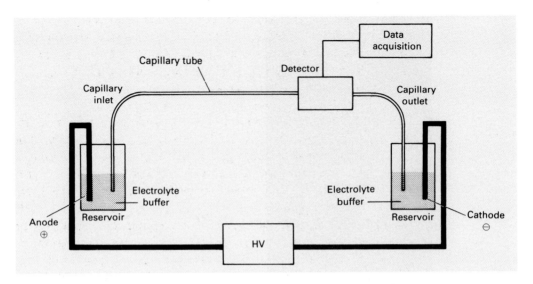

Fig. 10.17. Diagrammatic representation of a typical capillary electrophoresis apparatus.

From these equations it can be seen, first, that the column length plays no role in separation efficiency, but that it has an important influence on migration time and hence analysis time, and, secondly, high separation efficiencies are best achieved through the use of high voltages (μ and D are dictated by the solute and are not easily manipulated).

It therefore appears that the ideal situation is to apply as high a voltage as possible to as short a capillary as possible. However, there are practical limits to this approach. As the capillary length is reduced, the amount of heat that must be dissipated increases owing to the decreasing electrical resistance of the capillary. At the same time the surface area available for heat dissipations is decreasing. Therefore at some point significant thermal effect will occur, placing a practical limit on how short a tube can be used. Also the higher the voltage that is applied, the greater the current, and therefore the heat generated. In practical terms a compromise between voltage used and capillary length is required. Voltages of 10–50 kV with capillaries of 50–100 cm are commonly used.

The basic apparatus for CE is shown diagrammatically in Fig. 10.17. A small plug of sample solution (typically 5–30 μm^3) is introduced into the anode end of a fused silica capillary tube containing an appropriate buffer. Sample application is carried out in one of two ways: by high voltage injection or by pressure injection.

- *High voltage injection.* With the high voltage switched off, the buffer reservoir at the positive electrode is replaced by a reservoir containing the sample, and a plug of sample (e.g. 5–30 μm^3 of a 1 mg cm^{-3} solution) is introduced into the capillary by briefly applying high voltage. The sample reservoir is then removed, the buffer reservoir replaced, voltage again applied and the separation is then commenced.

- *Pressure injection.* The capillary is removed from the anodic buffer reservoir and inserted through an air-tight seal into the sample solution. A second tube provides pressure to the sample solution, which forces the sample into the capillary. The capillary is then removed, replaced in the anodic buffer and a voltage applied to initiate electrophoresis.

A high voltage (up to 50 kV) is then put across the capillary tube and component molecules in the injected sample migrate at different rates along the length of the capillary tube. Electrophoretic migration causes the movement of charged molecules in solution towards an electrode of opposite charge. Owing to this electrophoretic migration, positive and negative sample molecules migrate at different rates. However, although analytes are separated by electrophoretic migration, they are all drawn towards the cathode by electroendosmosis (Section 10.1). Since this flow is quite strong, the rate of electroendosmotic flow usually being much greater than the electrophoretic velocity of the analytes, all ions, regardless of charge sign, and neutral species are carried towards the cathode. Positively charged molecules reach the cathode first because the combination of electrophoretic migration and electroosmotic flow cause them to move fastest. As the separated molecules approach the cathode, they pass through a viewing window where they are detected by an ultraviolet monitor that transmits a signal to a recorder, integrator or computer. Typical run times are between 10 and 30 min. A typical capillary electrophoretograph is shown in Fig. 10.18.

This free solution method is the simplest and most widely practised mode of capillary electrophoresis. However, while the generation of ionised groups on the capillary wall is advantageous via the introduction of electroendosmotic flow, it can also sometimes be a disadvantage. For example, protein adsorption to the capillary wall can occur with cationic groups on protein surfaces binding to the ionised silanols. This can lead to smearing of the protein as it passes through the capillary (recognised as peak broadening) or, worse, complete loss of protein due to total adsorption on the walls. Some workers therefore use coated tubes where a neutral coating group has been used to block the silanol groups. This of course eliminates electroendosmotic flow. Therefore, during electrophoresis in coated capillaries, neutral species are immobile while acid species migrate to the anode and basic species to the cathode. Since detection normally takes place at only one end of the capillary, only one class of species can be detected at a time in an analysis using a coated capillary.

A range of variations on this basic technique also exist. For example, as seen above, in normal CE neutral molecules do not separate but rather travel as a single band. However, separation of neutral molecules can be achieved by including a surfactant such as SDS with the buffer. Above a certain concentration some surfactant molecules agglomerate and form micelles, which, under the influence of an applied electric field, will migrate towards the appropriate electrode. Solutes will interact and partition with the moving micelles. If a solute interacts strongly it will reach the detector later than one which partitions to a lesser degree. This method is known as micellular electrokinetic

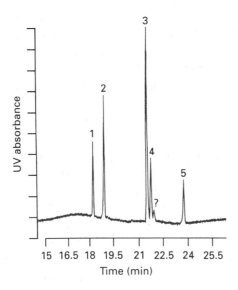

Fig. 10.18. Capillary electrophoresis of five structurally related peptides. Column length was 100 cm and the separation voltage 50 kV. Peptides were detected by their ultraviolet absorbance at 200 nm.

Peptide	
1	Lys-Arg-Pro-Pro-Gly-Phe-Ser-Pro-Phe-Arg
2	Met-Lys-Arg-Pro-Pro-Gly-Phe-Ser-Pro-Phe-Arg
3	Arg-Pro-Pro-Gly-Phe-Ser-Pro-Phe-Arg
4	Ser-Arg-Pro-Pro-Gly-Phe-Ser-Pro-Phe-Arg
5	Ile-Ser-Arg-Pro-Pro-Gly-Phe-Ser-Pro-Phe-Arg

(Courtesy of Patrick Camilleri and George Okafo, GSK Ltd.)

capillary electrophoresis (MECC). Since ionic solutes will also migrate under the applied field, separation by MECC is due to a combination of both electrophoresis and chromatography.

Original developments in CE concentrated on the separation of peptides and proteins, but in recent years CE has been successfully applied to the separation of a range of other biological molecules. The following provides a few examples.

- In the past, peptide analysis has been performed routinely using reversed-phase HPLC, achieving separation based on hydrophobicity differences between peptides. Peptide separation by CE is now also routinely carried out, and is particularly useful, for example as a means of quality (purity) control for peptides and proteins produced by preparative HPLC. Fig. 10.18 shows the impressive separation that can be achieved for peptides with very similar structures.
- High purity synthetic oligodeoxyribonucleotides are necessary for a range of applications including use as hybridisation probes in diagnostic and gene

cloning experiments, use as primers for DNA sequencing and the polymerase chain reaction (PCR), use in site-directed mutagenesis and use as antisense therapeutics. CE can provide a rapid method for analysing the purity of such samples. For example, analysis of an 18-mer antisense oligonucleotide containing contaminant fragments (8-mer to 17-mer) can be achieved in only 5 min.

- Point mutations in DNA, such as occur in a range of human diseases, can be identified by CE.
- CE can be used to quantify DNA. For example, CE analysis of PCR products from HIV-I allowed the identification of between 200 000 and 500 000 viral particles per cubic centimetre of serum.
- Chiral compounds can be resolved using CE. Most work has been carried in free solution using cyclodextrins as chiral selectors.
- A range of small molecules, drug and metabolites can be measured in physiological solutions such as urine and serum. These include amino acids (over 50 are found in urine), nucleotides, nucleosides, bases, anions such as chloride and sulphate (NO_2^- and NO_3^- can be separated in human plasma) and cations such as Ca^{2+} and Fe^{3+}.

10.6 MICROCHIP ELECTROPHORESIS

The further miniaturisation of electrophoretic systems has led to the development of microchip electrophoresis, which has many advantages over conventional electrophoresis methods, allowing very high speed analyses at very low sample sizes. For example, microchip analysis can often be completed in tens of seconds whereas capillary electrophoresis (CE) can take 20 min and conventional gel electrophoresis at least 2 h. Using new detection systems, such as laser-induced fluorescence, picomole to attomole (10^{-18} moles) sensitivity can be achieved, which is at least two orders of magnitude greater than for conventional CE. Detection systems for molecules that do not fluoresce include electrochemical detectors (Section 11.3.3), pulsed amperometric detection (PAD), and sinusoidal voltometry. All these detection techniques offer high sensitivity, are ideally suited to miniaturisation, are very low cost, and all are highly compatible with advanced micromachining and microfabrication (see below) technologies. Finally, the applied voltage required is only a few volts, which eliminates the need for the high voltages used by CE.

The manufacturing process that produces microchips is called microfabrication. The process etches precise and reproducible capillary-like channels (typically, 50 μm wide and 10 μm deep; slightly smaller than a strand of human hair) on the surface of sheets of quartz, glass or plastic. A second sheet is then fused on top of the first sheet, turning the etched channels into closed microfluidic channels. The end of each channel connects to a reservoir through which fluids are introduced/removed. Typically, the size of chips can be as small as 2 cm². Basically the microchip provides an electrophoretic system similar to CE but with more flexibility.

Current developments of this technology are based on integrating functions other than just separation into the chip. For example, sample extraction, pre-concentration of samples prior to separation, PCR amplification of DNA samples using infrared-mediated thermocycling for rapid on-chip amplification, and the extraction of separated molecules using microchamber-bound solid phases are all examples of where further functions have been built into a microchip elec-trophoresis system. An interface has also been developed for microchip elec-trophoresis–mass spectrometry (MCE–MS) where drugs have been separated by MCE and then identified by MS.

10.7 SUGGESTIONS FOR FURTHER READING

ALTRIA, K. D. (1996). *Capillary Electrophoresis Guide Book*. Humana Press, Totowa, NJ. (Detailed theory and practical procedures for the analysis of proteins, nucleic acids and metabolites.)

HAMES, B. D. and RICKWOOD, D. (2002). *Gel Electrophoresis of Proteins: A Practical Approach*, 3rd edn. Oxford University Press, Oxford. (Detailed theory and practical procedures for the electrophoresis of proteins.)

WALKER, J. M. (2002). *The Protein Protocols Handbook*, 2nd edn. Humana Press, Totowa, NJ. (Detailed theory and laboratory protocols for a range of electrophoretic techniques and blotting procedures.)

Chapter 11

Chromatographic techniques

11.1 PRINCIPLES OF CHROMATOGRAPHY

11.1.1 Distribution coefficients

The Russian botanist Mikhail Tswett is credited with the original development of a separation technique that we now recognise as a form of chromatography. In 1903 he reported the successful separation of a mixture of plant pigments using a column of calcium carbonate. In the process he became the first scientist to recognise that chlorophyll was not a single chemical compound. Modern chromatographic techniques take multiple forms, the majority of which can be automated and adapted to deal with large or very small amounts of the substances to be separated and purified.

The basis of all forms of chromatography is the distribution or partition coefficient (K_d), which describes the way in which a compound (the analyte) distributes between two immiscible phases. For two such phases A and B, the value for this coefficient is a constant at a given temperature and is given by the expression:

$$\frac{\text{concentration in phase A}}{\text{concentration in phase B}} = K_d \qquad (11.1)$$

The term effective distribution coefficient is defined as the total amount, as distinct from the concentration, of analyte present in one phase divided by the total amount present in the other phase. It is in fact the distribution coefficient multiplied by the ratio of the volumes of the two phases present. If the distribution coefficient of an analyte between two phases A and B is 1, and if this analyte is distributed between $10\,cm^3$ of A and $1\,cm^3$ of B, the concentration in the two phases will be the same, but the total amount of the analyte in phase A will be 10 times the amount in phase B.

All chromatographic systems consist of the stationary phase, which may be a solid, gel, liquid or a solid/liquid mixture that is immobilised, and the mobile phase, which may be liquid or gaseous, and which is passed over or through the stationary phase after the mixture of analytes to be separated has been applied to the stationary phase. During the chromatographic separation the analytes continuously pass back and forth between the two phases so that differences in their distribution coefficients result in their separation.

11.1.2 **Modes of chromatography**

Chromatographic separations may be carried out in one of two modes:

- *Column chromatography:* In this mode the stationary phase is packed into a glass or metal column. The mixture of analytes is then applied and the mobile phase, commonly referred to as the eluent, passed through the column either by gravity feed or by use of a pumping system or applied gas pressure. This is the most commonly used mode of chromatography from an analytical biochemical point of view. The stationary phase is either coated onto discrete small particles (the matrix) and packed into the column or applied as a thin film to the inside wall of the column. As the eluent flows through the column the analytes separate on the basis of their distribution coefficients and emerge individually in the eluate as it leaves the column.
- *Thin-layer or planar chromatography:* In this mode the stationary phase attached to a suitable matrix is coated thinly onto a glass, plastic or metal foil plate. The mixture of analytes is applied as a spot or band near the edge of the coated plate and the mobile liquid phase passed across the plate, held either horizontally or vertically, by capillary action, causing the analytes to migrate at characteristic rates to the opposite end. This mode of chromatography has the practical advantage over column chromatography that a number of samples can be studied simultaneously. Planar chromatography is simple to carry out but has been largely superseded by high performance liquid chromatography (HPLC) for many applications. However, it continues to find extensive use in the fields of peptide mapping and natural products research.

Principles of column chromatography

The principle of a column chromatographic separation may be illustrated by considering a column packed with a solid granular stationary phase to a height of 5 cm, surrounded by the mobile liquid phase of which there is 1 cm³ per cm of column, as shown in Fig. 11.1. If 32 µg of an analyte is added to the column in 1 cm³ of mobile phase, then, as this 1 cm³ moves on to the column to occupy position A, 1 cm³ of mobile phase will leave the base of the column. If the analyte has an effective distribution coefficient of 1, it will distribute itself equally between the solid and liquid phases (stage 1). If a further 1 cm³ of mobile phase is introduced on to the column, the mobile phase in section A will move down to B, taking 16 µg of the analyte with it, leaving 16 µg at A (stage 2). At both A and B, a redistribution of the analyte will occur so that there is 8 µg in the mobile phase and 8 µg in the solid phase. The addition of a further 1 cm³ of mobile phase to the column displaces the mobile phase in A to B and that in B to C, giving the distribution of the analyte as shown in stage 3. Addition of a further 1 cm³ of mobile phase leads to the distribution shown at stage 4, and a further 1 cm³ of mobile phase leads to the distribution shown at stage 5. It is apparent that, after a relatively small number of equilibrations, the analyte distributes itself symmetrically within a band. It is equally apparent that if a mixture of two analytes, one having a

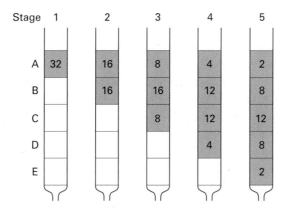

Fig. 11.1. Principle of a column chromatographic separation.

distribution coefficient of 1, the other a distribution coefficient of 100, was added to the column it would separate rapidly into distinct bands. In a real chromatographic column a very large number of equilibrations occur as the mobile phase passes down the column as a result of more mobile phase being added constantly to the top of the column. The outcome is that each analyte emerges in a distinct band from the column.

Basic column chromatographic components

A typical column chromatographic system using a gas or liquid mobile phase consists of the following components:

- *A stationary phase:* Chosen to be appropriate for the analytes to be separated.
- *A column:* This may be either of the conventional type, filled with the matrix coated with the stationary phase, or of the microbore type, in which the stationary phase is coated directly on the inside wall.
- *A mobile phase and delivery system:* Chosen to complement the stationary phase and hence to discriminate between the sample analytes and to deliver a constant rate of flow into the column.
- *An injector system:* To deliver test samples to the top of the column in a reproducible manner.
- *A detector and chart recorder:* To give a continuous record of the presence of the analytes in the eluate as it emerges from the column. Detection is usually based on the measurement of a physical parameter such as visible or ultraviolet absorption or fluorescence. A peak on the chart recorder represents each separated analyte.
- *A fraction collector:* For collecting the separated analytes for further biochemical studies.

Column liquid chromatography can be subdivided according to the back-pressure generated within the column during the separation process. Low pressure liquid chromatography (LPLC) generates pressures of less than 5 bar

(1 bar $= 14.5$ lbf in$^{-2} = 0.1$ MPa), since there is little resistance to eluent flow owing to the physical nature of the stationary phase. Gas–liquid chromatography also falls into this category. Medium pressure liquid chromatography (MPLC) generates pressures of between 6 and 50 bar and high pressure liquid chromatography (HPLC) pressures in excess of 50 bar. In practice the distinctions between MPLC and HPLC are often blurred and their equipment and procedures are virtually identical. Both give excellent resolutions and hence the term high performance liquid chromatography is preferred for both of them, since it better describes the chromatographic characteristics of the techniques and avoids the misconception that it is the high pressure that is fundamentally responsible for the high performance chromatography.

11.1.3 Selection of stationary and mobile phases

Successful chromatographic separations depend upon the correct choice of stationary and mobile phases so that the analytes to be separated have different distribution coefficients. This may be achieved by setting up one of the following:

- *Adsorption equilibrium:*   This is between a stationary solid phase and a mobile liquid phase (adsorption chromatography; hydrophobic interaction chromatography).
- *Partition equilibrium:*   This is between a stationary liquid phase and a mobile liquid or gas phase (partition chromatography; perfusion chromatography; ion-pair chromatography; chiral chromatography; gas–liquid chromatography).
- *Ion-exchange equilibrium:*   This is between a stationary, solid ion-exchanger and mobile, liquid electrolyte phase (ion-exchange chromatography; chromatofocusing; membrane chromatography).
- *Exclusion equilibrium:*   This is between a liquid phase trapped inside the pores of a stationary porous structure and the same mobile liquid phase (molecular exclusion or gel filtration).
- *Binding equilibrium:*   This is between a stationary immobilised ligand and a mobile liquid phase (affinity chromatography; immunoaffinity chromatography; lectin affinity chromatography; metal chelate affinity chromatography; dye–ligand chromatography; covalent chromatography).

In practice it is quite common for two or more of these equilibria to be involved simultaneously in a particular chromatographic separation.

11.1.4 Analyte development and elution

Analyte development and elution relates to the separation of the mixture of analytes applied to the stationary phase by the mobile phase and their elution from the column. Column chromatographic techniques can be subdivided on the basis of the development and elution modes.

- In zonal development, the analytes in the sample are separated on the basis of their distribution coefficients between the stationary and mobile phases. The sample is dissolved in a suitable solvent and applied to the stationary phase as a narrow, discrete band. Mobile phase, normally consisting of an organic solvent or a mixture of solvents often incorporating a buffered aqueous system, is then allowed to flow continuously over the stationary phase, resulting in the progressive separation and elution of the sample analytes. If the composition of the mobile phase is constant, the process is said to be isocratic elution. To facilitate separation, however, the composition of the mobile phase may be gradually changed, for example with respect to pH, salt concentration or polarity. This is referred to as gradient elution. The composition of the mobile phase may be changed continuously or in a stepwise manner. Successful zonal development results in the elution of pure samples of all the analytes. It is the most common form of chromatography.

- In displacement or affinity development, the analytes in the sample are separated on the basis of their affinity for the stationary phase. The sample of analytes dissolved in a suitable solvent is applied to the stationary phase as a discrete band. The analytes bind to the stationary phase with a strength determined by their affinity constant for the phase. The analytes are then selectively eluted by using a mobile phase containing a specific solute that has a higher affinity for the stationary phase than have the analytes in the sample. Thus, as the mobile phase is added, this agent displaces the analytes from the stationary phase in a competitive fashion, resulting in their repetitive binding and displacement along the stationary phase and eventual elution from the column in the order of their affinity for the stationary phase, the one with the lowest affinity being eluted first.

- In frontal development, the sample is continuously added to the stationary phase, thereby forcing the analytes along the stationary phase in the order of their affinity for it. The analyte with the lowest affinity accumulates at the front of the moving sample band and, whilst a pure sample of it can be isolated, pure samples of the other analytes cannot. In practice, the technique is effectively restricted to the analysis of a single trace impurity in an otherwise pure sample.

11.2 CHROMATOGRAPHIC PERFORMANCE PARAMETERS

11.2.1 Introduction

The successful chromatographic separation of analytes in a mixture depends upon the selection of the most appropriate process of chromatography followed by the optimisation of the experimental conditions associated with the separation. Optimisation requires an understanding of the processes that are occurring during the development and elution, and of the calculation of a number of experimental parameters characterising the behaviour of each analyte in the mixture.

In any chromatographic separation two processes occur concurrently to affect the behaviour of each analyte and hence the success of the separation of the analytes from each other. The first involves the basic mechanisms defining the

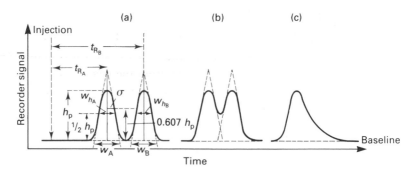

Fig. 11.2. (a) Chromatograph of two analytes showing complete resolution and the calculation of retention times; (b) chromatograph of two analytes showing incomplete resolution (fused peaks); (c) chromatograph of an analyte showing excessive tailing.

chromatographic process such as adsorption, partition, ion exchange, ion pairing and molecular exclusion. These mechanisms involve the unique kinetic and thermodynamic processes that characterise the interaction of each analyte with the stationary phase. The second general process defines the other processes, such as diffusion, which tend to oppose the separation and which result in non-ideal behaviour of each analyte. These processes are manifest as a broadening and tailing of each analyte band. The analytical challenge is to minimise these secondary processes.

11.2.2 Retention time and elution volume

A chromatograph is the pictorial record of the detector response as a function of elution volume or retention time. It consists of a series of peaks or bands, ideally symmetrical in shape, representing the elution of individual analytes, as shown in Fig. 11.2. The retention time t_R for each analyte has two components. The first is the time it takes the analyte molecules to pass through the free spaces between the particles of the matrix coated with the stationary phase. This time is referred to as the dead time, t_M. The volume of the free space is referred to as the column void volume, V_0. The value of t_M will be the same for all analytes and can be measured by using an analyte that does not interact with the stationary phase but simply spends all of the elution time in the mobile phase travelling through the void volume. The second component is the time the stationary phase retains the analyte, referred to as the adjusted retention time, t'_R. This time is characteristic of the analyte and is the difference between the observed retention time and the dead time:

$$t'_R = t_R - t_M \qquad\qquad\qquad\qquad\qquad (11.2)$$

It is common practice to relate the retention time t_R or t'_R for an analyte to a reference internal or external standard (Section 11.2.5). In such cases the relative retention time is often calculated. It is simply the retention time for the analyte divided by that for the standard.

11.2.3 Capacity factor

One of the most important parameters in chromatography is the capacity factor, k' (also called retention factor and capacity ratio). It is simply the additional time that the analyte takes to elute from the column relative to an unretained or, excluded analyte that does not interact with the stationary phase and which, by definition, has a k' value of 0. Thus:

$$k' = \frac{t_R - t_M}{t_M} = \frac{t'_R}{t_M} \tag{11.3}$$

It is apparent from this equation that if the analyte spends an equal time in the stationary and mobile phases, its t_R would equal $2t_M$ and its k' would be 1, whilst if it spent four times as long in the stationary phase as the mobile phase t_R would equal $5t_M$ so that k' would equal $(5t_M - t_M)/t_M = 4$. Note that k' has no units.

If an analyte has a k' of 4 it follows that there will be four times the amount of analyte in the stationary phase than in the mobile phase at any point in the column at any time. It is evident, therefore, that k' is related to the distribution coefficient of the analyte (equation 11.1), which was defined as the relative concentrations of the analyte between the two phases. Since amount and concentration are related by volume, we can write:

$$k' = \frac{t'_R}{t_M} = \frac{M_S}{M_M} = K_d \times \frac{V_S}{V_M} \tag{11.4}$$

where M_S is the mass of analyte in the stationary phase, M_M is the mass of analyte in the mobile phase, V_S is the volume of stationary phase, and V_M is the volume of mobile phase.

The ratio V_S/V_M is referred to as the volumetric phase ratio, β. Hence:

$$k' = K_d\beta \tag{11.5}$$

Thus the capacity factor for an analyte will increase with both the distribution coefficient between the two phases and the volume of the stationary phase. k' values normally range from 1 to 10. Capacity factors are important because they are independent of the physical dimensions of the column and the rate of flow of mobile phase through it. They can therefore be used to compare the behaviour of an analyte in different chromatographic systems. They are also a reflection of the selectivity of the system that in turn is a measure of its inherent ability to discriminate between two analytes. Such selectivity is expressed by the selectivity or separation factor, α, which can also be viewed as simply the relative retention ratio for the two analytes:

$$\alpha = \frac{k'_A}{k'_B} = \frac{K_{d_A}}{K_{d_B}} = \frac{t'_{R_A}}{t'_{R_B}} \tag{11.6}$$

The selectivity factor is influenced by the chemical nature of the stationary and mobile phases. Some chromatographic mechanisms are inherently highly selective. Good examples are affinity chromatography (Section 11.8) and chiral chromatography (Section 11.5.5).

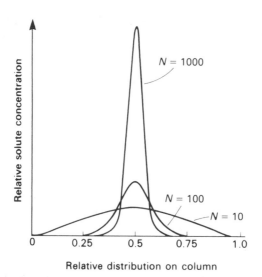

Fig. 11.3. Relationship between the number of theoretical plates (N) and the shape of the analyte peak.

11.2.4 Plate height and resolution

Plate height

Chromatography columns are considered to consist of a number of adjacent zones in each of which there is sufficient space for an analyte to completely equilibrate between the two phases. Each zone is called a theoretical plate (of which there are N in total in the column). The length of column containing one theoretical plate is referred to as the plate height, H, which has units of length normally in micrometres. The numerical value of both N and H for a particular column is expressed by reference to a particular analyte. Plate height is simply related to the width of the analyte peak (Fig. 11.3), expressed in terms of its standard deviation σ, and the distance it travelled within the column, x. Specifically:

$$H = \frac{\sigma^2}{x} \tag{11.7}$$

For symmetrical Gaussian peaks, the base width is equal to 4σ and the peak width at the point of inflection, w_i is equal to 2σ. Hence the value of H can be calculated from the chromatograph by measuring the peak width. The number of theoretical plates in the whole column of length L is equal to L divided by the plate height:

$$N = \frac{L}{H} = \frac{Lx}{\sigma^2} \tag{11.8}$$

If the position of a peak emerging from the column is such that $x = L$, from knowledge of the fact that the width of the peak at its base, w, obtained from tangents drawn to the two steepest parts of the peak, is equal to 4σ (this is a basic property of all Gaussian peaks) hence $\sigma = w/4$ and equation 11.8 can therefore be converted to:

$$N = \frac{L^2}{\sigma^2} = \frac{16L^2}{w^2} \tag{11.9}$$

If both L and w are measured in units of time rather than length, then equation 11.9 becomes:

$$N = 16(t_R/w)^2 \tag{11.10a}$$

Rather than expressing N in terms of the peak base width, it is possible to express it in terms of the peak width at half height ($w_{\frac{1}{2}}$) and this has the practical advantage that this is more easily measured:

$$N = 5.54(t_R/w_{\frac{1}{2}})^2 \tag{11.10b}$$

Equations 11.9 and 11.10a,b represent alternative ways to calculate the column efficiency in theoretical plates. The value of N, which has no units, can be as high as 50 000 to 100 000 per metre for efficient columns and the corresponding value of H can be as little as a few micrometres. The smaller the plate height (the larger the value of N), the narrower is the analyte peak (Fig. 11.3).

Peak broadening

A number of processes oppose the formation of a narrow analyte peak thereby increasing the plate height:

- *Application of the sample to the column:* It takes a finite time to apply the analyte mixture to the column, so that the part of the sample applied first will already be moving along the column by the time the final part is applied. The part of the sample applied first will elute at the front of the peak.
- *Longitudinal diffusion:* Fick's law of diffusion states that an analyte will diffuse from a region of high concentration to one of low concentration at a rate determined by the concentration gradient between the two regions and the diffusion coefficient (P) of the analyte. Thus the analyte within a narrow band will tend to diffuse outwards from the centre of the band, resulting in band broadening.
- *Multiple pathways:* The random packing of the particles in the column results in many routes between the particles for both mobile phase and analytes. These pathways will vary in length and hence elution time. The smaller the particle size the less serious is this problem and in open tubular columns the phenomenon is totally absent, which is one of the reasons why they give shorter elution times and better resolution than packed columns.
- *Equilibration time between the two phases:* It takes a finite time for each analyte in the test sample to equilibrate between the stationary and mobile phases as it passes down the column. As a direct consequence of the distribution coefficient, K_d, some of each analyte is retained by the stationary

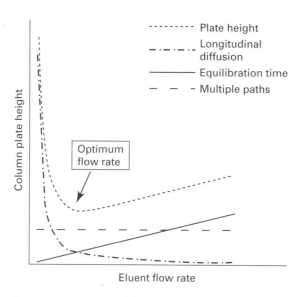

Fig. 11.4. van Deemter plot showing that the influence of flow rate on plate height is the net result of its influence on longitudinal diffusion, equilibration time and multiple pathways.

phase, whilst the remainder stays in the mobile phase and continues its passage down the column. This partitioning automatically results in some spreading of each analyte band. Equilibration time, and hence band broadening, is also influenced by the particle size of the stationary phase. The smaller the size, the less time it takes to establish equilibration. This is one of the reasons why HPLC gives better resolution than conventional LPLC.

Two of these four factors promoting the broadening of the analyte band are influenced by the flow rate of the eluent through the column. Longitudinal diffusion, defined by Fick's law, is inversely proportional to flow rate, whilst equilibration time due to the partitioning of the analyte is directly proportional to flow rate. These two factors together with that of the multiple pathways factor determine the value of the plate height for a particular column and, as previously stated, plate height determines the width of the analyte peak. The precise relationship between the three factors and plate height is expressed by the van Deemter equation (equation 11.11), which is shown graphically in Fig. 11.4.

$$H = A + \frac{B}{u_x} + Cu_x \hspace{3cm} (11.11)$$

where u_x is the flow rate of the eluent and A, B and C are constants for a particular column and stationary phase relating to multiple paths, longitudinal diffusion and equilibration time, respectively.

Fig. 11.4 gives a clear demonstration of the importance of establishing the optimum flow rate for a particular column. Longitudinal diffusion is much faster in a gas than in a liquid and as a consequence flow rates are higher in gas chromatography than in liquid chromatography.

As previously stated, the width of an analyte peak is expressed in terms of the standard deviation σ, which is half the peak width at the point of inflexion ($0.607 h_p$, where h_p is the peak height; Fig. 11.2). It can be shown that $\sigma = \sqrt{2Pt_R}$, where P is the diffusion coefficient of the analyte, i.e. a measure of the rate at which the analyte moves randomly in the mobile phase from a region of high concentration to one of lower concentration. It has units of m^2s^{-1}. Since the value of σ is proportional to the square root of t_R it follows that if the elution time increases by a factor of 4 the width of the peak will double. Thus the longer it takes a given analyte to elute the wider will be its peak. For this reason, increasing the column length is not the preferred way to improve resolution.

Asymmetric peaks

In some chromatographic separations, the ideal Gaussian-shaped peaks are not obtained, but rather asymmetrical peaks are produced. In cases where there is a gradual rise at the front of the peak and a sharp fall after the peak, the phenomenon is known as fronting. The most common cause of fronting is overloading the column so that reducing the amount of mixture applied to the column often resolves the problem. In cases where the rise in the peak is normal but the tail is protracted, the phenomenon is known as tailing (Fig. 11.2). The probable explanation for tailing is the retention of analyte by a few active sites on the stationary phase, commonly on the inert support matrix. Such sites strongly adsorb molecules of the analyte and only slowly release them. This problem can be overcome by chemically removing the sites, frequently hydroxyl groups, by treating the matrix with a silanising reagent such as hexamethyldisilazine. This process is sometimes referred to as capping. Peak asymmetry is usually expressed as the ratio of the width of the peak from the centre of the peak at $0.1 h_p$.

Resolution

The success of a chromatographic separation is judged by the ability of the system to resolve one analyte peak from another. Resolution (R_S) is defined as the ratio of the difference in retention time (Δt_R) between the two peaks (t_{RA} and t_{RB}) to the mean (w_{av}) of their base widths (w_A and w_B):

$$R_S = \frac{\Delta t_R}{w_{av}} = \frac{2(t_{RA} - t_{RB})}{w_A + w_B} \tag{11.12}$$

When $R_S = 1.0$, the separation of the two peaks is 97.7% complete (thus the overlap is 2.3%). When $R_S = 1.5$ the overlap is reduced to 0.2%. Unresolved peaks are referred to as fused peaks (Fig. 11.2). Provided the overlap is not excessive, the analysis of the individual peaks can be made on the assumption that their characteristics are not affected by the incomplete resolution.

Resolution is influenced by column efficiency, selectivity factor and capacity factors according to the equation:

$$R_S = \left[\frac{\sqrt{N}}{4}\left(\frac{\alpha - 1}{\alpha}\right)\right]\left[\frac{k'_2}{1 + k'_{av}}\right] \tag{11.13}$$

where k'_2 is the capacity factor for the longest retained peak and k'_{av} is the mean capacity factor for the two analytes.

Equation 11.13 is one of the most important in chromatography as it enables a rationale approach to be taken to the improvement of the resolution between the analytes. For example, it can be seen that resolution increases with $\sqrt{N}$. Since N is linked to the length of the column, doubling the length of the column will increase resolution by $\sqrt{2}$, i.e. by a factor of 1.4. Since both capacity factors and selectivity factors are linked to retention times and retention volumes, altering the nature of the two phases or their relative volumes will impact on resolution. Capacity factors are also dependent upon distribution coefficients, which in turn are temperature dependent; hence altering the column temperature may improve resolution.

The capacity of a particular chromatographic separation is a measure of the amount of material that can be resolved into its components without causing peak overlap or fronting. Ion-exchange chromatography (Section 11.6) and chromatofocusing (Section 11.6.3) have a high capacity, which is why they are often used in the earlier stages of a purification process.

11.2.5 Qualitative and quantitative analysis

Chromatographic analysis can be carried out on either a qualitative or a quantitative basis.

Qualitative analysis   The objective of this approach is to confirm the presence of a specific analyte in a test sample. This is achieved on the evidence of:

- A comparison of the retention time (R_f in thin-layer chromatography mode) of the peaks in the chromatograph with that of an authentic reference sample of the test analyte obtained under identical chromatographic conditions. Confirmation of the presence of the analyte in the sample can be obtained by spiking a second portion of the test sample with a known amount of the authentic compound. This should result in a single peak with the predicted increase in area.
- The use of either a mass spectrometer or nuclear magnetic resonance (NMR) spectrometer as a detector so that structural evidence for the identity of the analyte responsible for the peak can be obtained.

Quantitative analysis   The objective of this approach is to confirm the presence of a specific analyte in a test sample and to quantify its amount. Quantification is achieved on the basis of peak area coupled with an appropriate calibration graph. The area of each peak in a chromatograph can be shown to be proportional to the amount of the analyte producing the peak. The area of the peak may be determined by measuring the height of the peak (h_p) and its width at half the

Example 1 CALCULATION OF RESOLUTION OF TWO ANALYTES

Question

Two analytes A and B were separated on a 25 cm long column. The observed retention times were 7 min 20 s and 8 min 20 s, respectively. The base peak width for analyte B was 10 s. When a reference compound, which was completely excluded from the stationary phase under the same elution conditions, was studied, its retention time was 1 min 20 s. What was the resolution of the two analytes?

Answer

In order to calculate the required resolution, it is first necessary to calculate other chromatographic parameters.

(i) The adjusted retention time for A and B based on equation 11.2: $t'_R = t_R - t_M$

For analyte A

$t'_R = 440 - 80 = 360\,s$

For analyte B

$t'_R = 500 - 80 = 420\,s$

(ii) The capacity factor for A and B based on equation 11.3: $k' = t_R/t_M$

For analyte A

$k'_A = 360/80 = 4.5$

For analyte B

$k'_B = 420/80 = 5.25$

(iii) The selectivity factor for the two analytes based on equation 11.5: $\alpha = k'_B/k'_A$

$\alpha = 5.25/4.5 = 1.167$

(iv) The number of theoretical plates in the column; based on equation 11.10:
$N = (t_R/w)^2$

For analyte B

$N = (420/10)^2 = 1764$

(v) The resolution of the two analytes based on equation 11.13:

$R_S = (\sqrt{N}/4)\,[(\alpha - 1)/\alpha)]\,[k'_B/(1+k'_{av})]$ gives

$R_s = (\sqrt{1764}/4)(0.167/1.167)(5.25/1+4.875) = 1.34$

Discussion

From the earlier discussion on resolution, it is evident that a resolution of 1.34 is such as to give a peak separation of greater than 99%. If there were an analytical need to increase this separation it would be possible to calculate the length of column required to double the resolution. Since resolution is proportional to the square root of N, to double the resolution the number of theoretical plates in the column must be increased four-fold, i.e. to $4 \times 1764 = 7056$. The plate height in the column $H = L/N$, i.e. $250/1764 = 0.14\,mm$. Hence, to get 7056 plates in the column, its length must be increased to $0.14 \times 7056 = 987.84\,mm$ or 98.78 cm.

height (w_h) (Fig. 11.2). The product of these dimensions is taken to be equal to the area of the peak. This procedure is time consuming when complex and/or a large number of analyses are involved and dedicated integrators or microcomputers best perform the calculations. These can be programmed to compute retention time and peak area and to relate them to those of a reference standard, enabling relative retention ratios and relative peak area ratios to be calculated. These may be used to identify a particular analyte and to quantify it using previously obtained and stored calibration data. The data system can also be used to correct problems inherent in the chromatographic system. Such problems can arise either from the characteristics of the detector or from the efficiency of the separation process. Problems that are attributable to the detector are baseline drift, where the detector signal gradually changes with time, and baseline noise, which is a series of rapid minor fluctuations in detector signal, commonly the result of the operator using too high a detector sensitivity or possibly an electronic fault.

Internal standard

Quantification of a given analyte is based on the construction of a calibration curve obtained using a pure, authentic sample of the analyte. The construction of the calibration curve is carried out using the general principles discussed in Section 1.6.6. Most commonly the calibration curve is based on the use of relative peak areas obtained using an internal standard that has been subject to any preliminary extraction procedures adopted for the test samples. The standard must be carefully chosen to have similar physical and structural characteristics to those of the test analyte, and in practice is frequently an isomer or structural analogue of the analyte. Ideally, it should have a retention time close to that of the analyte but such that the resolution is greater than 99.5%.

External standard

An alternative approach to the use of an internal standard is the use of an external standard. In this method the standard is added to the test sample immediately before the sample is applied to the chromatographic column. It is therefore not taken through any preliminary extraction procedure and cannot compensate for variations in the efficiency of the extraction procedure. This method is valid only in those cases where the recovery of the analyte from the test sample is virtually quantitative and in those cases where there are no short-term fluctuations in detector response.

11.2.6 Sample preparation

Solvent extraction

Whilst chromatographic techniques are designed to separate mixtures of analytes this does not mean that attention need not be paid to the preliminary purification (clean up) of the test sample before it is applied to the column. On the contrary, it is clear that, for quantitative work using HPLC techniques in particular, such preliminary action is essential, particularly if the test analyte(s) is in a complex matrix such as plasma, urine, cell homogenate or microbiological culture medium. The extraction and purification of the components from a cell homogenate is often a complex multistage process. The associated principles for protein purification are discussed in Section 8.3. For some forms of analysis, for example the analysis of drugs in biological fluids, sample preparation is relatively easy. The most common clean-up technique is solvent extraction. This is based on the extraction of the analytes from aqueous mixtures using a low boiling water-immiscible solvent such as diethylether or dichloromethane. The technique is another example of the application of the principle of partition coefficients. Since organic compounds that are weak electrolytes, such as acids and bases, can exist in ionised or unionised forms depending upon their pK_a and the prevailing pH, the pH of the test sample must be adjusted to the appropriate value to permit the extraction of the unionised species. Organic solvents such as diethylether and dichloromethane also extract a significant quantity of water and, in general, this should be removed from the extract, for example by the addition of an anhydrous salt such as sodium sulphate or magnesium sulphate, before it is evaporated to dryness (often under nitrogen or *in vacuo*), dissolved in the minimum volume of an appropriate solvent such as methanol or acetonitrile, and applied to the column. This solvent extraction procedure tends to lack selectivity and is often unsatisfactory for the HPLC analysis of compounds in the range of ng cm^{-3} or less. It can sometimes be improved by the technique of ion-pairing (Section 11.3.2).

Solid-phase extraction

The alternative to solvent extraction is solid-phase extraction. Its advantage over simple solvent extraction is that it exhibits greater selectivity, mainly because it is a form of chromatography. The test solution is passed through a small (few millimetres in length) disposable column (cartridge) packed with relatively large particles of a bonded silica similar to those used for HPLC (Section 11.3.2). These selectively adsorb the analyte(s) under investigation and ideally allow interfering compounds to pass through. Preliminary thought has to be given to the particular bonded silica selected and the test sample should be treated with agents such as trichloroacetic acid, perchloric acid or organic solvents such as acetonitrile to deproteinise it so that the opportunity for protein binding of the analyte(s) is minimised. The pH of the test solution should also be adjusted to maximise the retention of the analyte. Once the test solution has been passed through the column, either by simple gravity feed or by the application of a slight vacuum to the receiver vessel, the column is washed with water to remove final traces of contaminants and the adsorbed analyte(s) recovered by elution with a small volume of an organic solvent such as methanol or acetonitrile. The extract is evaporated to dryness (under nitrogen or *in vacuo*) and the residue dissolved in the minimum volume of an appropriate solvent prior to chromatographic analysis. Several commercial forms of this solid-phase extraction technique are available that facilitate the simultaneous treatment of a large number of test samples and the term pipette tip chromatography coined to describe it.

Column switching

A more sophisticated procedure for sample preparation, particularly suited to the analysis of analytes in very low concentrations in complex mixtures by HPLC, is the technique of column switching. In this technique, the test solution is applied to a preliminary short column similar to the type used in solid-phase extraction. Once the test analyte has been adsorbed and impurities washed through the column, the analyte is eluted with a suitable organic solvent and the column eluate transferred directly to an analytical HPLC column. Technically this is not easy to achieve and requires several pumps and switching valves and is therefore expensive. One of the main problems with the technique is that, unless all interfering compounds are eluted from the preliminary column before the adsorbed analyte is switched to the analytical column, they will eventually accumulate in the analytical column and reduce its resolving power. Nevertheless, the technique has achieved many very difficult resolutions.

Supercritical fluid extraction

Supercritical fluid extraction (SFE) exploits the fact that gases such as carbon dioxide exist as a liquid under certain critical conditions. In the case of carbon dioxide, these conditions are 31.1 °C and 7.38 MPa and the resultant liquid carbon dioxide can be used as the extraction solvent, behaving as a low polarity solvent comparable to hexane. By altering the physical conditions of the extract, the carbon dioxide can be made to revert to a gas, thus simplifying the recovery of the extracted analytes.

Sample derivatisation

Some functional groups, especially hydroxyl, present in a test analyte may compromise the quality of its behaviour in a chromatographic system. The technique of analyte pre- or post-column derivatisation may facilitate better chromatographic separation and detection by masking these functional groups. Common derivatisation reagents are shown in Table 11.1.

11.3 LIQUID CHROMATOGRAPHY (LPLC AND HPLC)

11.3.1 Low pressure liquid chromatography (LPLC)

Columns

The column is invariably made of glass and is of a length and diameter appropriate to the amount of material to be separated. It should have a means of supporting the stationary phase as near to the base of the column as possible in order to minimise the dead space below the column support in which post-column mixing of separated analytes could occur. Commercial columns possess either a porous glass plate fused onto the base of the column or a suitable device for supporting a replaceable nylon net, which in turn supports the stationary phase. Capillary tubing normally leads the eluate from the column to the detector and/or fraction collection system. For some chromatographic separations, it is necessary for the temperature of the column to be raised or lowered during the separation. This is most simply achieved by jacketing the column so that water from a thermostatically controlled

Table 11.1 Examples of derivatising agents

Analyte	Reagent
A. Pre-column	
Ultraviolet detection	
Alcohols, amines, phenols	3,5-Dinitrobenzoyl chloride
Amino acids, peptides	Phenylisothiocyanate, dansyl chloride
Carbohydrates	Benzoyl chloride
Carboxylic acids	1-*p*-Nitrobenzyl-*N*,*N*′-diisopropylisourea
Fatty acids, phospholipids	Phenacyl bromide, naphthacyl bromide
Electrochemical detection	
Aldehydes, ketones	2,4-Dinitrophenylhydrazine
Amines, amino acids	*o*-Phthalaldehyde, fluorodinitrobenzene
Carboxylic acids	*p*-Aminophenol
Fluorescent detection	
Amino acids, amines, peptides	Dansyl chloride, dabsyl chloride, fluoroescamine, *o*-phthalaldehyde
Carboxylic acids	4-Bromomethyl-7-methoxycoumarin
Carbonyl compounds	Dansylhydrazine
B. Post-column	
Ultraviolet detection	
Amino acids	Phenylisothiocyanate
Carbohydrates	Orcinol and sulphuric acid
Penicillins	Imidazole and mercuric chloride
Fluorescent detection	
Amino acids	*o*-Phthalaldehyde, fluorescamine, 6-aminoquinolyl-*N*-hydroxysuccinimidyl carbamate

bath, set at the required working temperature, may be pumped around the outside of the column. More sophisticated methods include placing the column in a heating block or in a thermostatically controlled oven.

Matrix materials

The selection of a matrix for a particular stationary phase is vital to the successful chromatographic use of the phase. Generally speaking, a matrix needs to have:

- high mechanical stability to encourage good flow rates and to minimise pressure drop along the column;
- good chemical stability;
- functional groups to facilitate the attachment of the stationary phase;
- high capacity, i.e. density of functional groups to minimise bed volume;
- availability in a range of particle sizes; in addition some forms of chromatography require a matrix with a porous structure, in which case the pores need to be of the correct size and shape;
- an inert surface to minimise the non-selective adsorption of analytes and hence peak tailing.

In practice, the six most commonly used types of matrix are:

- *Agarose:* A polysaccharide made up of D-galactose and 3,6-anhydrogalactose units. The unbranched polysaccharide chains are cross-linked with agents such as 2,3-dibromopropanol to give gels that are stable in the pH range 3–14. They have good flow properties and are hydrophilic but they should never be allowed to dry out otherwise they undergo irreversible change. Commercial examples include Sepharose and Bio-Gel A.

- *Cellulose:* A polysaccharide of β-1–4-linked D-glucose units. For matrix use it is cross-linked with epichlorohydrin, the extent of cross-linking dictating the pore size. It is available in bead, microgranular and fibrous forms, has good pH stability and flow properties, and is highly hydrophilic. It is commonly used in ion-exchange chromatography.

- *Dextran:* A polysaccharide consisting of α-1–6-linked D-glucose units. For matrix use it is cross-linked with epichlorohydrin but is less stable to acid hydrolysis than are cellulose matrices. It is stable up to pH 12 and is hydrophilic. Commercial examples include Sephadex.

- *Polyacrylamide:* A polymer of acrylamide cross-linked with N,N'-methylene-bis-acrylamide. It is stable in the pH range 2–11. Commercial examples include Bio-Gel P.

- *Polystyrene:* A polymer of styrene cross-linked with divinylbenzene. Polystyrene matrices have good stability over all pH ranges and are most commonly used for exclusion and ion-exchange chromatography. They have relatively low hydrophilicities.

- *Silica:* A polymeric material produced from orthosilicic acid. The numerous silanol ($Si-OH$) groups make it hydrophilic. When derivatised, excess silanol groups can be capped by treatment with trichloromethylsilane. The stability of silica matrices is confined to the pH range 3–8. It is commonly used in perfusion chromatography. Closely related to the silica matrices is controlled pore glass. It is chemically inert but, like the silicas, tends to dissolve when the pH is above 8.

Stationary phases

The chemical nature of the stationary phase depends upon the particular form of chromatography to be carried out. Full details are given in later sections of this chapter. Most stationary phases are available attached to the matrices in a range of sizes and shapes. Both properties are important because they influence the flow rate and resolution characteristics. The larger the particle, the faster the flow rate but, conversely, the smaller the particle the larger the surface area-to-volume ratio and potentially the greater the resolving power. In practice a balance has to be struck. The best packing characteristics are given by spherical particles and most stationary phases now have a spherical or approximately spherical shape. Particle size is commonly expressed by a mesh size, which is a measure of the openings per square inch in a sieve; hence the larger the mesh size, the smaller is the particle. An 80–100 mesh (0.18–0.15 mm) or 100–120 mesh (0.075–0.038 mm) is most common

for routine use, whereas a 200–400 mesh (0.075–0.38 mm) is used for higher resolution work.

Column packing

Packing a column is normally carried out by gently pouring a slurry of the stationary phase attached to its matrix in the mobile phase into a column that has its
outlet closed, whilst the upper part of the slurry in the column is gently tapped to
ensure that no air bubbles are trapped and that the packing settles evenly. Poor
column packing gives rise to uneven flow (channelling) and reduced resolution.
The slurry is added until the required height is obtained. Once the required
column height has been obtained, the flow of mobile phase through the packed
column is started by opening the outlet, and continued until the packing has completely settled. This whole process generally requires considerable practice to
achieve reproducible results. To prevent the surface of the packed material from
being disturbed by the addition of mobile phase and the sample to the column, it is
normal to place a suitable protection device, such as nylon or rayon gauze, on the
top surface of the column. Some commercial columns possess an adaptor and
plunger, which serve the dual purpose of protecting the surface of the column and
providing an inlet (often capillary tubing) to carry the mobile phase to the column
surface. Once a column has been prepared, it is imperative that no part of it should
be allowed to run dry; hence a layer of mobile phase should always be maintained
above the column surface.

Application of sample

Several methods are available for the application of the sample to the top of the
prepared column:

- *Direct application to top of column bed:*   A simple way is to drain the mobile
  phase from above the column into the column bed by opening the flow outlet.
  The sample is then carefully applied by pipette and it too is allowed to run into
  the column. A small volume of mobile phase is then applied in a similar
  manner to wash remaining traces of the sample into the bed. Mobile phase is
  then carefully added to the column to a height of 2–5 cm and its flow started so
  that the height of the phase above the packed column is maintained at 2–5 cm.
- *Use of a sucrose density:*   An alternative procedure, which avoids the necessity
  to drain the column to the surface of the bed, is to increase the density of the
  sample by the addition of sucrose to a concentration of about 1%. When this
  solution is layered onto the liquid above the column bed, it will automatically
  sink to the surface of the column and hence be quickly passed into the column.
  This method of sample application is satisfactory, provided that the presence
  of sucrose does not interfere with the separation and subsequent analysis of
  the sample.
- *Use of a peristaltic pump:*   A third method involves the use of capillary tubing
  and/or syringe or peristaltic pump to pass the sample directly to the column
  surface. This method is the most satisfactory of the three possibilities.

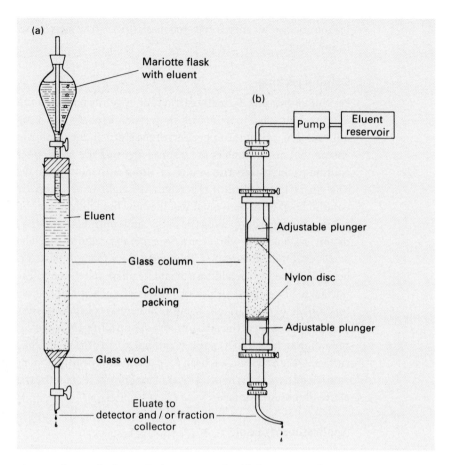

Fig. 11.5. Forms of columns for low pressure liquid chromatography.

In all cases, care must be taken to avoid overloading the column with sample, otherwise irregular separation and fronting will occur. It is also advantageous to apply the sample in as small a volume of solvent as possible because this ensures an initial tight band of material when the separation commences.

Column development and analyte elution

The components of the applied sample are separated by the continuous passage of the mobile phase through the column. This is referred to as column development. The separated analytes are then removed from the column by elution. During the development and elution process it is essential that the flow of mobile phase is maintained at a constant rate. This is best achieved by the use of either a Mariotte flask (Fig. 11.5) or a peristaltic pump, the most common form of which is the roller type (Fig. 11.6). Isocratic elution, using a single liquid as the mobile phase, or gradient elution may be used. In order to produce a suitable gradient, two or more eluents have to be mixed in the correct proportions prior to their entering the column. This may be achieved by the use of either gradient mixers (Fig. 11.7) or

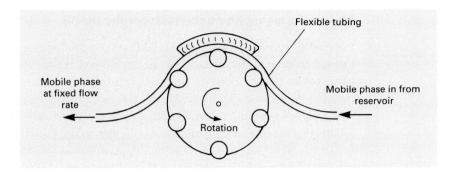

Fig. 11.6. Simple peristaltic pump commonly used in low pressure liquid chromatography.

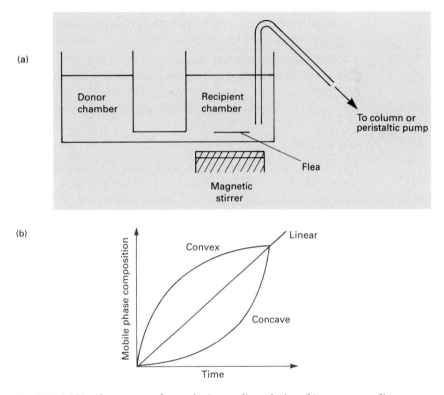

Fig. 11.7. (a) Simple apparatus for producing gradient elution; (b) common gradient shapes.

two or more peristaltic pumps programmed to deliver the separate eluents at predetermined rates into a mixing area before application to the column. Convex gradients give better resolution initially whereas concave gradients give better resolution at the end.

The methods for the detection and collection of the individual analytes as they emerge in the eluate are similar to those employed for HPLC (Section 11.3.2).

11.3.2 **High performance liquid chromatography (HPLC)**

It is evident from equations 11.1 to 11.12 that the resolving power of a chromatographic column increases with column length and the number of theoretical plates per unit length. However, there are practical limits to the length of a column owing to the problem of peak broadening (Section 11.2.4). As the number of theoretical plates in the column is related to the surface area of the stationary phase, it follows that the smaller the particle size of the stationary phase, the better the resolution, in part because it reduces the equilibration time of the analyte between the stationary and mobile phases (Section 11.2.4). Unfortunately, the smaller the particle size, the greater is the resistance to the flow of the mobile phase for a given flow rate. This resistance creates a back-pressure in the column that may be sufficient to cause the structure of the matrix to collapse, thereby actually reducing eluent flow and impairing resolution. This problem has been solved by the development of small particle size stationary phases that can withstand these pressures. This development, which has occurred in adsorption, partition, ion-exchange, exclusion and affinity chromatography, has resulted in faster and better resolution and explains why HPLC has emerged as the most popular, powerful and versatile form of chromatography. Many commercially available HPLC systems are microprocessor controlled to allow dedicated, continuous chromatographic separations.

Columns

Conventional columns (Fig. 11.8) used for HPLC are generally made of stainless steel and are manufactured so that they can withstand pressures of up to 5.5×10^7 Pa. The columns are generally 3–50 cm long and approximately 4 mm internal diameter, with flow rates of 1–3 cm^3 min^{-1}. Microbore or open tubular columns have an internal diameter of 1–2 mm and are generally 25–50 cm long. They can sustain flow rates of 5–20 mm^3 min^{-1}. Microbore columns have three important advantages over conventional columns:

- reduced eluent consumption owing to the slower flow rates,
- ideal for interfacing with a mass spectrometer owing to the reduced flow rate,
- increased sensitivity owing to the higher concentration of analytes that can be used.

Matrices and stationary phases

Three forms of matrix/stationary phase material are available, based on a rigid solid, as opposed to gel, structure as the materials need to withstand the high pressures generated in the column. All forms involve approximately spherical particles of a uniform size to minimize space for diffusion and hence band broadening to occur. The three forms are:

- *Microporous supports:*   In which micropores ramify through the particles, which are generally 5–10 mm in diameter.
- *Pellicular (superficially porous) supports:*   In which porous particles are coated onto an inert solid core such as a glass bead of about 40 mm in diameter.

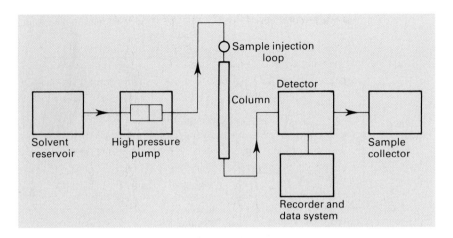

Fig. 11.8. Components of an isocratic HPLC system. For gradient elution two reservoirs and two pumps are used with liquid phase mixing before entry to the sample injection loop.

- *Bonded phases:*   In which the stationary phase is chemically bonded onto an inert support such as silica.

For adsorption chromatography, adsorbents such as silica and alumina are available as microporous or pellicular forms with a range of particle sizes. Pellicular systems generally have a high efficiency but low sample capacity and therefore microporous supports are preferred.

In partition chromatographic systems, the stationary phase may be coated onto the inert microporous or pellicular support. One disadvantage of supports coated with liquid stationary phases is that the mobile phase may gradually wash off the liquid phase. To overcome this problem, bonded phases have been developed in which the supporting material is silica.

Many different types of ion exchanger suitable for HPLC are available. The cross-linked microporous polystyrene resins are widely used. Pellicular resin forms are also available, as are bonded-phase exchangers covalently bonded to a cross-linked silicone network. These resins are classed as hard gels and readily withstand the pressures generated during analysis.

The stationary phases for exclusion separations are generally based on silica, polymethacrylate, polyvinylacetate, polyvinylchloride or on cross-linked dextran or agarose. All are available in a range of pore sizes. They are generally used where the eluent is an organic system. The supports for affinity separations are similar to those for exclusion separations.

Application of sample

The application of the sample onto a HPLC column in the correct way is a particularly important factor in achieving successful separations. The most common technique is the use of a loop injector (Fig. 11.9). This consists of a metal loop, of fixed small volume, that can be filled with the sample. The eluent from the pump is then channelled through the loop by means of a valve switching system and the

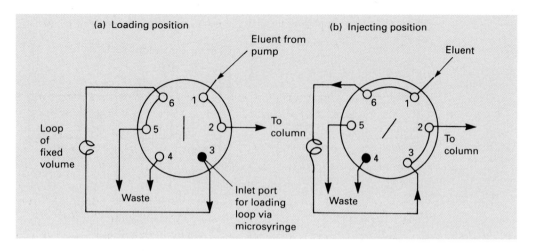

Fig. 11.9. HPLC loop injector: the loop is loaded (a) via port 3, with excess sample going to waste via port 5. In this position the eluent from the pump passes to the column via ports 1 and 2. In the injecting position (b), eluent flow is directed through the loop via ports 1 and 6 and then onto the column.

sample flushed onto the column via the loop outlet without interruption of the flow of eluent to the column.

Repeated application of highly impure samples such as sera, urine, plasma or whole blood, which have preferably been deproteinated, may eventually cause the column to lose its resolving power. To prevent this occurrence, a guard column is often installed between the injector and the column. This guard column is a short (1–2 cm) column of the same internal diameter and packed with material similar to that present in the analytical column. The packing in the guard column preferentially retains contaminating material and can be replaced at regular intervals.

Mobile phases

The choice of mobile phase to be used in any separation depends on the type of separation to be achieved. Isocratic elution may be made with a single pump, using a single eluent or two or more eluents pre-mixed in fixed proportions. Gradient elution generally uses separate pumps to deliver two eluents in proportions predetermined by a gradient programmer. All eluents for use in HPLC systems must be specially purified because traces of impurities can affect the column and interfere with the detection system. This is particularly the case if the detection system is based on the measurement of absorbance changes below 200 nm. Pure eluents for use in HPLC systems are available commercially, but even with these a 1–5 mm microfilter is generally introduced into the system prior to the pump. It is also essential that all eluents be degassed before use otherwise gassing (the presence of air bubbles in the eluent) tends to occur in most pumps. Gassing, which tends to be particularly bad for eluents containing aqueous methanol and ethanol, can alter column resolution and interfere with the continuous monitoring of the eluate. Degassing of the eluent may be carried out in several ways: by warming, by stirring vigorously with a magnetic stirrer, by applying a vacuum, by ultrasonication, and by bubbling helium gas through the eluent reservoir.

Pumps

Pumping systems for delivery of the eluent are one of the most important features of HPLC systems. The main features of a good pumping system are that it is capable of outputs of at least 5×10^7 Pa and ideally there must be no pulses (i.e. cyclical variations in pressure) as this may affect the detector response. There must be a flow capability of at least $10 \, cm^3 \, min^{-1}$ and up to $100 \, cm^3 \, min^{-1}$ for preparative separations.

Constant displacement pumps maintain a constant flow rate through the column irrespective of changing conditions within the column. One form of constant displacement pump is a motor-driven syringe-type pump that delivers a fixed volume of eluent onto the column by a piston driven by a motor. The constant volume syringe pump contains a screw-jack driven by a stepper motor. On the delivery stroke, the piston is driven at a constant rate, displacing eluent onto the column at the same rate. Two one-way valves control eluent flow in the chamber (Fig. 11.10a). The reciprocating pump is the most commonly used form of constant displacement pump. A motorized crank drives the piston, and check valves regulate entry of eluent to the column. On the compression stroke, eluent is forced from the pump chamber onto the column. During the return stroke, the exit check valve closes and eluent is drawn in via the entry valve to the pump chamber ready to be pumped onto the column on the next compression stroke (Fig. 11.10b). Such pumps produce small pulses of flow and pulse dampeners are usually incorporated into the system to minimise this pulsing effect. All constant displacement pumps have in-built safety cut-out mechanisms so that if the pressure within the column changes from pre-set limits the pump is inactivated automatically.

11.3.3 **Detectors**

Since the quantity of material applied to a LPLC or HPLC column is normally very small, it is imperative that the sensitivity of the detector system is sufficiently high and stable to respond to the low concentrations of each analyte in the eluate. The most commonly used detectors are as follows:

- *Variable wavelength detectors:* These are based upon ultraviolet–visible spectrophotometry. These types of detector are capable of measuring absorbances down to 190 nm and can give full-scale deflection (AUFS) for as little as 0.001 absorbance units. They have a sensitivity of the order of $5 \times 10^{-10} \, g \, cm^{-3}$ and a linear range of 10^5. All spectrophotometric detectors use continuous flow cells with a small internal volume (typically $8 \, mm^3$) and optical path length of 10 mm that allow the continuous monitoring of the column eluate.
- *Scanning wavelength detectors:* These have the facility to record the complete absorption spectrum of each analyte, thus aiding identification. Such

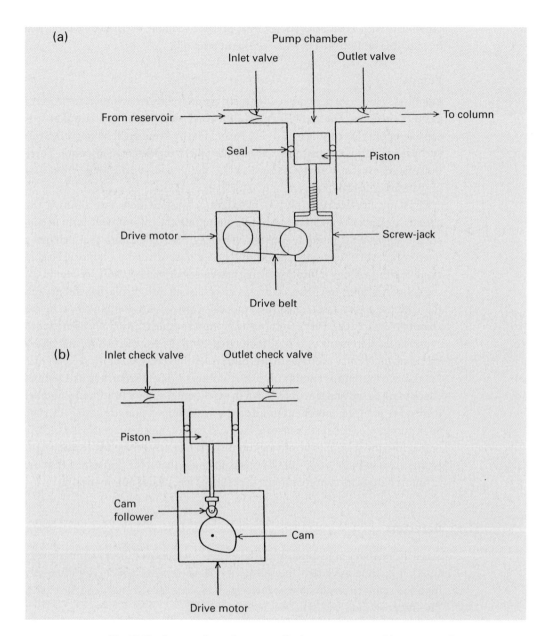

Fig. 11.10. Commonly used constant displacement pumps: (a) constant volume;
(b) reciprocating. In both types, the down stroke of the piston closes the outlet valve and
opens the inlet valve to release eluent into the pump chamber. The upstroke of the piston
closes the inlet valve and opens the outlet valve to release the eluent onto the column.
(Reproduced with permission from R. Newton (1982), Instrumentation for HPLC, in *HPLC
in Food Analysis*, R. Macrae (ed.), Academic Press, London.)

opportunities are possible either by temporarily stopping the eluent flow or by
the use of diode array techniques, which allow a scan of the complete
spectrum of the eluate within 0.01 s and its display as a three-dimensional
plot on a computer screen in real time (Fig. 11.11).

(a)

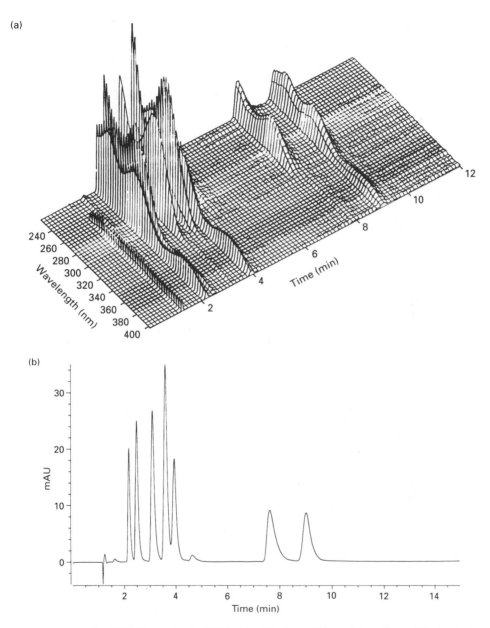

(b)

Fig. 11.11. Separation by HPLC of the dihydropyridine calcium channel blocker lacidipine and its metabolites. Column: ODS Hypercil. Eluent: methanol/acetonitrile/water (66%, 5%, 29%, by vol.) acidified to pH 3.5 with 1% formic acid. Flow rate: 1 cm³ min⁻¹. Column temperature: 40 °C. As recorded (a) by a diode array detector and (b) by an ultraviolet detector. (Reproduced by permission of GlaxoSmithKline, Stevenage.)

- *Fluorescence detectors:*   These are extremely valuable for HPLC because of their greater light sensitivity (10^{-12} g cm^{-3}) than ultraviolet detectors but they have a slightly reduced linear range (10^4). However, the technique is limited by the fact that relatively few analytes fluoresce. Pre-derivatisation of the test sample can broaden the applications of the technique.

- *Electrochemical detectors:*   These are selective for electroactive analytes and are potentially highly sensitive. Two types are available, amperometric and coulometric, the principles of which are similar. A flow cell is fitted with two electrodes: a stable counter electrode (Ag/AgCl or calomel, see Section 1.5.1) and a working electrode. A constant potential is applied to the working electrode at such a value that, as an analyte flows through the flow cell, molecules of the analyte at the electrode surface undergo either an oxidation or a reduction reaction, resulting in a current flow between the two electrodes (Section 1.5.1). The size of the current is recorded to give the chromatograph. The potential applied to the counter electrode is sufficient to ensure that the current detected gives a full-scale deflection on the recorder within the working analyte range. The two types of detector differ in the extent of conversion of the analyte at the detector surface and on balance amperometric detectors are preferred, since they have a higher sensitivity (10^{-12} g cm^{-3} as opposed to 10^{-8} g cm^{-3}) and greater linear range (10^5 as opposed to 10^4). For reduction reactions the working electrode is normally mercury, and for oxidative reactions carbon or a carbon composite. Analytes capable of undergoing oxidation include hydrocarbons, amines, amides, phenols, di- and triazines, phenothiazines, catecholamines and quinolines. Analytes capable of undergoing reduction include alkenes, esters, ketones, aldehydes, ethers, azo and nitro compounds. The eluent should of course be free from traces of compounds capable of responding to the detector.
- *Mass spectrometer detector:*   This enables the analyte to be detected and its structure determined simultaneously. The technical problems associated with the logistics of removing the bulk of the mobile phase before the sample is introduced into the mass spectrometer have been resolved in a number of ways that are discussed in detail in Chapter 9. Analytes may be detected by total ion current (TIC) (Section 9.4.1) or selected ion monitoring (SIM) (Section 9.5.7). An advantage of mass spectrometry detection is that it affords a mechanism for the identification of overlapping peaks. If there is a suspicion that a large peak is masking a smaller peak then the presence of a minor analyte can be confirmed by SIM, provided that the minor and major analytes have a unique molecular ion or fragment ion.
- *NMR spectrometer detector:*   This gives structural information about the analyte that is complementary to that obtained via HPLC–MS.
- *Refractive index detector:*   This relies on a change in the refractive index of the eluate as analytes emerge from the column. Its great advantage is that it will respond to any analyte in any eluent, changes in refractive index being either positive or negative. Its limitation is its relatively modest sensitivity (10^{-7} g cm^{-3}) but it is commonly used in the analysis of carbohydrates.
- *Evaporative light-scattering detector (ELSD):*   This relies on the vaporisation of the eluate, evaporation of the eluent and the quantification of the analyte by light scattering. The eluate emerging from the column is combined with a flow of air or nitrogen to form an aerosol; the eluent is then evaporated

from the aerosol by passage through an evaporator and the emerging dry particles of analyte irradiated with a light source and the scattered light detected by a photodiode. The intensity of the scattered light is determined by the quantity of analyte present and its particle size. It is independent of the analyte's spectroscopic properties and hence does not require the presence of a chromophoric group or any prior derivatisation of the analyte. It can quantify analytes in flow rates of up to $5\,cm^3\,min^{-1}$. Appropriate calibration gives good, stable quantification of the analyte with no baseline drift. It is an attractive method for the detection of fatty acids, lipids and carbohydrates.

The sensitivity of ultraviolet absorption, fluorescence and electrochemical detectors can often be increased significantly by the process of derivatisation, whereby the analyte is converted pre- or post-column to a chemical derivative. Examples are given in Table 11.1.

Fraction collectors

For studies in which the analyte in the eluate is to be collected and studied further, the eluate has to be divided into fractions. Two approaches are available to achieve this objective: either the eluate can be continuously monitored and the fraction containing a particular analyte collected, or the eluate can be divided into small ($1–10\,cm^3$) fractions, which are subsequently analysed and those containing a particular analyte bulked together. Automatic fraction collectors are designed either to collect a selected volume of eluate or to collect the eluate for a predetermined period of time before a new collection tube is placed in position automatically. The volume of eluate in each fraction may be determined in one of several ways. There may be a siphoning or similar system to deliver a predetermined volume into each tube, or there may be an electronic means of allowing a predetermined number of drops of eluate to enter each tube. This latter method has the slight disadvantage that if the composition of the eluate changes (e.g. during gradient elution), so too may its surface tension and hence droplet size, so that the actual volume collected also changes. A further possibility is that the eluate is allowed to enter each tube for a fixed time interval. In this case, if the flow rate through the column varies, so too will the volume of each fraction, but this is unusual and, in practice, fixed-time collectors are the most common.

11.3.4 **Fast protein liquid chromatography (FPLC)**

The wide applicability, speed and sensitivity of HPLC has resulted in it becoming the most popular form of chromatography and virtually all types of biological molecules have been assayed or purified using the technique. HPLC has had a particular impact on the separation of amino acids, peptides and proteins. Instruments dedicated to the separation of proteins have given rise to the technique of fast protein liquid chromatography (FPLC). There are no unique principles associated with FPLC, it is simply based on reversed-phase, affinity, exclusion, hydrophobic interaction and ion-exchange chromatography, and chromatofocusing. Mainly aqueous-based elution systems are used with special high capacity stationary phases of similar diameter to those used in conventional HPLC. However, the operating pressure (1–2 MPa) is lower than conventional HPLC. Microbore glass-lined stainless steel columns enable very small amounts of sample to be used, with separation taking as little as a few minutes. The technique enables such complex mixtures as tryptic digests of proteins and the culture supernatant of microorganisms to be applied directly to the column, but protein mixtures from cell extracts still need some form of preliminary fractionation (Section 8.3.3) prior to study.

11.3.5 Capillary electrochromatography

Capillary electrochromatography (CEC) is effectively a hybrid of HPLC and capillary electrophoresis (CE). As its name implies, it is carried out in capillary columns in which the stationary phase is either attached to an inert support and packed in the capillary or is coated directly onto the walls of the capillary. As in capillary electrophoresis, a potential is applied across the walls of the capillary, generating solvent flow by electroosmosis (Section 10.1). This electroosmotic flow (EOF) drives the solvent and the analytes in the applied sample through the capillary column. As the analytes move along the capillary they are subject to the opposing forces of EOF and distribution between the mobile and stationary phases. They will therefore be separated partly on the basis of differences in their distribution coefficients, K_d, between the two phases exactly as in all other forms of chromatography, and partly on the basis of differences in their electrophoretic mobility as in capillary electrophoresis. The consequence is that the capacity factor, k', characteristic of chromatography, is not valid in CEC.

The stationary phases used are similar to those of HPLC based on silica matrices. The mobile phase is generally an organic–aqueous system containing an electrolyte. The EOF is generated at the solid/liquid interface. The silica surface is negatively charged owing to deprotonisation of silanol groups and hence the mobile phase molecules carry a net positive charge, thereby forming an electrical double layer. The positively charged molecules near the surface of the silica induce similar changes in the nearby molecules. These molecules migrate towards the negative electrode under the influence of the applied field, dragging the bulk of the mobile phase with them. The velocity of the EOF is determined by a number of factors, including the size of the applied field and the viscosity and dielectric constant of the mobile phase. It is significantly slower in packed capillary columns than in the open tube variety.

The instrumentation for CEC is similar to that for CE except that both ends of the column are pressurised to ensure no pressure drop. Columns measuring 50 cm × 100 μm are commonly used and, because flow is produced by electroosmosis rather than applied pressure, smaller sized particles (1.5–5 μm) can be used than with HPLC, with the result that the column efficiency is much higher in CEC and the resolution time shorter than in HPLC.

11.3.6 Perfusion chromatography

The high resolution achieved by HPLC is based on the use of small diameter particles for the stationary phase. However, this high resolution is achieved at the cost of the generation of high pressures, relatively low flow rates and the constraints the high pressure imposes on the instrumentation. Perfusion chromatography overcomes some of these limitations by the use of small particles (10–50 μm diameter) that have channels of approximately 1 μm diameter running through them that allow the use of high flow rates without the generation of high pressures. The high flow rates result in small plate heights (Section 11.2.4) and hence high resolution in very short separation times. The particles are made of polystyrene-divinylbenzene and are available under the trade name POROS. Two types of pore are available: through pores that are long (up to 8000 Å (800 nm)) and diffusive pores that are shorter (up to 1000 Å (100 nm)). The stationary phase is coated to the particles, including the surface of the pores. The eluent perfuses through the pores, allowing the analyte to equilibrate rapidly with the stationary phase. By comparison, the microporous particles used in HPLC have a much smaller diameter pore, hence the greater back-pressure. All the forms of stationary phase used for the various form of chromatography are available for perfusion chromatography. The technique uses the same type of instrumentation as HPLC and FPLC. Protein separations in as short a time as 1 min can be achieved.

11.3.7 Membrane chromatography

An alternative to perfusion chromatography as a solution to the inherent limitations of HPLC is membrane chromatography. This avoids the use of small particles by using porous membranes stacked on top of each other and onto which the stationary phase is coated. The pores in the membrane are large, allowing free passage to the eluent and analyte. Equilibration is fast owing to the large surface area of each membrane, allowing high flow rates (up to 10 cm^3 min^{-1}) to be used. The membranes are contained in a cartridge that substitutes for the column in a conventional HPLC system.

11.4 ADSORPTION CHROMATOGRAPHY

11.4.1 Principle

This is the classic form of chromatography, which is based upon the principle that certain solid materials, collectively known as adsorbents, have the ability to hold molecules at their surface. This adsorption process, which involves weak, non-ionic attractive forces of the van der Waals and hydrogen-bonding type, occur at specific adsorption sites. These sites have the ability to discriminate between types of molecules and are occupied by molecules of either the eluent or of the analytes in proportions determined by their relative strength of interaction. As eluent is constantly passed down the column, differences in these binding strengths eventually lead to the separation of the analytes. The strength of interaction of a particular analyte with the binding sites depends upon the functional groups present in its structure. Hydroxyl and aromatic groups, for example, tend to increase interaction with the adsorption surface. In general, the strength of adsorption is influenced more by the presence of specific functional groups than by the overall molecular size of the analyte because only a specific group rather than the whole molecule can interact with the adsorption site.

Silica is a typical adsorbent. It has silanol (Si—OH) groups on its surface, which are slightly acidic and can interact with polar functional groups of the analyte or eluent. The topology (arrangement) of these silanol groups in different commercial preparations of silica explains their different separation properties. Other commonly used adsorbents are alumina and carbon. Adsorbents based on carbon, alumina or silica are available for low pressure chromatography and for HPLC. The silicas are acidic and good for the separation of basic materials whereas the aluminas are more basic and better suited for the resolution of acidic materials.

In general, an eluent with a polarity comparable to that of the most polar analyte in the mixture is chosen. Thus alcohols would be selected if the analytes contained hydroxyl groups, acetone or esters would be selected for analytes containing carbonyl groups, and hydrocarbons such as hexane, heptane and toluene for analytes that are predominantly non-polar. Mixtures of solvents are commonly used in the context of gradient elution. The presence of small amounts of water in the mobile phase is often beneficial when silica is used as the stationary phase, as the water molecules selectively block the more active silanol groups, leaving a more selective population of weaker binding sites.

Adsorption chromatography is most commonly used to separate non-ionic, water-insoluble compounds such as triglycerides, vitamins and many drugs.

11.4.2 Hydroxylapatite chromatography

Crystalline hydroxylapatite ($Ca_{10}(PO_4)_6(OH)_2$) is an adsorbent used to separate mixtures of proteins or nucleic acids. The mechanism of adsorption is not fully understood but is thought to involve both the calcium ions and phosphate ions on the surface and to involve dipole–dipole interactions and possibly electrostatic attractions. One of the most important applications of hydroxylapatite chromatography is the separation of single-stranded DNA from double-stranded DNA. Both forms of DNA bind at low phosphate buffer concentrations but, as the buffer concentration is increased, single-stranded DNA is selectively desorbed. As the buffer concentration is increased further, double-stranded DNA is released. This behaviour is exploited in the technique of Cot analysis (Section 5.3.4).

The affinity of double-stranded DNA for hydroxylapatite is so high that it can be selectively removed from RNA and proteins in cell extracts by use of this type of chromatography.

Hydroxylapatite is available commercially in a range of forms suitable for LPLC and HPLC. These include crystalline or spheroidal hydroxylapatite and forms bonded to an agarose matrix. The adsorption capacity of all these forms is maximal around neutral pH and the conditions usually include 20 mM phosphate buffer for the adsorption process. Elution is achieved by increasing the phosphate buffer concentration to 500 mM.

11.4.3 Hydrophobic interaction chromatography

This type of chromatography was developed to purify proteins by exploiting their surface hydrophobicity, which is related to the presence of non-polar amino acid residues. Groups of hydrophobic residues are scattered over the surface of proteins in a way that gives characteristic properties to each protein. In aqueous solution, these hydrophobic regions on the protein are covered with an ordered layer of water molecules that effectively mask the hydrophobic groups. These groups can, however, be exposed by the addition of salt ions, which preferentially take up the ordered water molecules. The exposed hydrophobic regions can then interact with each other. In hydrophobic interaction chromatography (HIC), the presence of hydrophobic groups attached to a suitable matrix facilitates protein–matrix interaction rather than facilitating protein–protein interaction. The most commonly used stationary phases are alkyl (ethyl to octyl) or phenyl groups attached to either polyamide-coated silicas or an agarose matrix. Commercial materials include: Phenyl Sepharose and Phenyl SPW, both for low pressure HIC; and Poly PROPYL Aspartamide, Bio-Gel TSK Phenyl and Spherogel TSK Phenyl for HPLC HIC.

Since HIC requires the presence of salting-out compounds such as ammonium sulphate to facilitate the exposure of the hydrophobic regions on the protein molecule, it is commonly used immediately after fractionation with ammonium sulphate as ammonium and sulphate ions are already present in the protein sample. To maximise the process, it is advantageous to adjust the pH of the protein sample to that of its isoelectric point. Once the proteins have been adsorbed onto the stationary phase, selective elution can be achieved in a number of ways, including the use of an eluent of gradually decreasing ionic strength or of increasing pH (this increases the hydrophilicity of the protein) (Fig. 11.12) or by selective displacement by a displacer that has a stronger affinity for the stationary phase than has the protein. Examples include non-ionic detergents such as Tween 20 and Triton X-100, aliphatic alcohols such as 1-butanol and ethylene glycol, and aliphatic amines such as 1-aminobutane. HIC has two advantages over reversed-phase HPLC. The first is that the use of aqueous elution conditions minimises protein denaturation. The second is that it has a high capacity. A limitation is that it gives only moderate resolution.

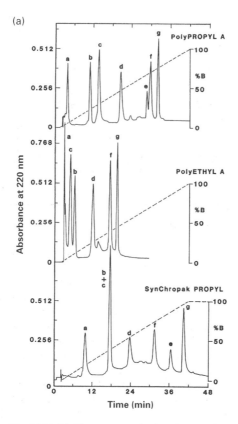

Fig. 11.12. (a) Chromatograph of a mixture of proteins separated by hydrophobic interaction chromatography using different stationary phases. A linear gradient elution program was used changing from 0 to 100% mobile phase B in 40 min. Mobile phase A: 1.8 M ammonium sulphate + 0.1 M potassium phosphate, pH 7.0. Mobile phase B: 0.1 M potassium phosphate, pH 7.0. Elution was monitored at 220 nm. (Reproduced with permission from K. Benedek (2003), High-Performance Interaction Chromatography, in *HPLC of Peptides and Proteins: Methods and Protocols* (Methods in Molecular Biology, **251**), M.-I. Aguilar (ed.), Humana Press, Totowa, NJ.)

11.5 PARTITION CHROMATOGRAPHY

11.5.1 Principle

Like other forms of chromatography, partition chromatography is based on differences in capacity factors, k', and distribution coefficients, K_d, of the analytes using liquid stationary and mobile phases. It can be subdivided into liquid–liquid chromatography, in which the liquid stationary phase is attached to a supporting matrix by purely physical means, and bonded-phase liquid chromatography, in which the stationary phase is covalently attached to the matrix. An example of liquid–liquid chromatography is one in which a water stationary phase is supported by a cellulose, starch or silica matrix, all of which have the ability to physically bind as much as 50% (w/v) water and remain free-flowing powders.

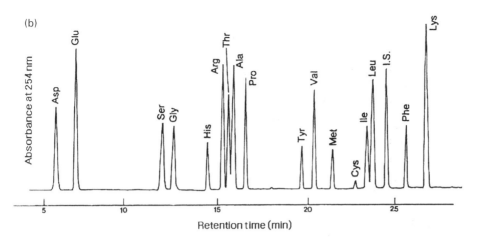

Fig. 11.12. (b) Chromatogram of the amino acids present in a hydrolysate of whole egg separated by reversed-phase chromatography. Egg proteins were hydrolysed with 6 M HCl at 145 °C for 4 h and then derivatised with phenylisothiocyanate to give the phenylthiocarbamyl derivatives (PTC). The derivatives were separated on a Nova-pak C_{18} column (300 mm × 3.9 mm internal diameter, 4 μm dimethyloctadecylsilyl-bonded amorphous silica, Waters) heated to 40 °C. A gradient elution program was used: 0–15 min solvent A (0.02 M phosphate buffer containing 5% methanol, 1.5% tetrahydrofuran, pH 6.8); 15–20 min 76% solvent A, 20% solvent B (solvent A: acetonitrile, 50:50, v/v), 4% solvent C (acetonitrile–water, 70:30, v/v); 20–30 min 70% solvent A, 20% solvent B, 10% solvent C with a flow rate of 1.2 cm³ min⁻¹ and detection at 254 nm. IS, internal standard (nor-leucine). (Reproduced with permission from H.-L. Woo (2001), Determination of amino acids in foods by reversed-phase high-performance liquid chromatography with new precolumn derivatives, butylthiocarbamyl, and benzylthiocarbamyl derivatives compared to the phenylthiocarbamyl derivative and ion-exchange chromatography, in *Amino Acid Analysis Protocols* (Methods in Molecular Biology, **159**), C. Cooper, N. Packer and K. Williams (eds.), Humana Press, Totowa, NJ.)

The advantages of this form of chromatography are that it is cheap, has a high capacity and has broad selectivity. Its disadvantage is that the elution process may gradually remove the stationary phase, thereby altering the chromatographic conditions. This problem is overcome by the bonded phases and this explains their more widespread use. Most bonded phases use silica as the matrix, which is derivatised to immobilise the stationary phase by reaction with an organochlorosilane:

$$-Si-OH + Cl-Si-(CH_3)_2R \quad \rightarrow \quad Si-O-Si-(CH_3)_2R + HCl$$

  silica   organo   derivatised silanol
            chlorosilane   group

Surplus silanol groups are removed by capping with chlorotrimethylsilane to improve the quality of the chromatography by decreasing tailing. There are two commonly used modes of partition chromatography that differ in the relative polarities of the stationary and mobile phases.

11.5.2 **Normal-phase liquid chromatography**

In this form of partition chromatography, the stationary phase is polar and the mobile phase relatively non-polar. The most popular stationary phase is an alkyl-amine bonded to silica. The mobile phase is generally an organic solvent such as hexane, heptane, dichloromethane or ethylacetate. These solvents form an elutropic series based on their polarity. Such a series in order of increasing polarity is as follows:

n-hexane $<$ cyclohexane $<$ trichloromethane $<$ dichloromethane $<$ tetrahydro-furan $<$ acetonitrile $<$ ethanol $<$ methanol $<$ ethanoic acid $<$ water

The mechanism of separation exploits the ability of the analyte to displace molecules of the mobile phase adsorbed as a monolayer on the surface of the station-ary phase, as well as the ability of the analyte to compete with mobile phase molecules in the formation of a bilayer on the stationary phase surface. The order of elution of analytes is such that the least polar is eluted first and the most polar last. Indeed, polar analytes generally require gradient elution with a mobile phase of increasing polarity, generally achieved by the use of methanol or dioxane. The main applications of normal-phase liquid chromatography are its use to separate analytes that have low water solubility and those that are not amenable to reversed-phase liquid chromatography.

11.5.3 **Reversed-phase liquid chromatography**

In this form of liquid chromatography, the stationary phase is non-polar and the mobile phase relatively polar, hence the name 'reversed phase'. By far the most commonly used type is the bonded-phase form, in which alkylsilane groups are chemically attached to silica. Butyl (C_4), octyl (C_8) and octadecyl (C_{18}) silane groups are most commonly used (Table 11.2). The mobile phase is commonly water or aqueous buffers, methanol, acetonitrile, or tetrahydrofuran or mixtures of them. The organic solvent is referred to as an organic modifier. Reversed-phase liquid chromatography differs from most other forms of chromatography in that the stationary phase is essentially inert and only non-polar (hydrophobic) inter-actions with analytes are possible.

Reversed-phase separation of analytes is determined principally by the charac-teristics of the mobile phase and probably involves a combination of adsorption and partition mechanisms. It is believed to have many similarities to hydrophobic interaction chromatography. No simple model has been described to explain reversed-phase chromatography but the solvophobic theory is the one most widely considered. It is based on the consideration of the balance of free energy and entropy changes associated with bonding of the analyte with the stationary phase and with the mobile phase. The attraction of the reversed-phase technique is that small changes in the mobile phase composition such as the addition of salts, change of pH or the amount of organic solvent, profoundly affect the separ-ation characteristics. Moreover, the technique is sensitive to temperature change such that a 10 deg.C increase approximately halves the capacity factor, k'. In

Table 11.2	Examples of silica-bonded phases for reversed-phase HPLC	
Product	Particle size (μm)	Pore size (Å)
μBondapak octadecyl	10	70
μBondapak phenyl	10	125
μBondapak CN	10	125
μBondapak NH$_2$	10	80
Zorbax octadecyl	6	70
Zorbax octyl	6	70
Zorbax NH$_2$	6	70
Discovery octyl	5	180
Supelcosil LC-octadecyl	5	120
Supelcosil LC-301 methyl	5	300
Supelcosil LC-308 octyl	5	300

1 Å = 0.1 nm.

reversed-phase chromatography, polar analytes elute first and non-polar analytes last. Non-polar analytes may need gradient elution using increasing proportions of a low polarity solvent such as hexane.

Reversed-phase HPLC is probably the most widely used form of chromatography mainly because of its flexibility and high resolution. It is widely used to analyse drugs and their metabolites, insecticide and pesticide residues, and amino acids and peptides. It is also now widely applied to proteins by using FPLC (Fig. 11.12). Octadecylsilane (ODS) phases bind proteins more tightly than do octyl- or methylsilane phases and are therefore more likely to cause protein denaturation because of the more extreme conditions required for the elution of the protein. In non-aqueous form, reversed-phase chromatography can be used to separate lipophilic compounds such as fats.

11.5.4 Ion-pair reversed-phase liquid chromatography

Although the separation of some highly polar compounds, such as amino acids, peptides, organic acids and the catecholamines, is commonly undertaken by reversed-phase chromatography, it is sometimes possible to achieve improved separation by one of two possible approaches:

- *Ion suppression:* The ionisation of the compound is suppressed by using a mobile phase with an appropriately high or low pH. For weak acid analytes, for example, an acidified mobile phase would be used.
- *Ion-pairing:* A counter ion that has a charge opposite to that of the analytes to be separated is added to the mobile phase so that the resulting ion-pair has sufficient lipophilic character to be retained by the non-polar stationary phase of a reversed-phase system. Thus, to aid the separation of acidic organic compounds (RCOOH), which would be present as their conjugate anions, a quaternary alkylamine ion such as tetrabutylammonium would be used as the

counter ion, whereas for the separation of bases (RNH_2), which would be present as cations, an alkyl sulphonate such as sodium heptanesulphonate would be used:

$$RCOO^- \; + \; R_4'N^+ \; \rightleftharpoons \; [RCOO^-N^+R_4']$$

carboxylic   counter   ion-pair

acid anion   cation

$$RN^+H_3 \; + \; R'SO_3^- \; \rightleftharpoons \; RH_3N^+ \; {}^-O_3SR']$$

conjugate   counter   ion-pair

acid of   anion

weak base

where R' is an appropriate aliphatic group. The mechanism by which ion-pairing results in better separation is not clear but two theories have been proposed. The first suggests that the ion-pair behaves as a single neutral species, whilst the second suggests that an active ion-exchange surface is produced in which the counter ion, which has considerable lipophilic properties, and the ions to be separated are adsorbed by the hydrophobic, non-polar stationary phase. In practice, the success of the ion-pairing approach is variable and somewhat empirical. The size of the counter ion, its concentration and the pH of the solution are all factors that may profoundly influence the outcome of the separation.

Octyl- and octadecylsilane-bonded phases are used most commonly in conjunction with a water/methanol or water/acetonitrile mobile phase. One of the advantages of ion-pair reversed-phase chromatography is that, if the sample to be resolved contains a mixture of non-ionic and ionic compounds, the two groups of compounds can be separated simultaneously because the ion-pair reagent does not affect the chromatography of the non-ionic species. This is not true of ion-exchange chromatography.

11.5.5 Chiral chromatography

Chiral compounds either contain at least one asymmetric carbon atom (chiral centre) or are molecularly asymmetric. They exist in two enantiomorphic forms (enantiomers), related as object and mirror images, that have the same physical and chemical properties and differ only in their interaction with plane-polarised light such that one is dextrorotatory ($+$) and the other laevorotatory ($-$). There are a number of conventions for indicating the spatial configuration, as opposed to optical properties, of enantiomers. The classical D and L system for monosaccharides and amino acids cannot be applied easily to other structures and the Cahn–Ingold–Prelog system, which assigns R (Latin, *rectus*) or S (Latin, *sinister*) configurations to an enantiomer, is of more general use. Until recently it has not been possible to resolve mixtures of enantiomers and this has created problems for the pharmaceutical industry in its development and clinical use of drugs, many of which are chiral, for although enantiomers have identical chemical and physical properties they are distinguishable biologically. Thus they differ in their ability to interact with the receptors involved in a range of physiological responses and they are often metabolised and excreted at different rates.

Chromatographic techniques have now been developed that allow mixtures of enantiomers to be resolved. One of these techniques is based on the fact that diastereoisomers, which are optical isomers that do not have an object–image relationship, have different physical properties even though they contain identical functional groups. They can therefore be separated by conventional chromatographic techniques, most commonly reversed-phase chromatography. The diastereoisomer approach requires that the enantiomers contain a function group that can be derivatised by a chemically and optically pure chiral derivatising agent (CDA) that converts them to a mixture of diastereoisomers:

$$(R + S) \quad + \quad R' \quad \rightleftharpoons \quad RR' + SR'$$

mixture of	chiral	mixture of
enantiomers	derivatising	diastereoisomers
	agent	

Examples of CDAs include the R or S form of the following:

For amines	N-trifluoroacetyl-1-prolylchloride, α-phenylbutyric anhydride
For alcohols	2-Phenylpropionyl chloride, 1-phenylethylisothiocyanate
For ketones	2,2,2-Trifluoro-1-pentylethylhydrazine
For aliphatic and alicyclic acids	1-Menthol, desoxyephedrine

Although this approach to chiral resolution is relatively simple, it is essential that the derivatisation process is rapid and quantitative. Very often this is not the case and this has restricted its use. An alternative approach to the resolution problem is to use a chiral mobile phase. In this technique a transient diastereomeric complex is formed between the enantiomers and the chiral mobile phase agent. Examples of chiral mobile phase agents include albumin, α_1-acid glycoprotein, α-, β- and γ-cyclodextrins, camphor-10-sulphonic acid and N-benzoxycarbonylglycyl-L-proline, all of which are used with a reversed-phase chromatographic system.

The most successful approach to chiral chromatography, however, has been the use of a chiral stationary phase. This is based upon the principle that the need for a three-point interaction between the stationary phase (working as a chiral discriminator) and the enantiomer would allow the resolution of racemic mixtures due to the different spatial arrangement of the functional groups at the chiral centre in the enantiomers. One such successful approach uses Pirkle phases, based on dinitrobenzoyl derivatives of amino acids, such as phenylglycine, that are bonded to silica. These phases are thought to function by allowing transient formation of enantiomer–stationary phase complexes by bonding such as hydrogen bonding and van der Waals forces. Elution is generally by the reversed-phase technique. Alternative chiral stationary phases include triacetylcellulose and various cyclodextrins bonded to silica. These cyclodextrins are cyclic oligosaccharides that have an open truncated conical structure 6–8 Å (0.6–0.8 nm) wide at their base. Their inner surface is predominantly hydrophobic, but secondary hydroxyl groups are located around the wide rim of the cone. β-Cyclodextrin has 7 gluco-pyranose units and contains 35 chiral centres and α-cyclodextrin has 6 glucopyra-nose units, 30 chiral centres and is smaller than β-cyclodextrin. Collectively they are referred to as chiral cavity phases because they rely on the ability of the enan-tiomer to enter the three-dimensional cyclodextrin cage while at the same time presenting functional groups and hence the chiral centre for interaction with hydroxyl groups on the cone rim. Enantiomers possessing a five-, six- or seven-membered aromatic ring have been resolved by this approach in conjunction with reversed-phase elution. Another approach is the use of the macrocyclic antibiotics vancomycin and teicoplanin as chiral stationary phases. Vancomycin has 18 chiral centres and teicoplanin 23. Both have been used successfully in chiral separations using normal and reversed-phase separations.

Since proteins are optically active, they can in principle be used as a chiral sta-tionary phase. Bovine serum albumin and α_1-acid glycoprotein (AGP) have been evaluated and found to be successful for a wide range of separations, but their mechanism of chiral separation is poorly understood. Both albumin and α_1-acid glycoprotein occur in plasma and have long been known to bind drugs. Albumin has at least two distinct binding sites to which acidic and basic drugs may bind. α_1-Acid glycoprotein has a single drug-binding site restricted to the binding of basic drugs such as propranolol. These protein chiral phases are used in conjunc-tion with aqueous buffers and cannot be used at extremes of pH or in the presence of organic solvents.

11.6 ION-EXCHANGE CHROMATOGRAPHY

11.6.1 Principle

This form of chromatography relies on the attraction between oppositely charged particles. Many biological materials, for example amino acids and proteins, have ionisable groups that may carry a net positive or negative charge. The net charge exhibited by these compounds is dependent on their pK_a values and on the pre-vailing pH of the solution in accordance with the Henderson–Hasselbalch equa-tion (Section 1.4.2, equations 1.8a,b and 1.9a,b). Ion-exchange chromatography is frequently chosen for the separation and purification of proteins, peptides, nucleic acids, polynucleotides and other charged molecules, mainly because of its high resolving power and high capacity.

There are two types of ion exchanger, namely cation and anion exchangers. Cation exchangers possess negatively charged groups and these will attract posi-tively charged cations. These exchangers are also called acidic ion exchangers because their negative charges result from the ionisation of acidic groups. Anion exchangers have positively charged groups that will attract negatively charged anions. The term basic ion exchangers is also used to describe these exchangers, as positive charges generally result from the association of protons with basic groups.

The ion-exchange mechanism is thought to be composed of five distinct steps:

- *Diffusion of the ion to the exchanger surface:* This occurs very quickly in homogeneous solutions.
- *Diffusion of the ion through the matrix structure of the exchanger to the exchange site:* This is dependent upon the degree of cross-linkage of the exchanger and the concentration of the solution. This process is thought to be the feature that controls the rate of the whole ion-exchange process.
- *Exchange of ions at the exchange site:* This is thought to occur instantaneously and to be an equilibrium process:

Cation exchanger:

$$RSO_3^-\dots \qquad Na^+ \qquad + \quad N^+H_3R' \quad \rightleftharpoons \quad RSO_3^-\dots N^+H_3R' + \qquad Na^+$$

| exchanger | counter ion | charged ion to be exchanged | bound ion | exchanged ion |

Anion exchanger:

$$(R)_4N^+\dots Cl^- + {}^-OOCR' \rightleftharpoons (R)_4N^+\dots {}^-OOCR' + \qquad Cl^-$$

The more highly charged the ionised molecule to be exchanged, the tighter it binds to the exchanger and the less readily it is displaced by other ions.

- *Diffusion of the exchanged ion through the exchanger to the surface.*
- *Selective desorption by the eluent and diffusion of the molecule into the external eluent:* The selective desorption of the bound ion is achieved by changes in pH and/or ionic concentration or by affinity elution. In the latter case an ion that has a greater affinity for the exchanger than has the bound ion is introduced into the system.

11.6.2 **Materials and applications**

Low pressure ion-exchange chromatography can be carried out using a variety of matrices and ionic groups. Matrices used include polystyrene, cellulose and agarose. Functional ionic groups include sulphonate ($-SO_3^-$) and quaternary ammonium ($-N^+R_3$), both of which are strong exchangers because they are totally ionised at all normal working pH values, and carboxylate ($-COO^-$) and diethyl-ammonium ($-HN^+(CH_2CH_3)_2$), both of which are termed weak exchangers because they are ionised over only a narrow range of pH values. Examples are given in Table 11.3. Bonded-phase ion-exchangers suitable for HPLC, containing a wide range of ionic groups, are available in pellicular and porous forms. The porous

Table 11.3   Examples of commonly used ion exchangers

Type	Functional groups	Functional group name	Matrices
Weakly acidic (cation exchanger)	$-COO^-$ $-CH_2COO^-$	Carboxy Carboxymethyl	Agarose Cellulose Dextran Polyacrylate
Strongly acidic (cation exchanger)	$-SO_3^-$ $-CH_2SO_3^-$ $-CH_2CH_2CH_2SO_3^-$	Sulpho Sulphomethyl Sulphopropyl	Cellulose Dextran Polystyrene Polyacrylate
Weakly basic (anion exchanger)	$-CH_2CH_2N^+H_3$ $-CH_2CH_2N^+H(CH_2CH_3)_2$	Aminoethyl Diethylaminoethyl	Agarose Cellulose Dextran Polystyrene Polyacrylate
Strongly basic (anion exchanger)	$-CH_2N^+(CH_3)_3$ $-CH_2CH_2N^+(CH_2CH_3)_3$ $-CH_2N^+(CH_3)_2$ $\quad\lvert$ $\quad CH_2CH_2OH$ $-CH_2CH_2N^+(CH_2CH_3)_2$ $\quad\lvert$ $\quad CH_2CH(OH)CH_3$	Trimethylaminomethyl Triethylaminoethyl Dimethyl-2-hydroxyethyl-aminomethyl Diethyl-2-hydroxypropyl-aminoethyl	Cellulose Dextran Polystyrene

variety is based on polystyrene, porous silica or hydrophilic polyethers, and is particularly valuable for the separation of proteins. They have a particle diameter of 5–25 μm. Most HPLC ion exchangers are stable up to 60 °C and separations are often carried out at this temperature, owing to the fact that the raised temperature decreases the viscosity of the mobile phase and thereby increases the efficiency of the separation.

Exchange capacity

All exchangers are characterised by a total exchange capacity, which is defined as the number of milliequivalents of exchangeable ions available, either per gram of dried exchanger or per unit volume of hydrated resin. Sometimes available capacity is also used to express the available capacity for an arbitrarily chosen molecule such as haemoglobin. These exchange capacities give an indication of the degree of substitution of the exchanger and are therefore a helpful guide in deciding on the scale of a particular application.

Choice of exchanger

The choice of the ion exchanger depends upon the stability of the test analytes, their relative molecular mass and the specific requirements of the separation. Many biological analytes, especially proteins, are stable within only a fairly narrow pH range so the exchanger selected must operate within this range. Generally, if an analyte is most stable below its isoionic point (giving it a net positive charge), a cation exchanger should be used, whereas if it is most stable above its isoionic point (giving it a net negative charge) an anion exchanger should be used. Either type of exchanger may be used to separate analytes that are stable over a wide range of pH. The choice between a strong and weak exchanger also depends on analyte stability and the effect of pH on analyte charge. Weak electrolytes requiring a very low or high pH for ionisation can be separated only on strong exchangers, as only they operate over a wide pH range. In contrast, for strong electrolytes, weak exchangers are advantageous for a number of reasons, including a reduced tendency to cause sample denaturation, their inability to bind weakly charged impurities and their enhanced elution characteristics. Although the degree of cross-linking of an exchanger does not influence the ion-exchange mechanism, it does influence its capacity. The relative molecular mass and hence size of the sample component therefore determines which specific exchanger should be used.

Eluent pH

The pH of the buffer selected as eluent should be at least one pH unit above or below the isoionic point of the analytes to be separated. In general, cationic buffers such as Tris, pyridine and alkylamines are used in conjunction with anion exchangers, and anionic buffers such as acetate, barbiturate and phosphate are used with cation exchangers. The precise initial buffer pH and ionic strength should be such as just to allow the binding of the sample components to the exchanger. Equally, a buffer of the lowest ionic strength that effects elution should initially be used for the subsequent elution of the analytes. This ensures that initially the minimum numbers of contaminants bind to the exchanger and that subsequently the maximum number of these impurities remains on the column. The amount of sample that can be applied to a column is dependent upon the size of the column and the capacity of the exchanger. Generally, if isocratic elution is to be used, the sample volume should be 1–5% of the bed volume. If, however, gradient elution is to be used, the initial conditions chosen are such that the exchanger binds all the test analytes at the top of the column. In this case the sample volume is not important and large volumes of dilute solution can be applied, thereby effectively introducing a concentration stage.

Elution

Gradient elution is far more common than isocratic elution. Continuous or stepwise pH and ionic strength gradients may be employed but continuous gradients tend to give better resolution with less peak tailing. Generally, with an anion exchanger, the pH gradient decreases and the ionic strength increases, whereas for cation exchangers both the pH and ionic gradients increase during the elution.

11.6.3 **Chromatofocusing**

The principle of chromatofocusing is similar to that of isoelectric focusing (Section 10.3.4). A linear pH gradient is generated in the column by initially

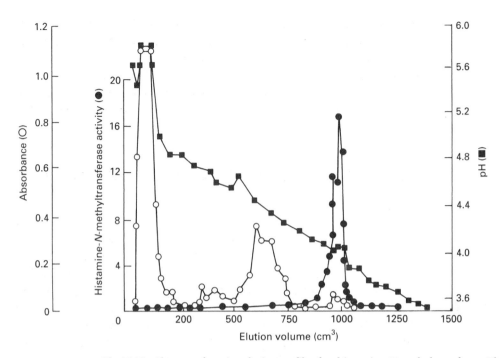

Fig. 11.13. Chromatofocusing elution profile of rat histamine-N-methyltransferase. The partially purified sample (approximately 130 mg protein) was applied to a polybuffer exchanger column (62 cm × 1.6 cm), previously equilibrated with 25 mM piperazine-HCl at pH 5.5; 5 cm³ of the eluent Polybuffer™74, pH 3.5, preceded the sample. Elution was carried out at a flow rate of 20 cm³ h⁻¹. The fractions (5 cm³) were assayed for pH (■), histamine-N-methyltransferase activity (●) expressed as extracted d.p.m. × 10⁻⁴ per 2.5 cm³ chloroform, and absorbance at 600 nm (○) measured after reaction with Coomassie Brilliant Blue. (Reproduced with permission from M. J. York (1982), The purification and kinetic properties of histamine-N-methyl transferase, M.Phil. thesis, University of Hertfordshire.)

pre-equilibrating an anion exchanger to a particular pH, and then running an amphoteric buffer, which has even buffering capacity over a range of pH and a starting pH lower than that at which the column was pre-equilibrated, through the column for a predetermined time. The result is the formation of a pH gradient that is 3–4 pH units lower at the top of the column than at the bottom. If a protein in a starting buffer of a pH similar to that prevailing at the top of the column is added to this pH gradient, it will migrate down the column as a cation, encountering an increasing pH, until it reaches a pH corresponding to its isoelectric point. Just beyond this point it will become an anion and will be able to bind to the positive groups of the exchanger. As the elution with the starting buffer continues, the prevailing pH along the column will be gradually lowered, causing the bound protein to become a cation and binding to cease. The protein will continue its movement down the column until once again it encounters a pH slightly above its isoelectric point, when again it will bind. This process is repeated continuously until the protein is eluted at a pH slightly above its isoelectric point (Fig. 11.13).

Proteins in a mixture added to the column would elute in the order of their isoelectric points. If more of the protein mixture were added to the top of the column during this elution process each protein would automatically catch up with its identical protein in the initial mixture, thereby producing a focusing effect and enabling large volumes to be applied to the column with no deleterious effect to resolution. Thus the technique has a high capacity. Chromatofocusing gives a good resolution of quite complex mixtures of proteins, provided that there are discrete differences in their isoelectric points. Proteins possessing very similar isoelectric points tend to be poorly resolved.

11.7 MOLECULAR EXCLUSION (GEL FILTRATION) CHROMATOGRAPHY

11.7.1 Principle

This chromatographic technique for the separation of molecules on the basis of their molecular size and shape exploits the molecular sieve properties of a variety of porous materials. Probably the most commonly used of such materials is a group of polymeric organic compounds that possess a three-dimensional network of pores that confers gel properties upon them. The term gel filtration is used to describe the separation of molecules of varying molecular size using these gel materials. Porous glass granules have also been used as molecular sieves and the term controlled-pore glass chromatography introduced to describe this separation technique. The terms exclusion or permeation chromatography describe all molecular separation processes using molecular sieves. This section is devoted mainly to gel filtration, as its principles and applications are best documented.

The general principle of exclusion chromatography is quite simple. A column of gel particles or porous glass granules is in equilibrium with a suitable mobile phase for the analytes to be separated. Large analytes that are completely excluded from the pores will pass through the interstitial spaces between the gel particles and will appear in the eluate first. Smaller analytes will be distributed between the mobile phase inside and outside the gel particles and will therefore pass through the column at a slower rate, hence appearing last in the eluate. Three stages in such a column are represented diagrammatically in Fig. 11.14.

The mobile phase trapped by a gel is available to an analyte to an extent that is dependent upon the porosity of the gel particle and the size of the analyte molecule. Thus the distribution of an analyte in a column of a gel is determined solely by the total volume of mobile phase, both inside and outside the gel particles, that is available to it. For a given type of gel, the distribution coefficient, K_d, of a particular analyte between the inner and outer mobile phase is a function of its molecular size. If the analyte is large and completely excluded from the mobile phase within the gel, $K_d = 0$ whereas, if the analyte is sufficiently small to gain complete access to the inner mobile phase, $K_d = 1$. Due to variation in pore size between individual gel particles, there is some inner mobile phase that will be available and some that will not be available to analytes of intermediate size; hence K_d values vary between 0 and 1. It is this complete variation of K_d between these two limits that makes it possible to separate analytes within a narrow molecular size range on a given gel.

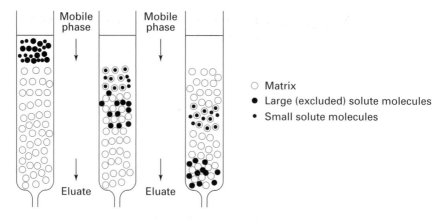

Fig. 11.14. Separation of different size molecules by exclusion chromatography. Large (excluded) molecules are eluted first in the void volume.

For two analytes of different relative molecular mass and K_d values, K'_d and K''_d, the difference in their elution volumes, V_S, can be shown to be:

$$V_S = (K'_d - K''_d) V_i \qquad (11.14)$$

where V_i is the inner volume within the gel available to a compound whose $K_d = 1$.

In practice, deviations from ideal behaviour, for example owing to poor packing of the column, make it advisable to reduce the sample volume below the value of V_S because the ratio between sample volume and inside gel volume affects both the sharpness of the separation and the degree of dilution of the sample.

11.7.2 Materials and applications

Gels that are commonly used for LPLC include dextrans, agarose, polyacrylamide, polyacryloylmorphine and polystyrene. The materials for HPLC and FPLC need to be more rigid to withstand the higher working pressures and are based on cross-linked dextrans, agarose, polystyrene, polyvinylchloride, polyvinylalcohol, poly-methacrylate or rigid controlled-pore glasses or silicas (Table 11.4). Some of these materials, such as those based on polystyrene, can be used only with non-aqueous systems.

Exclusion chromatography requires a single mobile phase and isocratic elution. It is most commonly used with ultraviolet absorption spectrophotometric detect-ors. Exclusion chromatography columns tend to be longer than those for other forms of chromatography in order to increase the amount of stationary phase and hence pore volume.

Applications

Purification   The main application of exclusion chromatography is in the purifi-cation of biological macromolecules by facilitating their separation from larger and smaller molecules. Viruses, enzymes, hormones, antibodies, nucleic acids and

Table 11.4 Stationary phases commonly used for exclusion chromatography

Polymer	Trade name	Fractionation range[a] ($M_r \times 10^{-3}$)
Low pressure liquid chromatography		
Dextran	Sephadex	
	G-10	<0.7
	G-25	1–5
	G-50	1.5–30
	G-100	4–150
	G-200	5–600
Dextran, cross-linked	Sephacryl	
	S-100	1–100
	S-200	5–250
	S-300	10–1500
	S-400	20–8000
Agarose	Sepharose	
	6B	10–4000
	4B	60–20000
	2B	70–40000
Polyacrylamide	Bio-Gel	
	P-2	0.1–1.8
	P-6	1–6
	P-30	2.5–40
	P-100	5–100
	P-300	60–400
High performance liquid chromatography (HPLC and FPLC)		
Polyvinylchloride	Fractogel	
	TSK HW-40	0.1–10
	TSK HW-55	1–700
	TSK HW-65	50–5000
	TSK HW-75	500–50000
Dextran linked to cross-linked agarose	Superdex	
	75	3–70
	200	10–600

[a] Determined for globular proteins. The range is approximately the same for single-stranded nucleic acids and smaller for fibrous proteins and double-stranded DNA.

polysaccharides have all been separated and purified by the use of appropriate gels or glass granules.

Relative molecular mass determination   The elution volumes of globular proteins are determined largely by their relative molecular mass (M_r). It has been shown that, over a considerable range of M_r values, the elution volume or K_d is an

Example 2 **ESTIMATION OF RELATIVE MOLECULAR MASS**

Question

The relative molecular mass (M_r) of a protein was investigated by exclusion chromatography using a Sephacryl S300 column and using aldolase, catalase, ferritin, thyroglobulin and Blue Dextran as standard. The following elution data were obtained.

	M_r	Retention volume V_r (cm^3)
Aldolase	158 000	22.5
Catalase	210 000	21.4
Ferritin	444 000	18.2
Thyroglobulin	669 000	16.4
Blue Dextran	2 000 000	13.6
Unknown		19.5

What is the approximate M_r of the unknown protein?

Answer

A plot of the logarithm of the relative molecular mass of individual proteins versus their retention volume has a linear section from which it can be deduced that the unknown protein with a retention volume of 19.5 cm^3 must have a relative molecular mass of 330 000.

approximately linear function of the logarithm of M_r. Hence the construction of a calibration curve, with proteins of a similar shape and known M_r, enables the M_r values of other proteins, even in crude preparations, to be estimated.

Solution concentration   Solutions of high M_r substances can be concentrated by the addition of dry Sephadex G-25 (coarse). The swelling gel absorbs water and low M_r substances, whereas the high M_r substances remain in solution. After 10 min the gel is removed by centrifugation, leaving the high M_r material in a solution whose concentration has increased but whose pH and ionic strength are unaltered.

Desalting   By use of a column of Sephadex G-25, solutions of high M_r compounds may be desalted. The high M_r compounds move with the void volume, whereas the low M_r compounds are distributed between the mobile and stationary phases and hence move slowly. This method of desalting is faster and more efficient than dialysis. Applications include removal of phenol from nucleic acid preparations, ammonium sulphate from protein preparations and salt from samples eluted from ion-exchange chromatography columns.

11.7.3 **Molecular imprinting**

This innovative form of chromatography has similarities with size exclusion chromatography. In molecular imprinting, the stationary phase is prepared by polymerising a suitable monomer in the presence of a cross-linking reagent and the specific analyte or one closely related to it, for which the phase is required. The chosen compound is referred to as the template. The resulting polymer is finely ground, sieved and washed with an organic solvent to remove the template. Its subsequent use as a stationary phase is based upon the fact that the polymer contains cavities with a molecular shape similar to that of the template and hence will selectively retain the test analyte from a mixture when the sample is eluted with an appropriate mobile phase. The technique has been successfully applied to the separation of a wide range of natural products.

11.8 AFFINITY CHROMATOGRAPHY

11.8.1 Principle

Separation and purification by affinity chromatography is unlike most other forms of chromatography and such techniques as electrophoresis and centrifugation in that it does not rely on differences in the physical properties of the molecules to be separated. Instead, it exploits the unique property of extremely specific biological interactions to achieve separation and purification. As a consequence, affinity chromatography is theoretically capable of giving absolute purification, even from complex mixtures, in a single process. The technique was originally developed for the purification of enzymes, but it has since been extended to nucleotides, nucleic acids, immunoglobulins, membrane receptors and even to whole cells and cell fragments.

The technique requires that the material to be isolated is capable of binding reversibly to a specific ligand that is attached to an insoluble matrix:

$$
\underset{\text{macromolecule}}{\text{M}} \quad + \quad \underset{\substack{\text{ligand} \\ \text{(attached} \\ \text{to matrix)}}}{\text{L}} \quad \underset{k_{-1}}{\overset{k_{+1}}{\rightleftharpoons}} \quad \underset{\text{complex}}{\text{ML}}
$$

Under the correct experimental conditions, when a complex mixture containing the specific compound to be purified is added to the immobilised ligand, generally contained in a conventional chromatography column, only that compound will bind to the ligand. All other compounds can therefore be washed away and the compound subsequently recovered by displacement from the ligand (Fig. 11.15). The method requires a detailed preliminary knowledge of the structure and biological specificity of the compound to be purified so that the separation conditions that are most likely to be successful may be carefully planned. In the case of an enzyme, the ligand may be the substrate, a competitive reversible inhibitor or an allosteric activator. The conditions chosen would normally be those that are optimal for enzyme–ligand binding. Since the success of the method relies on the reversible formation of the complex and on the numerical values of the first-order rate constants k_{+1} and k_{-1}, as the enzyme is added progressively to the

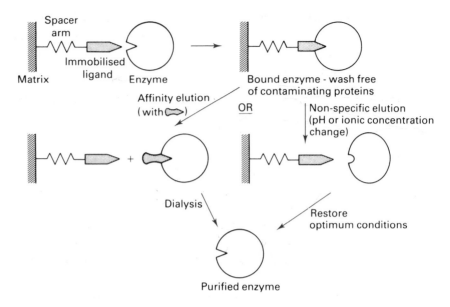

Fig. 11.15. Principle of purification of an enzyme by affinity chromatography.

insolubilised ligand in a column, the enzyme molecules will be stimulated to bind and a dynamic situation develops in which the concentration of the complex and the strength of the binding increase. It is because of this progressive increase in effectiveness during the addition of the sample to the column that column procedures are invariably more successful than batch-type methods. Nevertheless, alternative forms have been developed and are particularly suitable for large-scale work. They include the following:

- *Affinity precipitation:* The ligand is attached to a soluble carrier that can be subsequently precipitated by, for example, a pH change.
- *Affinity partitioning:* The ligand is attached to a water-soluble polymer such as polyethylene glycol, which, with the ligand bound, preferentially partitions into an aqueous polymer phase that is in equilibrium with a pure aqueous phase.

In all cases, for effective chromatography, the association constant, K_a, for the complex should be in the region 10^4 to 10^8 M.

11.8.2 Materials and applications

Matrix

An ideal matrix for affinity chromatography must have the following characteristics:

- possess suitable and sufficient chemical groups to which the ligand may be covalently coupled and it must be stable under the conditions of the attachment,

- be stable during binding of the macromolecule and its subsequent elution,
- interact only weakly with other macromolecules to minimise non-specific adsorption,
- exhibit good flow properties.

In practice, particles that are uniform, spherical and rigid are used. The most common ones are the cross-linked dextrans and agarose, polyacrylamide, poly-methacrylate, polystyrene, cellulose and porous glass and silica.

Ligand

The chemical nature of a ligand is dictated by the biological specificity of the compound to be purified. In practice it is sometimes possible to select a ligand that displays absolute specificity in that it will bind exclusively to one particular compound. More commonly, it is possible to select a ligand that displays group selectivity in that it will bind to a closely related group of compounds that possess a similar in-built chemical specificity. An example of the latter type of ligand is 5'-AMP, which can bind reversibly to many NAD^+-dependent dehydrogenases because it is structurally similar to part of the NAD^+ molecule. It is essential that the ligand possesses a suitable chemical group that will not be involved in the reversible binding of the ligand to the macromolecule, but which can be used to attach the ligand to the matrix. The most common of such groups are $-NH_2$, -COOH, -SH and -OH (phenolic and alcoholic).

To prevent the attachment of the ligand to the matrix interfering with its ability to bind the macromolecule, it is generally advantageous to interpose a spacer arm between the ligand and the matrix. The optimum length of this spacer arm is 6–10 carbon atoms or their equivalent. In some cases, the chemical nature of this spacer is critical to the success of separation. Some spacers are purely hydrophobic, most commonly consisting of methylene groups; others are hydrophilic, possessing carbonyl or imido groups. Spacers are most important for small immobilised ligands but generally are not necessary for macromolecular ligands (e.g. in immunoaffinity chromatography, Section 11.8.4) as their binding site for the mobile macromolecule is well displaced from the matrix.

The most common method of attachment of the ligand to the matrix involves the preliminary treatment of the matrix with cyanogen bromide (CNBr) (Fig. 11.16). The reaction conditions and the relative proportion of the reagents will determine the number of ligand molecules that can be attached to each matrix particle. Alternative coupling procedures involve the use of bis-epoxides, N,N'-disubstituted carbodiimides, sulphonyl chloride, sodium periodate, N-hydroxysuccinimide esters and dichlorotriazines. Many pre-activated matrices, prepared using these coupling reagents, are available commercially.

A range of different spacer arms is used. Examples include 1,6-diaminohexane, 6-aminohexanoic acid and 1,4-bis(2,3-epoxypropoxy)butane. Several supports of the agarose, dextran and polyacrylamide type are commercially available with a variety of spacer arms and ligands pre-attached ready for immediate use. Examples of ligands are given in Table 11.5.

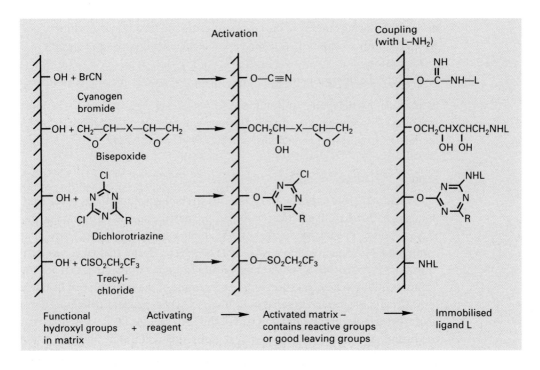

Fig. 11.16. Examples of coupling reactions used to immobilise ligands (L) for affinity chromatography. If a spacer arm is to be introduced between the immobilised ligand and the matrix, the coupling chemistry is similar.

Table 11.5 Examples of group-specific ligands commonly used in affinity chromatography

Ligand	Affinity
Nucleotides	
5'-AMP	NAD$^+$-dependent dehydrogenases, some kinases
2',5'-ADP	NADP$^+$-dependent dehydrogenases
Calmodulin	Calmodulin-binding enzymes
Avidin	Biotin-containing enzymes
Fatty acids	Fatty-acid-binding proteins
Heparin	Lipoproteins, lipases, coagulation factors, DNA polymerases, steroid receptor proteins, growth factors, serine protease inhibitors
Proteins A and G	Immunoglobulins
Concanavalin A	Glycoproteins containing α-D-mannopyranosyl and α-D-glucopyranosyl residues
Soybean lectin	Glycoproteins containing N-acetyl- α-(or β)-D-galactopyranosyl residues
Phenylboronate	Glycoproteins
Poly(A)	RNA containing poly(U) sequences, some RNA-specific proteins
Lysine	rRNA
Cibacron Blue F3G-A	Nucleotide-requiring enzymes, coagulation factors

Practical procedure

The procedure for affinity chromatography is similar to that used in other forms of liquid chromatography. The ligand-treated matrix suspended in buffer is packed into a column in the normal way for the particular type of support. The buffer used must contain any cofactors, such as metal ions, necessary for ligand–macromolecule interaction. Once the sample has been applied and the macromolecule bound, the column is eluted with more buffer to remove non-specifically bound contaminants.

The purified compound is recovered from the ligand by either specific or non-specific elution. Non-specific elution may be achieved by a change in either pH or ionic strength. pH shift elution using dilute acetic acid or ammonium hydroxide results from a change in the state of ionisation of groups in the ligand and/or the macromolecule that are critical to ligand–macromolecule binding. A change in ionic strength, not necessarily with a concomitant change in pH, also causes elution owing to a disruption of the ligand–macromolecule interaction; 1 M NaCl is frequently used for this purpose. If elution is achieved by a pH change, the pH of the collected fractions must be readjusted to the optimum value to minimise the opportunity for protein denaturation. Specific elution involves the addition of a high concentration of substrate, or reversible inhibitor of the macromolecule if it is an enzyme, or the addition of ligands for which the purified compound has a higher affinity than it has for the immobilised ligand. The purified compound is eventually recovered in a buffered solution that may be contaminated with eluting agents or high concentrations of salt and these must be removed by techniques such as exclusion chromatography before the isolation is complete.

Applications

Many enzymes and other proteins, including receptor proteins and immunoglobulins, have been purified by affinity chromatography. The application of the technique is limited only by the availability of immobilised ligands. The principles have been extended to nucleic acids and have made a considerable contribution to developments in molecular biology. Messenger RNA, for example, is routinely isolated by selective hybridisation on poly(U)-Sepharose 4B by exploiting its poly(A) tail. Immobilised single-stranded DNA can be used to isolate complementary RNA and DNA. Whilst this separation can be achieved on columns, it is usually performed using single-stranded DNA immobilised on nitrocellulose filters. Immobilised nucleotides are useful for the isolation of proteins involved in nucleic acid metabolism.

A valuable development of affinity chromatography is its use for the separation of a mixture of cells into homogeneous populations. The technique relies on the antigenic properties of the cell surface or the chemical nature of exposed carbohydrate residues on the cell surface or on a specific membrane receptor–ligand interaction. The immobilised ligands used include protein A, which binds to the Fc region of IgG (Section 7.1), a lectin or the specific ligand for a membrane receptor.

11.8.3 Lectin affinity chromatography

The lectins are a group of proteins produced by animals, plants and slime moulds that have the ability to bind carbohydrate and hence glycoproteins. They have a polymeric structure, most being tetrameric. Their subunits may be either identical, in which case they recognise a single specific saccharide, or of two types in which case they recognise two different saccharides. They all have a molecular mass in the range 40–400 kDa. Their ability to recognise and bind specific saccharides has made them highly valuable in the purification of glycoproteins, particularly membrane receptor proteins.

The most widely used lectins for lectin chromatography are those from leguminous plants (pea, castor bean, soybean) owing to their abundance. They can be immobilised to agarose matrices by conventional techniques and many are available commercially. If the nature of the saccharide component of a glycoprotein is not known, the lectin of choice is selected by a simple screening procedure. Once the glycoproteins have been bound to the immobilised lectin, elution can be achieved in a number of ways:

- by affinity elution using the simple monosaccharide for which the lectin has an affinity,
- by use of a borate buffer, which forms a complex with glycoproteins,
- by the careful change of pH (not below pH 3 or above pH 10),
- by the addition of a reagent such as ethylene glycol to reduce ligand hydrophobic interaction.

One of the attractions of lectin affinity chromatography is that it can be carried out in the presence of relatively high salt concentrations because it does not rely on ionic interactions. In principle, therefore, it can be applied directly after salt fractionation. It has also been used to separate mixtures of cells by taking advantage of the saccharide components of their outer membranes. Most lectin affinity chromatography has been carried out using conventional LPLC.

11.8.4 Immunoaffinity chromatography

The use of antibodies as the immobilised ligand has been exploited in the isolation and purification of a range of proteins including membrane proteins of viral origin. Monoclonal antibodies may be linked to agarose matrices by the cyanogen bromide technique. Protein binding to the immobilised antibody is achieved in neutral buffer solution containing moderate salt concentrations. Elution of the bound protein quite often requires forceful conditions because of the very tight binding with the antibody ($K_d = 10^{-8}$ to 10^{-12} M) and this may lead to protein denaturation. Examples of elution procedures include the use of high salt concentrations with or without the use of detergent and the use of urea or guanidine hydrochloride, both of which cause denaturation. The use of some other chaotropic agents (ions or small molecules that increase the water solubility of non-polar substances) such as thiocyanate, perchlorate and trifluoroacetate, or lowering the pH to about 3, may avoid denaturation.

11.8.5 Metal chelate chromatography (immobilised metal affinity chromatography)

This is a special form of affinity chromatography in which an immobilised metal ion such as Cu^{2+}, Zn^{2+}, Hg^{2+} or Cd^{2+} or a transition metal ion such as Co^{2+}, Ni^{2+} or Mn^{2+} is used to bind proteins selectively by reaction with the imidazole groups of histidine residues, thiol groups of cysteine residues and indole groups of tryptophan residues. The immobilisation of the protein involves the formation of a coordinate bond that must be sufficiently stable to allow protein attachment and retention during the elution of non-binding contaminating material. The subsequent release of the protein can be achieved either by simply lowering the pH, therefore destabilising the protein–metal complex, or by the use of complexing agents such as EDTA. Most commonly the metal atom is immobilised by attachment to an iminodiacetate- or tris(carboxymethyl)ethylenediamine-substituted agarose.

11.8.6 Dye–ligand chromatography

A number of triazine dyes that contain both conjugated rings and ionic groups, fortuitously have the ability to bind to some proteins. The term pseudo-ligands has therefore been used to describe the dyes. It is not possible to predict whether a particular protein will bind to a given dye as the interaction is not specific but is thought to involve interaction with ligand-binding domains via both ionic and hydrophobic forces. Dye binding to proteins enhances their binding to materials such as Sepharose 4B and this is exploited in the purification process. The attraction of the technique is that the dyes are cheap, readily coupled to conventional matrices and are very stable. The most widely used dye is Cibacron Blue F3G-A. Dye selection for a particular protein purification is empirical and is made on a trial-and-error basis. Attachment of the protein to the immobilised dye is generally achieved at pH 7–8.5. Elution is most commonly brought about either by a salt gradient or by affinity (displacement) elution.

11.8.7 Covalent chromatography

This form of chromatography has been developed specifically to separate thiol (-SH)-containing proteins by exploiting their interaction with an immobilised ligand containing a disulphide group. The principle is illustrated in Fig. 11.17. The most commonly used ligand is a disulphide 2′-pyridyl group attached to an agarose matrix such as Sepharose 4B. On reaction with the thiol-containing protein, pyridine 2-thione is released. This process can be monitored spectrophotometrically at 343 nm, thereby allowing the adsorption of the protein to

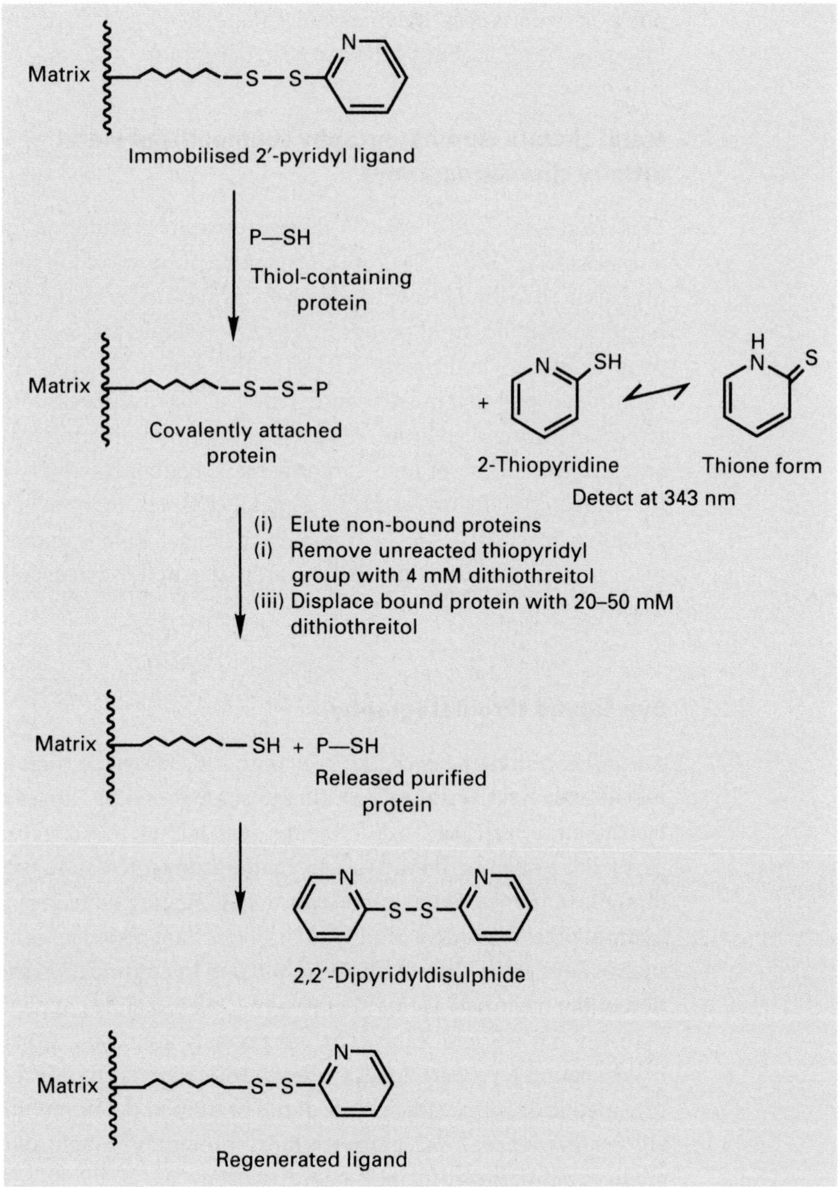

Fig. 11.17. Principle of purification of a protein (P-SH) by covalent chromatography.

be followed. Once the protein has been attached covalently to the matrix, non-thiol-containing contaminants are eluted and unreacted thiopyridyl groups removed by use of 4 mM dithiothreitol or mercaptoethanol. The protein is then released by displacement with a thiol-containing compound such as 20–50 mM dithiothreitol, reduced glutathione or cysteine. The matrix is regenerated by reaction with 2,2′-dipyridyldisulphide. The method has been used successfully for many proteins but its use is limited by its cost and the rather difficult regeneration stage. It can, however, be applied to very impure protein preparations.

11.9 GAS–LIQUID CHROMATOGRAPHY

11.9.1 Principle

The principles of gas–liquid chromatography (GLC or GC) are similar to those of LPLC and HPLC but the apparatus is significantly different. It exploits differences in the partition coefficients between a stationary liquid phase and a mobile gas phase of the volatilised analytes as they are carried through the column by the mobile gas phase. Its use is therefore confined to analytes that are volatile but thermally stable. The partition coefficients are inversely proportional to the volatility of the analytes so that the most volatile elute first. The temperature of the column is raised to 50–300 °C to facilitate analyte volatilisation. The stationary phase consists of a high boiling point liquid material such as silicone grease or wax that is either coated onto the internal wall of the column or supported on an inert granular solid and packed into the column. There is an optimum flow rate of the mobile gas phase for maximum column efficiency (minimum plate height, H). Very high resolutions are obtained (equations 11.8 to 11.12), hence the technique is very useful for the analysis of complex mixtures. GLC is a widely used for the qualitative and quantitative analysis of a large number of low polarity compounds because it has high sensitivity, reproducibility and speed of resolution. Analytically, it is a very powerful technique when coupled to mass spectrometry.

11.9.2 Apparatus and experimental procedure

The major components of a GLC system are:

- a column housed in an oven that can be temperature programmed,
- a sample inlet point,
- a carrier gas supply and control,
- a detector, amplifier and data recorder system (Fig. 11.18).

Columns

These are of two types:

- *Packed conventional columns:*   These consist of a coiled glass or stainless steel column 1–3 m long and 2–4 mm internal diameter. They are packed with stationary phase coated onto an inert silica support. Commonly used stationary phases include the polyethylene glycols (Carbowax 20M, very polar), methylphenyl- and methylvinylsilicone gums (OV17 and OV101, medium and non-polar respectively), Apiezon L (non-polar) and esters of adipic, succinic and phthalic acids. β-Cyclodextrin-based phases are available for chiral separations (Section 11.5.5). The most commonly used support is Celite (diatomaceous silica), which, because of the problem of support–sample interaction, is often treated so that the hydroxyl groups that occur in the Celite are modified. This is normally achieved by silanisation of the support with such compounds as hexamethyldisilazane. The support particles have an even

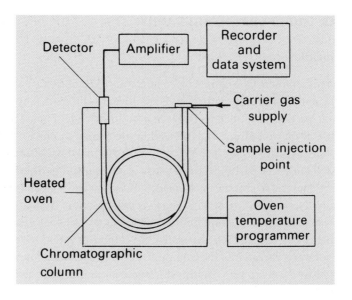

Fig. 11.18. Components of a GLC system.

size, which, for the majority of practical applications, is 60 to 80, 80 to 100, or 100 to 120 mesh (Section 11.3.1). Columns are dry-packed under a slight positive gaseous pressure and after packing must be conditioned for 24–48 h by heating to near the upper working temperature limit, whilst the carrier gas at normal flow rates is passed through the column. During this conditioning, the column should be disconnected from the detector to prevent its contamination. With good-quality liquid phases, column conditioning can be simplified to flushing with carrier gas at 100 °C.

● *Capillary (open tubular) columns:*   These are made of high quality fused quartz and are 10–100 m long and 0.1–1.0 mm internal diameter. They are of two types known as wall-coated open tubular (WCOT) and support-coated open tubular (SCOT), also known as porous layer open tubular (PLOT) columns, for adsorption work. In WCOT columns the stationary phase is thinly coated (0.1–5 μm) directly onto the walls of the capillary, whilst in SCOT columns the support matrix is bonded to the walls of the capillary column and the stationary phase coated onto the support. Commonly used stationary phases include polyethylene glycol (CP wax and DB wax, very polar) and methyl and phenyl-polysiloxanes (BP1, non-polar; BP10, medium polar). They are coated onto the supporting matrix to give a 1–25% loading, depending upon the analysis. The capacity of SCOT columns is considerably higher than that of WCOT columns.

The operating temperature for all types of column must be compatible with the stationary phase chosen for use. Too high a temperature results in excessive column bleed owing to the phase being volatilised off, contaminating the detector and giving an unstable recorder baseline. The working temperature range is chosen to give a balance between peak retention time and resolution. Column temperature is controlled to ±0.1 deg.C. Analyte partition coefficients are particularly sensitive to temperature so that analysis times may be regulated by adjustment of the column oven, which can be operated in one of two modes:

- *Isothermal analysis:*   Here a constant temperature is employed.
- *Temperature programming:*   The temperature is gradually increased to facilitate the separation of compounds of widely differing polarity or M_r. This, however, sometimes results in excessive bleed of the stationary phase as the temperature is raised, giving rise to baseline variation. Consequently some instruments have two identical columns and detectors, one set of which is used as a reference. The currents from the two detectors are opposed, hence, assuming equal bleed from both columns, the resulting current gives a steady baseline as the column temperature is raised. The choice of phase for analysis depends on the analytes under investigation and is best chosen after reference to the literature.

Application of sample

The majority of low and non-polar compounds are directly amenable to GLC, but other compounds possessing such polar groups as -OH, -NH$_2$ and -COOH are generally retained on the column for excessive periods of time if they are applied directly. Poor resolution and peak tailing usually accompany this excessive retention (Section 11.2.4). This problem can be overcome by derivatisation of the polar groups. This increases the volatility and effective distribution coefficients of the compounds. Methylation, silanisation and perfluoracylation are common derivatisation methods for fatty acids, carbohydrates and amino acids.

The test sample is dissolved in a suitable solvent such as acetone, heptane or methanol. Chlorinated organic solvents are generally avoided as they contaminate the detector. For packed and SCOT columns the sample is injected onto the column using a microsyringe through a septum in the injection port attached to the top of the column. Normally 0.1–10 mm^3 of solution is injected. It is common practice to maintain the injection region of the column at a slightly higher temperature (+20–50 °C) than the column itself as this helps to ensure rapid and complete volatilisation of the sample. Sample injection is automated in many commercial instruments as this improves the precision of the analysis. As there is only a small amount of stationary phase present in WCOT columns, only very small amounts of sample may be applied to the column. Consequently a splitter system has to be used at the sample injection port so that only a small fraction of the injected sample reaches the column. The remainder of the sample is vented to waste. The design of the splitter is critical in quantitative analyses in order to ensure that the ratio of sample applied to the column to sample vented is always the same.

Mobile phase

The mobile phase consists of an inert gas such as nitrogen for packed columns or helium or argon for capillary columns. The gas from a cylinder is pre-purified by passing through a variety of molecular sieves to remove oxygen, hydrocarbons and water vapour. It is then passed through the chromatography column at a flow

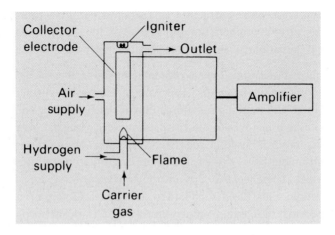

Fig. 11.19. GLC flame ionisation detector. The tip of the flame forms the anode and the collector electrode the cathode.

rate of 40–80 cm³ min⁻¹. A gas-flow controller is used to ensure a constant flow irrespective of the back-pressure and temperature of the column.

11.9.3 **Detectors**

Several types of detector are in common use in conjunction with GLC:

- *Flame ionisation detector (FID):*   This responds to almost all organic compounds. It has a minimum detection quantity of the order of $5 \times 10^{-12}\,\mathrm{g\,s^{-1}}$, a linear range of 10^7 and an upper temperature limit of $400\,°C$. A mixture of hydrogen and air is introduced into the detector to give a flame, the jet of which forms one electrode, whilst the other electrode is a brass or platinum wire mounted near the tip of the flame (Fig. 11.19). When the sample analytes emerge from the column they are ionised in the flame, resulting in an increased signal being passed to the recorder. The carrier gas passing through the column and the detector gives a small background signal, which can be offset electronically to give a stable baseline.

analyte $+ H_2 + O_2 \rightarrow$ combustion products $+ H_2O +$ ions $+$ radicals $+$ electrons
Σ (ions)⁻ $+ \Sigma$ (electrons)⁻ $\rightarrow$ current

- *Nitrogen–phosphorus detector (NPD) (also called a thermionic detector):*   This is similar in design to an FID but has a crystal of a sodium salt fused onto the electrode system, or a burner tip embedded in a ceramic tube containing a sodium salt or a rubidium chloride tip. The NPD has excellent selectivity towards nitrogen- and phosphorus-containing analytes and shows a poor response to analytes possessing neither of these two elements. Its linearity (10^5) and upper temperature limit $(300\,°C)$ are not quite as good as an FID but its detection limits $(10^{-14}\,\mathrm{g\,s^{-1}})$ are better. It is widely used in organophosphorus pesticide residue analysis.

- *Electron capture detector (ECD):*   This responds only to analytes that capture electrons, particularly halogen-containing compounds. This detector is widely used in the analysis of polychlorinated compounds, such as the pesticides DDT, dieldrin and aldrin. It has a very high sensitivity ($10^{-13}\,g\,s^{-1}$) and an upper temperature limit of $300\,°C$ but its linear range (10^2–10^4) is much lower than that of the FID. The detector works by means of a radioactive source (^{63}Ni) ionising the carrier gas and releasing an electron that gives a current across the electrodes when a suitable voltage is applied. When an electron-capturing analyte (generally one containing a halogen atom) emerges from the column, the ionised electrons are captured, the current drops and this change in current is recorded. The carrier gas most commonly used in conjunction with an ECD is nitrogen or an argon $+5\%$ methane mixture.
- *Flame photometric detector:*   This exploits the fact the P- and S-containing analytes emit light when they are burned in a FID-type detector. This light is detected and quantified. The detection limit is of the order of $1.0\,pg$ for P-containing compounds and $20\,pg$ for S-containing compounds.
- *Rapid scanning Fourier transform infrared detector:*   This records the infrared spectrum of the emerging analytes and can give structural as well as quantitative information about the analyte. Any analyte with an infrared spectrum can be detected with a detection limit of about $1\,ng$.
- *Mass spectrometer detector:*   This is a universal detector that gives a mass spectrum of the analyte and therefore gives both structural and quantitative data. Its detection limit is less than $1\,ng$ per scan. Analytes may be detected by a total ion current (TIC) (Section 9.4.1) trace that is non-selective, or by selected ion monitoring (SIM) (Section 9.5.7) that can be specific for a selected analyte. In cases where authentic samples of the test compounds are not available for calibration purposes or where the identity of the analytes is not known, a mass spectrometer is the best means of detecting and identifying the analyte. Special separators are available for removing the bulk of the carrier gas from the sample emerging from the column prior to its introduction in the mass spectrometer (Section 9.3).

The volatile solvent used to introduce the test sample onto the column gives rise to a solvent peak at the beginning of the chromatograph. The main forms of detector respond to this solvent with varying sensitivity, thereby affecting the detection and resolution of rapidly eluting analytes.

Most modern GLC systems are controlled by dedicated microcomputers capable of automating and optimising the experimental conditions, recording the calibration and test retention data, carrying out the statistical analysis, and displaying the outputs in colour graphics in real time.

11.9.4 **Applications**

Until the development of HPLC, GLC was probably the most commonly used form of chromatography. Its use nowadays is confined to volatile, non-polar compounds that do not need derivatisation. Analytes are characterised by their retention time or preferably by their retention time relative to a standard reference compound. In the analysis of compounds that form a homologous series, for example the methyl esters of the saturated fatty acids, there is a linear relationship between the logarithm of the retention time and the number of carbon atoms. There are similar but parallel calibration lines for mono- and di-unsaturated fatty acids. This can be exploited, for example, to identify an unknown fatty acid ester in a fat hydrolysate.

11.10 THIN-LAYER (PLANAR) CHROMATOGRAPHY

11.10.1 Principle

Although thin-layer chromatography (TLC) shares many theoretical principles with the various forms of column chromatography discussed so far, its practical format is quite different. The stationary phase is coated as a thin (0.25–2.0 mm) layer on a glass or metal foil plate commonly 5–20 cm square or rectangular. The test sample is applied as a spot or thin band near one end of the plate (origin) that is then placed in a reservoir of mobile phase that is allowed to pass over the plate, generally by simple capillary action. As there is little resistance to the flow, the front of the mobile phase moves rapidly across the layer. As it does so it transfers analytes in the test sample with it at a rate determined by their distribution coefficients between the mobile phase and the stationary phase. The stationary phase may be one of a variety of forms so that the separation process may be based on adsorption, partition, chiral, ion-exchange or molecular exclusion principles. Analyte movement ceases when the mobile phase front reaches the end of the layer or when the plate is removed from the mobile phase reservoir. The movement of a given analyte is characterised not by a retention time or volume but by a retardation factor (R_f) defined as follows:

$$R_f = \frac{\text{distance moved by the analyte from the origin}}{\text{distance moved by the mobile phase front from the origin}} \tag{11.15}$$

The performance of a thin-layer separation can be characterised by the number of theoretical plates (N), plate height (H) and capacity factor (k') that may be calculated according to the following equations:

$$N = 16(d_A/w)^2 \tag{11.16}$$

$$H = d_A/N \tag{11.17}$$

$$k' = (1 - R_f)/R_f = (d_f/d_A) - 1 \tag{11.18}$$

where d_A is the distance moved by the analyte from the origin, d_f is the distance moved by the mobile phase front from the origin, and w is the width of the analyte spot.

11.10.2 **Apparatus and experimental procedure**

Preparation of plates

The stationary phase is applied to the plate as a slurry, generally in water, using a plate spreader that allows a uniform layer of the required thickness to be deposited. Alternatively, pre-prepared plates are available commercially. For analytical separations the layer needs to be of the order of 0.25 mm thick and for preparative purposes about 2 mm. For all stationary phases except those for separations based on molecular exclusion, the coated plates are allowed to dry at room temperature before use. In the case of adsorption phases, this drying is achieved by heating the plate to 100–120 °C, since this temperature also serves to activate the adsorbent.

Application of sample

The sample dissolved in an organic solvent is applied by a micropipette about 2 cm from the edge of the plate. The solvent may be removed from the spot by gentle heating with an air dryer and more sample applied if necessary. Twelve to fifteen different samples can be applied as discrete spots on a single plate. For preparative purposes, the sample is applied as a band across the plate.

Plate development

The separation process takes place in a glass tank containing the mobile phase to a depth of about 1.5 cm. The tank is allowed to equilibrate for about 1 h with a glass lid on top. The plate is then placed vertically in the tank with the edge near the origin standing in the liquid. The lid is replaced and separation allowed to take place, generally within 20–30 min for analytical separations and up to 75–90 min for preparative separations. When the mobile phase front approaches the distant edge of the plate, the plate is removed from the tank and the separated analytes detected. The resolution of the analytes can be increased by the technique of two-dimensional development. In this technique the sample is applied as a single spot in one corner of the plate and the plate developed as previously. It is then dried, turned through 90° and developed in a second direction with a different mobile phase that has different K_d values for the analytes than had the first.

Detection of analytes

The separated analytes may be detected in a number of ways:

- by spraying the plate with a specific reagent that converts the analytes to a coloured product,
- by examining the plate under ultraviolet light, assuming that the analytes absorb in this region,
- by incorporating a fluorescent dye into the stationary phase so that when the plate is examined under ultraviolet light the analytes show as blue, green or black spots against a fluorescent background,

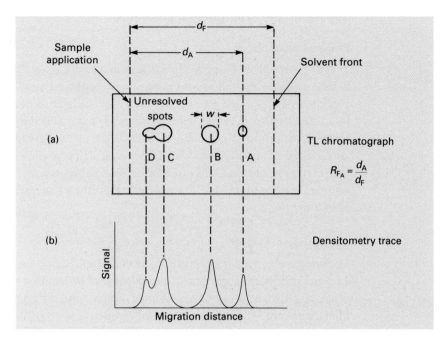

Fig. 11.20. (a) Thin-layer chromatograph of a mixture of analytes A to D; (b) the densitometer trace from which quantitative data can be calculated.

- by using radiolabelled analytes and subjecting the developed plate to autoradiography using an X-ray film or by scanning the plate with a radio-chromatograph scanner.

The amount of analyte present in each spot can best be measured using a precision densitometer. This measures the intensity of the spot in the visible or ultraviolet region and may simultaneously give a complete spectrum of the compound for identification purposes. The identification of unknown analytes is based on such data and on the comparison of the measured R_f value with those of reference compounds chromatographed alongside the test sample (Fig. 11.20).

11.10.3 Applications

The great attractions of TLC are its practical simplicity, low cost and ability to separate several test samples simultaneously. Its main disadvantages are the ease with which the layer may be damaged and its lack of good reproducibility. The consequence of these combined characteristics is that its use is currently confined to qualitative studies such as to check for the presence of a particular analyte. Examples include studies on natural products and peptide mapping. Further details can be found in the 'Suggestions for further reading' (Section 11.12).

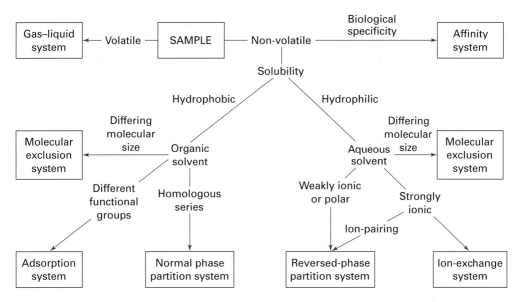

Fig. 11.21. Rationale for the choice of a chromatographic system.

11.11 **SELECTION OF A CHROMATOGRAPHIC SYSTEM**

It is possible to predict the type of system most likely to be applicable to the separation of compounds for which the physical characteristics are known (Fig. 11.21). The majority of chromatographic procedures exploit differences in physical properties of compounds, the exception being affinity chromatography, which is based on the specific ligand-binding properties of biological macromolecules. If this form of chromatography can be applied, it is the most likely to be successful. Volatile compounds are best separated by GLC, whereas non-volatile compounds that are soluble in organic solvents are generally best separated by either adsorption or normal-phase liquid chromatography. If the compounds have different functional groups, adsorption chromatography on silica with non-polar solvent is probably the better method. To separate low polarity compounds in a homologous series, normal-phase liquid systems are preferred. If water-soluble compounds are non-ionic or weakly ionic, reversed-phase liquid chromatography is preferable where a non-polar stationary phase such as a hydrocarbon is used together with a polar mobile phase such as water/acetonitrile or water/methanol mixtures. Water-soluble compounds that are strongly ionic are best separated by an ion-exchange system, using either an anionic or cationic resin, together with a suitable buffer system for elution. Ionic compounds can, however, be separated by reversed-phase partition systems by the technique of ion-pairing. Compounds differing in molecular size are best separated by molecular exclusion chromatography.

Whatever form of liquid chromatography is chosen for a particular biochemical study, the decision to use LPLC or HPLC depends on many factors including the availability of apparatus, cost, the scale of the separation, and whether the separation is to be qualitative or quantitative. The modern trend is to select HPLC, which is certainly capable of giving fast, accurate and precise data. Reversed-phase HPLC, in particular, is proving to be an extremely versatile technique. The application of HPLC techniques to protein separations, via FPLC, is also proving to be a quick, robust technique, particularly in cases where protein denaturation is not a problem. The simplicity of TLC and its facility to separate multiple samples simultaneously makes it attractive for routine, mainly quantitative separations.

11.12   SUGGESTIONS FOR FURTHER READING

MONDELLO, L., LEWIS, A. C. and BARTLE, K. D. (2002). *Multidimensional Chromatography*. Wiley, Chichester. (Discussion of such developments as the coupling of HPLC to GC and SCFC to GC; 2D GC and the applications of these techniques.)

SHERMA, J. and FRIED, B. (eds.) (2003). *Handbook of Thin-Layer Chromatography*, 3rd edn. Marcel Dekker, New York. (Detailed discussion of the principles, practice and applications of TLC to a wide range of biological applications.)

SIMPSON, N. J. K. (ed.) (2000). *Solid Phase Extraction – Principles, Techniques and Applications.* Marcel Dekker, New York. (Comprehensive coverage of this important analytical technique.)

VARIOUS AUTHORS. *Trends in Analytical Chemistry* (2002), **21**. (Whole volume of the journal devoted to a review of recent developments and applications of GC.)

Chapter 12

Spectroscopic techniques: I Atomic and molecular electronic spectroscopy

12.1 INTRODUCTION

12.1.1 Properties of electromagnetic radiation

The interaction of electromagnetic radiation with matter is essentially a quantum phenomenon and is dependent upon both the properties of the radiation and the appropriate structural parts of the material involved. This is not surprising, as the origin of the radiation is due to energy changes within the matter itself. An understanding of the properties of electromagnetic radiation and its interaction with matter leads to a recognition of the variety of types of spectra and consequently spectroscopic techniques and their application to the solution of biological problems. Also the transitions which occur within matter (see e.g. Section 12.1.2) are quantum phenomena and the spectra which arise from such transitions are, at least in principle, predictable. Table 12.1 shows the various interactions, with parts of matter, of the electromagnetic spectrum and corresponding wavelengths. The various parts of matter both give rise to and are affected by the radiation in the corresponding region of the spectrum.

Electromagnetic radiation (Fig. 12.1) is composed of both an electric vector and magnetic vector (which gives rise to the name), which oscillate in planes at right angles (normal) to each other and mutually at right angles to the direction of propagation.

12.1.2 Interaction with matter

Electromagnetic phenomena exhibit energy, frequency, wavelength and intensity. All these are interrelated and can be explained either in terms of waveforms or particles termed photons or quanta. These phenomena are best exemplified by considering electronic spectra. Electrons in either atoms or molecules may be distributed between several energy levels but principally reside in the lowest levels or ground state. In order for an electron to be promoted to a higher level (or excited state), energy must be put into the system and this gives rise to an absorption spectrum if the energy is derived from electromagnetic radiation. Only the exact amount of energy equivalent to the difference in energy level, in accordance with the rules of quantum mechanics, will be absorbed. This is termed one quantum of

Table 12.1 Interaction of electromagnetic radiation and the various parts or 'structures' of matter

Phenomenon	Region of spectrum	Wavelength
Nuclear	Gamma	0.1 nm
Inner electrons	X-rays	0.1–1.0 nm
Ionisation	Ultraviolet	0–200 nm
Valency electrons	Near ultraviolet and visible	200–800 nm
Molecular vibrations	Near infrared and infrared	0.8–25 μm
Rotation and electron spin orientation in magnetic fields	Microwaves	400 μm–30 cm
Nuclear spin orientation in magnetic fields	Radiowaves	100 cm and above

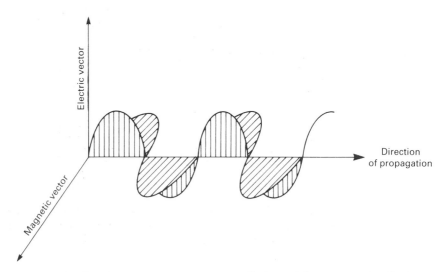

Fig. 12.1. The electric and magnetic vectors or 'oscillations' of electromagnetic radiation and the direction of propagation.

energy for a single-electron transition, and the absolute magnitude of each quantum will differ according to the difference in energy levels involved. When an electron falls from a higher to lower level, then exactly one quantum of energy is emitted from the system, giving rise to an emission spectrum. Energy in other forms may be put into the system; for example, the heating of metals achieves the promotion of electrons to higher energy levels and, if sufficient energy has been input, when they return to lower levels visible light is emitted. This gives rise to the effect of the glowing of heated metals.

Fig. 12.2a is a diagrammatic representation of electron transitions in the sodium atom. These transitions in most atoms give rise to relatively simple line spectra. The situation in molecules is somewhat more complicated, although the

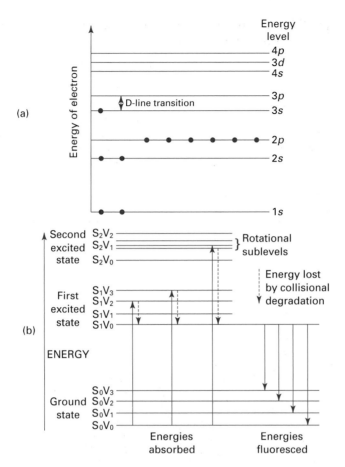

Fig. 12.2. Energy levels and transitions of electrons: (a) in the sodium atom and (b) in a fluorescent organic molecule. Note: for clarity, rotational sublevels have been indicated only for vibrational sublevel S_2V_1.

same basic principles apply, because more different kinds of energy level exist. Moreover the atoms in molecules may vibrate and rotate about a bond axis, which gives rise to vibrational and rotational sublevels. This situation is shown diagrammatically in Fig. 12.2b but, owing to the subdivision of energy levels in molecules, molecular spectra are usually observed as band spectra.

The energy change for an electron transition is defined in quantum terms by the following simple relation;

$$\Delta E = E_1 - E_2 = h\nu \tag{12.1}$$

where ΔE is the change in energy state of the electron or the energy of electromagnetic radiation absorbed or emitted by an atom or molecule, E_1 is the energy of the electron in its original state, E_2 is the energy of the electron in the final state, h is the Planck constant $(= 6.63 \times 10^{-34}\,\mathrm{J\,s})$, ν is the frequency of the electromagnetic radiation and is equal to the number of oscillations made by the wave in 1 s. It

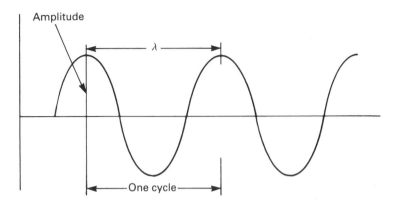

Fig. 12.3. Representation of terms in a single sinusoidal waveform. (The number of cycles occurring in unit time (second) is the frequency measured in hertz.)

therefore has units of reciprocal seconds (s^{-1}). One oscillation per second is called 1 Hz. Frequency is related to wavelength (λ) by the relationship $\nu = c/\lambda$ where c is the speed of light ($3 \times 10^8\,\mathrm{ms}^{-1}$ in a vacum). The wavelength of electromagnetic radiation is equal to $c\bar{\nu}$, where $\bar{\nu}$ is the wave number of electromagnetic radiation in waves cm^{-1} (kaysers). Fig. 12.3 shows some of the interrelationships. It should be noted that wavelength should be expressed in submultiples of a metre, i.e. nanometre (nm), micrometre (μm), centimetre (cm) etc. (not ångströms (Å) or mμ or μ) and frequency expressed in hertz (not cycles s^{-1}).

In Fig. 12.2a,b, electron transitions in atoms or molecules give rise to the electronic spectra generally observed as absorption, emission or fluorescence phenomena (Section 12.5) in the ultraviolet and visible regions of the electromagnetic spectrum. The basic quantum relationships hold for other regions also. Of course, different energy transitions occur in these other regions and these will be indicated as each appropriate part of the system is dealt with.

In the following subsections, each region of the electromagnetic spectrum is treated in terms of the interaction involved, instrumentation used and application to appropriate biological problems. The treatment is unequal, however, and some sections are presented in considerably more detail to reflect usage.

12.2 γ-RAY SPECTROSCOPY AND γ-RAY RESONANCE SPECTROSCOPY

12.2.1 Principles

γ-Rays are of nuclear origin, but they are also part of the electromagnetic spectrum and so, in principle, it is possible to develop spectroscopic methods involving them. Owing to their considerable penetrating power, the main applications in a biological context are in imaging but also in radiotherapy. The rays arise from energy transitions occurring within the nucleus, the mechanisms of which are not described here. For further details, see the literature cited in Section 12.11.

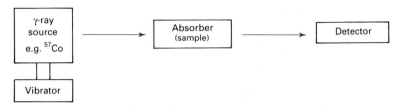

Fig. 12.4. Layout of a simple Mössbauer spectrometer.

An important application of γ-ray emission spectroscopy is the use of the element technicium, Tc, which does not occur naturally but is a product of the nuclear industry. This element may be used for medical studies because, if it is complexed to a compound that is preferentially concentrated in specific biological tissues, particularly bone, liver or brain, its location can be determined by its emission spectrum. The emitted radiation is detected using a device known as a γ-camera, enabling the shape and structure of the tissue under study to be investigated. Despite the name given to the instrument, in this type of application the technique is essentially spectroscopic.

Nuclear γ-resonance, the so-called Mössbauer effect, was discovered in 1957. Many isotopes exhibit the effect but the main emphasis appears to have centred around the ^{57}Fe isotope. Although the applications have been somewhat limited, there is considerable potential for the study of biologically important metal-containing complexes.

12.2.2 **Mössbauer spectroscopy**

Principles

The γ-ray energy from a radioactive nucleus may be modulated by giving a Doppler velocity to the source. The Doppler effect (observed in all waveforms, sound and electromagnetic) is recognised as the apparent change in frequency that occurs when the source is moving relative to the detector (observer). The change in frequency is proportional to the source velocity and any velocity may be chosen to give the required frequency. γ-Rays of discrete energy can be absorbed resonantly by appropriate nuclei. The source used is usually ^{57}Co; this emits a range of γ-rays with different energies, an appropriate one of which may be selected. The selected ray is then modulated by the imposed Doppler phenomenon.

Instrumentation

Fig. 12.4 shows a very simplified diagram of the arrangement required to perform Mössbauer spectroscopy. Usually, because of the energies and wavelengths involved, the Doppler velocity can be imposed by rapidly vibrating the ^{57}Co source.

Applications

The major application of this technique is in the study of the coordination of metal atoms by ligands of an appropriate complexing agent. Model compounds have been investigated, enabling a better understanding of how certain metals of biological importance are affected by changes in the binding properties of the ligand either by chemical modification or because of local environment differences. An example is sickle cell anaemia, where, compared with normal haemoglobin, the iron atom is distorted out of the plane of the haem moiety.

12.3 X-RAY SPECTROSCOPY

12.3.1 Principles

Whereas γ-rays are of nuclear origin, X-rays arise from displacement of inner, extranuclear electrons. The electrons, with principle quantum numbers 1, 2 and 3, in an atom can be imagined to occupy shells – K, L and M, respectively. Should a bombarding electron from an external source have sufficient energy to displace a K shell (innermost) electron in a target atom, then this vacancy is filled within a time span of 10^{-4} s by an L shell electron and an X-ray of appropriate wavelength is emitted. The energy transition from L to K is, of course, governed by quantum rules and $E = h\upsilon$ must be satisfied; hence the frequency and wavelength of the emitted X-ray are determined.

X-rays can be absorbed by matter and this gives rise to X-ray absorption spectra. The rules applying to the relationship between an incident beam of monochromatic X-radiation (I_0) and the transmitted portion I, are similar to the Beer–Lambert case described in Section 12.4.1. If μ is the linear absorption coefficient of the absorbing material then

$$I = I_0 e^{-\mu x} \tag{12.2}$$

where x is the thickness of the absorber.

If X-rays have wavelength shorter than the so-called K absorption edge of an atom, then it is possible for the incident radiation to dislodge K electrons. This then results in the emission of X-rays (because of K electron displacement) of a frequency different from that of the incident ray. The phenomenon is called X-ray fluorescence and gives rise to X-ray fluorescence analysis (XRFA). The general principles of fluorescence are considered in Section 12.5.

12.3.2 Instrumentation and applications

A suitable X-ray source is required that can be focused into the specimen chamber where the substance under test is excited by the incident beam. A monochromator is required also to disperse the fluorescent (emitted) radiation and finally a suitable detector and data-processing facilities are needed. Fig. 12.5 is a simple representation of the required layout.

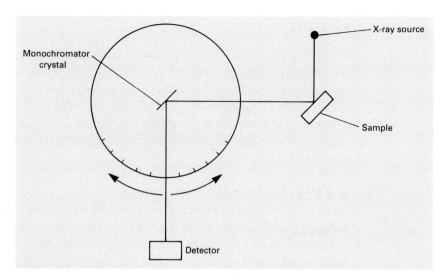

Fig. 12.5. X-ray fluorescence analysis. Dispersion of fluorescent X-rays may be detected at various angles.

The technique has wide applications in forensic science and environmental pollution studies because it enables many elements to be detected and concentrations measured. Of course the analysis is essentially concerned with elements but can be a useful adjunct to, for example, the detection and measurement of trace elements in fertilisers. Such elements may well find their way into the food chain, with possible toxic consequences if they potentially interfere with normal metabolism. An example of such an application would be the study of the uptake of lead in plants at various distances from, say, a heavily used thoroughfare.

Absorption and emission spectra are obtained in ways similar to those described below for the ultraviolet/visible region of the electromagnetic spectrum (Section 12.4). A clinical application for performing bone densitometry measurements involves either single-photon or dual energy X-ray absorptiometry (DEXA). These studies are useful for monitoring hormone replacement therapy (HRT) in female patients. X-ray spectrometers obviously require a more rigorous approach to the incorporation of safety features, but the essential requirements of source, monochromator and detector are the same.

12.4 **ULTRAVIOLET AND VISIBLE LIGHT SPECTROSCOPY**

These regions of the electromagnetic spectrum and their associated techniques are probably the most widely used, for both routine analytical work and research into biological problems. The energy transitions that occur here are exactly those described in Section 12.1.2. It is convenient, however, to deal here with the appropriate laws related to the absorption of 'light', that region of the electromagnetic spectrum for which these laws were developed.

12.4.1 **Principles**

The Beer–Lambert law is a combination of two laws, each dealing separately with the absorption of light, related to the concentration of the absorber (the substance responsible for absorbing the light) and the pathlength or thickness of the layer (related to the absolute amount of the absorber). Provided an absorbing substance is partially transparent it will transmit a portion of the incident radiation. The ratio of the intensities of transmitted and incident light gives the transmittance, T, expressed as:

$$T = I/I_0 \tag{12.3}$$

where I_0 is the intensity of incident radiation and I is the intensity of transmitted radiation. (Note: intensity = number of photons interacting in unit time (seconds).)

A 100% value of T represents a totally transparent substance, with no radiation being absorbed, whereas a zero value of T represents a totally opaque substance, which, in effect, represents complete absorption. For intermediate values we can define the absorbance (A) or extinction (E), which is given by the logarithm (base 10) of the reciprocal of the transmittance:

$$A = E = \log(1/T) = \log(I_0/I) \; \text{transmitted} \tag{12.4}$$

Absorbance used to be called optical density (OD) but continued use of this term should be discouraged. Also, as absorbance is a logarithm it is by definition unitless and has a range of values from 0 ($\equiv 100\% T$) to ∞ ($\equiv 0\% T$). However, the use of the term 'absorbance' is incorrect when the measurement is based on light scattering rather than absorption. This situation is commonly encountered in the estimation of bacterial cell numbers or measurements on isolated organelles. It is for this reason that microbiologists continue to use the term optical density for cell count studies. In such studies the more correct term is attenuance, symbol D. Attenuance reduces to absorbance when there is negligible light scattering.

It is now possible to define the Beer–Lambert law, which, as described above, states that the absorbance is proportional to both the concentration of absorber and thickness of the layer, as

$$A = \epsilon_\lambda cl \tag{12.5}$$

where ϵ_λ is the molar absorbance coefficient (or molar extinction coefficient) for the absorber at wavelength λ, c is the concentration of absorbing solution, and l is the pathlength through the solution (or thickness).

In the strictest use of SI units the concentration should be expressed as $mol\,m^{-3}$ (which is not molar) and the pathlength in metres. As A is unitless this would give units for ϵ_λ as $mol^{-1}\,m^2$ (derived from $1/(mol\,m^{-3}\,m)$), if equation 12.5 is rearranged to give $\epsilon_\lambda = A/(cl)$). This is to be expected, as the value of the absorbance is also dependent upon the area of illumination by the incident radiation. As this area is identical for both sample and reference it can be ignored in any calculations. However, more practical units for ϵ_λ are $dm^3\,mol^{-1}\,cm^{-1}$, which conform to the definition of molarity (despite being incoherent in SI terms) and the common use of 1 cm pathlength cuvettes (see Section 1.2.2). Sometimes molar absorbance coefficients are extremely large and in such cases a more convenient way of expressing values is to quote the absorbance of a 1 cm thick sample of a 1% solution of the absorbant. This is distinguished by writing the coefficient as $A_{1cm}^{1\%}$.

Example 1 CALCULATION OF MOLAR EXTINCTION COEFFICIENT

Question

An aliquot of a solution containing a light-absorbing substance at a concentration of 5 g dm^{-3}, was placed in a 2 cm light path cuvette. The cuvette was placed in a spectrophotometer and a beam of light of wavelength λ was passed through the cuvette containing the solution. A transmission value of 80% was recorded.

What is (i) the absorbance of the solution, and (ii) the molar extinction coefficient if the molecular mass of the substance is known to be 410?

Answer

(i) As the concentration is given in terms of absolute mass per unit volume, it is necessary to find a 'specific extinction coefficient', ϵ_s.

The transmission, T, is expressed as the percentage $100 \times I_t$, of the incident light I_0;

$$T = 80\% = 100 \times \frac{I_t}{I_0}$$

If $I_0 \equiv 100\%$ of the light, then

$I_t \equiv 80\%$

$$\frac{I_t}{I_0} = \frac{80}{100} = 0.8$$

Absorbance $= A = \log(1/T) = \log(1/0.8) = \log(1.25) = 0.0969$

$A = \epsilon_s \times c \times \ell = \epsilon_s \times 5 \times 2$

Therefore,

$$\epsilon_s = \frac{0.0969}{10} = 9.69 \times 10^{-3} \, \mathrm{g^{-1} \, dm^3 \, cm^{-1}}$$

(ii) As the specific extinction coefficient relates to 'per gram', the molar extinction coefficient is obtained simply by multiplying by the relative molecular mass. Hence,

$\epsilon_s \times 410 = \epsilon_\lambda$

$9.69 \times 10^{-3} \times 410 = 3.973 \, \mathrm{(mol \, dm^{-3})^{-1} cm^{-1}}$

12.4.2 Instrumentation

What material is used in the optical parts of the instrument depends on the wavelength used. In the ultraviolet region it is necessary to use prisms, gratings, reflectors and cuvettes made of silica. Above 350 nm wavelength, borosilicate glass may be used but also there are now some plastic materials (e.g. disposable cuvettes) available that are transparent over virtually the whole of the visible region and into the near ultraviolet.

Wavelength selection is obviously of crucial importance. In the visible region where the analyte may not absorb, but can be readily modified chemically to produce a coloured product, coloured filters may be used that absorb all but a certain limited range of wavelengths. This limited range is known as the bandwidth of the filter. The methods that use filter selectors and depend on the production of a coloured compound are the basis of colorimetry; such methods give moderate accuracy, as even the best filters (interference types) do not have particularly narrow bandwidths. The usual procedure is to use two optically matched cuvettes, one containing a blank in which all the materials are mixed except the sample under test, an equivalent volume of solvent being added to this mixture, and the other containing the coloured material to be measured. It is necessary to standardise or zero the instrument using the blank, change cuvettes and read the absorbance. The best analytical procedure requires the zero to be reset between each measurement as colorimeters, and some filters, are influenced by temperature changes. It is also good practice to work from the most dilute (least colour) to the most concentrated because even if the cuvette is rinsed between each measurement the possibility of carryover should be minimised. Table 12.2 shows a number of commonly used colorimetric assays.

If the wavelength is selected using prisms or gratings, the technique is called spectrophotometry. In both colorimetry and spectrophotometry, the usual procedure is to prepare a set of standards and produce a concentration versus absorbance calibration curve, which is linear because it is a Beer–Lambert plot. Absorbances of unknowns are then measured and the concentration interpolated from the linear region of the plot. Interpolation is critical because:

- one should never extrapolate beyond the region for which any instrument has been calibrated,
- particularly in colorimetry, a phenomenon known as the Job effect (see below) occurs.

If we continue to take measurements beyond the colour reagent limit, it is observed that the linearity of the Beer–Lambert calibration does not continue indefinitely but forms a plateau, at a point which indicates that there is insufficient reagent to produce any more colour. This phenomenon is known as the Job effect. To extrapolate beyond the linear portion of the curve, therefore, would potentially introduce enormous errors. Furthermore, if a particular sample gives a very high absorbance reading, it is incorrect procedure merely to dilute that sample. This achieves nothing as all the materials in the sample are diluted to the same extent. The correct procedure is to return to the original material and dilute that appropriately and then perform all the steps required to produce colour.

If high precision is not required and the absorbances of the test and standard are close in value, the Beer–Lambert linear relation may be assumed for this experiment and an approximate concentration obtained from the simple relationship:

Table 12.2   Common colorimetric assays

Substance	Reagent	Wavelength (nm)
Inorganic phosphate	Ammonium molybdate; H_2SO_4; 1,2,4-amino-naphthol; $NaHSO_3$, Na_2SO_3	600
Amino acids	(a) Ninhydrin	570 (proline 420)
	(b) Cupric salts	620
Peptide bonds	Biuret (alkaline tartrate buffer, cupric salt)	540
Phenols, tyrosine	Folin (phosphomolybdate, phosphotungstate, cupric salt)	660 or 750 (750 more sensitive)
Protein	(a) Folin	660
	(b) Biuret	540
	(c) BCA reagent (bicinchoninic acid)	562
	(d) Coomassie Brilliant Blue	595
Carbohydrate	(a) Phenol, H_2SO_4	Varies, e.g. glucose 490, xylose 480
	(b) Anthrone (anthrone, H_2SO_4)	620 or 625
Reducing sugars	Dinitrosalicylate, alkaline tartrate buffer	540
Pentoses	(a) Bial (orcinol, ethanol, $FeCl_3$, HCl)	665
	(b) Cysteine, H_2SO_4	380–415
Hexoses	(a) Carbazole, ethanol, H_2SO_4	540 or 440
	(b) Cysteine, H_2SO_4	380–415
	(c) Arsenomolybdate	Usually 500–570
Glucose	Glucose oxidase, peroxidase, o-dianisidine, phosphate buffer	420
Ketohexose	(a) Resorcinol, thiourea, ethanoic acid, HCl	520
	(b) Carbazole, ethanol, cysteine, H_2SO_4	560
	(c) Diphenylamine, ethanol, ethanoic acid, HCl	635
Hexosamines	Ehrlich (dimethylaminobenzaldehyde, ethanol, HCl)	530
DNA	Diphenylamine	595
RNA	Bial (orcinol, ethanol, $FeCl_3$, HCl)	665
α-Oxo acids	Dinitrophenylhydrazine, Na_2CO_3, ethyl acetate	435
Sterols	Liebermann–Burchardt reagent (acetic anhydride, H_2SO_4, chloroform)	625
Steroid hormones	Liebermann–Burchardt reagent	425
Cholesterol	Cholesterol oxidase, peroxidase, 4-amino-antipyrine, phenol	500

$$\text{concentration} = \frac{\text{test absorbance}}{\text{standard absorbance}} \qquad (12.6)$$

Of course, such an assumption for individual experiments is valid only if the Beer–Lambert relationship has been established for that particular reaction on a previous occasion.

It is important to note that, when plotting calibration curves, despite the fact that the Beer–Lambert relationship implies that there is zero absorbance at zero concentration, and that the instrument is physically zeroed, it is wrong to force the drawn line through zero. This would be to give greater credence to this point than any other and assume an unjustified level of precision. The best straight line should be drawn through the points by regression methods (Section 1.6.6).

A further point to note is that the accuracy of the instrument is not uniform throughout the transmission range. The final measurement is an electrical one involving a galvanometer. The maximum accuracy can be shown to occur at 36.8% transmission, and between 20% and 80% the relative error is about $\pm 2\%$. Owing to the nature of galvanometric measurements, the errors at low and high absorbance can be large. This indicates that the analysis should be designed to give absorbance readings in the middle of the range of the transmission scale.

In a colorimeter, the bandwidth of the wavelengths is determined by the filter. A filter that appears red to the human eye is transmitting red light and absorbing almost everything else. This kind of filter would be used to examine blue solutions as they would absorb red light. In general the filter should be of a colour complementary to that of the solution under test.

The arrangement in such an instrument can be very simple, consisting merely of a light source (lamp), filter, cuvette and photosensitive detector to collect the transmitted light. Another detector is required to measure the incident light, or a single detector is used to measure incident and transmitted light alternately. This latter design is both cheaper and analytically better as it eliminates variation between detectors.

The spectrophotometer is a much more sophisticated instrument. A photometer is a device for measuring 'light' and 'spectro' implies the whole range of continuous wavelengths that the light source is capable of producing. The detector in the photometer is generally a photocell in which a sensitive surface receives photons and a current is generated that is proportional to the intensity of the light beam reaching the surface. In instruments for measuring ultraviolet/visible light, two lamps are usually required: one, a tungsten filament lamp, produces wavelengths in the visible regions; the second, a hydrogen or deuterium lamp, is suitable for the ultraviolet. There is a switchover point, usually at 350 nm, although often both lamps are lit all the time that an instrument is in use if both ultraviolet and visible are to be used. The 'switch' in the latter case is then just a mechanical means of directing the appropriate beam along the optical axis, using mirrors or lenses. Mirrors are more frequently used, owing to cheapness and the fact that less light is lost, due to chromatic aberration, in a reflectance than a refraction system. The arrangement may be very simple, as in a colorimeter, but this really defeats the object of the instrument. Fig. 12.6a shows the optical arrangement in a single-beam instrument. Here, first the blank and then the sample must be moved into the beam, adjustments made and readings taken. Fig. 12.6b illustrates the double-beam device. In this arrangement the beam is split into two parts, one passing through the blank, or reference, at the same time as the other part passes through the sample. This approach obviates any problems of variation in light intensity, as both

(a)

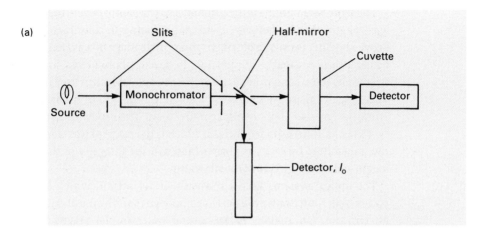

(b)

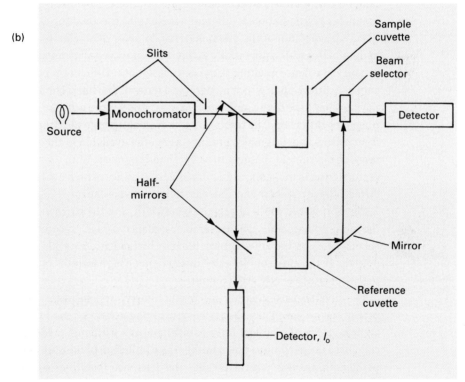

Fig. 12.6. Optical arrangements in (a) a simple single-beam spectrophotometer and (b) a double-beam spectrophotometer.

reference and sample would be affected equally. The resultant measured absorbance is the difference between the two transmitted beams of light recorded by the matched detectors. Multibeam instruments are available that allow the simultaneous recording of absorbance changes at two or more predetermined wavelengths.

The light or radiation emitted from the source lamps covers the whole range of wavelengths that the lamp is capable of producing. In colorimeters, as described above, the filter is used to obtain an appropriate range of wavelengths within the bandwidth it is capable of selecting. In spectrophotometers the bandwidth is selected by the monochromator, which is the optical system used in these devices. Theoretically, these systems select a single wavelength of monochromatic radiation, the emergent light being a parallel beam. The bandwidth here is defined as twice the half-intensity bandwidth, which is the range of wavelengths for which the transmitted intensity is greater than half the intensity of the chosen wavelength and it is a function of the slit width.

The optical systems used are usually either prisms, which split the multi-wavelength source radiation into its component parts by the phenomenon known as refraction (an analogy is the natural water-droplet prisms that produce a rainbow), or gratings, which achieve the same thing by diffraction. Refraction occurs because radiation of different wavelengths travels along different paths in the denser medium of the prism material. In order that velocity conservation is maintained overall, a potentially slower-moving wavepacket must travel a shorter distance in a dense medium than does a faster one. Diffraction occurs by reflectance at a surface upon which is engraved a series of fine lines. The distance apart of the lines has to be of the same order of magnitude as the wavelength of the radiation being diffracted. The resolution of wavelengths is greater from gratings than from prisms and, originally, gratings were only available in the most expensive research instruments because they were hand engraved. With the advent of photoreproduction in the semiconductor industry, gratings of high quality can be reproduced in large numbers and hence are now relatively cheap.

The optical slit width affects the bandwidth, and the narrower the slit width the more reproducible are measured absorbance values. In contrast, sensitivity becomes less as the slit narrows, because less radiation travels through to the detector. In the most sophisticated instruments, a high level of control is available to the operator, usually via a computer.

The cuvettes used in either spectrophotometry or colorimetry are an integral part of the system. They should be optically matched for the most precise and accurate work, the optical faces parallel and the pathlengths identical. In flow cells, used in continuous flow systems, the parallelism of the optical faces and the pathlength are less critical because the reference (baseline) solution and the sample both occupy the same cell successively in time. Microcells are available for limited specimens and the extreme of this is the microscale spectophotometer, where a very narrow parallel beam of monochromatic radiation passes through the microcell and then enters a microscope optical system.

The major advantage of the spectrophotometer, however, is the facility to scan the wavelength range over both ultraviolet and visible and obtain absorption spectra. These are plots of absorbance versus wavelength and a typical example is shown in Fig. 12.7. This shows the extent of absorbance (absorption peaks) at various wavelengths for reduced cytochrome c. Absorption spectra in the ultraviolet (200–400) and visible (400–700) nm ranges arise owing to the kinds of

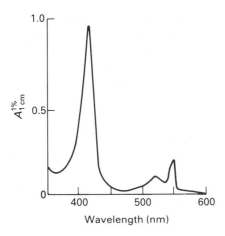

Fig. 12.7. Absolute absoption spectrum of reduced cytochrome *c*.

electron transitions described above (Section 12.1.2), usually the delocalised π-bonding electrons of carbon–carbon double bonds and the lone pairs of nitrogen and oxygen. The wavelengths of light absorbed are determined by the actual electronic transitions occurring and hence specific absorption peaks may be related to known molecular substructures. The term chromophore relates to a specific part of the molecule that independently gives rise to distinct parts of an absorption spectrum. Conjugation of double bonds lowers the energy (lower frequency) required for electronic transitions and hence causes an increase in the wavelength at which a chromophore absorbs. This phenomenon is termed a bathochromic shift. Conversely a decrease in conjugation (e.g. protonation of an aromatic ring nitrogen) causes a hypsochromic shift to lower wavelength. Changes in peak maxima (increase or decrease in absorbance) can also occur. A hyperchromic shift describes an increase and a hypsochromic shift a decrease in absorption maximum.

There are a number of specialised types of spectrophotometer available other than those already mentioned above. Recording spectrophotometers are usually capable of both scanning a predetermined spectrum (the prism or grating angle is changed by a motor-driven system, thereby emitting a continuously changing bandwidth along the optical axis) and monitoring changes at a predetermined wavelength. Although data are commonly recorded on a chart as hard copy, the more sophisticated devices capture and store data in computer systems and in some cases computer control is an option. Variable chart and scanning speeds and absorbance scale expansion are available. It is also possible to incorporate automatic cell changers and measurement at predetermined time intervals for time-dependent changes (e.g. kinetic studies, see Section 15.2.2). Measurement at the temperature of liquid nitrogen ($-196\,^\circ$C) increases the resolution, owing to the reduced thermal motion of the molecules. The absorbance generally increases also as the apparent pathlength is increased, because of internal reflections occurring in the frozen sample. Reflectance instruments measure the radiation absorbed when a light beam is reflected by the sample, for example pastes and suspensions of microorganisms that are too opaque to transmit the radiation. In such cases, internal reflection and refraction is occurring and hence the true pathlength is unknown; the strict Beer–Lambert law is therefore inapplicable, making quantification difficult. A reference reflecting surface is required and magnesium oxide is frequently used.

12.4.3 Applications

Qualitative and quantitative analysis

Qualitative analysis may be performed in the ultraviolet/visible regions to identify certain classes of compound both in the pure state and in biological mixtures, for example proteins, nucleic acids, cytochromes and chlorophylls. The technique may also be used to indicate chemical structures and intermediates occurring in a system. The most precise analysis, however, is obtained by infrared methods.

Quantitative analysis may be performed by making use of the fact that certain chromophores, for example the aromatic amino acids in proteins and the heterocyclic bases in nucleic acids, absorb at specific wavelengths. Proteins may be measured at 280 nm and nucleic acids at 260 nm, although corrections are usually necessary to account for interfering substances. Such corrections commonly require the measurement of the absorbance, by the interfering substance, at a wavelength remote from that for the compound under test, plus a knowledge of the absorbance at the test wavelength. If the ratio of the absorbances of the interfering substance is known for the remote and test wavelengths then the correction is simple, for example (Section 8.3.2) the $A_{280/260}$ ratio for proteins in the presence of nucleic acid. More sophisticated algebraic techniques are available for the more complicated cases, for example R. A. Morton's and D. W. Stubbs' correction for the amount of vitamin A in saponified oils.

The amounts of substances with overlapping spectra, such as chlorophylls a and b in diethylether may be estimated if their extinction coefficients are known at two different wavelengths. For n components absorbance data are required at n wavelengths.

A phenomenon known as Rayleigh light scattering (Section 12.7) occurs with moderate concentrations of some biological macromolecules (e.g. large DNA fragments) measured at 260 nm. This introduces an interference leading to error but may be accounted for by measuring the scattering in a region of the spectrum where DNA does not absorb, for example at 330–430 nm.

Difference spectra

A difference spectrum is the difference between two absorption spectra. There are essentially two ways in which difference spectra may be obtained: first, indirectly, by subtraction of one absolute spectrum from another (Fig. 12.8a); secondly, directly, by placing one compound in the reference cell and the other in the test cuvette (Fig. 12.8b). Fig. 12.8a shows the two absolute spectra of ubiquinone and ubiquinol and differences in absorbance may be calculated at wavelength points

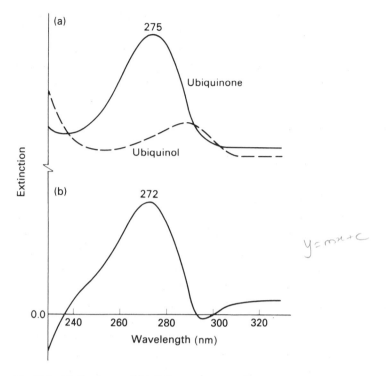

Fig. 12.8. (a) Absolute and (b) difference spectra of ubiquinone and ubiquinol.

with suitable regular intervals between them. The resultant absorbance values may then be plotted at the same wavelength points. Fig. 12.8b shows this difference spectrum, which is obviously the same, although obtained in a different manner. Difference spectrophotometry has the advantage of enabling the detection of small absorbance changes in a system with a high background absorbance. An example of this kind of investigation is the measurement of changes in the oxidation state of components of the respiratory chain in intact mitochondria and chloroplasts.

The following important observations should be made:

- Difference spectra may contain negative absorbance values.
- Both absorption maxima and minima may be displaced and extinction coefficients are different from those of absolute absorption peaks.
- There are points of zero absorbance in the difference spectrum, equivalent to those wavelengths where both the reduced and oxidised forms of the compound exhibit identical absorbances (isobestic points) and which may be used for checking for the presence of interfering substances.

A more complex example is that of the cytochrome a_3–CO complex minus cytochrome a_3, the difference spectrum being obtained by using anaerobic bacteria in the reference cuvette and the same system complexed with CO in the sample or

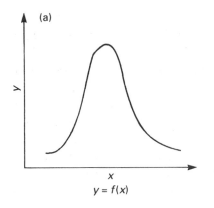

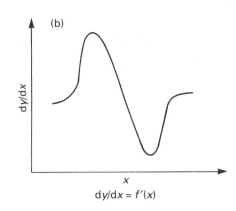

Fig. 12.9. First-differential spectra.

test cuvette. Cytochrome a_3 is the terminal electron carrier and is the only component in the system that reacts with carbon monoxide.

Frequently the term difference spectrum refers specifically to the absolute reduced spectrum minus the absolute oxidised spectrum, for example the difference spectrum of cytochrome c corresponds to the cytochrome c_{red} minus cytochrome c_{ox} difference spectrum. A similar difference spectrum may be obtained for a suspension of mitochondria using the so-called reversal technique. This involves measuring the change in absorbance at each wavelength when the preparation passes from the aerobic to the anaerobic state. The resultant spectrum obtained is a combined difference spectrum, for the cytochromes a, a_3, b, c, c_1 and NAD^+ and flavoprotein. Shoulders on peaks observed in difference spectra obtained at room temperature may be resolved into distinct peaks at $-196\,°C$ by measuring low temperature difference spectra.

An alternative to low temperature studies of unresolved absorption spectra (difference or absolute) is a purely mathematical one and is termed differential spectroscopy. If the algebraic relationship that governs the shape of a symmetrical peak is known then it may be differentiated and the differential plotted against the original variable. An ideal example is shown in Fig. 12.9a,b.

Almost always the algebraic relationship is unknown. However, the results may be readily obtained by digital computer techniques by sampling the curve at small intervals of the x-axis (wavelength). This process gives $\Delta y/\Delta x$ or $\Delta abs/\Delta \lambda$. If the $\Delta \lambda$ intervals were infinitesimally small, the limiting value would be dy/dx. Furthermore, higher order differential spectra may be obtained by feeding the data back to the processor chip as many times as are required. The value of higher-order calculations is in many cases dubious but second-order differential spectra (d^2y/dx^2) solve a number of otherwise intractable problems and instruments are commercially available, with the facility for making the calculations. The binding of a monoclonal antibody to its antigen may be monitored using second-order differential spectroscopy.

Binding spectra

Binding spectra or substrate binding spectra may be used to study the extent of interaction between an enzyme and its substrate. The binding of a substrate to a haem group containing a ferric ion in the high spin state perturbs the spectrum by displacing the ligand water from the sixth position of the ferric ion, causing it to change to the low spin state. The process may be followed spectrophotometrically. An example of this is the binding of a drug (substrate) to liver microsomal mono-oxygenase (mixed function oxidase), which causes a blue shift of the cytochrome P450 component of the enzyme from 420 nm to 390 nm (a hypsochromic shift).

Valuable structural studies may be performed on some particular biological macromolecules such as proteins and nucleic acids. In proteins, the spectrum of a chromophore depends largely on the polarity of the microenvironment. A change in the polarity of a solvent in which the protein is dissolved changes the spectrum of a particular amino acid chromophore without changing the conformation of the protein. This phenomenon is known as solvent perturbation and obviously, to be accessible to the solvent, the amino acid residue must be on the surface of the protein. Solvents or solutions miscible with water must be used and examples are dimethylsulphoxide, dioxane, glycerol, mannitol, sucrose and polyethylene glycol.

The aromatic amino acids are powerful chromophores in the ultraviolet. Processes such as denaturation (unfolding) of a polypeptide chain by pH, temperature and ionic strength can be monitored as more of these residues become exposed to the incident radiation.

Many other processes may be followed, particularly if the amino acid residue tyrosine is involved, for example protein–protein binding, protein–metal or protein–small molecule interactions. The range may be extended by the use of reporter group techniques in which an artificial chromophore is attached to the appropriate region of the protein.

In nucleic acid studies, solvent perturbation may be used to estimate the number of unpaired bases in RNA. If normal water is replaced by 50% ^2H_2O as solvent the ^2H_2O only changes the spectral components due to unpaired nucleotides. Also the denaturation of the helical structure of DNA in solution may be investigated when the double-stranded DNA is heated through its melting temperature (Section 5.2.3). The extinction at 260 nm increases (hyperchromic shift) on denaturation and decreases again (hypochromic shift) on renaturation, which occurs on cooling. Effects on the secondary structure of DNA by pH and ionic strength may be studied in a similar way.

Action spectra

In certain situations an action spectrum may be shown as a plot of a physiological (non-extinction) parameter against wavelength. In many complex biological systems such a spectrum often corresponds to the absorption spectrum of a single key compound. An example is the plotting of the rate of oxygen evolution by green plant tissue against the wavelength of light used to irradiate the system. This results in a graph similar to the spectrum of the chlorophylls.

Example 2 CALCULATION OF CONCENTRATION AND ABSORBANCE

Question

If a solution containing ATP is found to have an absorbance of 0.17 in a 1 cm cuvette and the molar extinction coefficient is $1.54 \times 10^4 \, (mol \, dm^{-3})^{-1} cm^{-1}$, what is

(i) the concentration of ATP solution,

(ii) the transmission of the solution in a 1 cm cuvette and

(iii) the absorbance of a 2.5×10^{-2} mM solution of ATP in a 4 cm cuvette?

Answer

(i) The concentration is found by the direct application of the Beer–Lambert Law.

$$A = \log\left(\frac{I_0}{I_t}\right) = \epsilon_\lambda \, c\ell$$

$$0.17 = 1.54 \times 10^4 \times c \times 1$$

Therefore,

$$c = [ATP] = \frac{0.17}{1.54 \times 10^4 \times 1} = 1.104 \times 10^{-5} \, M$$

(ii) $A = \log\left(\dfrac{I_0}{I_t}\right) = \log\left(\dfrac{1}{T}\right)$

Therefore,

$$0.17 = \log\left(\frac{1}{T}\right)$$

$$\frac{1}{T} = \text{antilog} \, (0.17) = 1.4791$$

and $T = 0.676$ or 67.6%

(iii) As we have a value of the molar extinction coefficient we must convert the given concentration to mol dm^{-3} (M).

Hence

2.5×10^{-2} mmol $dm^{-3} = 2.5 \times 10^{-5} \, M$

Then

absorbance $= A = \epsilon_m \times c \times \ell$

or

$A = 1.54 \times 10^4 \times 2.5 \times 10^{-5} \times 4 = 1.54$

As an aside, it is worth recalling that absorbance (because it is a logarithm) is unitless by definition. This is clearly demonstrated by performing 'quantity algebra' on the units of each term.

e.g. $\epsilon_\lambda \, (mol \, dm^{-3})^{-1} cm^{-1}$

$c \, (mol \, dm^{-3})^{-1} M$

ℓ cm

Hence,

$$\epsilon_\lambda \times c \times \ell \equiv (mol\,dm^{-3})^{-1}\,cm^{-1} \times (mol\,dm^{-3})^{-1} \times cm$$

and all units cancel.

12.5 **SPECTROFLUORIMETRY**

12.5.1 **Principles**

Fluorescence is an emission phenomenon, the energy transition from a higher to lower state within the molecule concerned being measured by the detection of this emitted radiation rather than the absorption. In order for the transition from higher to lower states to occur, an earlier excitation event, for example caused by absorption of electromagnetic radiation, must have taken place. The wavelength(s) of absorbed radiation must be at lower values (higher energy) than the emitted (fluoresced) wavelength. The difference between these two wavelengths is known as the Stokes shift and in general the best results are obtained from compounds involving large shifts. It is possible for a compound to absorb (be excited) in the ultraviolet region and emit or fluoresce in the visible.

In Fig. 12.2b an example of the various permissible energy levels is shown. Most electrons will occupy the ground state S_0V_0 at room temperature. Elevation to a higher energy level, S_1, S_2, etc., may be achieved by absorption of electromagnetic energy (photons) in less than 10^{-15} s. Energy may be lost very rapidly (as heat) by collision degradation, resulting in minimal vibrational energy in the lowest excited state, S_1V_0. Electrons in this state return to the ground state in less than 10^{-8} s, the emitted energy being manifested as fluorescence. Many organic molecules absorb in the ultraviolet/visible regions but do not fluoresce. Fortunately, of those that do, many are of biological interest. Also, although a knowledge of the structure of an organic molecule may allow predictions about its absorption spectrum, this is not true with fluorescence. Aliphatic molecules, which are usually flexible, tend to photodissociate rather than fluoresce, whereas aromatic compounds with delocalised π-electrons sometimes fluoresce.

The emitted radiation appears as band spectra because there are many closely related values (for the wavelengths) dependent upon the final vibrational and rotational energy levels attained. These band spectra are usually independent of the wavelength of the exciting radiation and have a mirror image relationship with the absorption peak with the greatest wavelength.

An associated phenomenon is phosphorescence, but this emission has long decay times and usually persists when the exciting energy is no longer applied. Phosphorescence arises as a result of intersystem crossing to the lowest triplet state. This light emission usually occurs at longer wavelengths than does fluorescence.

Fluorescence spectra give information about events that occur in less than 10^{-8} s. The ratio:

$$Q = \frac{quanta\ fluoresced}{quanta\ absorbed} \tag{12.7}$$

gives Q as the quantum efficiency and is usually independent of the exciting wavelength. At low concentrations, the intensity of fluorescence (I_f) is related to the intensity of the incident radiation (I_0) by:

$$I_f = 2.3 I_0 \epsilon_\lambda \, cdQ, \qquad \text{i.e. } I_f \alpha \, c \tag{12.8}$$

where c is the concentration of the fluorescing solution (molar), d is the light path in fluorescing solution (cm), and ϵ_λ is the molar extinction coefficient for the absorbing material at wavelength λ ($dm^3 mol^{-1} cm^{-1}$).

The technique of spectrofluorimetry is most accurate at very low concentrations, whereas absorption spectrophotometry is least accurate at these concentrations. For example, 100 pg of catecholamines or NADH may be measured fluorimetrically, whereas absorption spectrophotometry requires 100 μg each of the catecholamines serotonin and adrenaline. This is due to increased sensitivity, which is easily adjustable over a large range by amplification of the detector signal. The technique allows great spectral selectivity because, owing to the Stokes shift, two monochromators may be used, one for the exciting wavelength and the other for the emitted fluorescence. Although no reference cuvette is required, a calibration curve must be obtained.

Susceptibility to pH, temperature, solvent polarity and the inability to predict whether a particular compound will fluoresce, are disadvantages but the major one is the phenomenon of quenching. This occurs because energy that might have been emitted as fluorescence is lost to other molecules by collisional interaction. This partly explains the increased sensitivity and accuracy in low concentrations because there are fewer molecules, and hence collisions, although the effects of solvent must not be neglected. Many materials such as detergents, stopcock grease, filter paper and some tissues may cause interference by the release of fluorescing agents.

12.5.2 Instrumentation

The direct relationship between fluorescence intensity and concentration allows relatively simple electronics and optics to be used. Two monochromators may be employed, the first (M_1) for selecting the excitation wavelength. Fluorescence emission occurs in all possible directions and one direction (90°) is chosen and the second monochromator (M_2) is used for determination of the fluorescence spectrum. The radiation source is generally either a mercury lamp or a xenon arc, excitation wavelengths frequently being selected in the ultraviolet region and the emission wavelengths in the visible region. The detector is usually a sensitive photocell, for example a red-sensitive photomultiplier for wavelengths greater than 500 nm. Temperature control is required for accurate work as the intensity of fluorescence may vary between 10% and 50% for a 10 deg.C change at approximately 25 °C.

Two approaches are possible for the illumination of the sample: the simplest is the basic 90° illumination (Fig. 12.10), the alternative approach being front-face

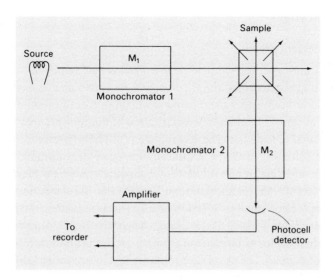

Fig. 12.10. The basic component of a spectrofluorimeter set up for 90° illumination.

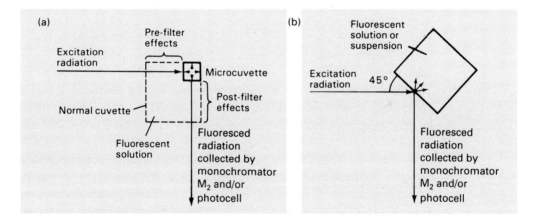

Fig. 12.11. Reduction of filter effects using (a) microcuvettes and (b) front-face illumination.

illumination (FFI; Fig. 12.11), which obviates pre- and postfilter effects. These latter effects arise owing to the absorption of radiation prior to it reaching the fluorescent molecules (prefilter absorption) and the reduction in the amount of emitted radiation escaping from the cuvette (postfilter effects). Such effects are more evident in concentrated solutions, and the use of microcuvettes (containing less material) can be of value (Fig. 12.11a). FFI is essential for examining suspensions, and cuvettes with only one optical face are required. Excitation and emission occur at the same face but generally the technique is somewhat less sensitive than 90° illumination.

12.5.3 **Applications**

Fluorescent probes

Applications of the technique are many and varied, despite the fact that relatively few compounds exhibit the phenomenon. A compound may have its fluorescence and absorption spectra compared as an aid to identification; the effects of pH, solvent composition and the polarisation of fluorescence may all contribute to structural elucidation. The measurement of phosphorescence and phosphorescence lifetimes can also be of value in compound identification.

The detection of non-fluorescent compounds may be achieved by coupling a fluorescent probe (or fluor) in a similar way to the use of reporter groups in absorption spectrophotometry (Section 12.4.3). This is termed extrinsic fluorescence as distinct from intrinsic fluorescence, where the native compound exhibits the property due to the presence of aromatic groups in amino acid side-chains in the case of proteins. The use of such probes is valuable in both qualitative and quantitative analysis. For instance, amino acids and peptides separated by chromatography or electrophoresis may be identified by coupling to their primary amino groups either dansyl chloride or o-phthalaldehyde (Section 8.4.2). The latter conjugates fluoresce intensely blue and the total oligopeptide fingerprint may be determined on only 10^{-5} g of protein. If the separation methods are used in column form, then quantification is possible by forming derivatives post-column. Acridine orange is an extrinsic fluor that can be used to determine the strandedness of polynucleotides as the Stokes shifts differ between conjugates of single- and double-stranded polynucleotides, which fluoresce red and green, respectively. The fluor should be tightly bound at a specific site, its fluorescence should be sensitive to environmental changes and it should not have adverse effects on the system being studied. Some structures of fluorescent probes are shown in Fig. 12.12.

The major use of fluorimetry in biochemistry is in quantitative determination of materials present in concentrations too low for absorption spectrophotometry. Assays of vitamin B_1 in foodstuffs, NADH, hormones, drugs, pesticides, carcinogens, chlorophyll, cholesterol, porphyrins and some metal ions indicate the range. Self- and contaminant quenching can be determined by adding a known quantity of a standard to an unknown quantity of a pure compound and measuring the fluorescence before and after the addition.

Ca^{2+} may be measured in the cytoplasm by the chelating agent Quin-2, which preferentially binds the metal. The fluorescence increases about five-fold on binding. More sensitive probes for this analysis are Fura-2 and Indo-1. Quin-1 is a chelating agent that may be used as a fluorescent probe to monitor intracellular pH changes in the range 5–9. Over this range, there is a 30-fold increase in fluorescence.

Enzyme assays and kinetic analysis

The general principles of enzyme assays, which are discussed in Section 15.2.2, often rely on the use of spectrofluorimetric assays. An example is the anion of

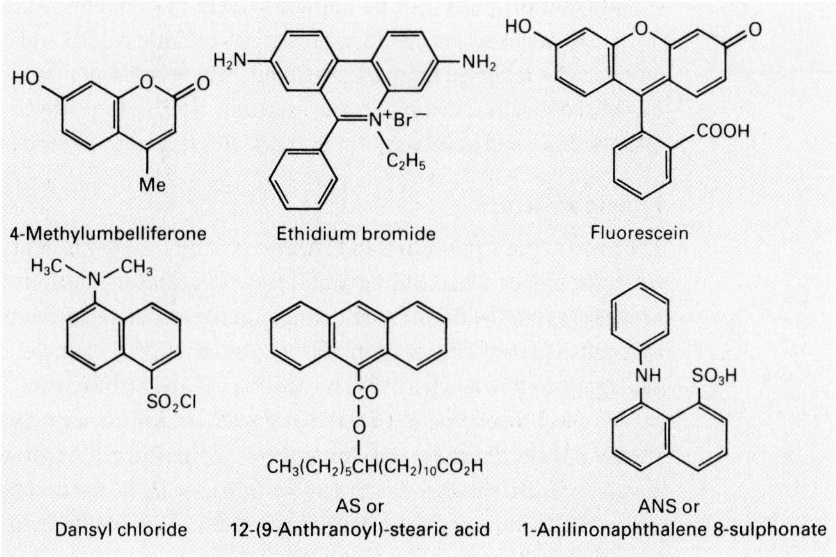

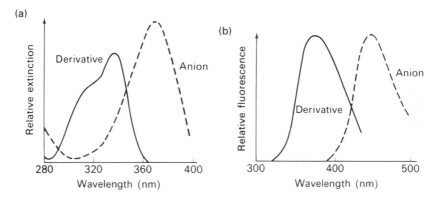

Fig. 12.12. Structure of some fluorescent probes.

Fig. 12.13. Spectra of the methylumbelliferone anion and derivatives of 4-methyl-umbelliferone at pH 10: (a) absorption spectra; (b) fluorescence spectra.

4-methylumbelliferone, which fluoresces at 450 nm. Its rate of appearance may be monitored when it is produced as a result of enzymic action on an ether or ester derivative of the fluor. The enzymes used are group-specific hydrolases and their kinetics may be studied by fluorescence measurement; Fig. 12.13a,b shows typical absorption and fluorescence spectra. Irradiation is usually at 350–400 nm wavelength and virtually all the fluorescence measured between 450 nm and 500 nm is due to the anion product. It is claimed that one molecule of β-galactosidase may be detected when it acts on fluorescein bis(β-D-galactopyranoside) as substrate because the sensitivity of the method is so great. Hence actual numbers of molecules in a single bacterial cell may be determined, as may the synthesis of the enzyme in individual cells in a population.

Spectrofluorimetry can be applied widely in metabolic studies where NAD$^+$ forms are involved as cofactors. This arises because NADH and NADPH fluoresce, whereas the oxidised equivalents do not. Therefore redox processses may be followed kinetically *in vitro* at concentrations similar to those encountered *in vivo*, and also followed in intact cells or organelles (e.g. mitochondria).

Protein structure

The presence of tryptophan and FAD as cofactors allows proteins to exhibit intrinsic fluorescence. The binding and release of cofactors, inhibitors, substrates etc., at sites close to the fluor, cause changes in the associated fluorescence spectra and as a consequence information about conformational changes, denaturation and aggregation may be gleaned. The absence of an intrinsic fluor can be overcome by coupling a suitable extrinsic fluor such as anilino-napthalene 8-sulphonate (ANS), dansyl chloride and derivatives of fluorescein or rhodamine. A recent development of the use of extrinsic fluors has been the use of the green fluorescent protein (GFP) of *Aequorea victoria* as the fluor. GFP has an intrinsic strong green fluorescence that requires no additional cofactors. By genetic engineering techniques, chimeras of GFP and the test protein can be produced without altering the normal functioning of the latter. Ligand-induced changes in the conformation of the test protein will be reflected in the fluorescence of the GFP. Similar studies can be carried out using the red fluorescent protein isolated from *Discosoma striata* (see Section 16.3.2).

Membrane structure

The fluorescent properties of a molecule are affected by its mobility and environment, particularly the polarity of the latter. These effects in the vicinity of a fluorescent probe may be monitored by measuring changes in fluorescence. Various probes having charged and hydrophobic regions (ANS and *N*-methyl-2-anilino-6-naphthalene sulphonate (MNS)) and hence able to orient themselves across lipid/aqueous interfaces may be used to study membrane structure and gain information about the properties of such interfaces. Incorporation of phospholipids containing 12-(9-anthroanoyl)-stearic acid and 2-(9-anthroanoyl)-palmitic acid into membranes yields information about the regions 0.5 nm and 1.5 nm, respectively, from the phosphate head groups of the lipid bilayer. The basic membrane structure and also the effects of temperature and certain biological phenomena may be studied. Changes in mitochondrial membranes during energy transduction have also been monitored using an ANS probe.

Fluorescence recovery after bleaching (FRAP)

If a fluor is exposed to a pulse of high intensity radiation it may be irreversibly bleached, i.e. permanently lose its ability to fluoresce. Fluorescently labelled phospholipids incorporated into a biological membrane may be subjected to this treatment and then the motion of such entities (in the membrane) can be studied by monitoring (with low intensity radiation) the re-emergence of fluorescence as the bleached and unbleached molecules interdiffuse. Applications include the lateral motion of extrinsically labelled rhodopsin in the photoreceptor membrane, the study of polymerisation of proteins such as actin and the diffusion of fluorescently labelled proteins microinjected into cells (see also Section 16.3.3).

Fluorescence resonance energy transfer

In a number of cases energy may be transferred, by fluorescence resonance energy transfer (FRET), from a donor to an acceptor fluor, provided there is overlap between the donor fluorescence spectrum and the acceptor absorption spectrum. The fluors must also be closely situated and transfer efficiency is related to spatial separation. This efficiency may be measured either as quenching of the donor fluorescence by acceptor or as the intensities of fluorescence of acceptor when the latter is irradiated both in the presence and in the absence of the donor.

Intrinsic fluors such as tryptophan or extrinsic ones attached to amino acids, -SH groups, sugars or fluorescent analogues of substrates, inhibitors, cofactors or phospholipids may be employed in energy transfer experiments to deduce distances within protein molecules. Accuracy is limited to about ± 0.5 nm and determinations include the localisation of metals in metalloproteins, the measurement of the extent of conformational changes in enzymes and receptors when substrate or ligand binding occurs (Section 16.3.2), the distances between various pairs of proteins in the ribosome and the three-dimensional structure of transfer RNAs.

Fluorescence polarisation and depolarisation

The excitation wavelengths used may be polarised by introducing a suitable polariser between the first monochromator (M_1) and the sample. The emitted radiation may be totally unpolarised or partially polarised and may be detected by using a second polariser between the emission monochromator (M_2) and the detector.

Molecular rotations affect fluorescence depolarisation: for instance, the rotation of an absorber chromophore and energy transfer between chromophores increase the depolarisation effect. High concentrations of chromophore and high viscosity of the solvent result in the measurement of mainly energy transfer. At low concentrations and low viscosity the effects of molecular motion predominate.

The mobility of whole molecules, or parts thereof, may be investigated using this technique. The lifetimes of intrinsic fluors of proteins and nucleic acids are usually too short, as these biological macromolecules move relatively slowly. Hence extrinsic fluors are frequently used in these studies. Examples of such studies include the binding of fluorescent substrates, the binding of inhibitors and cofactors to enzymes and receptors (Section 16.3.2), reduction of mobility (increase of overall mass and hence inertia); and the antigen/antibody complexation reaction. The association and dissociation of multisubunit proteins, such as lactate dehydrogenase and chymotrypsin, and the viscosity of living cells may also be measured.

An interesting historical aside involves the use of highly viscous glycerol to slow down the rotation and translation of large molecules in depolarisation experiments. It was knowledge of this totally unconnected fact that gave the clue to the use of glycerol as a matrix in fast atom bombardment mass spectrometry.

Microspectrofluorimetry

In this technique a microscope is combined with a spectrofluorimeter equipped with fibre optics to enable the examination of single bacterial cells binding fluorescent antibodies and also the fluorescent intensity of subcellular structures. The extra amount of nucleic acid that tends to be present in malignant cells will take up more of the fluorescent probe acridine orange than do normal cells. This observation may be used to detect malignant cells in biopsy tissue.

The fluorescence-activated cell sorter

This system, described in Section 7.8.5, makes use of the light emitted by cells carrying a fluorescently labelled antibody to trigger their physical separation from unlabelled cells as they flow through a fine capillary (Section 16.3.2).

Fluorescence immunoassay

These methods are dealt with extensively in Section 7.7.6 but are worthy of a brief mention here.

Several immunoassays have been developed using fluorescent probes to label either antigen or antibody. The binding of a labelled hapten by an antibody may alter the intensity of fluorescence, thus enabling the complex formation to be monitored. Changes in polarisation methods applied to immunoassay have been mentioned above. A major disadvantage of either of these approaches is the high background fluorescence that often accompanies the process and interferes with the measurement. The most promising development in this area is time-resolved fluorescence immunoassay. Two approaches have been combined to reduce the effects of background fluorescence and hence increase the sensitivity. First, europium chelates are usually used as the fluor, as they have large Stokes shifts and long-lived fluorescence. Secondly, a fluorimeter has been designed that delays the measurement of the emitted light by 400 μs, during which time the non-specific background fluorescence has almost completely decayed. Such an approach has led to the development of dissociation-enhanced lanthanide fluoroimmunoassay (DELFIA).

Multicomponent analysis by synchronous luminescence spectrometry

Despite its name this is really a fluorescence technique and allows the simultaneous analysis of multicomponent mixtures without the need to resort to the use of rather complicated algorithms and sophisticated computer techniques. For this reason it is included in this section.

In conventional luminescence spectrometry an emission spectrum is monitored by scanning the emission wavelength λ_{em} whilst the luminescent (fluorescent) compound is excited at a fixed excitation wavelength λ_{exc}. Conversely an excitation spectrum is obtained by scanning λ_{exc} whilst the emission is monitored at a fixed λ_{em}.

A combined method involves scanning both λ_{em} and λ_{exc} together, i.e. varying both simultaneously or synchronously. This is feasible despite the loss of constant excitation energy employed in the conventional method.

The luminescence intensity, I_s, is obtained from equation 12.9, the right-hand side of which is derived from the Beer–Lambert law:

$$I_s = KcdE_X(\lambda - \Delta\lambda)E_M(\lambda) \tag{12.9}$$

where K is an aggregate constant; c is concentration of analyte; d is the optical pathlength; λ is the emission wavelength; $E_M(\lambda)$ is the emission spectrum; $E_X(\lambda - \Delta\lambda)$ is related to the experimentally determined exitation spectrum, which involves excitation at a wavelength λ'. It is a specific requirement of this technique that the difference between excitation and emission wavelengths remains fixed, i.e. $\Delta\lambda = \lambda - \lambda'$. Hence $\lambda' = \lambda - \Delta\lambda$ in the expression above. It is often convenient in practice to choose $\Delta\lambda$ to be the same as the Stokes shift.

A number of advantages of the method are that complex spectra may be reduced to a single peak, spectral bands are generally narrowed, a spectral range is produced (this is of particular advantage to the analytical scientist as against the requirements of the purist spectroscopist); and spectra of multicomponent systems may be simplified. In addition, multiplicity of scan rates for both monochromators allows for considerable variability in the operation of the technique.

Amongst the applications of the technique is the measurement of the fluorescence associated with benzo(a)pyrene (BP) molecules covalently attached to nucleic acids, both DNA and RNA, isolated from the epidermis of BP-treated mice. The measurements were made at 77 K in frozen aqueous solutions by use of a photon-counting fluorimeter operating in synchronous scanning mode. A $\Delta\lambda$ of 28 nm was chosen, which corresponds to the Stokes shift for the fluorescence of bound BP. Other applications have involved the measurement of the carcinogenic polycyclic hydrocarbon dibenz(a,h)anthracene in extracts of cigarette smoke, resolution of tyrosine and tryptophan in proteins and polypeptides, and quantitative determination of hallucinogens (e.g. LSD). Derivative spectra may also be obtained, enabling the resolution of phenylalanine, tyrosine and tryptophan in admixture, protein mixtures, and catecholamines. The method offers potential for applications in clinical analysis.

12.6 CIRCULAR DICHROISM SPECTROSCOPY

12.6.1 Principles

It has been known for some time that optical isomers (isomers whose mirror images are non-superimposable) possess the property of allowing the rotation of plane-polarised light. Electromagnetic radiation oscillates in all possible directions and it is possible to select preferentially waves oscillating in a single plane. This is achieved using a polarising material such as Polaroid or a nicol prism. The technique of polarimetry essentially measures the angle through which the plane of polarisation is changed after such light is passed through a solution containing

Example 3 FLUORIMETRIC ASSAYS AND QUENCHING

Question

A metabolite M was isolated from cerebrospinal fluid (CSF). After excitation at $\lambda_1 = 280$ nm the material fluoresced at $\lambda_2 = 360$ nm.

Using a standard spectrofluorimeter:

  (i) the instrument scale was set to zero with solvent (e.g. buffer) and the 100% mark using a pure sample of M as standard (conc. 100 ng/100 cm^{-3}),

 (ii) a blank was measured on a solution containing all the components except M and gave a reading of 11.2%,

(iii) an extract including M gave a total fluorescence measurement of 67%,

(iv) an overall fluorescence reading of 92% was observed when the extract above had an amount of pure M added, as internal standard, to give an equivalent concentration of 1 μg dm^{-3}. (Note this concentration is equivalent to 100 ng 100 cm^{-3}.)

Calculate the concentration of M in the sample of CSF in μg dm^{-3} and the proportion of quenching, if any. Also state the Stokes shift for the assay.

Answer

The best way to proceed is to define the individual intensities.

    Let I_s be the 100% value due to the standard.
    Let I_b be the 11.2% value due to the blank.
    Let I_t be the 67% value due to the total fluorescence.
    Let I_f be the 92% value due to the overall fluorescence when sample is 'spiked' with internal standard.
    Let I_u be the 55.8% value due to the blank correction $I_t - I_b$ (67 − 11.2).
    Let I_{as} be the 25% value due to the 'quenched' internal standard $I_f - I_t$ (92 − 67).

Then

$$\frac{\text{assay fluorescence of unknown}}{\text{assay fluorescence of int. std}} = \frac{\text{amount of unknown}}{\text{amount of int. std}}$$

$$\frac{I_u}{I_{as}} = \frac{\text{amount of unknown}}{1\ \mu\text{g dm}^{-3}}$$

$$\text{amount of unknown} = \frac{I_u \times 1\ \mu\text{g dm}^{-3}}{I_{as}} = \frac{55.8}{25} = 2.2\ \mu\text{g dm}^{-3}$$

The degree of quenching is found as follows:

    pure standard gives $I_s = 100\%$
    equivalent amount of standard in assay $I_{as} = 25\%$

Hence, quenching,

$$Q = 100 \times \left(\frac{100 - 25}{100}\right) = 75\%$$

The value of the Stokes shift is the difference between the emission and excitation wavelengths,

$$\Delta\lambda = \lambda_2 - \lambda_1 = 360 - 280 = 80\ \text{nm}$$

a chiral (optically active) substance. Optical rotary dispersion (ORD) spectroscopy is a technique for measuring this ability to rotate the plane of polarisation, as a function of the wavelength. However, such chiral substances may also absorb the plane-polarised radiation at certain wavelengths. In such cases the chromophore is termed an optically active chromophore or chiral centre, as it may only be part of a complex molecule. The technique of ORD has been largely supplanted by circular dichroism (CD) spectroscopy, which gives rather better information about the three-dimensional structure of macromolecules containing chiral centres. In CD, circularly polarised light is used and this is obtained by superimposing two plane-polarised light waves of the same wavelengths and amplitudes but differing in phase by one quarter of a wavelength and in their planes of polarisation by 90°. Just as plane-polarised light may be left (L) or right (R) handed, so can circularly polarised light. Whether R or L circularly polarised light is produced depends on the relative positions of the peaks of the two plane-polarised waves.

The asymmetry inherent in the structure of chiral molecules or centres interacts differently with polarised light. Not only are the R and L waves of plane-polarised light differentially absorbed and refracted, resulting in a beam in a different plane (the basis of polarimetry), but in the case of circularly polarised light a similar differential interaction occurs. In the latter case, the resultant beam, after having passed through the sample, is a recombination of the R and L components to give an emergent beam of elliptically polarised light. In polarimetry the specific rotation $[\alpha]_\lambda$ would be measured, whereas in CD spectroscopy it is the ellipticity, θ, which is measured:

$$\theta = 2.303\,\Delta A$$
$$= 33\,\Delta A \text{ degrees} \tag{12.10}$$

where ΔA is the difference in absorption between R and L components.

A CD spectrum is usually a plot of ellipticity versus wavelength and information regarding the structure of certain entities may be gleaned from it.

12.6.2 **Instrumentation**

The basic layout of a CD spectrometer is shown in Fig. 12.14. Both L and R circularly polarised light may be produced alternately, from a single monochromator, by the passage of plane-polarised light through an electrooptic modulator. This modulator is a crystal that, when subjected to alternating currents, transmits either the R or the L component, depending on the polarity of the electric field to which it is exposed. The photomultiplier detector produces a voltage proportional to the ellipticity of the resultant beam emerging from the sample container.

12.6.3 **Applications**

The major application of CD is the study of conformation of biological macromolecules and complements data generated from nuclear magnetic resonance experiments (Chapter 13).

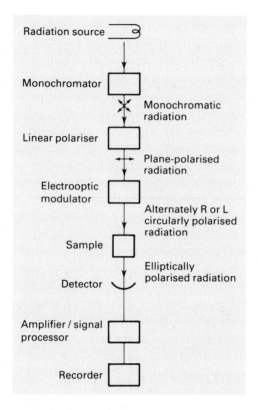

Fig. 12.14. The main components of a CD spectrometer.

Proteins

Information can be gained about the relative proportions of secondary structure, α-helical, β-sheet and random coil, in solution. The application of CD to tertiary structure is limited, owing to inadequate theoretical understanding of the influences of different parts of these molecules at this level of structure. The CD spectra of poly-L-amino acids have been obtained and are used as standards for calculating the percentage of each form of secondary structure in proteins. Curve-fitting procedures using computer processing have been used to apply the method to unknown proteins.

One of the most important benefits to be gained from CD spectroscopy is the study of conformational changes during, or because of, interactions with other entities. Examples are the determination of binding constants of substrates, cofactors, inhibitors or activators of virtually any enzyme. The binding of the inhibitor 3-cytidilic acid to the active site of pancreatic ribonuclease changes the CD spectrum of a remotely situated tyrosine residue. The binding of this inhibitor must therefore cause a conformational change in a distant part of the enzyme. CD spectroscopy is very sensitive and may be used to monitor the conversion of α- and β-structures to random coil (a major event of the denaturation process).

Nucleic acids

It is possible to calculate the CD spectrum of a single strand of DNA from the known nearest-neighbour frequency. Experimentally determined deviations from this calculated spectrum are indicative of a variation in structure, for example double strandedness. The CD spectrum of double-stranded DNA appears to be independent of the base composition in the range of wavelengths usually used.

A large increase in the CD spectrum of mononucleotides is observed when they link to form even short oligonucleotide chains. This observation provides evidence that hydrophobic interactions between stacked bases are important in stabilising the double-stranded structure of DNA.

All nucleotides exhibit chiral properties, and their CD is greatly increased on the adoption of a helical conformation. Hence the technique may be used to study structural changes in nucleic acids, for example loss of helicity of single-stranded DNA as a function of temperature and pH, structural changes on the binding of cations and proteins, transfer RNA–amino acid binding, transitions between single- and double-stranded DNA, DNA histone interactions in chromatin, the structure of ribosomal RNA in the ribosomes, and the interaction of double-stranded DNA and intercalating drugs.

12.7 **TURBIDIMETRY AND NEPHELOMETRY**

The two similar techniques of turbidimetry and nephelometry are both associated with the estimation of the concentrations of dilute suspensions. In turbidimetry, the apparent absorption of radiation by the suspension is measured. The apparent absorption should be measured at a wavelength where *true* absorption is not occurring; hence the Beer–Lambert law does not apply in turbidimetry. When radiation is passed through a transparent medium, for example a solution in a cuvette, one or both of two distinct physical phenomena might occur. In the case of extinction, true absorption of energy occurs and allows changes in the energy states of electrons, magnetic conditions, molecular vibrations, etc. The medium through which the radiation is passing, and in which the absorption is occurring, is termed optically empty, when this is the only phenomenon occurring. However, in the case of a suspension, a quite distinct radiative phenomenon may occur in which the light is scattered by the suspended particles. This scattering is due to reflection and refraction and gives rise to the Tyndall effect; it occurs in all directions and is an example of the more general Rayleigh scattering.

In turbidimetry the incident and transmitted radiation may be measured in an ordinary colorimeter or spectrophotometer, but the contribution of true absorption, if any, is small and the Beer–Lambert law is not strictly applicable as it holds only for very thin layers or very dilute suspensions.

The scattered light or Tyndall light may also be measured, usually at right angles (normal) to the incident radiation. This gives the Tyndall ratio, which is the ratio of the Tyndall intensity to that of the incident radiation. If this ratio is measured directly, a Tyndall meter would be used. If, however, the Tyndall intensity is compared with that of a standard suspension of known concentration, then the instrument is known as a nephelometer (measures cloudiness). The concentrations of suspensions of microorganisms may be obtained using nephelometry and those of proteins and some other biological macromolecules by turbidimetry (Section 12.4.1).

These techniques are difficult to use but in experienced hands can be of value. The relationship between energy input (incident radiation) and measured output (transmitted or scattered), however, is complicated and non-linear. It should be noted that these techniques are not strictly spectroscopic but are included here for completeness.

12.8 LUMINOMETRY

12.8.1 Principles

The emission and radiative techniques discussed above all depend on some physical phenomenon within the molecules concerned. The phenomenon also depends on the prior input of energy, frequently obtained from electromagnetic radiation. The radiative phenomenon luminescence arises in a different way. Although it is essentially the emission of electromagnetic radiation in the visible region (i.e. light), it arises as the result of a chemical reaction. Luminometry is the technique used to measure this luminescence, and, although not a spectrophotometric technique, it is included for completeness as it is an important method in biological science.

Chemiluminescence occurs as a result of excited electrons relaxing to the ground state (see Fig. 12.2b). The prior excitation arises as a result of a chemical reaction that yields a fluorescent product, and the chemiluminescent spectrum of a reaction such as luminol with oxygen to produce 3-aminophthalate is the same as the fluorescent spectrum of the product. A similar phenomenon is bioluminescence, so-called because the light emission arises from an enzyme-catalysed reaction (Section 15.2.2) usually involving luciferase. The colour of the light emitted in the latter case depends on the source of the enzyme and varies between 560 nm (greenish yellow) and 620 nm (red) wavelengths. This method has the distinct advantage of high sensitivity, as a result of the reaction having a high quantum yield – 100% under favourable conditions.

12.8.2 Instrumentation

It is not electromagnetic radiation that is the source of the excitation energy, hence no monochromator is required. Luminometry can therefore be performed with relatively simple photometers. Two minor complications are the need to amplify the output signal prior to recording and the need to maintain fairly strict temperature control. This control is necessary owing to the sensitivity of reactions to temperature, particularly in the case of enzyme-catalysed reactions.

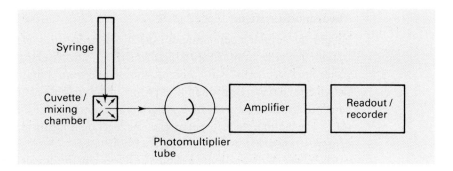

Fig. 12.15. Diagram of the main components of a simple luminometer.

Fig. 12.15 shows the layout of the main components. The reactants are introduced into a suitable light-protected reaction vessel in which adequate mixing takes place. The emitted light is collected by a photomultiplier tube, which is connected to a direct current amplifier with a wide range of sensitivity and linear response.

12.8.3 Applications

The firefly luciferase system

Details for the firefly luciferase system are given in Section 15.2.2. ATP concentration may be measured in an assay that is rapid to carry out and whose accuracy is comparable to spectrophotometric and fluorimetric assays. The sensitivity is, however, vastly increased, having a limit of detection of 10^{-15} M and a linear range of 10^{-12} to 10^{-6} M ATP. The concentrations of ADP, AMP and cyclic AMP may also be determined using appropriate enzymes, for example pyruvate kinase for ADP $\rightarrow$ ATP, adenylate kinase for AMP $\rightarrow$ ADP, and phosphodiesterase for cyclic AMP $\rightarrow$ AMP. In principle, all the enzymes and metabolites involved in ATP interconversion reactions may be assayed by this method. Examples are the enzymes creatine kinase, hexokinase and ATP sulphurase, and the substrates creatine phosphate, glucose, GTP, phosphoenolpyruvate and 1,3-diphosphoglycerate.

The bacterial luciferase system

Details of the bacterial luciferase system also are given in Section 15.2.2. The determination of nicotinamide adenine dinucleotides (and phosphates) and flavin mononucleotides, in their reduced states (i.e. NADH, NADPH and $FMNH_2$) may be made in assays which use this system. A concentration range of 10^{-9} to 10^{-12} M is achievable, which is much more sensitive than the corresponding spectrophotometric and fluorimetric assays, although the NADPH assay is less sensitive than the NADH assay by a factor of about 20. The method can be applied to a whole range of coupled enzyme reaction systems of the redox type that involve these nucleotides as coenzymes.

The aequorin system

Despite the development of calcium-specific electrodes, the calcium ion concentration may be determined with high sensitivity, intracellularly, using the phosphoprotein aequorin. The protein is isolated from luminescent medusae (jellyfish) and is practically non-fluorescent. In the presence of Ca^{2+}, however, it is converted from its natural yellow reflective colour to the blue fluorescent protein (BFP). The bioluminescent spectrum of the reaction is identical with the fluorescent spectrum of BFP:2Ca^{2+} but different from BFP:Ca^{2+}.

Ease of use, high sensitivity to, and relative specificity for, calcium and the non-toxicity of aequorin to living cells are advantages. The disadvantages are the scarcity of the protein, its large molecular size, consumption during the reaction and the non-linearity of the light emission relative to calcium concentration. Also the reaction is sensitive to its chemical environment and the limited speed in which it can respond to rapid changes in calcium concentration, for example influx and efflux in certain cell types.

Chemiluminescence

Luminol and its derivatives can undergo chemiluminescent reactions with high efficiency. For instance, enzymically generated H_2O_2 may be detected by the emission of light at 430 nm wavelength in the presence of luminol and microperoxidase (Section 15.2.2).

Competitive binding assays may be used to determine low concentrations of hormones, drugs and metabolites in biological fluids. Such assays depend on the ability of proteins such as antibodies and cell receptors to bind specific ligands with high affinity. Competition between labelled and unlabelled ligand for appropriate sites on the binding compound occurs. If the concentration of the binding compound is known, i.e. the number of available sites is known and a limited but known concentration of labelled ligand is introduced, then under saturation conditions all sites are occupied and the concentration of unlabelled ligand can be determined. Use of labelled ligand allows the concentration of only binding compound (the number of sites) to be determined. A variety of labels, including radio-isotopes, is in common use, enabling the fractions in the bound and free states to be distinguished. Labelling with a luminol derivative, completing the binding reaction, separating bound and free fractions allows the protein to be assayed by its chemiluminescence. The system must be calibrated using standards and, under the most favourable conditions, 10^{-12} M of a compound may be determined.

Whilst polymorphonuclear leukocytes are phagocytosing, singlet molecular oxygen is produced that exhibits chemiluminescence. The effects of pharmacological and toxicological agents on these and other phagocytic cells can be studied by monitoring this luminescence.

12.9 ATOMIC SPECTROSCOPY

All of the methods described above, with the exception of nuclear phenomena in the γ- and X-ray regions, have dealt essentially with molecular spectroscopy.

The general theory of electron transitions was discussed in Section 12.1.2 and for simplicity the phenomena were described mainly in atomic terms, although the extension to molecules is not too difficult. It was indicated above (Section 12.1.2) that, in general, molecules give rise to band spectra and atoms to clearly defined line spectra. These lines can be observed by eye either as light, associated with a particular wavelength, which are atomic emission spectra or black lines against a bright background, which are atomic absorption spectra. Some elements, particularly metals, have an important role to play in biological systems, whether as simple cofactors in enzymes, the central atom in biological macromolecules such as iron in haemoglobin or magnesium in chlorophyll, or as toxic substances that affect metabolism. Use of atomic spectroscopy will enable data to be obtained that are important in understanding the biological roles of these elements.

In a spectrum of an element, the wavelengths at which absorption or emission are observed are associated with transitions where the minimal energy change occurs. For example, in Fig. 12.2a is shown the $3s$–$3p$, or D-line transition in the sodium atom that gives rise to the emission of orange light. When electron transitions occur in an atom they are limited by the availability of an empty orbital or level. An orbital or level could not be overfilled without contravening the Pauli exclusion principle. In order for energy changes to be minimal, transitions tend to occur between levels close together in energy terms. These limitations mean that emission and absorption lines are absolutely characteristic of the element concerned. At least for simple atoms it is theoretically possible to deduce their electronic structure from their line spectra. The wavelengths emitted from excited atoms may be identified using a spectroscope, spectrograph or a direct reading spectrophotometer that uses as detectors the human eye, a photographic plate or a photoelectric cell, respectively.

In general, and in contrast to molecular spectroscopy, atom concentrations are not measured directly in solution. The atoms have to be volatilised either in a flame or electrothermally in an oven. In this state the elements will readily emit or absorb monochromatic radiation at the appropriate wavelength. Usually nebulisers (atomisers) will be used to spray the standard or test solution into the flame through which the light is passed. Alternatively the light beam is passed, in an oven, through a cavity containing the vaporised material.

12.9.1 Principles of atomic flame spectrometry

This technique takes advantage of the properties described above to determine the amounts of a specific element that may be present. The emission of light is measured by emission flame spectrophotometry and absorption by atomic absorption flame spectrophotometry.

The energy absorbed or emitted is proportional to the number of atoms in the optical path. In the case of emission it is strictly the number of excited atoms, but under reproducible standard conditions this will be the same as that for a calibrating standard. Flame instability, variation in temperature and composition of the flame make standard conditions difficult to achieve. Sodium gives high backgrounds and hence should be measured first and then a similar amount added to all other standards. Excess hydrochloric is usually added as chloride compounds are often the most volatile salts. Calcium and magnesium emissions are enhanced by the addition of alkali metals and suppressed by addition of phosphate, silicate and aluminate (by the formation of non-dissociable salts). This suppression effect may be relieved by the addition of lanthanum and strontium salts. Cyclic analysis may be performed that involves the estimation of each interfering substance in a mixture and then the standards for each component in the mixture are 'doped' with each interfering substance. The process is repeated (usually only two to three cycles are necessary) with refined estimates of interfering substance, until self-consistent values are obtained for each component; this implies minimal interference effects resulting from the concentrations approaching those in the unknown sample.

Flame instability requires that assays are carried out in triplicate and it is advantageous to bracket a determination of an unknown with measurements of the same standard to achieve the greatest accuracy. The use of lithium as an internal standard improves the technique. Polythene bottles should be used for storage if possible, as metal ions are both absorbed and released by glass.

Biological samples are usually converted to ash prior to the determination of metals. This can be done dry if sublimation losses are prevented. Wet ashing (in solution) is often used; this employs an oxidative digestion similar to the Kjeldahl method (see Section 8.3.2).

12.9.2 Instrumentation

Atomic emission spectrophotometry

The nebulisers used are usually of the type that involves passing a stream of air over a capillary tube whose other end dips into the solution under test. Larger droplets tend not to remain in the hottest part of the flame long enough, in direct injection systems, for their constituents to be volatilised and hence are allowed to settle out in a cloud chamber. Combustion of air and natural gas gives a temperature of 1500 °C, which is adequate for sodium determination. Calcium is better assayed at 2000 to 2500 °C and magnesium and iron require 2500 °C, obtained from an air/acetylene gas mixture. Bandwidth selection using a filter device may be used for routine analyses of moderate accuracy. More accurate measurements require a monochromator. The best accuracy achieves a resolution of 0.1–0.2 nm over the range 200–1000 nm. Table 12.3 lists the wavelengths used for a number of metals, together with their detection limits. Detectors are often of the photocell type but flame instability limits their value as their potential accuracy is not realised. Multichannel polychromators allow the emission of up to six elements at one time to be measured. The basic layout of an atomic (flame) emission spectrophotometer is shown in Fig. 12.16.

Atomic absorption spectrophotometry

In these instruments either a double monochromator with a source of white light or a hollow cathode discharge lamp is used to produce radiation in a very narrow

Table 12.3 The detection limits for various elements in emission and absorption flame spectrophotometry, flameless absorption spectrophotometry, and ion-selective electrodes

| Element | Emission | | Absorption | | | Ion-selective electrode: detection limit (p.p.m.) |
	Detection limit (p.p.m.)	Wavelength (nm)	Detection limit (p.p.m.) Flame	Flameless	Wavelength (nm)	
Calcium	0.005	442.7	0.1	0.00007	442.7	0.02
Copper	0.1	324.8	0.1	0.0001	324.8	0.0006
Iron	0.5	372.0	0.2	0.0001	248.3	
Lead			0.5	0.0002	283.3	0.21
Lithium	0.001	670.7	0.03	0.0001	670.7	
Magnesium	0.1	285.2	0.01	0.00001	285.2	
Manganese	0.02	403.3	0.05	0.00004	279.5	
Mercury			10.0	0.018	253.8	
Potassium	0.001	766.5	0.03	0.00003	766.5	0.04
Sodium	0.0001	589.0	0.03	0.00001	589.0	0.02
Strontium	0.01	460.7	0.06	0.0001	460.9	

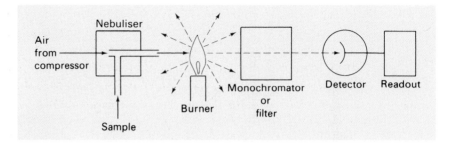

Fig. 12.16. The main components of an atomic emission (flame) spectrophotometer.

bandwidth. Discharge lamps emit radiation at a wavelength specific for the element being assayed. This specificity can be obtained only from a pure sample of the element that is excited electrically to produce an arc spectrum of that element, and electrodeless discharge lamps are now available. Nebulisers and burners are similar to the emission devices but 10 cm flames are often used to obtain an increased optical length. Both single and double beam instruments are available, the latter often incorporating a chopper to give intermittent pulses and prevent stray light from the flame reaching the detector. The most useful wavelength range is 190–850 nm.

Flameless instruments

A flameless atomic absorption spectrophotometer incorporates a graphite tube as an oven, which may be heated electrothermally to 3000 °C. Monochromatic light specific to the element being assayed is produced either by a hollow cathode discharge lamp or an electrodeless discharge lamp. The graphite tube forms an optical cavity, in which the sample resides and through which the monochromatic radiation is passed. Absorption is measured continuously as the temperature is raised and computer methods allow the superimposition of absorption and temperature profiles, with time, to be produced. This approach allows optimum conditions to be determined for future analyses. The flameless technique is 100 times more sensitive than flame methods and has the distinct advantage of being able to be automated as the inherent dangers of using combustible gases have been eliminated.

12.9.3 Applications

Sodium and potassium may be assayed at concentrations of a few parts per million (< 5) using simple filter photometers. The more sophisticated emission flame spectrophotometers may be used to assay some 20 elements in biological samples, the most common being calcium, magnesium and manganese. Absorption flame spectrophotometers are usually more sensitive than emission types and can usually detect < 1 p.p.m. of each of more than 20 elements. Exceptions to this are the alkali metals. Relative precision is about 1% in a working range of 20–200 times the detection limit (Table 12.3).

The techniques were widely used in clinical laboratories, for the determination of metals in body fluids. However, the technique has been largely superseded by the use of ion-selective electrodes (ISEs). These are amenable to automation and measurements can be carried out on very small samples (Sections 1.5.2 and 1.7.2). These determinations aid diagnosis and are valuable in the monitoring of many therapeutic regimes. In physiological and pharmacological research, sodium, potassium, calcium, magnesium, cadmium and zinc may be measured directly, but copper, lead, iron and mercury require prior extraction from the biological source. The methods are also widely used in element determination in soil and plant materials and, after suitable ashing procedures, may be used for metals in macromolecules, organelles, cells and tissues.

12.9.4 Atomic fluorescence spectrophotometry

Prior excitation of atoms by electromagnetic radiation rather than by thermal energy is required (cf. molecular fluorescence, Section 12.8.1). Atoms are again required to be in the vapour state: the phenomenon is not observed in solution as it is with molecules. The source beam must be intense but less spectrally pure than that required for atomic absorption spectrophotometry, as only the resonant wavelengths will be absorbed and lead to fluorescence. Direct emission from the flame being recorded by the detector must be avoided and this may be achieved by modulation of the detector amplifier to the same frequency as that of the primary source. Although limited to only a few metals, the extreme sensitivity achievable in appropriate cases makes it better than comparable methods. For example, zinc and cadmium may be detected at levels as low as 1 and 2 parts per 10^{10}, respectively.

12.10 LASERS

Laser is an acronym for *l*ight *a*mplification by *s*timulated *e*mission of *r*adiation. A detailed explanation of how laser light is generated is not possible here. A simple view is that electromagnetic radiation used as the excitation agent can be considered as the input of photons to an absorbing material. This results in elevation of an electron to a higher energy level as described above (Section 12.1.2). If, whilst the electron is in an excited state, another photon of precisely the correct energy arrives, then, instead of the electron being promoted to an even higher energy level, it returns to its original ground state. This return is accompanied by the emission of two coherent photons. These photons have associated wavelengths that are exactly in phase, hence the term coherent. A laser-producing material has to be pumped and this is often achieved by surrounding the material with a rapidly flashing high intensity flash tube that gives an ample supply of suitable photons.

The emitted, coherent light has considerable advantages, but in particular it can be produced with zero bandwidth, i.e. unique invariant wavelengths can be selected to excite molecules or atoms in a very precise way. It is also possible to generate, from appropriate sources, groups of selected wavelengths should this be required. Various applications are under development in spectroscopic and spectrophotometric methods that take advantage of the spectral purity of laser light.

An important application is the laser reflectance method for determining complementary DNA (cDNA) in nucleic acid studies. The use of reverse transcriptase and DNA polymerase (see Section 6.2.5) allows the nucleotide sequence corresponding to the primary sequence of a peptide fragment or protein to be synthesised. Chain growth occurs at the 3′ end from a primer section, and chain termination occurs when a dideoxynucleotide is incorporated into the growing complementary strand (Chapter 5). Four 'channels' are required, each containing primer, all four deoxynucleoside triphosphates and one of each of the four dideoxy compounds. In each of the four channels, chain termination occurs at different points. Also, at the 5′ end of the primers a different fluorescent label is attached that has no influence on the subsequent reactions but can be used to identify uniquely components of the resulting mixtures in each channel. Mixtures are separated by gel electrophoresis (see Section 10.2.2) in which distance travelled in the gel is effectively inversely proportional to the mass of the fragment. The gel is illuminated with a narrow beam of laser light and fluorescent emission from each label is measured (a different wavelength is emitted from each label). The band on the gel can be identified by including, to interrupt the emitted beam, a rotating filter disc that contains four sectors, each of which allows only one fluorescent wavelength to pass. By design, which fluor relates to which dideoxy terminator is known and mobility, position and amount are determined. The system can be automated and avoids the use of radioisotopes. It is reliable and precise, and data interpretation can be done by computer.

12.11 SUGGESTIONS FOR FURTHER READING

BRAND, L. and JOHNSON, M. L. (eds.) (1997). *Fluorescence Spectroscopy.* Methods in Enzymology vol. 278. Academic Press, San Diego. (An authoritative coverage of the applications of the form of spectroscopy in biochemistry.)

HARWOOD, L. M. and CLARIDGE, D. W. (1997). *Introduction to Organic Spectroscopy.* Oxford Chemistry Primers no. 43. Oxford University Press, Oxford. (A good text for studying some of the principles of spectroscopy in greater depth.)

HOLLAS, J. M. (2002). *Basic Atomic and Molecular Spectroscopy.* Wiley/RSC, London. (Contains many worked examples that are ideal for self-directed study.)

PAVIA, D. L., LAMPMANN, N. G. M. and KRIZ, G. S. (2001). *Introduction to Spectroscopy,* 3rd edn. Harcourt, New York. (Good coverage of all the techniques with many worked examples.)

Chapter 13

Spectroscopic techniques: II Vibrational spectroscopy and electron and nuclear spin orientation in magnetic fields

13.1 INTRODUCTION

In Chapter 12 it was established that the electromagnetic spectrum was a continuum of frequencies from the high energy γ-rays of nuclear origin to the long wavelength region of the radiofrequencies. The energy associated with the spectrum decreases as it is traversed from the high to low frequency regions, according to the rules of quantum theory. There is therefore no obvious logical dividing point where this overall spectrum may be split. The split presented in this text is one of convenience. The justification is purely pragmatic and is based on 'common practice'. The biologist or biomedical scientist, having isolated a 'new' material (compound), is faced, initially, with the requirement to identify this isolate. Amongst the spectroscopic and spectrometric techniques available, assuming sufficient pure material has been obtained, the first analytical procedures to be used would, in practice, involve the methods described in this chapter. There are two important reasons for this approach: first, a considerable amount of information is obtained from a 'single' analysis and, secondly, the techniques are non-destructive. In view of the latter reason, replicate analyses may be performed in many cases, to improve signal-to-noise ratios, and precious samples can be recovered that may then be subjected to other analytical investigations.

In Chapter 9 the mass spectrometric techniques are encountered. These techniques give information different from and complementary to the spectroscopic ones. They have the distinct advantage of being considerably more sensitive and hence the investigator, often faced with having too small a sample to make use of the spectroscopic techniques, is forced to use mass spectrometry. However, it is essential to recognise that the spectroscopic techniques give information that is not available from mass spectrometry alone. Also, a disadvantage with mass spectrometry is that the technique is destructive and some of the sample is lost during the analytical procedure, although, with the most sensitive systems now available, the loss is probably insignificant. In many situations the amount of sample destroyed during analysis is less than losses arising from sample transfer!

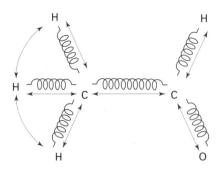

Fig. 13.1. Possible vibrations in acetaldehyde.

13.2 INFRARED AND RAMAN SPECTROSCOPY

13.2.1 Principles

With reference to the introductory statement of Section 13.1, the region of the electromagnetic spectrum, ranging from γ-rays to the near ultraviolet/visible (0.1–800 nm), contains frequencies that are sufficiently energetic to cause electron transitions, and the highest energy γ-rays are associated with nuclear transitions. From the near infrared region onwards there is insufficient energy to effect transitions of the kind alluded to above. Over the portion of the electromagnetic spectrum encompassing the range 0.8–25 μm the phenomena involve 'bond vibrations'. The term must be interpreted in a rather wider sense than just uniform oscillations and taken to include bending deformations as well.

Infrared and Raman

These two spectroscopic methods are complementary, giving similar information, but the criteria for the phenomena to occur are different for each type. It is also true that, for asymmetric molecules, absorptions will give rise to both types and virtually the same information could be gained from either. However, for symmetrical molecules having a centre of symmetry, the fundamental frequencies that appear in the Raman do not appear in the infrared and vice versa. The two methods are then truly complementary.

The reasons are the two different mechanisms on which the two types depend. Both are indicated in Fig. 13.1 for a simple molecule, acetaldehyde. For the purposes of this discussion the bonds between atoms can be considered as flexible springs so that the atoms are in constant vibrational motion, i.e. the molecule is not fixed and rigid.

Bonds can either stretch or deform (bend) and theory predicts that if a molecule contains n atoms there will be $3n - 6$ fundamental vibrations in total. Of these, $2n - 5$ cause bond deformations and $n - 1$ cause bond stretching. In Table 13.1 are listed the most important fundamental frequencies observed in acetaldehyde molecules.

The region of the electromagnetic spectrum ranges from the red end of the visible to the microwave lengths. Energy is input by irradiating in the appropriate

Table 13.1 Some fundamental frequencies associated with vibrations in acetaldehyde

Functional group	Vibration type	Frequency (cm^{-1})
$-CH_3$	Bending	1460
		1365
$-C-C-$	Stretching	1165
$-C=O$	Stretching	1730
$-C-H$ (in CH_3)	Stretching	2960
		2870
$-C-H$ (in CHO)	Stretching	2720

region with electromagnetic radiation. The criterion for an infrared spectrum is that there is a change in dipole moment, i.e. a change in charge displacement. Conversely, if there is a change in the polarisability of the molecule, a portion of the scattered radiation will have a frequency different from that of the incident radiation. These different frequencies constitute Raman spectra. It should be noted that more information can be gained about oscillations in molecules by proceeding even further into the microwave region and using microwave spectroscopy.

The fundamental frequencies observed are characteristic of the functional groups concerned and are absolutely specific. This gives rise to the term fingerprint for the infrared pattern obtained. As the number of functional groups increases in more complex molecules, the absorption bands in the infrared patterns become more difficult to assign. However, group frequencies arise that help to simplify interpretation. These groups of certain bands regularly appear near the same wavelength and may be assigned to specific molecular groupings, just as particular chromophores absorb in the ultraviolet and visible regions. Such group frequencies are extremely valuable in structural diagnosis. It should be noted that, in infrared spectra, which are vibrational spectra, it is usual to work in frequency units, hertz (Hz), rather than wavelength.

The frequency associated with a particular group varies slightly, owing to the influence of the molecular environment. This is extremely useful in structural biochemistry studies as it is possible to distinguish between $C-H$ vibrations in methylene (-CH_2) and methyl groups (-CH_3). Decrease in wavelength also occurs when double bonds are formed as the stretching frequency increases.

13.2.2 Instrumentation

The most common source is a Nichrome alloy coil heated to incandescence. This region of the electromagnetic spectrum contains the heat waves. Samples of solids are either prepared in mulls such as nujol and held as layers between salt planes such as NaCl or pressed into KBr discs. Non-covalent materials must be used for sample containment and also in the optics, as these materials are transparent to infrared.

Detectors are of the heat recognition type. The Golay cell contains gas or liquid whose expansion is registered when the energy is absorbed. Thermal detectors such as thermocouples can also be employed. Analysis using a Michelson interferometer allows Fourier transform infrared spectroscopy (FT–IR) to be performed. This instrument involves fixed and rotating mirrors that split the incident beam into two. The beams are recombined after passage through the sample but as the two pathlengths are different, interference patterns arise that may be analysed by Fourier transform methods (see Section 13.4.1 for consideration of FT methods). The Beer–Lambert law applies in all cases except complex mixtures, where more complicated mathematical procedures are required.

13.2.3 Applications

The use of infrared and Raman spectroscopy is mainly in biochemical research for intermediate-sized molecules such as drugs, metabolic intermediates and substrates. Examples are the identification of substances such as penicillin and its derivatives, small peptides and environmental pollutants. It is an ideal and rapid method for measuring certain contaminants in foodstuffs and can be coupled to a gas–liquid chromatograph (GC–IR) when it is also frequently used for the analysis of drug metabolites (Section 11.9.3). Fig. 13.2 shows the major bands of an FT–IR spectrum of the drug phenacetin. Gas analysis is rapid, particularly for measuring different concentrations of gases such as CO_2, CO and CH≡CH (acetylene) in biological samples. Use in the study of photosynthesis and respiration in plants is valuable, particularly for CO_2 metabolism.

13.3 ELECTRON SPIN RESONANCE SPECTROSCOPY

13.3.1 Magnetic phenomena

Prior to any detailed discussion of electron spin resonance (ESR) and nuclear magnetic resonance (NMR) (Section 13.4) methods it is worth while considering the more general phenomena applicable to both.

An important consideration is magnetism and how it arises. All substances are magnetic, and magnetism arises from the motion of charged particles. This motion is controlled by internal forces in a system and, for the purposes of this discussion, the major contribution to magnetism in molecules is due to the spin of the charged particle.

Consider the situation in the chemical bonds of a molecule where electrons (negatively charged) have the property of spin controlled by strict quantum rules. The simplest view of the chemical bond is that of paired electrons with opposite spins. It is true that in many chemical systems the electrons may become delocalised, i.e. lose their association with a particular atom, but the essential argument still applies in that for pairs of electrons in molecular orbitals the spins must be opposite (no two electrons can have all the quantum numbers identical: the Pauli principle). Each of these spinning electronic charges generates a magnetic effect,

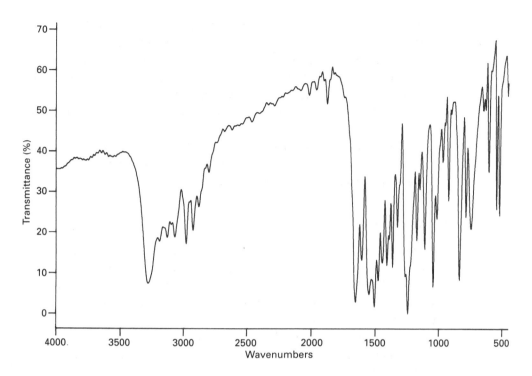

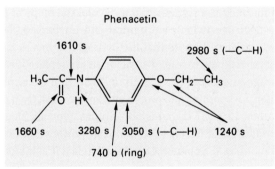

Fig. 13.2. FT–IR spectrum of phenacetin. Bands at the appropriate frequencies (cm^{-1}) are shown, indicating the bonds with which they are associated and the type (s, stretching; b, bending or deformation).

but in electron pairs the effect is almost self-cancelling. The mathematical considerations do not in general apply exactly in molecules but in atoms a value for magnetic susceptibility may be calculated and is of the order of -10^{-6} g^{-1}. This is diamagnetism, possessed by all substances because all substances contain the miniscule magnets, i.e. electrons. Diamagnetism is temperature independent.

If an electron is unpaired there is no counterbalancing opposing spin and the magnetic susceptibility is of the order of $+10^{-3}$ to $+10^{-4}$ g^{-1}. In cases where this possibility arises, the underlying diamagnetism is so small by comparison that it is irrelevant and the free electron case gives rise to paramagnetism. Free electrons can arise in a number of examples, the most notable of which is in the structure of certain metals such as iron, cobalt and nickel. These metals exhibit an extreme case of paramagnetism that is termed ferromagnetism and are the materials from which permanent magnets, with which everyone is familiar, can be made. Some crystal structures allow free electrons to exist but free radicals (free electron entities) are probably the most important systems in biological investigations.

The way in which a substance behaves in an externally applied magnetic field allows us to distinguish between diamagnetism and paramagnetism. A paramagnetic material is attracted by an external magnetic field and a diamagnetic substance is rejected. This principle is employed in the GUOY balance, which allows the quantification of the magnetic effects. A balance pan is suspended between the poles of a suitable electromagnet (to supply the external field). The substance under test is weighed in air with the current switched off. The same sample is then reweighed with the current on, the result being that a paramagnetic substance apparently weighs more and a diamagnetic substance apparently less.

Exactly similar arguments can be made regarding atomic nuclei. Of course, it is not now the extranuclear electrons but the subnuclear particles that are the spinning charged particles. Strictly speaking (because of interchangeability) it is the number of nucleons (protons plus neutrons) that determine whether a species will exhibit nuclear paramagnetism. It is beyond the scope of this discussion to explore why neutrons (which are neutral and uncharged; Section 14.1.1) are involved. It is sufficient to note that the hydrogen atoms in a molecule exhibit residual nuclear magnetism and, if some or all are replaced by deuterium, then there is no magnetism from the deuterium. Hydrogen contains a single proton, whereas deuterium contains one proton and one neutron (two nucleons, an even number). Carbon-12 (^{12}C) contains six protons plus six neutrons – an even number, no residual magnetism. ^{13}C contains six protons (because it is carbon) but seven neutrons, an odd number of nucleons; hence it exhibits residual nuclear magnetism.

13.3.2 **The resonance condition**

In both ESR and NMR techniques (Section 13.4) two possible energy states exist for either electronic or nuclear magnetism in the presence of an external magnetic field:

- *Low energy state E_1:*   The field generated by the spinning charged particle lies with, or is parallel to, the external field.
- *High energy state E_2:*   The field generated by the spinning charged particle lies against, or is antiparallel to, the external field.

The resonance condition is satisfied when the transition from the low to high energy states occurs and equation 13.1 is satisfied (see below). Energy must be absorbed for these transitions to occur: one quantum or $h\nu$ (where h is the Planck constant). In the appropriate external magnetic fields it is shown that the frequency of applied radiation, v, occurs in the microwave region for ESR (sometimes called electron paramagnetic resonance (EPR)) and the radiofrequency region for NMR (sometimes called nuclear paramagnetic resonance). In both techniques, two possibilities exist for determining the absorption of electromagnetic energy (at the resonance point):

- either a constant frequency is employed and the external magnetic field swept; or
- a constant external magnetic field is used and the appropriate region of the spectrum swept.

For technical reasons the more commonly employed option is the first, but the same results would be obtained if either option were chosen.

13.3.3 **Principles**

The quantum of energy required to cause the resonance condition to be satisfied, and transition between energy states in an ESR experiment, may be quantified as

$$h v = g \beta H \tag{13.1}$$

where g is the spectroscopic splitting factor (a constant), β is magnetic moment of the electron (termed the Bohr magneton), and H is the strength of the applied external field.

The frequency of the absorbed microwave radiation is a function of the paramagnetic species β and the applied magnetic field strength H (equation 13.1). This indicates that either may be varied to the same effect. The absorption of the energy is recorded as a peak in the ESR spectrum and is indicative of the presence of a paramagnetic species. The area under the peak is proportional to the concentration of that species, strictly the number of unpaired electron spins. Calibration of the instrument with known standards allows the concentration to be calculated. The standard, containing a known number of spins, must have the same line shape as the unknown for a reliable comparison to be made. Examples of standards are solutions of peroxylamine disulphonate or the solid 1,1-diphenyl-2'-picryl-hydrazyl (DPHH). The solid standard contains 1.53×10^{21} unpaired spins per gram in the pure state and may be diluted by admixture with carbon black in order to give lower concentrations.

For a delocalised electron (some free radicals), $g = 2.0023$ but for localised electrons, for example in transition metal atoms, g varies and its precise value gives information about the nature of the bonding in the environment of the unpaired electron within the molecule. When resonance occurs, the absorption peak is broadened owing to spin–lattice interactions, i.e. the interaction of the unpaired electron with the rest of the molecule. This gives further information about the structure of the molecule.

High resolution ESR may be performed by examining the hyperfine splitting of the absorption peak, which is caused by interaction of the unpaired electron with adjacent nuclei. This yields information about the spatial location of atoms in the molecule. Proton (^{1}H) hyperfine splitting for free radicals occurs in the region of 0 to 3×10^{-3} tesla (1 tesla = 10^4 gauss and is a measure of the magnetic induction, which is linearly related to the magnetic field strength) and yields data analogous to those obtained in high resolution NMR. In fact a considerable improvement in the effective resolution of an ESR spectrum may be achieved by using the electron nuclear double resonance (ENDOR) technique. In this approach the sample is irradiated simultaneously with microwaves for ESR and RF (radio frequency) for NMR. The RF signal is swept for a fixed point of the ESR spectrum. The output display is the ESR signal height versus swept nuclear RF. The approach is particularly useful when there is a large variety of nuclear levels that broaden the normal electron resonance line. A similar but different technique is electron double resonance (ELDOR), in which the sample is irradiated with two microwave frequencies. One is used for observation of the ESR signal at some point in the spectrum, whilst the other is used to sweep other parts of the spectrum. This is used to display the ESR signal as a function of the difference of the two microwave frequencies. ELDOR finds use in the separation of overlapping multiradical spectra and to study relaxation phenomena, for example chemical spin exchange.

13.3.4 Instrumentation

Fig. 13.3 is a diagram of the main components of an ESR instrument. The field strengths generated by the electromagnets are of the order of 50 to 500 millitesla, and variations of less than 1 in 10^6 are required for highest accuracy. The monochromatic microwave radiation is produced in the Klystron oscillator, the wavelength being of the order of 3×10^{-2} m (9000 MHz).

The samples are required to be in the solid state; hence biological samples are usually frozen in liquid nitrogen. The first-order differential (dA/dH) is usually plotted against H, not A versus H. Hence a plot similar to that in Fig. 12.9 is obtained and this shape is called a 'line' in ESR spectroscopy. Generally there are relatively few unpaired electrons in a molecule, resulting in fewer than 10 lines, which are not closely spaced.

13.3.5 Applications

Metalloproteins

ESR spectroscopy is one of the main methods used to study metalloproteins, particularly those containing molybdenum (xanthine oxidase), copper (cytochrome oxidase and copper blue enzymes) and iron (cytochrome, ferredoxin). Both copper and non-haem iron, which do not absorb in the ultraviolet/visible regions, possess ESR absorption peaks in one of their oxidation states. The appearance and disappearance of their ESR signals are used to monitor their activity in the multi-enzyme systems of intact mitochondria and chloroplasts, as well as in isolated enzymes. In metalloproteins there exists a specific stereochemical structure whereby a characteristic number of ligands (frequently amino acid residues of the

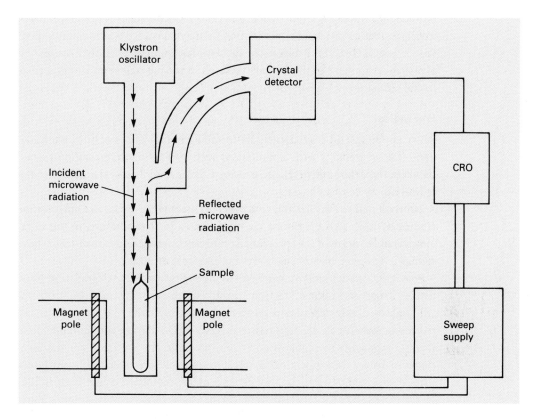

Fig. 13.3. Diagram of an ESR spectrometer. CRO, cathode ray oscilloscope.

protein) are coordinated to the metal. ESR studies show that the structural geometry is frequently distorted from that of model systems and the distortion may be related to biological function.

Spin labels

Spin labels are stable and unreactive free radicals used as reporter groups or probes. The procedure of spin labelling is the attachment of these probes to biological molecules that lack unpaired electrons. The label can be attached to either a substrate or a ligand. Often the spin label contains the nitric oxide moiety. These labels enable the study of events that occur with a frequency of 10^7 to $10^{11}\,s^{-1}$. If the motion is restricted in some directions, only anisotropic motion (movement in the same direction) may be studied, for example in membrane-rigid spin label in bilayers. Here the label is attached so that the NO group lies parallel to the long axis of the lipid.

Intramolecular motions and lateral diffusion of lipid through the membrane may be observed and measured. This study is achieved by either (i) concentrating the spin-labelled lipids into one region of the bilayer, or (ii) randomly incorporating, usually into model membranes. The diffusion of the spin labels allows them to come into contact with each other and causes line broadening in the spectrum. Another label used to study lipid motion in bilayers is 2,2,6,6-tetramethylpiperidine-1-oxyl (TEMPOL). Labelling of glycerophosphatides with this compound allows measurement of the flip rate between inner and outer surfaces as well as lateral diffusion.

Free radicals

Spin trapping is a process whereby an unstable free radical has stability conferred upon it by reacting it with a compound such as 5,5-dimethylpyrroline-1-oxide (DMPO). Hyperfine splittings are observed that depend upon the nature of the radical R'.

Molecules in the triplet (phosphorescent) state (Section 12.5.1) may also be studied by ESR. This gives data complementary to that obtained in the ultraviolet/visible region of the spectrum. For instance, free radicals due to the triplet state of tryptophan have been observed in cataractous lenses.

Free radicals are found in many metabolic pathways and as degradation products of drugs and toxins. Electron transfer mechanisms in mitochondria and chloroplasts involve paramagnetic species, for example the Fe $-$ S centres. Other redox processes involving the flavin derivatives FAD, FMN and semiquinones lend themselves readily to exploration by this approach. The $g = 2.003$ signal is associated mainly with mitochondria, but different cell lines show different intensities. This phenomenon is also dependent on metabolic state. Factors that increase metabolic activity also lead to an increase in organic radical signal. Many studies have involved the free radical polymer melanin and the ascorbyl radical. The latter has been used to study the effects of certain drugs on sperm maturation.

Carcinogenesis is an area where free radicals have been implicated and where their study has been of value. There is, in general, a lower concentration of free radicals in tumours than in normal tissues. Also a concentration gradient is observed, being higher in the peripheral non-necrotic surface layers than in the inner regions of the tumour. The free radicals may, of course, initiate the neoplasia. The development of implanted tumours in mice has also been studied. Chemical carcinogens are in many cases associated with generation of free radicals. An example is the prediction of carcinogenicity of certain polycyclic hydrocarbons. Polycyclic hydrocarbons arise by the successive linking of benzene rings along ring edges. Examples of such compounds are naphthalene (two rings), and anthracene and phenanthrene (three rings). As more rings are added the structures become increasingly complicated. As these compounds possess 'aromatic' character it becomes increasingly possible for the free electron of the radical to be accommodated, i.e. these kinds of radicals become more stable and therefore possibly more long lived. The fact that they may survive for extended periods of time allows more damage to be done. Many of the precursors of these radicals exist in natural sources such as coal tar, tobacco smoke and other products of combustion, hence the environmental risk.

Another source of free radicals is the irradiation, for example with γ-rays, of biological material. For instance -S $-$ S- cross-linkages in proteins may be identified by irradiating the protein, and the free radical produced has the free electron localised in the -S — S- region. Another major application in this area is examining irradiated foodstuffs for residual free radicals. The technique can be used to establish whether or not the packed foodstuff has been irradiated. A similar biomedical/environmental application involves the study of hard biological materials such as bone or teeth. When such materials are exposed to ionising radiation, energy is stored in them and this energy may give rise to the production of free radicals. Clearly ESR may be used to detect these radicals and is used in 'dose assessment' in nuclear radiation accidents.

Metabolic studies

Many metabolic studies have made use of ESR. Examples are the metabolism of drugs, processes occurring in the microsomes of the liver, peroxidation mechanisms and the free radical products of oxygen. Superoxide dismutases scavenge oxygen-related (dioxygenyl) free radicals O_2^+ (that have been associated, for example, with inflammation and ageing). Nitric oxide, NO, as an independent entity, operates as a physiological messenger regulating the nervous, immune and cardiovascular systems. It has been implicated in septic (toxic) shock, hypertension, stroke and neurodegenerative diseases. Although NO is involved in normal synaptic transmission, excess levels are neurotoxic. Superoxide dismutase attenuates the neurotoxicity by removal of O_2^+, hence limiting its availability for reaction with NO to produce peroxynitrite.

13.4 NUCLEAR MAGNETIC RESONANCE SPECTROSCOPY

The essential background theory of the phenomena that allow NMR to occur has been dealt with in Section 13.3.1. The miniscule magnets involved here are nucleons (in effect protons) rather than electrons. The specific principles, instrumentation and applications are treated below.

13.4.1 Principles

Again there is considerable similarity with ESR. Most studies involve the use of ^{1}H (hence the term proton magnetic resonance (PMR) but ^{13}C, ^{15}N and ^{31}P isotopes are used in biochemical studies.

The resonance condition in NMR is satisfied in an external magnetic field of several hundred millitesla, with absorptions occurring in the region of radiowave 40 MHz frequency for resonance of the ^{1}H nucleus. The actual field scanned is small compared with the total field applied and the radio frequencies absorbed are specifically stated on such spectra.

The molecular environment of a proton governs the value of the applied external field at which the nucleus resonates. This is recorded as the chemical shift (τ) and is measured relative to an internal standard, frequently tetramethylsilane (TMS), whose structure $(CH_3)_4Si$ contains 12 identical protons. The chemical shift arises from the applied field inducing secondary fields (15×10^{-4} to 20×10^{-4} tesla) at the proton by interacting with the adjacent bonding electrons. If the induced field opposes the applied field, the latter will have to be at a slightly higher value for resonance to occur. Alternatively, if the induced and applied fields are aligned the latter is required to be at a lower value for resonance. In the opposing field case, the nucleus is said to be shielded, the magnitude of the shielding being proportional to the electron-withdrawing power of proximal substituents. In the aligned field case, the nucleus is said to be deshielded. The field axis may be calibrated in units on a scale from 0 to 10, with TMS at the maximum value. The type of proton may thus be identified by the absorption peak position, i.e. its chemical shift and the area under each peak being proportional to the number of such protons in a particular group. Fig. 13.4 is a simplified diagram of an ethyl alcohol spectrum in which there are three methyl, two methylene (methene) and one alcohol group protons. The peaks appear in the area proportions 3:2:1.

High resolution NMR yields further structural information derived from the observation of hyperfine splitting. This arises owing to spin–spin splitting or coupling, owing to the interaction of bonding electrons with like or different spins, and may extend to nuclei four or five bonds apart. It is shown as fine-structure splitting of peaks already separated by chemical shifts. NMR spectra are of great value in elucidating chemical structures. Both qualitative and quantitative information may be obtained, and hyperfine splitting yields information about the near-neighbour environment of a nucleus. The advances in computing power have made possible many of the more advanced NMR techniques. Weak signals may be enhanced by running many scans and accumulating the data; baseline noise, which is random, then tends to cancel out whereas the real signal increases. This approach significantly improves the signal-to-noise ratio and the method is known as computer averaging of transients or CAT scanning. On combining CAT scanning with the very rapid acquisition and data processing of pulse-acquire/ Fourier transform methods, very powerful tools become available. In addition the facile manipulation of data postacquisition and the generation of difference spectra has dramatically improved the usefulness and applicability of the basic technique.

Despite the value and continued use of what might be termed 'conventional' proton NMR, much more structural information may be obtained by resorting to pulsed input, of the radio frequency energy, and subjecting the resulting output to computer analysis by Fourier transform. This approach has given rise to a wide variety of procedures that allow the production of multidimensional spectra (four-dimensional in the most sophisticated experiments), ^{13}C and other odd-isotope NMR spectra and the determination of multiplicities and scan images.

In common with all of the spectroscopic techniques already discussed, the energy is input in the form of electromagnetic radiation and 'entities' are promoted from lower to higher states. The 'entities' are electrons in the ultraviolet/visible techniques, bond oscillations and deformations in the infrared, Raman and microwave techniques and magnetic spin orientations in ESR and NMR. All these processes follow the strict quantum rules already described. Clearly (after a certain, albeit short, time span) the entities that were previously promoted to the higher states may return to the original condition. The general term for this process is relaxation. A very simple example is observable in the ultraviolet/visible region,

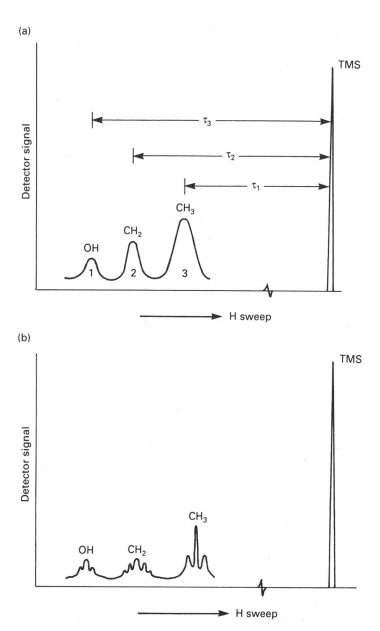

Fig. 13.4. NMR spectrum of ethyl alcohol (a) at low resolution and (b) at high resolution. The latter resolved only in very pure samples. TMS, trimethylsilane.

where an absorption spectrum arises when the energy is input and absorbed and an emission spectrum when the system relaxes.

Pulse-acquire and Fourier transform methods

A number of approaches to the method used for the production of spectra exists but mainly one of two options is used. In 'conventional' spectroscopy the electromagnetic energy is supplied, from the source, as a continuously changing frequency over a preselected spectral range. The response is detected by an appropriate device and whether the scan is from shorter to longer wavelength (higher to lower frequency), or the reverse, is irrelevant. The essential point is that the change is smooth and regular between fixed limits. The alternative is to put all the energy, i.e. all the resonant frequencies between the fixed limits, in at the same time. This is achieved by irradiating the sample with a broadband pulse of all these frequencies at one go. The output is, of course, also measured simultaneously and the observed result is, in general, a very complicated interference pattern. Fortunately these patterns are amenable to analysis by Fourier transform methods, which, although being quite complicated mathematical procedures, can be performed readily using modern computer facilities and appear transparent to the user.

The approaches differ with the spectroscopic technique. As indicated in Section 13.2.2, FT–IR involves the method of interferometry and the interferograph that results arises from observation of the frequencies which pass through the sample and are not absorbed. What is detected in FT–NMR is known as the free induction decay (FID). This is akin to the emission spectrum referred to in ultraviolet/visible methods in that the FID arises from the excited species re-emitting the absorbed frequencies. The discussion so far has, for the sake of simplicity, attempted to describe the observed phenomena in terms of single entities, i.e. single nuclei. In a real sample of material in which bulk magnetism may be observed, this arises from the accumulation of all the miniscule nuclear magnets. It may be demonstrated using Boltzmann statistics that, when the sample is placed in an external magnetic field, at thermal equilibrium there will be a slight excess of spins, the so-called α-spins, aligned or parallel with this field. Note that this is the normal low energy condition, the high energy state being that of the antiparallel β-spins. This gives rise to the bulk magnetisation vector, $\boldsymbol{M}$, and, by agreed convention, it is taken to lie along the z-axis of a three-dimensional Cartesian coordinate system, the z-axis being parallel to the direction of the external magnetic field. The magnetic induction of the external field is designated B_0. Now consider the input of a pulse of the appropriate radio frequency (RF) radiation. Recall that this is electromagnetic radiation comprising an electric and a magnetic vector. The magnetic vector of the RF radiation has an associated magnetic field whose magnetic induction may be designated B_1. If the transmitter coils supplying the pulse of RF radiation are arranged so that B_1 is perpendicular to the z-axis along which the bulk magnetisation vector, $\boldsymbol{M}$, lies, then $\boldsymbol{M}$ will be rotated through an angle θ towards the x–y plane. The value of θ depends upon the magnitude of the B_1 field and the duration of the pulse. Fig. 13.5a,b is a diagrammatic representation of this process, with $\theta = \pi/2$ for simplicity (see 'Multidimensional NMR', below, for further explanation). The cumulative spins comprising $\boldsymbol{M}$ are no longer parallel to the external magnetic field, i.e. $\boldsymbol{M}$ no longer lies along the z-axis. In the absence of a further pulse of RF radiation the system will relax, M returning to lie along the z-axis. It is this return or relaxation, which is first-order exponential, that gives rise to the free induction decay alluded to above and data are acquired during the decay period. As described, this would be known as a simple pulse-acquire experiment. Multipulse RF input, possibly at different angles, gives rise to a large array of

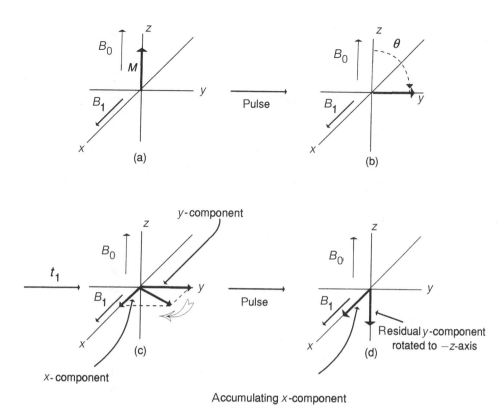

Fig. 13.5. Rotation of magnetism during radio frequency pulses.

different experiments, resulting in the production of extremely valuable data. Two relaxation processes are important in NMR and associated techniques. The first-order exponential decay observed in FID arises from energy dissipation by spin–lattice or longitudinal relaxation. In this situation the energy is lost to the matrix (surroundings). The time span for this process is designated T_1. An alternative process is spin–spin or transverse relaxation with time span T_2, where energy is dissipated between spins rather than the environment. T_1 is always greater than or equal to T_2 and for small organic molecules they are equal.

It is beyond the scope of this text to examine the specific details of the Fourier transform method. It is sufficient to recognise that the mathematical procedure effects the translation of a signal in the time domain to a corresponding 'peak' in the frequency domain. For a sine wave of single frequency, v Hz (cycles per second), 1 cycle is mapped in $1/v$ seconds. The ordinary sine wave is normally shown in the time domain as a portion of an infinite cycle of oscillations of constant amplitude. The frequency appears as a single peak in the frequency domain, also of fixed amplitude. Fig. 13.6a shows the effect of the translation between domains for a single sine wave and Fig. 13.6b that for the single FID pattern. All complicated interference patterns may be separated into their constituent sine and cosine waves by Fourier analysis and transformed between domains. Fig. 13.7

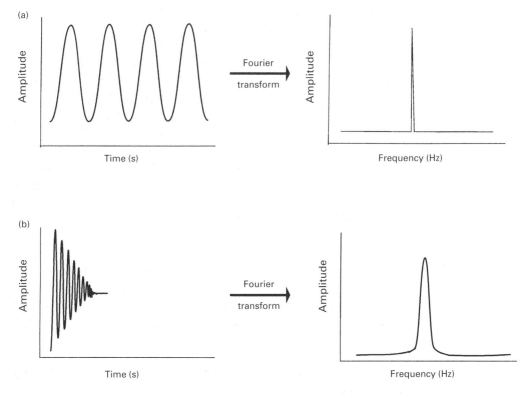

Fig. 13.6. Diagrammatic representation of the Fourier transformation of a single frequency sine wave and single FID. (a) Sine wave, (b) single free induction decay.

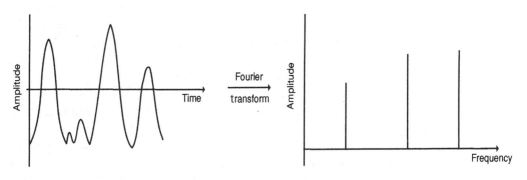

Fig. 13.7. FT of a three-sine-wave combination.

shows the transform of a waveform comprising three sine waves of different frequency and amplitude.

The time domain oscillograph representing the FID from a real NMR experiment would of course be much more complicated, as it would comprise many more contributory sine and cosine waves. These would be extracted, transformed to the frequency domain and presented as peaks in a spectrum.

In Section 13.3.2 it was indicated that spins or spinning nuclei generate magnetic fields that may extend their influence through space. Proximal neighbours are subject to this influence, directly, and the general term for this phenomenon is dipolar interaction. If the signal intensity of a resonance is observed to change when the state of a near neighbour is perturbed from the equilibrium, then what is being seen is an example of the nuclear Overhauser effect (NOE). This effect is of profound importance in the elucidation of the three-dimensional stereochemistry of the molecular species under investigation. The magnetic influences encountered in the dipolar interaction are transmitted through space over a limited distance and for the NOE to be observed the distance between nuclei must be of the order of about 0.4 nm or less. Clearly this spatial constraint enables information to be gained about the three-dimensional geometry of the molecule being examined when considered together with scalar coupling (spin–spin coupling) information, this being the influence whose effects occur through bonds.

It is possible to saturate spins in a given population (the perturbation) with a selective 90° irradiation, giving ample time for the acquisition of proton spectra involving ^1H–^1H interactions giving rise to NOE enhancements. By performing a second irradiation at a point in the RF spectrum that is remote from any resonant frequencies, off-resonance irradiation, a control spectrum (no NOEs produced) is generated that may be subtracted from the previously acquired one, resulting in the cancelling out of any signals that are not NOE enhancements. The results obtained are referred to as steady-state NOEs and the method is termed the NOE difference experiment.

One of the main advantages to be gained from the use of pulse-acquire/Fourier transform methods coupled to signal averaging, together with the development of high field magnets, is the ability to obtain ^{13}C NMR spectra. This isotope of carbon exists in low abundance, 1.108%, and compared to the essentially 100% abundance of ^1H it may be recognised that, in general, signal intensities are likely to be low. Despite the advances described above, about 10 times the amount of sample, in most cases, is required for ^{13}C NMR spectra as compared with that for ^1H spectra.

Owing to the low abundance of the ^{13}C nucleus, the chance of finding two such species next to each other in a molecule is very small. This is considered in more detail in Chapter 9. In consequence of this, ^{13}C–^{13}C interactions (homonuclear couplings) do not arise. It is true that ^1H–^{13}C interaction (heteronuclear coupling) is possible but, for technical reasons such as band overlap, it is usual to generate decoupled spectra. The result is that, in general, ^{13}C spectra are very much simpler and cleaner and have improved signal-to-noise ratios (albeit with higher sample loadings) compared with their proton resonance counterparts. There are clear advantages in this approach but at least one considerable disadvantage. The ability to observe multiplicities has been lost, i.e. whether a particular ^{13}C is associated with a methyl (CH_3), methene (CH_2) or methyne (CH) group. Some of this information may be regained by performing the decoupling using off-resonance irradiation as in the NOE difference experiments described above. However, a method that has become routine is distortionless enhancement by polarisation transfer (DEPT). This method requires a multipulse excitation sequence at different angles, frequently 45°, 90° or 135°. Although interactions have been decoupled, in this situation the resonances exhibit positive or negative signal intensities, or signal phases, which are dependent on the number of protons directly attached to the carbon nucleus. For example, in a DEPT-135 experiment: CH and CH_3 are both positive; CH_2 is negative. Clearly a single DEPT-135 experiment would suffice if no methyl groups are present. DEPT signals for the above primary, secondary or tertiary carbons, from irradiations at 45° and 90°, are either positive or zero.

Multidimensional NMR

Consider further the processes described in Fig. 13.5a–d. The magnetisation vector M is originally aligned along the z-axis parallel to the vector direction of the external field, B_0. A pulse B_1 is applied, at right angles, i.e. parallel to the x-axis and M is rotated to the y-axis through 90°, provided the pulse is of sufficient magnitude and lasts for a sufficient time (Fig. 13.5a,b). Apart from the decay process this vector will precess (rotate) in the x–y plane, towards the x-axis (Fig. 13.5c) with a characteristic frequency, the Larmor frequency, during a period of time t_1. This is quite distinct from the decay process, FID, which overlaps it. At any point between the x- and y-axes the vector M may be resolved into components along these two axes. If, during t_1, a second B_1 pulse is applied then the component along the y-axis will again be rotated, in this instance towards the $-z$-axis. The component along the x-axis is unaffected because it is parallel to B_1. If the time t_1 is zero, i.e. there are immediately consecutive B_1 pulses, then M rotates from the z- to the y-axis with the first pulse and then immediately to the $-z$-axis with the second pulse. For $t_1 = 0$ there will be no x component as there has been no time available for it to be established. For values of $t_1 > 0$ a component of M along the x-axis will be established whose magnitude depends on the length of t_1. The longer t_1 the greater will be the magnitude of the x component because M will have moved nearer to this axis. By applying successive B_1 pulses with increasing lengths of t_1, an accumulated x component of magnetisation is produced and a series of FIDs may be measured and stored separately in the computer. The y- and $-z$-components are not measurable. This accumulation of FIDs gives rise to a second dimension in the time domain and each may be transformed by Fourier methods.

Two-dimensional frequency diagrams are produced as contour maps. Values on the diagonal correspond to chemical shifts, etc., that would have been shown in a one-dimensional experiment. It is the asymmetrical, off-diagonal information that is new. These data arise from the correlation of coupling interactions between nuclei, the main advantage being that the information is all gathered in one experiment, an achievement entirely dependent on the use of multipulse excitation. Proton–proton correlation gives rise to homonuclear correlation spectroscopy (COSY). Proton–carbon correlation gives rise to heteronuclear chemical shift correlation spectroscopy (hetero-COSY or HETCOR).

The achieved and potential sophistication of NMR experiments is quite phenomenal, allowing more useful two-dimensional and extension into three- and four-dimensional spectra. Considering again Fig. 13.5a–d (the COSY pulse

sequence), the second 90° pulse rotates the magnetisation vector along the
$-z$-axis. Various transverse components are removed by electronic control and
the vector in the $-z$ direction accumulates (cf. the process described above for the
COSY case). A third 90° pulse is then applied and produces magnetisation, which
can be measured. Repeat of the pulse sequence for varying (increasing) values of t_1
gives rise to changes that are observable during the final 90° pulse. The outcome is
a two-dimensional experiment that allows the detection of NOEs and is known as
nuclear Overhauser effect spectroscopy (NOESY). This can be improved upon yet
further by studying phenomena in the rotating frame coordinate system rather
than fixed Cartesian coordinates. Such an experiment involves rotating frame
nuclear Overhauser effect spectroscopy (ROESY). A significant problem is that, for
^{1}H NOESY NMR to be of value, all the NOEs should be resolved. In the study of biological macromolecules this becomes less likely with the increase in molecular
mass. The use of triple pulse sequences (three time variables) in conjunction with a
COSY or NOESY sequence generates a three-dimensional spectrum. This, in effect,
is a cube and is akin to stacking two-dimensional spectra one on top of the other.
Note that this is a near analogy and not a simple stacking procedure. In order to
achieve this it is necessary to incorporate into the molecule under investigation an
isotopically labelled nuclide such as ^{13}C or ^{15}N. A whole new range of interactions
between ^{1}H, ^{13}C and/or ^{15}N is now possible and adds extensively to the analytical
procedure. To obtain the resolution advantages of the four-dimensional spectrum,
both ^{13}C and ^{15}N must be incorporated, the heavy isotope of carbon being deliberately introduced at particular points in the carbon chain in order to be associated
with specific aliphatic hydrogens. Essentially, three separate two-dimensional
experiments are combined, the different interactions being ^{1}H–^{1}H, ^{1}H–^{13}C and
^{1}H–^{15}N. It is interesting to note that, in the four-dimensional case, the manipulation of the generated data by powerful computer techniques results in substantially improved resolution without a corresponding increase in complexity.

13.4.2 Instrumentation

The essential details of an NMR instrument are shown diagrammatically in
Fig. 13.8. It will be seen yet again that the layout is almost identical to that of ESR,
except that instead of a Klystron oscillator being present to generate microwave
radiation, two sets of coils, a transmitter and a receiver, are used for generation and
reception, respectively, of the appropriate RF. Samples in solution are contained in
sealed tubes, which are rotated rapidly in the cavity to eliminate irregularities and
imperfections; in this way an average and uniform signal is reflected to the receiver
to be processed and recorded. Solid state and high field NMR are more recent and
rapidly advancing techniques enable hitherto difficult or impossible investigations. The latest developments allow multidimensional NMR to be performed, per-
mitting even more sophisticated structural analyses to be carried out. Many of
these developments in instrumentation differ from the simple design shown in
Fig. 13.8 in terms of the geometric layout of the coils, for the multipulse methods
described above, sophisticated electronics and advanced computer facilities.

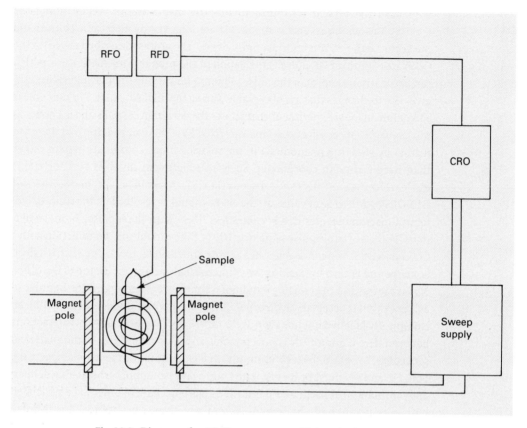

Fig. 13.8. Diagram of an NMR spectrometer. CRO, cathode ray oscilloscope; RFO, radio frequency oscillator; RFD, radio frequency detector.

13.4.3 **Applications**

Molecular structure determination

The study of molecular structure, conformational changes and certain types of kinetic investigation is the main use of NMR in the biological field. Most work is done in solution, and in order to eliminate solvent effects the equivalent deuterated solvent (for proton NMR) would be used. The use of the technique in drug metabolism studies is of increasing importance, particularly when coupled with infrared and X-ray diffraction data, which can then be used in molecular modelling methods using sophisticated computer techniques to try to elucidate drug action. Fig. 13.9 shows a high resolution proton resonance spectrum of phenacetin and, together with the FT–IR spectrum shown in Fig. 13.2, yields substantial structural information. For comparative purposes, the two-dimensional COSY spectrum of phenacetin is shown in Fig. 13.10, where contours along the diagonal give information equivalent to that shown in Fig. 13.9. The off-diagonal contours represent additional information; for explanation, see the legend to Fig. 13.10.

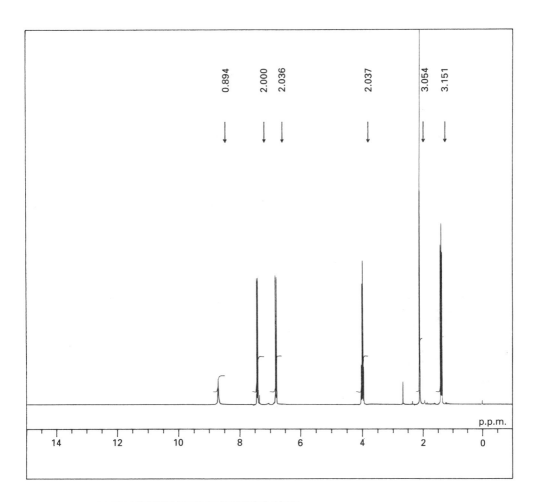

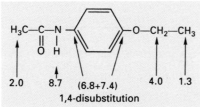

Fig. 13.9. NMR spectrum of phenacetin. The values associated with the downward-pointing arrows, shown slightly to the right of each peak in the upper diagram, indicate the approximate number of protons involved. In the lower diagram the shifts in p.p.m. are shown, indicating which proton is involved. The peak at 1.3 p.p.m. is a triplet because it is next to a -CH₂ group and that at 4.0 is a quadruplet because it is next to a -CH₃ group. The peaks at 6.8 and 7.4 p.p.m. are a pattern characteristic of 1,4 disubstitution in an aromatic ring.

(a)

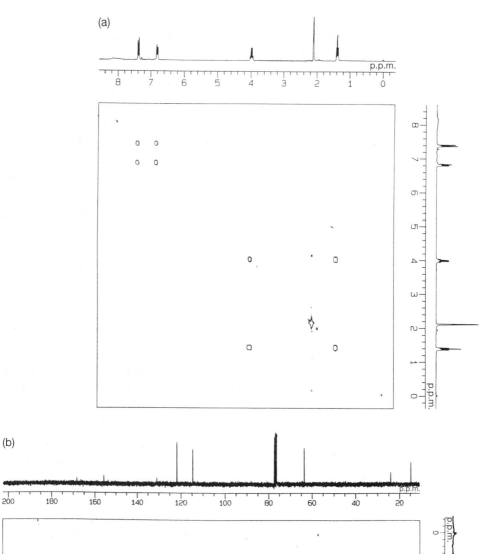

(b)

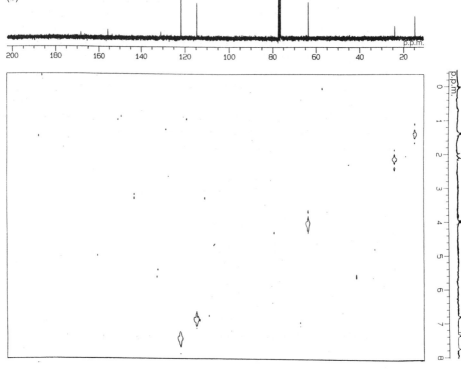

An examination of the scientific literature in the field shows a plethora of results for biological macromolecules using the whole battery of techniques described above. For peptide and protein structural studies the species tend to be arbitrarily divided into those with relative molecular mass less than 15 000 and those between 15 000 and 30 000. Low resolution NMR has been obtained on the *lac* repressor headpiece and bovine pancreatic trypsin inhibitor (BPTI). High resolution protein structures for antiviral protein BDS-1, the C3a and C5a inflammatory proteins, plastocyanin, thioredoxin, epidermal growth factor and the interleukins are some examples. The application of solid state NMR has been valuable in the study of, for example, Alzheimer's β-amyloid peptide and melanostatin. Much more specialised methods are required to extend the mass range beyond 30 000 but it is now possible and several antibodies have been investigated.

Structures in aqueous solution

A distinct advantage of NMR is its use in studying molecular behaviour in solution. Any particular state is averaged, of course, but often produces more useful

Fig. 13.10. Two-dimensional NMR spectra may be best imagined as looking down on a forest where all the trees (representing peaks in the spectrum) have been chopped off at the same fixed height. Taller trees would have thicker trunks at a given height. The equivalent is the larger contours observed which derive from larger peaks in the unidimensional spectra.

(a) This figure is the correlated (COSY) NMR spectrum of phenacetin showing the homonuclear ^{1}H–^{1}H interactions. The single spectra along each axis are identical and the contours along the diagonal of the two-dimensional map represent the 'birds-eye view' of the chopped-off peaks. The off-diagonal contours, which are symmetrically distributed as a mirror image about the diagonal, represent new information. As an example of the interpretation, place a rule horizontally at the 1.3 p.p.m. position of the right-hand spectrum (triplet) and another rule vertically at the 4.0 p.p.m. position on the top spectrum (quadruplet). Where these two rules intersect is the location of a contour which represents the interaction between protons located in adjacent -CH_2- and -CH_3 groups.

(b) This is the heteronuclear ^{13}C – ^{1}H correlation spectrum. The contours in the two-dimensional map here represent interactions between the nuclear magnets of ^{13}C and the associated protons. The ^{1}H spectrum lies vertically along the right-hand axis and the ^{13}C spectrum lies horizontally along the top. The contour positions are located as described in (a) above and the p.p.m. values and interactions are listed below.

^{13}C	^{1}H	Interaction	
14	1.3	CH_3-	(Ethyl–O)
24	2.1	CH_3-	(Acetyl)
63	4.0	CH_2-	Ethyl–O
115	6.8	Ring C	(Ethyl–O)
122	7.4	Ring C	(=N–H)
132	—	Ring C	(=N–H)
156	—	Ring C	(Ethyl–O)
167	—	=C=O	
	7.8	=N–H	

p.p.m.

A triplet observed at 77 p.p.m. is due to residual chloroform in the solvent.

information than the constrained structures available from X-ray crystallographic studies. Results of studies of protein folding are exemplified by ribonuclease A, cytochrome c, barnase, α-lactalbumin, lysozyme, ubiquitin and BPTI.

The techniques have been applied to the study of enzyme kinetics both *in vivo* and *in vitro*. Amongst the groups of enzymes studied are: chymotrypsin, trypsin, papain, pepsin, thermolysin; adenylate, creatinine and pyruvate kinases; alkaline phosphatase, ATPase and ribonuclease (Section 15.4.7). Other examples are glycogen phosphorylase, dihydrofolate reductase and triosephosphate isomerase.

Nucleic acids

Application to the nucleic acids includes not only a variety of structural studies of both DNA and RNA but additionally investigations of interactions between various drugs and DNA and between binding proteins and DNA. Sequence assignments in oligosaccharides have been obtained but work on intact glycoproteins has not been promising, particularly in multidimensional NMR, owing to the difficulty in deconvoluting the data. Interactions between proteins and lipid bilayers in membranes have been observed and the structure of certain membrane proteins has been related to their predicted biological function. Examples of such proteins are gramicidin A, bacteriorhodopsin and rhodopsin, phage coat proteins and alamethicin.

Phosphate metabolism

The isotope ^{31}P exhibits nuclear resonance and NMR has been used extensively in studies of phosphate metabolism. The relative and changing concentrations of AMP, ADP and ATP can be measured and hence their metabolism studied in living cells and tissues. Intracellular and extracellular inorganic phosphate concentrations may be measured in living cells and tissues also because the chemical shift of inorganic phosphate varies with pH.

Magnetic resonance imaging

The analytical applications described above may be extended into the clinical environment. Physiological material such as urine, blood and cerebrospinal fluid may be studied directly. Appropriate tissue biopsy samples are also amenable to examination. In such cases, biochemical phenomena are being observed. For instance, the measurement of metabolic concentrations at specific sites in tissues is possible. The extension to small whole animals in pharmacological investigations and the human subject has become possible with the advent of superconducting magnet technology and other improvements. ATP metabolism in healthy and unhealthy individuals and changes during exercise are measurable.

The major direct clinical application, however, is in imaging. Unfortunately, owing to the low energy transitions in the radio frequency region of the electromagnetic spectrum, NMR is a relatively insensitive technique. This imposes limitations and attention is focused almost exclusively on ^{1}H resonance in the development of magnetic resonance imaging (MRI). There are two important reasons for this:

first the proton is one of the more sensitive nuclides, and, secondly, it is present in biological systems in considerable abundance. However, not all types of proton in all molecular environments are easily studied. Those protons making a major contribution to the NMR response reside in compounds in rapid physical motion. By far the most important compound in this respect is water, which contains two protons and is a major constituent of biological systems. Lesser contributions from protons in other compounds are measurable in special circumstances.

In NMR, the resonance frequency of the particular nuclide contributing the magnetic spin is proportional to the strength of the applied external magnetic field. If an external magnetic field 'gradient' is applied then a range of resonant frequencies may be observed which reflects the spatial distribution of the spinning nuclei. Three major approaches are in wide use which result in (i) projection reconstruction, (ii) Fourier imaging and (iii) echo-planar imaging. For detailed consideration of these different methods the reader is referred to more specialised texts (see Section 13.5).

A particular advantage of MRI is that there is some flexibility in the choice of physical property that is imaged. The number of spins in a particular, defined spatial region gives rise to the spin density as a measurable parameter. This measure may be combined with measures of the principal relaxation times (T_1 and T_2) to give more meaningful results. The imaging of flux, as either bulk flow or localised diffusion, adds considerably to the options available. In terms of whole-body scanners the 'overall picture' is reconstructed from images generated in contiguous slices and clearly owes much to advances in computing power as well as magnetic resonance technology. Resolution and image contrast are major considerations for the technique and subject to continuing development. Equipment cost and data acquisition time remain other important issues affecting the development of MRI.

Water is distributed differently in different tissues but constitutes, in total, about 55% of body mass in the average human subject. In soft tissues the water distribution varies between 60% and 90% of the total mass. The differences in water content in white and grey matter in the brain and between normal tissue and most tumours generate sufficient contrast to enable high resolution images to be produced. Fig. 13.11 reproduces an MRI scan showing a vertical longitudinal section of the human head and brain. In adipose tissue the ^1H signal from lipids is measurable and the chemical shift differences for $-CH_2-$ are such that distinction from water may be made. Reproduced in Fig. 13.12 are photographs obtained from MRI scans of fat and thin patients in order that the distribution of adipose tissue may be compared. The thin patient represents the control in the experiment.

It is also possible to distinguish the different relaxation properties. Tissue water behaves quite differently from the pure substance. Transverse relaxation, T_2, does not generally follow a single exponential decay process whereas longitudinal relaxation, T_1, does. T_2 relaxations must be split into at least two exponential decays, having a typical value of 20–100 ms. For T_1 decays the range is 100–500 ms. These values are significantly less than for pure water and the differences may

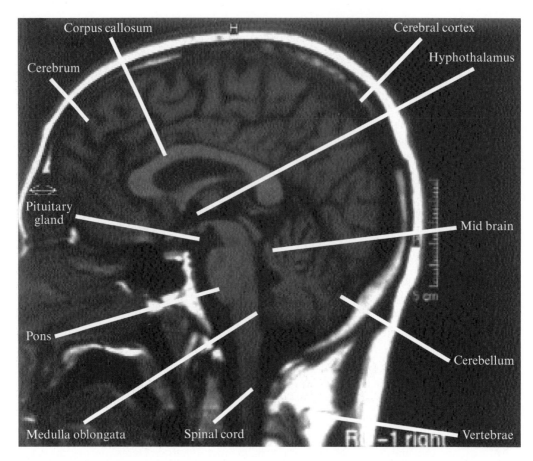

Fig. 13.11. Vertical longitudinal section through the human head by magnetic resonance imaging (MRI). The major features are identified and labelled, although specific items such as the pituitary gland and hypothalamus are barely visible. (This figure is modified from an MRI scan kindly donated by the Radiology Department of the Stepping Hill Hospital, Stockport, Cheshire.)

arise from the presence of hydrophilic macromolecules in the tissue environment. In the case of tumours, however, the T_1 values are elevated compared with normal tissue, adding a further important discriminator, although the elevation is less marked in human tumours compared with laboratory-grown material. Disadvantages with this approach are the overlap of values and also that elevated T_1 decays are not tumour specific but may also be evident in normal rapidly regenerating tissue. Other NMR parameters and observational differential diagnosis of the magnetic resonance image must also be taken into account. The shape, size and location of the abnormal image must be considered by the radiologist when making a diagnosis.

At present there is an almost bewildering array of options available in terms of different pulse sequences, scan protocols, and chemical shift and relaxation time data measurements that can be made. The procedures can be applied to

(a)

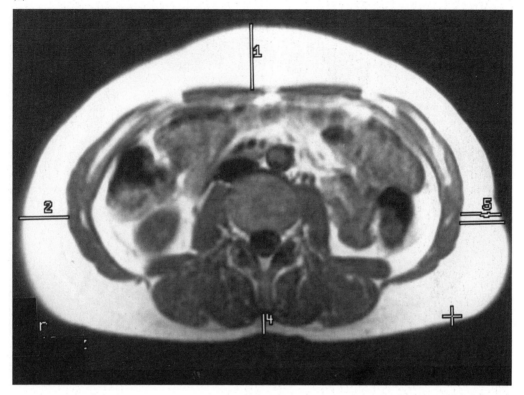

Fig. 13.12. (a) and (b) show MRI scans of transverse sections (contiguous slice) through the abdominal regions of 'fat' and 'obese' subjects. The fatty deposits are indicated by the intense white regions, the resonance arising from the protons of the methylene groups of long-chain fatty acids. (The scans are reproduced by kind permission of the Oxford Lipid Metabolism Group, Nuffield Department of Clinical Medicine, University of Oxford.)

three-dimensional and contiguous slice imaging of whole body or specific organ investigations on head, thorax, abdomen, liver, pancreas, kidney and musculo-skeletal regions. Use of contrast agents has enabled 'organ function' such as renal function to be explored, if the agent passes into the urine. If such an agent can be administered intravenously then exploration of blood flow, tissue perfusion, and transport across the blood/brain barrier may be investigated and also defects in vascular anatomy recognised. Contrast agents for use in MRI will generally be required to show paramagnetic properties. Clearly, as in other invasive methods, they must be non-toxic.

NMR and the associated technique of MRI offer the analytical biochemist and the clinician a phenomenal variety of procedures. Both types of application continue to challenge almost all alternative approaches. Clearly there are hazards associated with any technique but these magnetic resonance methods appear, on the basis of current knowledge, to be relatively safe, particularly with the absence of ionising radiation.

(b)

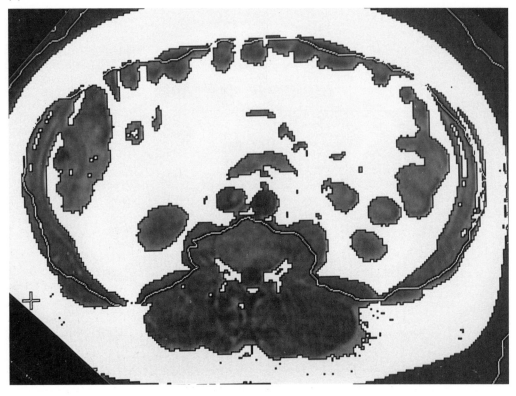

Fig. 13.12. (*Cont.*)

13.5 **SUGGESTIONS FOR FURTHER READING**

EVANS, J. N. S. (1995). *Biomolecular NMR Spectroscopy.* Oxford University Press, Oxford.
(Contains several excellent chapters on the application of NMR to the study of enzymes.)
REID, D. G. (1997). *Protein NMR Techniques.* Humana Press, Totawa, NJ. (Includes some good
examples of the application of single and multidimensional NMR to the study of proteins.)

Chapter 14

Radioisotope techniques

14.1 THE NATURE OF RADIOACTIVITY

14.1.1 Atomic structure

An atom is composed of a positively charged nucleus that is surrounded by a cloud of negatively charged electrons. The mass of an atom is concentrated in the nucleus, even though it accounts for only a small fraction of the total size of the atom. Atomic nuclei are composed of two major particles, protons and neutrons. Protons are positively charged particles with a mass approximately 1850 times greater than that of an orbital electron. The number of orbital electrons in an atom must be equal to the number of protons present in the nucleus, since the atom as a whole is electrically neutral. This number is known as the atomic number (Z). Neutrons are uncharged particles with a mass approximately equal to that of a proton. The sum of protons and neutrons in a given nucleus is the mass number (A). Thus

$$A = Z + N$$

where N is the number of neutrons present.

Since the number of neutrons in a nucleus is not related to the atomic number, it does not affect the chemical properties of the atom. Atoms of a given element may not necessarily contain the same number of neutrons. Atoms of a given element with different mass numbers (i.e. different numbers of neutrons) are called isotopes. Symbolically, a specific nuclear species is represented by a subscript number for the atomic number, and a superscript number for the mass number, followed by the symbol of the element. For example:

$$^{12}_{6}C \quad ^{14}_{6}C \quad ^{16}_{8}O \quad ^{18}_{8}O$$

However, in practice it is more conventional just to cite the mass number (e.g. ^{14}C). The number of isotopes of a given element varies: there are 3 isotopes of hydrogen, ^{1}H, ^{2}H and ^{3}H, 7 of carbon ^{10}C to ^{16}C inclusive, and 20 or more of some of the elements of high atomic number.

14.1.2 Atomic stability and radiation

In general, the ratio of neutrons to protons in the nucleus will determine whether an isotope of a given element is stable enough to exist in nature. Stable isotopes for

Table 14.1 Properties of different types of radiation

Alpha	Beta	Gamma, X-rays and Bremmstrahlung
Heavy charged particle	Light charged particle	Electromagnetic radiation (em)
More toxic than other forms of radiation	Toxicity same as em radiation per unit of energy	Toxicity same as beta radiation per unit of energy
Not penetrating	Penetration varies with source	Highly penetrating

elements with low atomic numbers tend to have an equal number of neutrons and protons, whereas stability for elements of higher atomic numbers is associated with a neutron:proton ratio in excess of 1. Unstable isotopes, or radioisotopes as they are more commonly known, are often produced artificially, but many occur in nature. Radioisotopes emit particles and/or electromagnetic radiation as a result of changes in the composition of the atomic nucleus. These processes, which are known as radioactive decay, arise, either directly or as a result of a decay series, in the production of a stable isotope.

14.1.3 Types of radioactive decay

There are several types of radioactive decay; only those most relevant to biochemists are considered below. A summary of properties is given in Table 14.1.

Decay by negatron emission

In this case a neutron is converted to a proton by the ejection of a negatively charged beta (β) particle called a negatron (β^-):

neutron $\rightarrow$ proton + negatron

To all intents and purposes a negatron is an electron, but the term negatron is preferred, although not always used, since it serves to emphasise the nuclear origin of the particle. As a result of negatron emission, the nucleus loses a neutron but gains a proton. The N/Z ratio therefore decreases while Z increases by 1 and A remains constant. An isotope frequently used in biological work that decays by negatron emission is ^{14}C.

$$^{14}_{6}C \rightarrow {}^{14}_{7}N + \beta^-$$

Negatron emission is very important to biochemists because many of the commonly used radionuclides decay by this mechanism. Examples are: ^{3}H and ^{14}C, which can be used to label any organic compound; ^{35}S used to label methionine, for example to study protein synthesis; and ^{32}P, a powerful tool in molecular biology when used as a nucleic acid label.

Decay by positron emission

Some isotopes decay by emitting positively charged β-particles referred to as positrons (β^+). This occurs when a proton is converted to a neutron:

proton $\rightarrow$ neutron + positron

Positrons are extremely unstable and have only a transient existence. Once they have dissipated their energy they interact with electrons and are annihilated. The mass and energy of the two particles are converted to two γ-rays emitted at 180° to each other. This phenomenon is frequently described as back-to-back emission.

As a result of positron emission the nucleus loses a proton and gains a neutron, the N/Z ratio increases, Z decreases by 1 and A remains constant. An example of an isotope decaying by positron emission is ^{22}Na:

$$^{22}_{11}\text{Na} \rightarrow ^{22}_{10}\text{Ne} + \beta^+$$

Positron emitters are detected by the same instruments used to detect γ-radiation. They are used in biological sciences to spectacular effect in brain scanning with the technique positron emission tomography (PET scanning) used to identify active and inactive areas of the brain.

Decay by alpha particle emission

Isotopes of elements with high atomic numbers frequently decay by emitting alpha (α) particles. An α-particle is a helium nucleus; it consists of two protons and two neutrons ($^4\text{He}^{2+}$). Emission of α-particles results in a considerable lightening of the nucleus, a decrease in atomic number of 2 and a decrease in the mass number of 4. Isotopes that decay by α-emission are not frequently encountered in biological work. Radium-226 (^{226}Ra) decays by α-emission to radon-222 (^{222}Rn), which is itself radioactive. Thus begins a complex decay series, which culminates in the formation of ^{206}Pb:

$$^{226}_{88}\text{Ra} \rightarrow ^4_2\text{He}^{2+} + ^{222}_{86}\text{Rn} \rightarrow \rightarrow \rightarrow ^{206}_{82}\text{Pb}$$

Alpha emitters are extremely toxic if ingested, due to the large mass and the ionising power of the atomic particle.

Electron capture

In this form of decay a proton captures an electron orbiting in the innermost K shell:

proton + electron $\rightarrow$ neutron + X-ray

The proton becomes a neutron and electromagnetic radiation (X-rays) is given out. Example:

$$^{125}_{53}\text{I} \rightarrow ^{125}_{52}\text{Te} + \text{X-ray}$$

Decay by emission of γ-rays

In contrast to emission of α- and β-particles, γ-emission involves electromagnetic radiation similar to, but with a shorter wavelength than, X-rays. These γ-rays result from a transformation in the nucleus of an atom (in contrast to X-rays, which are emitted as a consequence of excitation involving the orbital electrons of an atom) and frequently accompany α- and β-particle emission. Emission of γ-radiation in itself leads to no change in atomic number or mass.

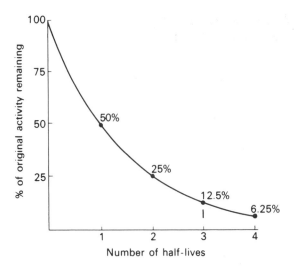

Fig. 14.1. Demonstration of the exponential nature of radioactive decay.

γ-Radiation has low ionising power but high penetration. For example, the γ-radiation from ^{60}Co will penetrate 15 cm of steel. The toxicity of γ-radiation is similar to that of X-rays.

Example:

$$^{131}_{53}I \rightarrow {}^{131}_{54}Xe + \beta^- + \gamma$$

14.1.4 Radioactive decay energy

The usual unit used in expressing energy levels associated with radioactive decay is the electron volt. (One electron volt (eV) is the energy acquired by one electron in accelerating through a potential difference of 1 V and is equivalent to 1.6×10^{-19} J.) For the majority of isotopes, the term million or mega electron volts (MeV) is more applicable. Isotopes emitting α-particles are normally the most energetic, falling in the range 4.0–8.0 MeV, whereas β- and γ-emitters generally have decay energies of less than 3.0 MeV.

14.1.5 Rate of radioactive decay

Radioactive decay is a spontaneous process and it occurs at a definite rate characteristic of the source. This rate always follows an exponential law. Thus the number of atoms disintegrating at any time is proportional to the number of atoms of the isotope (N) present at that time (t). Expressed mathematically, the exponential curve (Fig. 14.1) gives the equation.

$$-\frac{dN}{dt} \propto N$$

Table 14.2	Half-lives of some isotopes used in biological studies

Isotope	Half-life
^{3}H	12.26 years
^{14}C	5760 years
^{22}Na	2.58 years
^{32}P	14.20 days
^{33}P	25.4 days
^{35}S	87.20 days
^{42}K	12.40 h
^{45}Ca	165 days
^{59}Fe	45 days
^{125}I	60 days
^{131}I	8.05 days
^{135}I	9.7 h

$$\text{or} \quad -\frac{dN}{dt} = N \tag{14.1}$$

where λ is the decay constant, a characteristic of a given isotope defined as the fraction of an isotope decaying in unit time (t^{-1}). By integrating equation 14.1 it can be converted to a logarithmic form:

$$\ln\frac{N_t}{N_o} = -\lambda t \tag{14.2}$$

where N_t is the number of radioactive atoms present at time t, and N_o is the number of radioactive atoms orginally present. In practice it is more convenient to express the decay constant in terms of half-life $\left(t_{\frac{1}{2}}\right)$. This is defined as the time taken for the activity to fall from any value to half that value (Fig. 14.1). If N_t in equation 14.2 is equal to one-half of N_o then t will equal the half-life of the isotope. Thus

$$\ln\tfrac{1}{2} = -\lambda t_{\frac{1}{2}} \tag{14.3}$$

$$\text{or } 2.303 \log (1/2) = -\lambda t_{\frac{1}{2}} \tag{14.4}$$

$$\text{or } t_{\frac{1}{2}} = 0.693/\lambda \tag{14.5}$$

The values of $t_{\frac{1}{2}}$ vary widely from over 10^{19} years for lead-204 (^{204}Pb) to 3×10^{-7} s for polonium-212 (^{212}Po). The half-lives of some isotopes frequently used in biological work are given in Table 14.2. Note that two important elements, oxygen and nitrogen, are missing from the table. This is because the half-lives of radioactive isotopes of these elements are too short for most biological studies (^{15}O has a $t_{\frac{1}{2}}$ of 2.03 min, whereas ^{13}N has a $t_{\frac{1}{2}}$ of 10.00 min). The advantages and disadvantages of working with isotopes of differing half-lives are given in Table 14.3.

Table 14.3 The advantages and disadvantages of working with a short half-life isotope

Advantages	Disadvantages
High specific activity (see Section 14.3.4) makes the experiment more sensitive	Experimental design, isotope decays during time of experiment
Easier and cheaper to dispose of	Cost of replacement for further experiments
Lower doses likely (e.g. in diagnostic testing of human subjects)	Frequently need to calculate amount of activity remaining

Example 1 THE EFFECT OF HALF-LIFE

Question Given $\ln(N_t/N_o) = -\lambda t$ and that the half-life of ^{32}P is 14.2 days, how long would it take a solution containing 42 000 d.p.m. of ^{32}P to decay to 500 d.p.m.?

Answer Use equation 14.5 to calculate the value of λ. This gives a value of 0.0488 days^{-1}. Then use equation 14.2 to calculate the time taken for the counts to decrease. In this equation $N_o = 42\,000$ and $N_t = 500$. This gives a value for t of 90.8 days.

14.1.6 Units of radioactivity

The Système International d'Unités (SI system) uses the becquerel (Bq) as the unit of radioactivity. This is defined as one disintegration per second (1 d.p.s.). However, an older unit, not in the SI system and still frequently used is the curie (Ci). This is defined as the quantity of radioactive material in which the number of nuclear disintegrations per second is the same as that in 1 g of radium, namely 3.7×10^{10} (or 37 GBq, see Table 14.10). For biological purposes this unit is too large and the microcurie (μCi) and millicurie (mCi) are used. It is important to realise that the curie refers to the number of disintegrations actually occurring in a sample (i.e. d.p.s.) not to the disintegrations detected by the radiation counter, which will generally be only a proportion of the disintegrations occurring and are referred to as counts (i.e. c.p.s.).

Normally, in experiments with radioisotopes, a carrier of the stable isotope of the element is added. It therefore becomes necessary to express the amount of radioisotope present per unit mass. This is the specific activity. It may be expressed in a number of ways including disintegration rate (d.p.s. or d.p.m.), count rate (c.p.s. or c.p.m.) or curies (mCi or μCi) per unit of mass of mixture (units of mass are normally either moles or grams). An alternative method of expressing specific activity, which is not very frequently used, is atom percentage excess. This is defined as the number of radioactive atoms per total of 100 atoms of the compound. For quick reference, a list of units and definitions frequently used in radiobiology is provided in Table 14.10.

14.1.7 Interaction of radioactivity with matter

α-Particles

These particles have a very considerable energy (3–8 MeV) and all the particles from a given isotope have the same amount of energy. They react with matter in two ways. First, they may cause excitation. In this process energy is transferred from the α-particle to orbital electrons of neighbouring atoms, these electrons being elevated to higher orbitals. The α-particle continues on its path with its energy reduced by a little more than the amount transferred to the orbital electron. The excited electron eventually falls back to its original orbital, emitting energy as photons of light in the visible or near visible range. Secondly, α-particles may cause ionisation of atoms in their path. When this occurs the target orbital electron is removed completely. Thus the atom becomes ionised and forms an ion-pair, consisting of a positively charged ion and an electron. Because of their size, slow movement and double positive charge, α-particles frequently collide with atoms in their path. Therefore they cause intense ionisation and excitation and their energy is rapidly dissipated. Thus, despite their inital high energy, α-particles are not very penetrating.

Negatrons

Compared with α-particles, negatrons are very small and rapidly moving particles that carry a single negative charge. They interact with matter to cause ionisation and excitation exactly as with α-particles. However, due to their speed and size, they are less likely than α-particles to interact with matter and therefore are less ionising and more penetrating than α-radiation. Another difference between α-particles and negatrons is that, whereas for a given α-emitter all the particles have the same energy, negatrons are emitted over a range of energy, i.e. negatron emitters have a characteristic energy spectrum (see Fig. 14.5b). The maximum energy level (E_{max}) varies from one isotope to another, ranging from 0.018 MeV for ³H to 4.81 MeV for ³⁸Cl. The difference in E_{max} affects the penetration of the radiation: β-particles from ³H can travel only a few millimetres in air, whereas those from ³²P can penetrate over 1 m of air. The reason for negatrons of a given isotope being emitted within an energy range was explained by W. Pauli in 1931, when he postulated that each radioactive event occurs with an energy equivalent to E_{max} but that the energy is shared between a negatron and a neutrino. The proportion of total energy taken by the negatron and the neutrino varies for each disintegration. Neutrinos have no charge and negligible mass and do not interact with matter.

γ-Rays and X-rays

These rays (henceforth collectively referred to as γ-rays for simplicity) are electromagnetic radiation and therefore have no charge or mass. They rarely collide with neighbouring atoms and travel great distances before dissipating all their energy (i.e. they are highly penetrating). They interact with matter in many ways. The three most important ways lead to the production of secondary electrons, which in turn cause excitation and ionisation. In photoelectric absorption, low energy γ-rays interact with orbital electrons, transferring all their energy to the electron, which is then ejected as a photoelectron. The photoelectron subsequently behaves as a negatron. In contrast, Compton scattering, which is caused by medium energy γ-rays, results in only part of the energy being transferred to the target electron, which is ejected. The γ-ray is deflected and moves on with reduced energy. Again

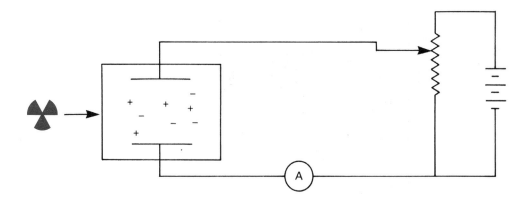

Fig. 14.2. Detection based on ionisation.

the ejected electron behaves as a negatron. Pair production results when very high energy γ-rays react with the nucleus of an atom and all the energy of the γ-ray is converted to a positron and a negatron.

When high atomic number materials absorb high energy β-particles, the absorber gives out a secondary radiation, an X-ray called Bremsstrahlung. For this reason, shields for ^{32}P use low atomic number materials such as Perspex.

14.2 DETECTION AND MEASUREMENT OF RADIOACTIVITY

There are three commonly used methods of detecting and quantifying radio-activity. These are based on the ionisation of gases, on the excitation of solids or solutions, and the ability of radioactivity to expose photographic emulsions, i.e. autoradiography.

14.2.1 Methods based upon gas ionisation

The effect of voltage upon ionisation

As a charged particle passes through a gas, its electrostatic field dislodges orbital electrons from atoms sufficiently close to its path and causes ionisation (Fig. 14.2). The ability to induce ionisation decreases in the order

$$\alpha > \beta > \gamma \qquad (10\,000:100:1)$$

Accordingly, α- and β-particles may be detected by gas ionisation methods, but these methods are poor for detecting γ-radiation. If ionisation occurs between a pair of electrodes enclosed in a suitable chamber, a pulse (current) flows, the magnitude of which is related to the applied potential and the number of radiation particles entering the chamber (Fig. 14.3). The various 'regions' shown in Fig. 14.3 will now be considered.

In the ionisation chamber region of the curve, each radioactive particle produces only one ion-pair per collision. Hence the currents are low, and very

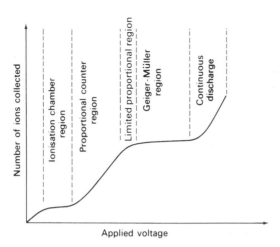

Fig. 14.3. Effect of voltage on pulse flow.

sensitive measuring devices are necessary. This method is little used in quantitative work, but various types of electroscopes, which operate on this principle, are useful in demonstrating the properties of radioactivity. At a higher voltage level than that of the simple ionisation chambers, electrons resulting from ionisation move towards the anode much more rapidly; consequently they cause secondary ionisation of gas in the chamber, resulting in the production of secondary ionisation electrons, which cause further ionisation and so on. Hence from the original event a whole torrent of electrons reaches the anode. This is the principle of gas amplification and is known as the Townsend avalanche effect, after its discoverer. As a consequence of this gas amplification, current flow is much greater. As can be seen in Fig. 14.3, in the proportional counter region the number of ion-pairs collected is directly proportional to the applied voltage until a certain voltage is reached, when a plateau occurs. Before the plateau is reached there is a region known as the limited proportional region, which is not often used in detection and quantification of radioactivity and hence will not be discussed.

The main drawback of counters that are manufactured to operate in the proportional region is that they require a very stable voltage supply because small fluctuations in voltage result in significant changes in amplification. Proportional counters are particularly useful for detection and quantification of α-emitting isotopes, but it should be noted that relatively few such isotopes are used in biological work.

In the Geiger–Müller region all radiation particles, including weak β-particles, induce complete ionisation of the gas in the chamber. Thus the size of the current is no longer dependent on the number of primary ions produced. Since maximal gas amplification is realised in this region, the size of the output pulse from the detector will remain the same over a considerable voltage range (the so-called Geiger–Müller plateau). The number of times this pulse is produced is measured rather than its size. Therefore it is not possible to discriminate between different isotopes using this type of counter.

Since it takes a finite time for the ion-pairs to travel to their respective electrodes, other ionising particles entering the tube during this time fail to produce ionisation and hence are not detected, thereby reducing the counting efficiency. This is referred to as the dead time of the tube and is normally 100 to 200 μs. When the ions reach the electrode they are neutralised. Inevitably some escape and produce their own ionisation avalanche. Thus, if unchecked, a Geiger–Müller tube would tend to give a continuous discharge. To overcome this, the tube is quenched by the addition of a suitable gas, which reduces the energy of the ions. Common quenching agents are ethanol, ethyl formate and the halogens.

Example 2 THE EFFECT OF DEAD TIME

Question

What do you think will happen to the counting efficiency of a Geiger–Müller counter as the count rate rises?

Answer

The efficiency will fall since there will be an increased likelihood that two or more β-particles will enter the tube during the dead time.

Instrumentation

Counters based on gas ionisation used to be the main method employed in the quantification of radioisotopes in biological samples. Currently, scintillation counting (Section 14.2.2) has virtually taken over. However, all laboratories use small hand-held radioactivity monitors based on gas ionisation, the end-window design being the most popular type (Fig. 14.4). These counters have a thin end-window made from aluminium and can detect β-radiation from high energy (^{32}P) and weak emitters (^{14}C), but are incapable of detecting ^{3}H because the radiation cannot penetrate the end-window. For the same reason they are not very efficient detectors of α-radiation.

End-window ionisation counters are used for routine monitoring of the radioactive laboratory to check for contamination. They are also useful in experimental situations where the presence or absence of radioactivity needs to be known rather than the absolute quantity, for example quick screening of radioactive gels prior to autoradiography or checking of chromatographic fractions for labelled components.

The inability of end-window counters to detect weak β-emitters presents a problem in biosciences because ^{3}H is a very commonly used radioisotope. The problem can be overcome by using a so-called windowless counter where a gas flow is used. These instruments are rather cumbersome and need to be carried around on an object that resembles a golf trolley. They are useful for mass screening of premises for ^{3}H contamination but are rarely used as routine. Most laboratories monitor for ^{3}H by doing a wipe test regularly, i.e. using wet tissues or cotton wool to take swabs for scintillation counting.

(a)

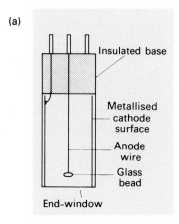

(b)

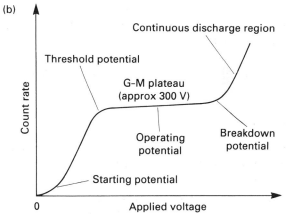

Fig. 14.4. (a) The Geiger–Müller (G–M) tube and (b) the effect of applied voltage on count rate.

14.2.2 **Methods based upon excitation**

As outlined in Section 14.1.7, radioactive isotopes interact with matter in two ways, causing ionisation, which forms the basis of Geiger–Müller counting, and excitation. The latter effect leads the excited compound (known as the fluor) to emit photons of light. This fluorescence can be detected and quantified. The process is known as scintillation and when the light is detected by a photomultiplier, forms the basis of scintillation counting. The electric pulse that results from the conversion of light energy to electrical energy in the photomultiplier is directly proportional to the energy of the original radioactive event. This is a considerable asset of scintillation counting, since it means that two, or even more, isotopes can be separately detected and measured in the same sample, provided they have sufficiently different emission energy spectra (see below). The mode of action of a photomultiplier is shown in Fig. 14.5.

In summary, scintillation counting provides information of two kinds:

● *Quantitative:*   The number of scintillations is proportional to the rate of decay of the sample, i.e. the amount of radioactivity.

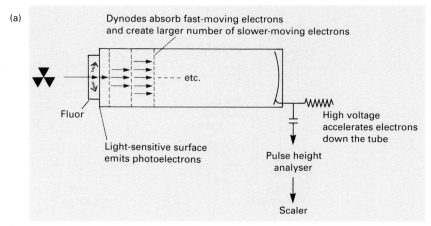

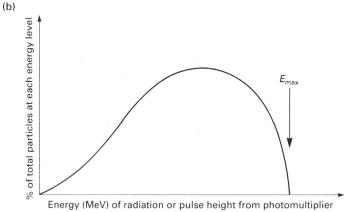

Fig. 14.5. (a) The mode of action of a photomultiplier and (b) the energy spectrum of a typical β-emitter.

● *Qualitative:* The intensity of light given out and therefore signal from the photomultiplier is proportional to the energy of radiation.

Types of scintillation counting

There are two types of scintillation counting, which are illustrated diagrammatically in Fig. 14.6. In solid scintillation counting the sample is placed adjacent to a crystal of fluorescent material. The crystal that is normally used for γ-isotopes is sodium iodide, whereas for α-emitters zinc sulphide crystals are preferred and for β-emitters organic scintillators such as anthracene are used. The crystals themselves are placed near to a photomultiplier, which in turn is connected to a high voltage supply and a scaler (Fig. 14.6a). Solid scintillation counting is particularly useful for γ-emitting isotopes. This is because, as explained in Section 14.1.7, these rays are electromagnetic radiation and collide only rarely with neighbouring atoms to cause ionisation or excitation. Clearly, in a crystal the atoms are densely packed, making collisions more likely. Conversely, solid scintillation counting is generally unsuitable for weak β-emitting isotopes such as ^{3}H and ^{14}C, because

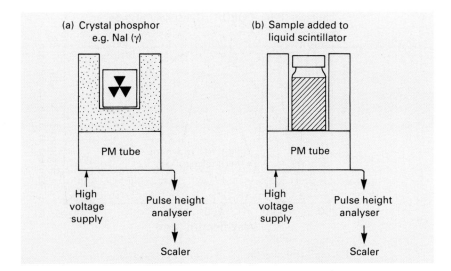

Fig. 14.6. Diagrammatic illustration of solid (a) and liquid (b) scintillation counting methods.

even the highest energy negatrons emitted by these isotopes would have hardly sufficient energy to penetrate the walls of the counting vials in which the samples are placed for counting. As many of the isotopes used in radioimmunoassay (Section 7.7) are γ-emitting isotopes, solid scintillation counting is frequently used in biological work.

In liquid scintillation counting (Fig. 14.6b), the sample is mixed with a scintillation cocktail containing a solvent and one or more fluors. This method is particularly useful in quantifying weak β-emitters such as ^{3}H, ^{14}C and ^{35}S, which are frequently used in biological work. For these isotopes, liquid scintillation counting is the usual method. Thus the remainder of this section will place particular emphasis on this technique, though it should be pointed out that most of what follows applies equally to solid scintillation counting used in the quantification of γ-emitters.

Energy transfer in liquid scintillation counting

A small number of organic solvents fluoresce when bombarded with radioactivity. The light emitted is of very short wavelength (Fig. 14.7) and is not efficiently detected by most photomultipliers. However, if a compound is dissolved that can accept the energy from the solvent and itself fluoresce at a longer wavelength, then the light can be more efficiently detected. Such a compound is known as a primary fluor and the most frequently used example is 2,5-diphenyloxazole (PPO). Unfortunately the light emitted by PPO is not always detected with very high efficiency (depending on the photomultiplier detector) but this can be overcome by including a secondary fluor or wavelength shifter such as 1,4-bis(5-phenyloxazol-2-yl)benzene (POPOP). Thus the energy transfer process becomes

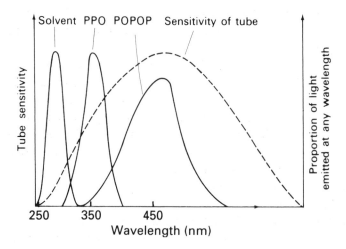

Fig. 14.7. Emission spectra of various fluors in relation to sensitivity of phototubes.

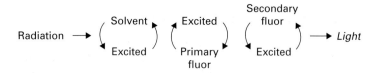

The question obviously arises as to why a primary fluor *and* a secondary fluor are necessary when it is the latter that emits light at the best wavelength for detection. The answer is simply that the solvent cannot transfer its energy directly to the secondary fluor.

PPO and POPOP were among the original fluors used in liquid scintillation counting and remain a favourite choice. However, compounds such as 2-(4'-*t*-butylphenyl)-5-(4"-biphenylyl)-1,3,4-oxadiazole (BUTYL-PBD) is a better primary fluor but is quite expensive and is affected by extremes of pH.

Most laboratories now buy their scintillation cocktails already prepared and there are many different makes and recipes on the market. Competition and an increasing awareness of health and safety mean that scintillation cocktails are gradually becoming less toxic and have a lower fire hazard. A final point: some cocktails (as just described) are designed for organic samples and others for aqueous samples (these cocktails include an emulsifier such as the detergent Triton X-100); it is important that the appropriate formulation is used.

Advantages of scintillation counting

The very fact that scintillation counting is widely used in biological work indicates that it has several advantages over gas ionisation counting. These advantages are listed below.

- The rapidity of fluorescence decay (10^{-9} s), which, when compared to dead time in a Geiger–Müller tube (10^{-4} s), means much higher count rates are possible.
- Much higher counting efficiencies particularly for low energy β-emitters; over 50% efficiency is routine in scintillation counting and efficiency can rise to over 90% for high energy emitters. This is partly due to the fact that the negatrons do not have to travel through air or pass through an end-window of a Geiger–Müller tube (thereby dissipating much of the energy before causing ionisation) but interact directly with the fluor; energy loss before the event that is counted is therefore minimal.
- The ability to accommodate samples of any type, including liquids, solids, suspensions and gels.
- The general ease of sample preparation (see below).
- The ability to count separately different isotopes in the same sample, which means dual labelling experiments can be carried out (see below).
- Scintillation counters are highly automated, hundreds of samples can be counted automatically and built-in computer facilities carry out many forms of data analysis, such as efficiency correction, graph plotting, radioimmunoassay calculations, etc.

Disadvantages of scintillation counting

It would not be reasonable, having outlined some of the advantages of scintillation counting, to disregard the disadvantages of the method. Fortunately, however, most of the inherent disadvantages have been overcome by improvement in instrument design. These disadvantages include the following.

- The cost per sample of scintillation counting is not insignificant; however, other factors including versatility, sensitivity, ease and accuracy outweigh this factor for most applications.
- At the high voltages applied to the photomultiplier, electronic events occur in the system that are independent of radioactivity but contribute to a high background count. This is referred to as photomultiplier noise and can be partially reduced by cooling the photomultipliers. Since temperature affects counting efficiency, cooling also presents a controlled temperature for counting, which may be useful. Low noise photomultipliers, however, have been designed to provide greater temperature stability in ambient temperature systems. Also the use of a pulse height analyser can be set so as to reject, electronically, most of the noise pulses that are of low energy (the threshold or gate setting). The disadvantage here is that this also rejects the low energy pulses resulting from low energy radioactivity (e.g. ^{3}H). Another method of reducing noise, which is incorporated into most scintillation counters, is to use coincidence counting. In this system two photomultipliers are used. These are set in coincidence such that only when a pulse is generated in both tubes at the same time is it allowed to pass to the scaler. The chances of this happening for a pulse generated by a radioactive event is very high compared to the chances of a noise event occurring in both

photomultipliers during the so-called resolution time of the system, which is commonly of the order of 20 ns. In general, this system reduces photomultiplier noise to a very low level.

- The greatest disadvantage of scintillation counting is quenching. This occurs when the energy transfer process described earlier suffers interference. Correcting for this quenching contributes significantly to the cost of scintillation counting. Quenching can be any one of three kinds.

  (i) *Optical quenching:* This occurs if inappropriate or dirty scintillation vials are used. These will absorb some of the light being emitted, before it reaches the photomultiplier.

  (ii) *Colour quenching:* This occurs if the sample is coloured and results in light emitted being absorbed within the scintillation cocktail before it leaves the sample vial. When colour quenching is known to be a major problem, it can be reduced, as outlined later.

  (iii) *Chemical quenching:* This form of quenching, which occurs when anything in the sample interferes with the transfer of energy from the solvent to the primary fluor or from the primary fluor to the secondary fluor, is the most difficult form of quenching to accommodate. In a series of homogeneous samples (e.g. $^{14}CO_2$ released during metabolism of $[^{14}C]$glucose and trapped in alkali, which is then added to the scintillation cocktail for counting), chemical quenching may not vary greatly from sample to sample. In these cases relative counting using sample counts per minute can be compared directly. However, in the majority of biological experiments using radioisotopes, such homogeneity of samples is unlikely and it is not sufficiently accurate to use relative counting (i.e. counts per minute). Instead, an appropriate method of standardisation must be used. This requires the determination of the counting efficiency of each sample and the conversion of counts per minute to absolute counts (i.e. disintegrations per minute), as described later. It should be noted that quenching is not such a great problem in solid (external) scintillation counting.

- *Chemiluminescence:* This can also cause problems during liquid scintillation counting. It results from chemical reactions between components of the samples to be counted and the scintillation cocktail, and produces light emission unrelated to excitation of the solvent and fluor system by radioactivity. These light emissions are generally low energy events and are rejected by the threshold setting of the photomultiplier in the same way as is photomultiplier noise. Chemiluminescence, when it is a problem, can usually be overcome by storing samples for some time before counting, to permit the chemiluminescence to decay. Many contemporaneous instruments are able to detect chemiluminescence and substract it or flag it on the printout.

- *Phospholuminescence:* This results from components of the sample, including the vial itself, absorbing light and re-emitting it. Unlike chemiluminescence,

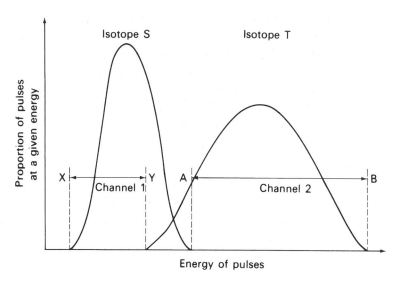

Fig. 14.8. Diagram to illustrate the principle of counting dual-labelled samples.

which is a once-only effect, phospholuminescence will occur on each exposure of a sample to light. Samples that are pigmented are most likely to phosphoresce. If this is a problem, samples should be adapted to dark prior to counting and the sample holder should be kept closed throughout the counting process.

Despite all the complications described above, scintillation counters are universal in biosciences departments. This is because the instruments have automated systems for calculating counting efficiency; in other words, the instruments do all the hard work!

Using scintillation counting for dual-labelled samples

A feature of the scintillation process is that the size of electric pulse produced by the conversion of light energy in the photomultiplier is related directly to the energy of the original radioactive event. Because different β-emitting isotopes have different energy spectra, it is possible to quantify two isotopes separately in a single sample, provided their energy spectra are sufficiently different. Examples of pairs of isotopes that have sufficiently different energy spectra are ^{3}H and ^{14}C, ^{3}H and ^{35}S, ^{3}H and ^{32}P, ^{14}C and ^{32}P, ^{35}S and ^{32}P. The principle of the method is illustrated in Fig. 14.8, where it can be seen that the spectra of two isotopes (S and T) overlap only slightly. By setting a pulse height analyser to reject all pulses of an energy below X (threshold X) and to reject all pulses of an energy above Y (window Y) and also to reject below a threshold of A and a window of B, it is possible to separate the two isotopes completely. A pulse height analyser set with a threshold and window for a particular isotope is known as a channel (e.g. a ^{3}H channel).

Most modern counters operate with a so-called multichannel analyser. These are based on an analogue-to-digital converter; electronic signals from the photomultiplier are converted to digital signals stored in a computer. Thus the entire energy spectrum is analysed simultaneously. This greatly facilitates multi-isotope counting and in particular allows the effect of quenching on dual-label counting to be assessed adequately.

Dual-label counting has proved to be useful in many aspects of molecular biology (e.g. nucleic acid hybridisation and transcription), metabolism (e.g. steroid synthesis) and drug development.

Determination of counting efficiency

As outlined above, a major problem encountered in scintillation counting is that of quenching, which makes it necessary to determine the counting efficiency of some, if not all, of the samples in a particular experiment. This can be done by one of several methods of standardisation, all of which apply to both solid and liquid scintillation counting, though again in this section emphasis is placed on the latter method.

Internal standardisation   The sample is counted (and gives a reading of, say, A c.p.m.), removed from the counter and a small amount of standard material of known disintegrations per minute (B d.p.m.) is added. The sample is then recounted (C c.p.m.) and the counting efficiency of the sample calculated:

$$\text{counting efficiency} = [100\,(C - A)/B]\,\% \tag{14.6}$$

It is obviously necessary in this method to use an internal standard (the spike) that contains the same isotope as the one being counted and also to ensure that the standard itself does not act as a quenching agent. Suitable ^{14}C-labelled standards include [^{14}C]toluene, [^{14}C]hexadecane, [^{3}H]benzoic acid and ^{3}H$_2$O (benzoic acid and water are themselves quenching agents and must be used in only very small amounts). Internal standardisation is simple and reliable and corrects adequately for all types of quenching. Carefully carried out, it is the most accurate way of correcting for quenching. On the other hand, it demands very accu-

---

Example 3 **THE INTERNAL STANDARD METHOD FOR CALCULATING COUNTING EFFICIENCY**

Question

An experimental sample of ^{3}H on a filter paper in scintillation fluid gave a count rate of 1450 c.p.m. in a liquid scintillation counter. The filter was removed and 5064 d.p.m. added to it. On recounting, the filter gave a reading of 2878 c.p.m. What was the d.p.m. of the experimental sample?

Answer

It is first necessary to use equation 14.6 to calculate the counting efficiency:

counting efficiency = [100(2878 − 1450)/5064]%

This gives a value of 28.2%. This value is then used to correct the original count figure, i.e.:

(1450/28.2)100 = 5142 d.p.m.

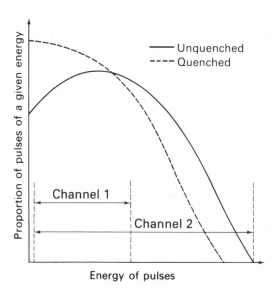

Fig. 14.9. The effect of quenching of a β-energy spectrum.

rate pipetting when the standard is added, and it is time consuming because each sample must be counted twice. It also means that the sample cannot be recounted in the event of error because it will be contaminated with the standard. Moreover, time elapses between the first and second count and changes in sample quenching characteristics can also occur, which can lead to considerable inaccuracies. However, it is the means by which the following two methods are calibrated.

Channels ratio   When a sample in a scintillation counter is quenched, the scintillation process is less efficient: less light is produced for a given quantum energy of radiation. Thus the energy spectrum for a quenched sample appears to be lower than for an unquenched sample (Fig. 14.9). The higher the degree of quenching, the more pronounced is the resulting decrease in the spectrum. This fact is made use of in the channels ratio method for determining counter efficiency. The method involves the preparation of a calibration curve based on counting in two channels that cover different, but overlapping, parts of the spectrum. As a sample is quenched, and the spectrum shifts to gradually lower apparent energies, the ratio of counts in each channel will vary. To prepare the standard curve, a set of quenched standards is counted: the absolute amount of radioactivity is known and therefore the efficiency of counting in each channel can easily be determined.

The efficiency is then plotted against channels ratio to form the standard curve (Fig. 14.10). Typical data for a set of ^{14}C quenched standards are given in Table 14.4. It is important to realise that a standard curve applies to only one set of circumstances – one radioisotope, counter and scintillation fluid.

Once the standard curve has been prepared, the efficiency of counting experimental samples can be determined. Samples are counted in the same two channels, the ratio is calculated, put into the graph and the efficiency read. In practice all

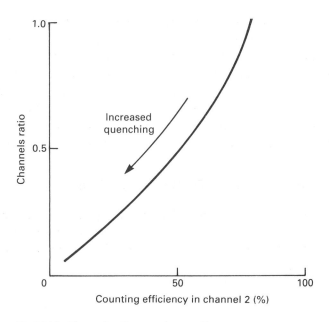

Fig. 14.10. Channels ratio quench correction curve.

Table 14.4 **Radioactivity recorded with gradually increasing quench in two channels of a scintillation counter**

| | c.p.m. | | Ratio | Counting efficiency |
Sample	Channel 1	Channel 2	Ch1 : Ch2	in channel 2 (%)
^{14}C standard (203 600 d.p.m.) unquenched	171 930	184 250	0.93	90.5
^{14}C standard (203 600 d.p.m.) with increasing quench	146 610	168 840	0.87	82.9
	94 240	135 090	0.70	66.3
	52 260	102 030	0.51	50.1
	16 030	58 320	0.27	28.6
	5 920	34 740	0.17	17.1
	2 060	20 270	0.10	9.9
	1 130	13 260	0.08	6.5

the data can be stored in the counter's computer and corrected values printed automatically.

Multichannel scintillation counters operate on the same principle but the whole shape and position of the spectrum is analysed. This is given a digital parameter that relates to counting efficiency. Manufacturers have developed their own titles for such parameters, for example LKB Instruments' Automatic Quench Compensation or Packard's Automatic Efficiency Control. These systems have greater precision than the two-channel approach, as the whole of the spectrum is used for analysis. The channels ratio method is suitable for all types and even high degrees of quenching. Furthermore, counting in more than one channel is simultaneous and this method is, therefore, less time consuming than either internal or external standardisation. It is also, in practice, an acceptably accurate method for determining counting efficiency, provided care is taken in the preparation of the calibration curve. However, it is notoriously inaccurate at low count rates, because the error on the counts per minute is high and there will be a larger error on the channels ratio because it is calculated from two values of the counts per minute. It is also inaccurate for very highly quenched samples. For these reasons the method that follows is most frequently the procedure of choice.

Example 4 CHANNELS RATIO EFFICIENCY CALCULATION

Question

The efficiency of counting 100 000 d.p.m. of a [^{14}C]leucine solution was estimated in a scintillation counter using two channels, A and B, in scintillation fluid containing increasing amounts of chloroform. The following data were obtained:

Chloroform (cm^3)	c.p.m. A	c.p.m. B
0	48 100	54 050
1	31 612	42 150
2	17 608	28 400
3	7 400	15 000

An unknown sample of [^{14}C]leucine gave the following data:

Channel A   1890 c.p.m.
Channel B   2700 c.p.m.

How much radioactivity is present in the unknown sample?

Answer

Plot efficiency in channel A or B (e.g. 48 000 × 100/100 000 or 54 050 × 100/100 000, then 31 612 × 100/100 000 or 42 150 × 100/100 000 etc.) against c.p.m. A/c.p.m. B (e.g. 48 000/54 050, then 31 612/42 150, etc.). Calculate c.p.m. A/c.p.m. B for the experimental sample (1890/2700), put this into your graph and read off the efficiency. Correct the c.p.m. in channel A or B (depending on which one you choose to calculate efficiencies) for the efficiency (e.g. 1980 × 100/26.5 if you used channel A (26.5% is the efficiency obtained from the graph of channels ratio against efficiency in channel A).

Try plotting two graphs (efficiency in A or B versus c.p.m. A/c.p.m. B) and work out the answer using both in turn; you should get the same answer of 7130 d.p.m. each time.

External standardisation   Instruments have a γ-emitting external standard built into the counter. Under the control of the counter each sample to be counted is exposed to this external source, which is automatically shifted from a lead shield to the counting chamber. The γ-radiation penetrates the vial and excites the scintillation fluid. The resulting spectrum is unique to the source and is significantly different from that produced by the sample in the vial. The γ-source

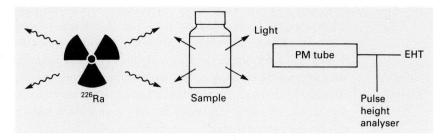

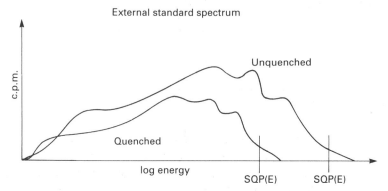

Fig. 14.11. The external standard for estimating counting efficiency. The external source irradiates the sample. The counter analyses the spectrum, which shifts to lower energies if the sample is quenched. The SQP(E), i.e. standard quench parameter (external), expressed without units, is derived from the energy axis and relates to the extent of quench. The greater the quench in the sample, the lower the SQP(E) and the lower the counting efficiency (see Table 14.5).

used (e.g. ^{137}Cs, ^{133}Ba or ^{226}Ra) varies according to the make of instrument. The spectrum obtained by ^{226}Ra is shown in Fig. 14.11.

Quenching agents present in the scintillation fluid will significantly affect the spectrum obtained. The instrument analyses this spectrum and assigns a quench parameter to it. The precise method used depends on the make of counter; LKB Instruments refer to a standard quench parameter for the external source (SQP(E)) based on a point on the energy axis (Fig. 14.11). Other manufacturers use slightly different approaches but the principle is the same: the spectrum for the external standard varies according to the degree of quench in the vial and, therefore, the efficiency of counting of the internal experimental sample.

As for the channels ratio method, a standard curve is required, i.e. a range of quenched standards is counted and the external standard spectrum analysed in each case. The resulting data (Table 14.5) are used to prepare a standard curve that is held in the instrument's computer. Unknown samples are then counted in the same way, the efficiency read from the standard curve and the sample counts corrected.

The external standard approach is now routine in most laboratories, the main advantage over the channels ratio method being that it is suited to samples with low count rates. However, it is not without disadvantages: a standard curve is required for each set of circumstances (as with the channels ratio) and the user can

Table 14.5 Recorded radioactivity from a ^{14}C standard sample with increasing quench detected by an external standard

Sample	c.p.m.	External quench parameter[a]	Counting efficiency (%)
^{14}C standard (203 600 d.p.m.) unquenched	194 930	810	95.7
^{14}C standard (203 600 d.p.m.) with increasing quench	146 141	422	93.5
	181 171	207	89.0
	167 731	126	82.4
	145 879	76	71.6
	126 913	55	62.3
	108 641	42	53.3
	96 103	37	47.2

[a] e.g. SQP(E), see Fig. 14.11.

be lulled into a false sense of security. The system is so highly automated that it is easy to lose sight of the basic principles and the method is not always appropriate. A case in point is the counting of ^3H precipitated onto filters counted in scintillation fluid. The external standard method will calculate the degree of quench in the fluid (which will probably be very low) but will not take into account the poor penetration of ^3H β-particles from the filter into the scintillation fluid: artificially high efficiencies will be recorded.

In all cases where an automated procedure for calculating counting efficiencies is employed it is prudent to count a few prepared samples in which the true amount of radioactivity is known.

Example 5 EXTERNAL STANDARD EFFICIENCY CALCULATIONS

Question

The efficiency of detecting ^{14}C in a scintillation counter was determined by counting a standard sample containing 105 071 d.p.m. at different degrees of quench analysed by the external standard approach:

c.p.m.	SQP
87 451	0.90
62 361	0.64
45 220	0.46
21 014	0.21

SQP, standard quench parameter.

An experimental sample gave 2026 c.p.m. at an SQP of 0.52. What is the true count rate?

Answer Plot the efficiency (e.g. (87 451 × 100/105 071)%) versus SQP. Obtain the efficiency (48%) for the experimental sample and correct 2026 to give an answer of 4221 d.p.m.

Sample preparation

It is impossible here to give details of all aspects of sample preparation for scintil-lation counting. However, major considerations are outlined below and the reader is referred to books cited in Section 14.7 for further details.

Sample vials   In solid scintillation counting, sample preparation is easy and only involves transferring the sample to a glass or plastic vial (or tube) compatible with the counter. In liquid scintillation counting, sample preparation is more complex and starts with a decision on the type of sample vial to be used. These may be glass, low potassium glass (with low levels of ^{40}K that reduce background count) or poly-ethylene. The last of these types are cheaper but are not suitable for cleaning and reuse, whereas glass vials can be reused many times provided they are thoroughly cleaned. Polyethylene vials give better light transfer and result in slightly higher counting efficiencies, but are inclined to exhibit more phosphorescence than do glass vials. The recent trend is towards mini-vials, which use far smaller volumes of expensive scintillation cocktails. Modern counters are able to accept many types of vial; the smallest vial possible should be used (within the obvious con-straints of sample volume) to save costs and in consideration of environmental issues, as scintillation fluids are toxic. Some counters are designed to accept very small samples in special polythene bags split into an array of many compart-ments; these are particularly useful to, for example, the pharmaceutical industry where there are laboratories that do large numbers of receptor binding assays.

Scintillation cocktails   Toluene-based cocktails are the most efficient, but will not accept aqueous samples, because toluene and water are immiscible and massive quenching results. Cocktails based on 1,4-dioxane and naphthalene that can accommodate up to 20% (v/v) water can be used, but they have largely been phased out due to toxicity. Emulsifier-based cocktails are the most frequently used for counting aqueous samples. They contain an emulsifier such as Triton X-100 and can accept up to 50% water (v/v); however, phase transitions occur from single phase to two phase or gel, as the water content increases. Accurate counting cannot be done if the samples are in the two-phase state. Many ready-made cock-tails are on the market and are sold with precise instructions regarding sample condition.

Volume of cocktail   It should be noted that the efficiency of scintillation counting varies with sample volume, though this is less of a problem in modern counters. Nevertheless, care should be taken that sample vials in a given series of counts contain the same volume of sample and that all instrument calibration is done using the same volume as for experimental samples.

Overcoming major colour quenching   If colour quenching is a problem it is possible to bleach samples before counting. Care should be taken, however, since bleach-ing agents such as hydrogen peroxide can give rise to chemiluminescence in some scintillation cocktails.

Table 14.6	Some isotopes suitable for Čerenkov counting		
Radioisotope	E_{max} (MeV)	% of spectrum above 0.5 MeV	Counting efficiency (%)
^{22}Na	1.39	60	30
^{32}P	1.71	80	40
^{36}Cl	0.71	30	10
^{42}K	3.5	90	80

Tissue solubilisers   Solid samples, such as plant and animal tissues, may be best counted after solubilisation by quaternary amines such as NCS solubiliser or Soluene. Not surprisingly these solutions are highly toxic and great care is required. The sample is added to the counting vial containing a small amount of solubiliser and digestion is allowed to proceed. When digestion is complete, scintillation cocktail is added and the sample counted. Again, chemiluminescence can be a problem with tissue solubilisers.

Combustion methods   A suitable alternative to bleaching of coloured samples or digestion of tissues is the use of combustion techniques. Here samples are combusted in an atmosphere of oxygen, usually in a commercially available combustion apparatus. Thus samples containing ^{14}C would be combusted to $^{14}CO_2$, which is collected in a trapping agent such as sodium hydroxide and then counted; ^3H-containing samples are converted to ^3H_2O for counting.

     As indicated earlier, only important considerations in sample preparation are discussed above and details are not given. However, it is worthy of comment that almost any type of radioactive sample containing β-emitting istopes can be prepared for counting in a liquid scintillation counter by one method or another, including cuttings from paper chromatographs or membrane filters, again illustrating the versatility and importance of this technique for quantifying radioactivity.

Čerenkov counting

The Čerenkov effect occurs when a particle passes through a substance with a speed higher than that of light passing through the same substance. If a β-emitter has a decay energy in excess of 0.5 MeV, then this causes water to emit a bluish white light usually referred to as Čerenkov light. It is possible to detect this light using a typical liquid scintillation counter.

     Since there is no requirement for organic solvents and fluors, this technique is relatively cheap, sample preparation is very easy, and there is no problem of chemical quenching. Table 14.6 lists some isotopes that are suitable for this detection method. Most work has been done on ^{32}P, which has 80% of its energy spectrum above the Čerenkov threshold and which can be detected at around 40% efficiency. It may be noted from Table 14.6 that, as the proportion of the energy spectrum above 0.5 MeV increases, so too does the detection efficiency.

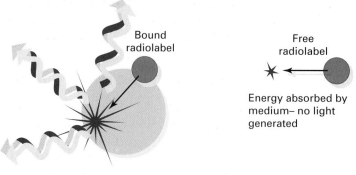

Bound
radiolabel

Free
radiolabel

Energy absorbed by
medium– no light
generated

Bead stimulated to emit light

Fig. 14.12. The concept behind SPA. (Reproduced by courtesy of Amersham Biosciences.)

Table 14.7	Advantages of scintillation proximity assay

Versatile: use with enzyme assays, receptors, any molecular interactions
Works with a range of appropriate isotopes such as ^{3}H, ^{14}C, ^{35}S and ^{33}P
No need for separation step (e.g. free from bound ligand)
Less manipulation therefore reduced toxicity
Amenable to automation

Scintillation proximity assay

Scintillation proximity assay (SPA) is an application of scintillation counting that facilitates automation and rapid throughput of experiments. It is therefore highly suited to work such as screening for biological activity in new drugs. The principle of SPA is illustrated in Fig. 14.12. SPA beads are constructed from polystyrene (or sometimes other materials) that combine a binding site for a molecule of interest with a scintillant. You need to remember that some types of radiation do not travel far, in particular β-particles from weak energy emitters such as ^{3}H and ^{14}C. If molecules containing such radioisotopes are in solution with a suspension of SPA beads, the radiation does not stimulate the scintillant in the beads and cannot be detected efficiently by a scintillation counter. This is because the radiation is absorbed by the solution; it does not reach the scintillant. If, on the other hand, the radioisotope becomes bound to the bead, it is close enough to stimulate the scintillant in the bead, so light is given out and the isotope is detected.

There are many applications of this technology such as enzyme assays and receptor binding, indeed any situation where we want to investigate the interaction between two molecules. Take receptor binding as an example. In this case a receptor for a particular ligand (such as a drug or hormone) is attached to the SPA beads. The ligand is radiolabelled and mixed with the beads. Any ligand that binds will stimulate the scintillant and be counted. If the researcher wishes to investigate chemicals that might interface with this binding (which is the mode of action of many medicines), they can be added at increasing concentration to study the effect and, for example, determine optimum dosage (see also Section 16.3.2).

A summary of the advantages of SPA technology is shown in Table 14.7.

14.2.3 Methods based upon exposure of photographic emulsions

Ionising radiation acts upon a photographic emulsion to produce a latent image much as does visible light. For a photograph, a radiation source, an object to be imaged and photographic emulsion are required. For an autoradiograph, a radiation source (i.e. radioactivity) emanating from within the material to be imaged (the object) is required, along with a sensitive emulsion. The emulsion consists of a large number of silver halide crystals embedded in a solid phase such as gelatin. As energy from the radioactive material is dissipated in the emulsion, the silver halide becomes negatively charged and is reduced to metallic silver, thus forming a particulate latent image. Photographic developers are designed to show these silver grains as a blackening of the film, and fixers remove any remaining silver halide. Thus a permanent image of the location of the original radioactive event remains.

This process, which is known as autoradiography, is very sensitive and has been used in a wide variety of biological experiments. These unusally involve a requirement to locate the distribution of radioactivity in biological specimens of different types. For instance, the sites of localisation of a radiolabelled drug throughout the body of an experimental animal can be determined by placing whole-body sections of the animal in close contact with a sensitive emulsion such as an X-ray plate. After a period of exposure, the plate, upon development, will show an image of the section in tissues and organs in which radioactivity was present. Similarly, radioactive metabolites isolated and separated by chromatographic or electrophoretic techniques during metabolic studies can be located on the chromatograph or electrophoretograph and the radioactive spots can subsequently be recovered for counting and identification.

The techniques of autoradiography (Fig. 14.13) have become more important with recent developments in molecular biology (Chapters 5 and 6). Consequently more detail is given below on some important aspects of the technique.

Suitable isotopes

In general, weak β-emitting isotopes (e.g. ^3H, ^{14}C and ^{35}S) are most suitable for autoradiography, particularly for cell and tissue localisation experiments. This is because, as a result of the low energy of the negatrons, the ionising track of the isotope will be short and a discrete image will result. This is particularly important when radioactivity associated with subcellular organelles is being located. For this, ^3H is the best radioisotope, since its energy will all be quickly dissipated within the emulsion. Electron microscopy can then be used to locate the image in the developed film. For location within whole organisms or tissues, either ^{14}C or ^3H is suitable; more energetic isotopes (e.g. ^{32}P) are less suitable because their higher energy negatrons produce much longer track lengths and result in less

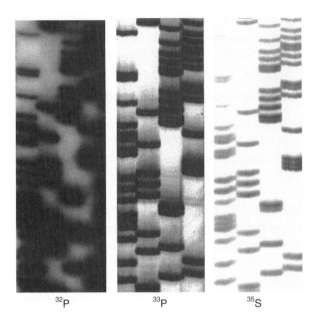

Fig. 14.13. Three autoradiograph showing the use of different radioisotopes in DNA sequencing. The isotope with the highest energy (^{32}P) leads to the poorest resolution because the radiation spreads out further, making the DNA bands appear thicker. The lowest energy radiation (from ^{35}S) gives the best resolution. (Reproduced with permission from M. W. Cunningham, A. Patel, A. C. Simmonds and D. Williams (2002), *In vitro* labelling of nucleic acids and proteins, in *Radioisotopes in Biology*, (2nd edn), R. J. Slaten (ed.), Oxford University Press, Oxford.)

discrete images that are not sufficiently discriminatory for microscopic location. Conversely, for location of, for example, DNA bands in an electrophoretic gel, ^{32}P is useful. In this case low energy ^{3}H negatrons would largely dissipate their energy within the gel (and in the wrapping around the gel, which is usually necessary to prevent the gel sticking to the emulsion), thereby reducing sensitivity to a low level. However, the more energetic ^{32}P negatrons will leave the gel and produce a strong image. If very thin gels are prepared, then ^{35}S or ^{14}C can be detected with high resolution, for example in DNA sequencing gels where ^{35}S is used as the label.

Choice of emulsion and film

A variety of emulsions is available with different packing densities of the silver halide crystals. Care must be taken to choose an emulsion suitable for the purposes of the experiment, since the sensitivity of the emulsion will affect the resolution obtained. Manufacturers' literature should be consulted and their advice sought if one is in any doubt. X-ray film is generally suitable for macroscopic samples such as whole-body sections of small mammals, chromatographs or electrophoretographs. When light or electron microscopic detection of the location of the image in the emulsion is required (cellular and subcellular localisation of radioactivity), very sensitive films are necessary, as is a very close apposition of sample and film. In these cases a stripping film technique can be used in which the film is supplied attached to a support. It is stripped from this and applied directly to the sample. Alternatively, liquid emulsions are prepared by melting strips of emulsion by heating them to around 60 °C. Then either the emulsion is poured onto the sample or the sample attached to a support is dipped into the emulsion. The emulsion is then allowed to set before being dried. Such a method is often referred to as a dipping-film method and is preferred when very thin films are required.

Background

Accidental exposure to light, chemicals in the sample, natural background radioactivity (particularly ^{40}K in glass) and even pressure applied during handling and storage of film will cause a background fog (i.e. latent image) on the developed film. This can be problematic, particularly in high resolution work (e.g. involving microscopy) and care must be taken at all times to minimise its effect. Background will always increase during exposure time, which should therefore always be kept to a minimum.

Time of exposure and film processing

The time of exposure depends upon the isotope, sample type, level of activity, film type and purpose of the experiment. The same applies to the processing of the film in order to display the image. Generally the process must be adapted to a given purpose, and a great deal of trial and error is often involved in arriving at the most suitable procedures.

Direct autoradiography

In direct autoradiography, the X-ray film or emulsion is placed as close as possible to the sample and exposed at any convenient temperature. Quantitative images are produced until saturation is reached. The approach provides high resolution but limited sensitivity: isotopes of energy equal to, or higher than, ^{14}C ($E_{max} = 0.156$ MeV) are required.

Fluorography

Many of the currently popular methods in molecular biology involve separation of macromolecules or fractions of macromolecules by gel electrophoresis (Sections 10.3 and 10.4). The separated macromolecules or fractions form bands in the electrophoretograph that must be located. This is often achieved by radio-labelling the macromolecules with ^3H or ^{14}C and subjecting the gel to autoradiography. Because these are weak β-emitters, much of their energy is lost in the gel and long exposure times are necessary even when very high specific activity sources are used. However, if a fluor (e.g. PPO or sodium silicate) is infiltrated into the gel, and the gel dried and then placed in contact with a preflashed film (see below), sensitivity can be increased by several orders of magnitude. This is because the negatrons emitted from the isotope will cause the fluor to become excited and emit light, which will react with the film. Thus use is made of both the ionising and the exciting effects of radioactivity in fluorography.

Intensifying screens

When ^{32}P-labelled or γ-isotope-labelled samples (e.g. [^{32}P] DNA or ^{125}I-labelled protein fractions in gels) are to be located, the opposite problem to that presented by low energy isotopes prevails. These much more penetrating particles and rays cause little reaction with the film as they penetrate right through it, producing a poor image. The image can be greatly improved by placing, on the other side of the film from the sample, a thick intensifying screen consisting of a solid phosphor. Negatrons penetrating the film cause the phosphor to fluoresce and emit light, which superimposes its image on the film. There is, therefore, an increase in sensitivity but a parallel reduction in resolution due to the spread of light emanating from the screen.

Low temperature exposure

If the energy of ionising radiation is converted to light (i.e. with fluorography or intensifying screens) the kinetics of the film's response are affected. The light is of low intensity and a back reaction occurs that cancels the forming latent image. Exposure at low temperature ($-70\,^\circ$C) slows this back reaction and will therefore provide higher sensitivity. There is no point in doing direct autoradiography at low temperature as the kinetics of the film response are different. There is nothing to be gained by exposing preflashed film (see below) at low temperature.

Preflashing

As described above, the response of a photographic emulsion to radiation is not linear and usually involves a slow initial phase (lag) followed by a linear phase. Sensitivity of films may be increased by preflashing. This involves a millisecond light flash prior to the sample being brought into juxtaposition with the film and is often used where high sensitivity is required or if results are to be quantified.

Quantification

As indicated earlier, autoradiography is usually used to locate rather than to quantify radioactivity. However, it is possible to obtain quantitative data directly from autoradiographs by using a densitometer, which records the intensity of the image. This in turn is related to the amount of radioactivity in the original sample. There are many varieties of densitometers available and the choice made will depend on the purpose of the experiment. Quantification is not reliable at low or high levels of exposure because of the lag phase (i.e. the back reaction, as described above) or saturation, respectively; however, preflashing combined with fluorography or intensifying screens obviates the problem for small amounts of radioactivity. In this case all photons contribute equally to the image of the pre-exposed film.

14.3 OTHER PRACTICAL ASPECTS OF COUNTING RADIOACTIVITY AND ANALYSIS OF DATA

14.3.1 Counter characteristics

Background count

Radiation counters of all types always register a count, even in the absence of radioactive material in the apparatus. This may be due to such sources as cosmic radiation, natural radioactivity in the vicinity, nearby X-ray generators, and/or circuit noises. By means of the various methods already outlined and the use of lead shielding, this background radiation may be considerably reduced, but its value must always be recorded and accounted for in all experiments. Some commercial instruments have automatic background subtraction facilities.

Dead time

At very high count rates in Geiger–Müller counting, counts are lost due to the dead time of the Geiger–Müller tube. Correction tables are available and these should be used when necessary to correct for lost counts. Dead time is not a problem in scintillation counting.

Geometry

When samples with an end-window ionisation counter, such as a Geiger–Müller tube, are compared, it is important to standardise the position of the sample in relation to the tube, otherwise the fraction of the emitted radiation entering the tube may vary and hence so will the observed count.

14.3.2 Sample and isotope characteristics

Self-absorption

Self-absorption is primarily a problem with low energy β-emitters: radiation is absorbed by the sample itself. Self-absorption can be a serious problem in the counting of low energy radioactivity by scintillation counting if the sample is particulate or is, for instance, stuck to a membrane filter. Care should be taken to ensure comparability of samples because the methods of standardisation outlined earlier will not correct for self-absorption effects. Where homogeneity is not possible, particulate samples should be digested or otherwise solubilised prior to counting. Self-absorption is a major problem with Geiger–Müller counting and significantly reduces sensitivity and reliability. It is very difficult to count low energy emitters reliably with these counters and this was a major factor in the switch to scintillation counting.

Half-life

The half-life of an isotope (Section 14.1.5) may be short and, if so, this must be allowed for in the analysis of data.

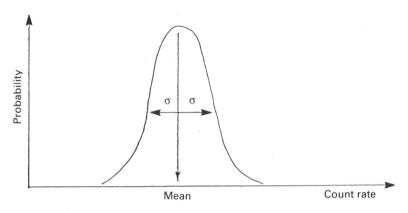

Fig. 14.14. The distribution of count rates around a mean, showing the standard deviation, σ.

Statistics

The emission of radioactivity is a random process. This can be demonstrated readily by making repeated measurements of the activity of a long-lived isotope, each for an identical period of time. The resulting counts will not be the same but will vary over a range of values, with clustering near the centre of the range. If a sufficiently large number of such measurements is made and the data are plotted, a normal distribution curve will be obtained. For a single count, there-fore, we cannot obtain a true count. Instead, we take the mean of a large number of counts as being very close to the true count. However, the accuracy of this mean will depend on the spread or standard deviation (σ) for the data. Statistical theory states that, for a normal distribution such as that shown in Fig. 14.14, 68.2% of values obtained lie ± 1 σ, and 95.5% lie ± 2 σ from the mean ($\bar{x}$) (Section 1.6.3).

Clearly, if we wish to compare samples, and in particular to state that two samples contain different amounts of radioactivity, then we need to take account of the counting statistics. Fortunately Poisson mathematics makes the task rela-tively easy as

$$\sigma = \sqrt{\text{total counts taken}} \tag{14.7a}$$

or

$$\sigma = \sqrt{\left(\frac{\text{count rate}}{\text{time}}\right)} \tag{14.7b}$$

Therefore to quote a figure with 95.5% certainty, state:

$$\text{total counts} \pm 2 \sqrt{\text{total counts}} \tag{14.8}$$

For example, if 1600 counts are recorded this can be expressed as 1600 ± 80. There is, therefore, a 95.5% chance that the true figure lies between 1520 and 1680.

When data are expressed as d.p.m. or c.p.m., again using 95.5% certainty, then

$$\text{error on count rate} = 2\sqrt{\left(\frac{\text{count rate}}{\text{time}}\right)} \qquad (14.9)$$

Using the same example, if the 1600 counts were obtained in 1 min:

$$\text{error on count rate} = 2\sqrt{\left(\frac{1600}{1}\right)} = 80$$

and therefore 1600 c.p.m. $\pm$ 80 c.p.m.

If the 1600 counts were obtained in 10 min:

$$\text{error on count rate} = 2\sqrt{\left(\frac{160}{10}\right)} = 8$$

and therefore 160 c.p.m. $\pm$ 8 c.p.m. Note that the error is the same. This is because effectively the same number of measurements, i.e. counts, has been taken in each case.

If we had recorded 160 counts in only 1 min, then:

$$\text{error on count rate} = 2\sqrt{\left(\frac{160}{1}\right)} = 25$$

and therefore 160 c.p.m. $\pm$ 25 c.p.m.

Consider these other simple examples for a series of 1 min counts:

counts = 100	$\sigma = \sqrt{100}$,	therefore $\pm$10% error at 68.2% certainty
counts = 1000	$\sigma = \sqrt{1000}$,	therefore $\pm$3% error at 68.2% certainty
counts = 10 000	$\sigma = \sqrt{10\,000}$,	therefore $\pm$1% error at 68.2% certainty

In summary, the counts per minute data become more accurate for *higher count rates* and/or *longer counting times*. It is common practice to count to 10 000 counts or for 10 min, whichever is the quicker, although for very low count rates longer counting times are required.

Example 6 ACCURACY OF COUNTING

Question

A sample recording 564 c.p.m. was counted over 10 min. What is the accuracy of the measurement for 95.5% confidence?

Answer

It is necessary to apply equation 14.9 to calculate the counting error:

counting error = $2\sqrt{564/10} = 15$

so the range in which the counts should fall with 95.5% confidence is 564$\pm$15.

14.3.3 Supply, storage and purity of radiolabelled compounds

There are several suppliers of radiolabelled compounds, the main ones being Amersham Biosciences plc., Du Pont, NEN and ICN. The suppliers usually include details of the best storage conditions and quality control data with their products. This is because several types of decomposition can occur; for example internal decomposition resulting from radioactive decay such as $^{14}C \rightarrow ^{14}N$, and external decomposition where emitted radiation is absorbed by other radioactive molecules, causing impurities. The extent to which decomposition occurs is dependent on many factors such as temperature, energy of radiation, concentration and the formulation of the compound. It is, therefore, imperative to store radioisotopes by the method recommended by the supplier and to maintain sterility of the stock. If necessary, chromatographic procedures will be required to check on the purity of the labelled compounds.

14.3.4 Specific activity

The specific activity of a radioisotope defines its radioactivity related to the amount of material (e.g. Bq mol^{-1}, Ci mmol^{-1} or d.p.m. μmol^{-1}). Suppliers offer a range of specific activities for their compound, the highest often being the most expensive. The advantages of using a very high specific activity are as follows:

- Products of a reaction using the labelled precursor can be produced at high specific activity (e.g. for DNA probes, see Section 5.10).
- Small quantities of radiolabelled compound can be added such that the equilibrium of metabolic concentrations is not unduly perturbed.
- Calculating the amount of substance required to make up radioactive solutions of known specific activity is simplified, as the contribution to concentration made by the stock radiolabelled solution is often negligible (see below).

Sometimes, however, it is not necessary to purchase the highest specific activity available. For example, enzyme assays *in vitro* often require a relatively high substrate concentration and so specific activity may need to be lowered. Consider the example below (for definitions of units, see Table 14.10):

[^{3}H]Leucine is purchased with a specific activity of 5.55 TBq mmol^{-1} (150 Ci mmol^{-1}) and a concentration of 9.25 MBq 250 mm^{-3} (250 μCi 250 mm^{-3}). A 10 cm^3 solution of 250 mM and 3.7 kBq cm^{-3} (0.1 μCi cm^{-3}) is required. It is made up as follows:

- 10 cm^3 at 3.7 kBq cm^{-3} is 37 kBq (1 μCi), therefore pipette 1 mm^3 of stock radioisotope into a vessel (or, to be more accurate, pipette 100 mm^3 of a ×100 dilution of stock in water).
- Add 2.5 cm^3 of a 1 M stock solution of cold leucine, and make up to 10 cm^3 with distilled water.

There is no need to take into account the amount of unlabelled leucine in the [^{3}H]leucine preparation; it is a negligible quantity due to the high specific activity. If necessary (e.g. to manipulate solutions of relatively low specific activity), however, the following formula can be applied:

$$W = Ma\left[(1/A') - (1/A)\right] \tag{14.10}$$

where W is the mass of cold carrier required (mg), M is the amount of radioactivity present (MBq), a is the molecular weight of the compound, A is the original specific activity (MBq mmol^{-1}), and A' is the required specific activity (MBq mmol^{-1}).

Example 7 MAKING UP A SOLUTION OF KNOWN ACTIVITY

Question

One litre of [^{3}H]uridine with a concentration of 100 μmol cm^{-3} and 50 000 c.p.m. cm^{-3} is required. If all measurements are made on a scintillation counter with an efficiency of 40%, how would you make up this solution if the purchased supply of [^{3}H]uridine has a specific activity of 20/Ci mol^{-1}?

[NB: M_r uridine = 244; 1 Ci = 22.2 × 10^{11} d.p.m.]

Repeat the calculation in becquerels.

Answer

This problem is similar to the leucine example given above. Correcting for the 48% counting efficiency: 50 000 c.p.m. is 125 000 d.p.m. Multiplying this by 10^3 for a litre gives a d.p.m. equivalent of 56.3 μCi (125 × 10^6/22.2 × 10^5 = 56.3 μCi). Given 20 Ci mol^{-1}, work out how many moles there are in 56.3 μCi (56.3/20 × 10^6 = 2.815 μmoles). 100 000 μmoles of uridine are required in a litre; from the molecular mass this is 24.4 g. The 2.815 μmoles from the radioactive input is only 0.685 mg and so can effectively be ignored. The answer is, therefore, 56.3 μCi (2.08 MBq) of [^{3}H]uridine plus 24.4 g of uridine.

14.3.5 The choice of radionuclide

This is a complex question depending on the precise requirements of the experiment. A summary of some of the key features of radioisotopes commonly used in biological work is shown in Table 14.8.

14.4 INHERENT ADVANTAGES AND RESTRICTIONS OF RADIOTRACER EXPERIMENTS

Perhaps the greatest advantage of radiotracer methods over most other chemical and physical methods is their sensitivity. For example, a dilution factor of 10^{12} can be tolerated without the detection of ^{3}H-labelled compounds being jeopardised. It is thus possible to detect the occurrence of metabolic substances that are normally present in tissues at such low concentrations as to defy the most sensitive chemical methods of identification. A second major advantage of using radiotracers is that they enable studies *in vivo* to be carried out to a far greater degree than can any other technique.

In spite of these significant advantages, certain restrictions have to be appreciated. First, although they undergo the same reactions, different isotopes may do so at different rates. This effect is known as the isotope effect. The different rates are approximately proportional to the differences in mass between the isotopes. The extreme case is the isotopes ^{1}H and ^{3}H, the effect being small for ^{12}C and ^{14}C and

Table 14.8	The relative merits of commonly used β-emitters	
Isotope	Advantages	Disadvantages
^{3}H	Safety High specific activity possible Wide choice of positions in organic compounds Very high resolution in autoradiography	Low efficiency of detection Isotope exchange with environment Isotope effect
^{14}C	Safety Wide choice of labelling position in organic compounds Good resolution in autoradiography	Low specific activity
^{35}S	High specific activity Good resolution in autoradiography	Short half-life Relatively long biological half-life
^{33}P	High specific activity Good resolution in autoradiography Less hazardous than ^{32}P	Lower specific activity than ^{32}P Less sensitive than ^{32}P Cost
^{32}P	Ease of detection High specific activity Short half-life simplifies disposal Čerenkov counting	Short half-life affects costs and experimental design External radiation hazard Poor resolution in autoradiography

Taken from *Radioisotopes in Biology, A Practical Approach*, 2nd edn, ed. R. J. Slater (2002), Oxford University Press, with permission.

almost insignificant for ^{33}P and ^{32}P. Secondly, the amount of activity employed must be kept to the minimum necessary to permit reasonable counting rates in the samples to be analysed, otherwise the radiation from the tracer may elicit a response from the experimental organism and hence distort the results. A third consideration is that, in order to administer the tracer, the normal chemical level of the compound in the organism is automatically exceeded. The results are therefore always open to question.

14.5 SAFETY ASPECTS

The greatest practical disadvantages of using radioisotopes is their toxicity: they produce ionising radiations. When absorbed, radiation causes ionisation and free radicals form that interact with the cell's macromolecules, causing mutation of DNA and hydrolysis of proteins. The toxicity of radiation is dependent not simply on the amount present but on the amount absorbed by the body, the energy of the absorbed radiation and its biological effect. There are, therefore, a series of additional units used to describe these parameters. Originally, radiation hazard was measured in terms of exposure, i.e. a quantity expressing the amount of ionisation in air. The unit of exposure is the roentgen (R), which is the amount of radiation that produces 1.61×10^{15} ion-pairs (kg air)$^{-1}$ (or 2.58×10^{-4} coulombs (kg air)$^{-1}$).

The amount of energy required to produce an ion-pair in air is 5.4×10^{-18} joules (J) and so the amount of energy absorbed by air with an exposure of 1 R is:

$$1.61 \times 10^{15} \times 5.4 \times 10^{-18} = 0.00869 \text{ J (kg air)}^{-1}$$

Although the roentgen has been used as a unit of radiation hazard, it is now considered inadequate for two reasons: first, it is defined with reference to X-rays (or γ-rays) only; and, secondly, the amount of ionisation or energy absorption in different types of material, including living tissue, is likely to be different from that in air.

The concept of radiation absorbed dose (rad) was introduced to overcome these restrictions. The rad is defined as the dose of radiation that gives an energy absorption of 0.01 J (kg absorber)$^{-1}$; this has now been changed to the gray, an SI unit, representing absorption of 1 J kg^{-1} (i.e. 100 rads).

The gray (Gy) is a useful unit, but it still does not adequately describe the hazard to living organisms. This is because different types of radiation are associated with differing degrees of biological hazard. It is, therefore, necessary to introduce a correction factor, known as the weighting factor (W), which is calculated by comparing the biological effects of any type of radiation with that of X-rays. The unit of absorbed dose, which takes into account the weighting factor is the sievert (Sv) and is known as the equivalent dose. Thus:

$$\text{equivalent dose (Sv)} = \text{Gy} \times W \tag{14.11}$$

The majority of isotopes used in biological research emit β-radiation. This is considered to have a biological effect that is very similar to X-rays and has a weighting factor of 1. Therefore, for β-radiation, Gy = Sv. Alpha particles, with their stronger ionising power, are much more toxic and have a weighting factor of 20. Therefore, for α-radiation, 1 Gy = 20 Sv. It is likely that, as our knowledge of the biological effectiveness of different forms of radiation progresses, so the quality factor for different types of radiation may change in the future. Absorbed dose from known sources can be calculated from knowledge of the rate of decay of the source, the energy of radiation, the penetrating power of the radiation and the distance between the source and the laboratory worker. As the radiation is emitted from a source in all directions, the level of irradiation is related to the area of a sphere, $4\pi r^2$. Thus the absorbed dose is inversely related to the square of the distance from the source (r); or, put another way, if the distance is doubled the dose is quartered. A useful formula is

$$\text{dose}_1 \times \text{distance}_1^2 = \text{dose}_2 \times \text{distance}_2^2 \tag{14.12}$$

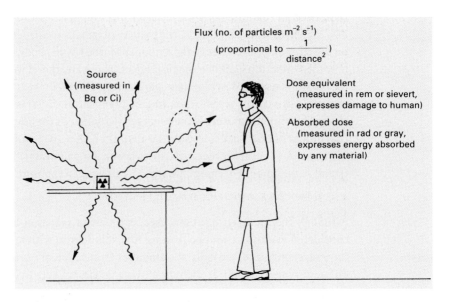

Fig. 14.15. The relationship between radioactivity of source and absorbed dose.

The relationship between radioactive source and absorbed dose is illustrated in Fig. 14.15.

The rate at which dose is delivered is referred to as the dose rate, expressed in Sv h^{-1}. It can be used to calculate your total dose. For example, a source may be delivering 10 μSv h^{-1}. If you worked with the source for 6 h, your total dose would be 60 μSv.

Currently the dose limit for workers exposed to radiation is 15 mSv in a year to the whole body, but this is rarely ever approached by biologists because the levels of radiation used are so low. Limits are set for individual organs. The most important of these to know are for hands (500 mSv year^{-1}) and for lens of the eye (150 mSv year^{-1}). Dose limits are constantly under review and, although dose limits are set, it is against internationally agreed guidelines to work to such a limit, i.e. to assume that all is satisfactory if the limit is not exceeded. Instead, the ALARA principle is applied, to work always to a dose limit that is as low as reasonably achievable. Work that may cause a worker to exceed three-tenths or one-tenth of the dose limit must be carried out in a controlled area or a supervised area, respectively. In practice, work in the biosciences rarely involves a worker receiving a measurable dose. Supervised areas are common but not always required (e.g. for ^{3}H or ^{14}C experiment). Controlled areas are required in only certain circumstances, for example for isotope stores or radioiodination work. A major problem, however, in biosciences is the internal radiation hazard. This is caused by radiation entering the body, for example by inhalation, ingestion, absorption or puncture. This is a likely source of hazard where work involves open sources, i.e. liquids and gases; most work in biology involves manipulations of radioactive liquids. Control of contamination is assisted by:

Table 14.9	Annual limits on intake (ALI) for some commonly used isotopes

Nuclide	ALI (MBq)
^3H	480
^{14}C	34
^{32}P	6.3
^{125}I	1.3

- complying with local rules, written by an employer,
- conscientious personal conduct in the laboratory,
- regular monitoring,
- carrying out work in some kind of containment.

Calculating the dose received following the ingestion of a radioisotope is complex. Detailed information is published by the International Commission on Radiological Protection and assessments, for example for experiments on human volunteers, can be obtained from the National Radiological Protection Board. However, one relatively simple concept is the annual limit on intake (ALI). The ingestion of one ALI results in a person receiving a dose limit to the whole body or to a particular organ. Some ALIs are shown in Table 14.9. Management of radiation protection is similar in most countries. In the USA, there is a Code of Federal Regulations. In the UK there is the Radiaoactive Substances Act (1993) and the Ionising Radiations Regulations (1999). Every institution requires certification (monitored by the Environmental Protection Agency in the USA or the Environment Agency in the UK) and employs a Radiation Protection Advisor.

When handling radioisotopes the rule is to:

- maximise the distance between yourself and the source,
- minimise the time of exposure and
- maintain shielding at all times.

14.6 APPLICATIONS OF RADIOISOTOPES IN THE BIOLOGICAL SCIENCES

14.6.1 Investigating aspects of metabolism

Metabolic pathways

Radioisotopes are frequently used for tracing metabolic pathways. This usually involves adding a radioactive substrate, taking samples of the experimental material at various times, extracting and chromatographically, or otherwise, separating the products. Radioactivity detectors can be attached to gas–liquid chromatography or high performance liquid chromatography columns to monitor radioactivity coming off the column during separation. Alternatively, radioactivity can be located on paper or thin-layer chromatography with either a

Geiger–Müller chromatograph scanner or with autoradiography. If it is suspected that a particular compound is metabolised by a particular pathway, then radioisotopes can also be used to confirm this. For instance, it is possible to predict the fate of individual carbon atoms of [^{14}C]acetate through the tricarboxylic acid, or Krebs, cycle. Methods have been developed whereby intermediates of the cycle can be isolated and the distribution of carbon within each intermediate can be ascertained. This is the so-called specific labelling pattern. Should the actual pattern coincide with the theoretical pattern, then this is very good evidence for the mode of operation of the Krebs cycle.

Another example of the use of radioisotopes to confirm the mode of operation, or otherwise, of a metabolic pathway is in studies carried out on glucose catabolism. There are numerous ways whereby glucose can be oxidised, the two most important ones in aerobic organisms being glycolysis followed by the Krebs cycle together with the pentose phosphate pathway. Frequently, organisms or tissues possess the necessary enzymes for both pathways to occur and it is of interest to establish the relative contribution of each to glucose oxidation. Both pathways involve the complete oxidation of glucose to carbon dioxide, but the origin of the carbon dioxide in terms of the six carbon atoms of glucose is different (at least in the initial stages of respiration of exogenously added substrate). Thus it is possible to trap the carbon dioxide evolved during the respiration of specifically labelled glucose (e.g. [6-^{14}C]glucose or [1-^{14}C]glucose in which only the C-6 atom is radioactive) and obtain an evaluation of the contribution of each pathway to glucose oxidation.

The use of radioisotopes in studying the operation of the Krebs cycle or in evaluating the pathway of glucose catabolism are just two examples of how such isotopes can be used to confirm metabolic pathways. Further details of these and other examples, including use of dual-labelling methods, can be found in the various texts recommended in Section 14.7.

Metabolic turnover times

Radioisotopes provide a convenient method of ascertaining turnover times for particular compounds. As an example, the turnover of proteins in rats will be considered. A group of rats is injected with a radioactive amino acid and left for 24 h, during which time most of the amino acid is assimilated into proteins. The rats are then killed at suitable time intervals and radioactivity in organs or tissues of interest is determined. In this way it is possible to ascertain the rate of metabolic turnover of protein. Using this sort of method, it has been shown that liver protein is turned over in 7–14 days, while skin and muscle protein is turned over every 8–12 weeks, and collagen is turned over at a rate of less than 10% per annum.

Studies of absorption, accumulation and translocation

Radioisotopes have been very widely used in the study of the mechanisms and rates of absorption, accumulation and translocation of inorganic and organic compounds by both plants and animals. Such experiments are generally simple to perform and can also yield evidence on the route of translocation and sites of accumulation of molecules of biological interest.

Pharmacological studies

Another field where radioisotopes are widely used is in the development of new drugs. This is a particularly complicated process, because, besides showing whether a drug has a desirable effect, much more must be ascertained before it can be used in the treatment of clinical conditions. For instance, the site of drug accumulation, the rate of accumulation, the rate of metabolism and the metabolic products must all be determined. In each of these areas of study, radiotracers are extremely useful, if not indispensable. For instance, autoradiography on whole sections of experimental animals (Section 14.2.3) yields information on the site and rate of accumulation, while typical techniques used in metabolic studies can be used to follow the rate and products of metabolism.

14.6.2 **Analytical applications**

Enzyme and ligand binding studies

Virtually any enzyme reaction can be assayed using radiotracer methods, as outlined in Section 15.2.2, provided that a radioactive form of the substrate is available. Radiotracer-based enzyme assays are more expensive than other methods, but frequently have the advantage of a higher degree of sensitivity. Radioisotopes have also been used in the study of the mechanism of enzyme action and in studies of ligand binding to membrane receptors (Section 16.3.1).

Isotope dilution analysis

There are many compounds present in living organisms that cannot be accurately assayed by conventional means because they are present in such low amounts and in mixtures of similar compounds. Isotope dilution analysis offers a convenient and accurate way of overcoming this problem and avoids the necessity of quantitative isolation. For instance, if the amount of iron in a protein preparation is to be determined, this may be difficult using normal methods, but it can be done if a source of ^{59}Fe is available. This is mixed with the protein and a sample of iron is subsequently isolated, assayed for total iron and the radioactivity determined.

If the original specific activity was 10 000 d.p.m. (10 mg)$^{-1}$ and the specific activity of the isolated iron was 9000 d.p.m. (10 mg)$^{-1}$ then the difference is due to the iron in the protein (x), i.e.

$$\frac{9000}{10} = \frac{10\ 000}{10 + x} \tag{14.13}$$

therefore $x = 1.1$ mg.

This technique is widely used in, for instance, studies on trace elements.

Example 8 ISOTOPE DILUTION CALCULATION

Question

To determine the nutritional quality of protein in a foodstuff the content of lysine was determined by isotope dilution analysis. To an acid hydrolysate of the protein (1 mg), 0.5 μmole of [³H]lysine (1 Ci mol⁻¹) was added. A sample of lysine was purified from the hydrolysate by chromatography and the specific activity determined by scintillation counting at 25% efficiency. The value obtained was 2071 c.p.m. μg⁻¹. What is the % (w/w) lysine content of soybean protein? 1 Ci = 22.2 × 10¹¹ d.p.m.; M_r lysine = 148.

Answer

To address this problem it is necessary to apply equation 14.13. Since the counting efficiency was only 25%, it is necessary to multiply the observed count by 4.

0.5 μmole of lysine = 74 μg. Hence, using equation 14.13, we get:

$(2071 \times 4)/1 = (22.2 \times 10^{11} \times 0.5 \times 10^{-6})/(74 + x)$

where x is the lysine content of the sample. From this equation, $x = 60$ μg or 6% of the 1 mg protein sample.

Radioimmunoassay

One of the most significant advances in biochemical techniques in recent years has been the development of the radioimmunoassay. This technique is discussed in Section 7.7 and is not elaborated upon here.

Radiodating

A quite different analytical use for radioisotopes is in the dating (i.e. determining the age) of rocks, fossils and sediments. In this technique it is assumed that the proportion of an element that is naturally radioactive has been the same throughout time. From the time of fossilisation or deposition the radioactive isotope will decay. By determining the amount of radioisotope remaining (or by examining the amount of a decay product) and from a knowledge of the half-life, it is possible to date the sample. For instance, if the radioisotope normally comprises 1% of the element and it is found that the sample actually contains 0.25% then two half-lives can be assumed to have elapsed since deposition. If the half-life is one million years then the sample can be dated as being two million years old.

For long-term dating, isotopes with long half-lives are necessary, such as ²³⁵U, ²³⁸U and ⁴⁰K, whereas for shorter-term dating ¹⁴C is widely used. It cannot be overemphasised that the assumptions made in radiodating are sweeping and hence palaeontologists and anthropologists who use this technique can give only approximate dates to their samples.

14.6.3 Other applications

Molecular biology techniques

Recent advances in molecular biology that have led to advances in genetic manipulation have depended heavily upon use of radioisotopes in DNA and RNA

Table 14.10   Units commonly used to describe radioactivity

Unit	Abbreviation	Definition
Counts per minute or second	c.p.m. c.p.s.	The *recorded* rate of decay
Disintegrations per minute or second	d.p.m. d.p.s.	The *actual* rate of decay
Curie	Ci	The number of d.p.s. equivalent to 1 g of radium (3.7×10^{10} d.p.s.)
Millicurie	mCi	$Ci \times 10^{-3}$ or 2.22×10^9 d.p.m.
Microcurie	μCi	$Ci \times 10^{-6}$ or 2.22×10^6 d.p.m.
Becquerel (SI unit)	Bq	1 d.p.s.
Terabecquerel (SI unit)	TBq	10^{12} Bq or 27.027 Ci
Gigabecquerel (SI unit)	GBq	10^9 Bq or 27.027 mCi
Megabecquerel (SI unit)	MBq	10^6 Bq or 27.027 μCi
Electron volt	eV	The energy attained by an electron accelerated through a potential difference of 1 volt. Equivalent to 1.6×10^{-19} J
Roentgen	R	The amount of radiation that produces 1.61×10^{15} ion-pairs kg^{-1}
Rad	rad	The dose that gives an energy absorption of 0.01 J kg^{-1}
Gray	Gy	The dose that gives an energy absorption of 1 J kg^{-1}. Thus 1 Gy = 100 rad
Rem	rem	The amount of radiation that gives a dose in humans equivalent to 1 rad of X-rays
Sievert	Sv	The amount of radiation that gives a dose in humans equivalent to 1 Gy of X-rays. Thus 1 Sv = 100 rem

sequencing, DNA replication, transcription, synthesis of complementary DNA, recombinant DNA technology and many similar studies. Many of these techniques are more fully discussed in Chapters 5 and 6.

Clinical diagnosis

Radioisotopes are very widely used in medicine, in particular for diagnostic tests. Lung function tests routinely made using xenon-133 (^{133}Xe) are particularly useful in diagnosis of malfunctions of lung ventilation. Kidney function tests using [^{133}I]iodohippuric acid are used in diagnoses of kidney infections, kidney blockages or imbalance of function between the two kidneys.

Various aspects of haematology are also studied by using radioisotopes. These include such aspects as blood cell lifetimes, blood volumes and blood circulation times, all of which may vary in particular clinical conditions.

Ecological studies

The bulk of radiotracer work is carried out in biochemical, clinical or pharmaco-logical laboratories; nevertheless, radiotracers are also of use to ecologists. In particular, migratory patterns and behaviour patterns of many animals can be monitored using radiotracers. Another ecological application is in the examination of food chains where the primary producers can be made radioactive and the path of radioactivity followed throughout the resulting food chain.

Sterilisation of food and equipment

Very strong γ-emitters are now widely used in the food industry for sterilisation of prepacked foods such as milk and meats. Normally either ^{60}C or ^{137}Ce is used, but care has to be taken in some cases to ensure that the food product itself is not affected in any way. Thus doses often have to be reduced to an extent where sterilisation is not complete but nevertheless food spoilage can be greatly reduced. ^{60}Co and ^{137}Ce are also used in sterilisation of plastic disposable equipment such as Petri dishes and syringes, and in sterilisation of drugs that are administered by injection.

Mutagens

Radioisotopes may cause mutations, particularly in microorganisms. In various microbiological studies mutants are desirable, especially in industrial microbiology. For instance, development of new strains of a microorganism that produce higher yields of a desired microbial product frequently involve mutagenesis by radioisotopes.

14.7 SUGGESTIONS FOR FURTHER READING

BILLINGTON, D., JAYSON, G. G. and MALTBY, P. J. (1992). *Radioisotopes*. Bios Scientific, Oxford. (A description of principles and applications in the biosciences, for undergraduates and research workers.)

CONNOR, K. J. and MCLINTOCK, I. S. (1994). *Radiation Protection Handbook for Laboratory Workers*. HHSC, Leeds. (A safety manual for laboratory work.)

SLATER, R. J. (1996). Radioisotopes in molecular biology. In *Molecular Biology and Molecular Medicine*, ed. R. A. Myers, pp. 209–219. VCH, New York. (A summary of the application of radioisotopes to molecular biology.)

SLATER, R. J.(2002). *Radioisotopes in Biology – A Practical Approach*, 2nd edn. Oxford University Press, Oxford. (A detailed account of the handling and use of radioactivity in biological research.)

Chapter 15

Enzymes

15.1 CHARACTERISTICS AND NOMENCLATURE

Enzymes are single- or multiple-chain proteins that act as biological catalysts with the ability to promote specific chemical reactions under the mild conditions that prevail in most living organisms. They have three distinctive characteristics:

- *Specificity:* Enzymes show a characteristic specificity for the reaction they promote and the substrates they can use. As a generalisation, anabolic enzymes show a higher specificity than catabolic ones. Bond specificity is characteristic of enzymes such as the peptidases and esterases that hydrolyse specific bond types. The specificity of these enzymes is determined by the presence of specific functional groups adjacent to the bond to be cleaved. Group specificity is characteristic of enzymes that promote a particular reaction on a structurally related group of substrates. As an example, the kinases catalyse the phosphorylation of substrates that have a common structural feature such as a particular amino acid (e.g. the tyrosine kinases) or sugar (e.g. hexokinase). Absolute or near-absolute specificity is characteristic of anabolic enzymes that catalyse one specific reaction. Enzymes may also display stereospecificity and be able to distinguish between optical and geometrical isomers of substrates or, in the case of the NAD^+- or $NADP^+$-requiring dehydrogenases, to distinguish between apparently identical hydrogen atoms located on opposite sides of the nicotinamide ring (see Section 15.4.4).
- *High catalytic rate:* Enzymes enhance the reaction rate by factors as high as 10^{12} relative to the non-enzyme-catalysed reaction. They achieve this high catalytic power by facilitating the formation of an energetically favoured transition state from substrate to product, thereby lowering the activation energy for the reaction. They do not alter the position of equilibrium of a reversible reaction but they do accelerate the establishment of the equilibrium position (see Section 15.3.5).
- *High capacity for regulation:* The activity of enzymes that control the rate of a particular metabolic pathway can be enhanced or reduced in response to changing intracellular and extracellular demands. A range of regulatory mechanisms operate to allow short-, medium- and long-term changes in activity. Examples include feedback inhibition, covalent modification and gene induction and repression (see Section 15.5.2).

Binding sites

Enzymes reversibly bind their substrate(s) at a specific binding site, generally known as the active or catalytic site, created by the specific three-dimensional structure of the protein molecule but consisting of a relatively small number of amino acid residues. The resulting enzyme–substrate complex promotes a chemical reaction, facilitated by specific amino acid residues in the catalytic site, resulting in the formation of the product. Different amino acid residues in the site may be involved in the binding of the substrate(s) in the correct stereo orientation and in promoting the chemical reaction. An enzyme may also contain regulatory or allosteric sites to which other molecules, commonly distinct from the substrate and often key metabolites such as ATP and AMP, can bind, inducing conformational changes in the active site and thereby enhancing or reducing the activity of the catalytic site. These regulatory molecules are termed effectors, and their regulatory site may be on either the same subunit as the catalytic site or a different subunit (see Section 15.3.3).

The binding of a substrate to an enzyme involves a number of weak, reversible forces including:

- ion-pairing (salt bridges) between ionised groups ($-NH_3^+$, $-COO^-$) within the substrate and oppositely charged groups within the catalytic site;
- hydrogen bonding between such groups as $-OH$, $-NH_2$, $-COOH$;
- interatomic van der Waals forces;
- hydrophobic interactions;
- cation-π interactions – electrostatic attraction between a cation, such as that of a protonated amino group within the substrate, and the negative electrostatic potential associated with the face of a simple π system typically provided by the aromatic side-chain of phenylalanine, tyrosine or tryptophan found in the catalytic site.

Cofactors

The catalytic properties of an enzyme are often dependent upon the presence of non-peptide molecules called cofactors or coenzymes. These may be either weakly or tightly bound to the enzyme, in the latter case they are referred to as a prosthetic group. Examples of coenzymes include NAD^+, $NADP^+$, FMN and FAD, whilst examples of prosthetic groups include haem and oligosaccharides, and simple metal ions such as Mg^{2+}, Fe^{2+} and Zn^{2+}. An enzyme lacking its cofactor is termed an apoenzyme, and the active enzyme with its cofactor the holoenzyme.

Nomenclature and classification

By international convention, each enzyme is classified into one of six groups on the basis of the type of chemical reaction that it catalyses. Each group is divided into subgroups according to the nature of the chemical group and coenzymes involved in the reaction. In accordance with the Enzyme Commission (EC) rules, each enzyme can be assigned a unique four-figure code and an unambiguous systematic name based upon the reaction catalysed. The six groups are:

- *Group 1:* Oxidoreductases, which transfer hydrogen or oxygen atoms or electrons from one substrate to another. The group includes the dehydrogenases, reductases, oxidases, dioxidases, hydroxylases, peroxidases and catalase;
- *Group 2:* Transferases, which transfer chemical groups between substrates. The group includes the kinases, aminotransferases, acetyltransferases, carbamyltransferases and phosphorylases.
- *Group 3:* Hydrolases, which catalyse the hydrolytic cleavage of bonds. The group includes the peptidases, esterases, phosphatases and sulphatases.
- *Group 4:* Lyases, which catalyse elimination reactions resulting in the formation of double bonds. The group includes adenylyl cyclase (also known adenylate cyclase), enolase and aldolase.
- *Group 5:* Isomerases, which interconvert isomers of various types by intramolecular rearrangements. The group includes phosphoglucomutase and glucose-6-phosphate isomerase;
- *Group 6:* Ligases (also called synthases), which catalyse covalent bond formation with the concomitant breakdown of a nucleoside triphosphate, commonly ATP. The group includes carbamoyl phosphate synthase and DNA ligase.

As an example of the operation of these rules consider the enzyme alcohol dehydrogenase that catalyses the reaction:

$$\text{alcohol} + NAD^+ \rightleftharpoons \text{aldehyde or ketone} + NADH + H^+$$

It has the systematic name alcohol:NAD oxidoreductase and the classification number $1:1:1:1$. The first 1 indicates that it is an oxidoreductase, the second 1 that it acts on a CH-OH donor, the third 1 that NAD^+ or $NADP^+$ is the acceptor and the fourth 1 that it is the first enzyme named in the 1:1:1 subgroup. Systematic names tend to be user-unfriendly and for day-to-day purposes recommended trivial names are preferred. When correctly used they give a reasonable indication of the reaction promoted by the enzyme in question but they fail to fully identify all the reactants involved. For example, glyceraldehydes-3-phosphate dehydrogenase fails to identify the involvement of orthophosphate and NAD^+ and phosphorylase kinase fails to convey the information that it is the b form of phosphorylase that is subject to phosphorylation involving ATP.

Isoenzymes

Some enzymes exist in multiple forms called isoenzymes or isoforms that differ in amino acid sequence. An example is lactate dehydrogenase (LD) (EC 1:1:1:27) that exists in five isoforms. LD is a tetramer that can be assembled from two subunits H (for heart) and M (for muscle). The five forms are therefore H4, H3M, H2M2, HM3 and M4, which can be separated by electrophoresis and shown to have different affinities for their substrates, lactate and pyruvate, and for analogues of these two compounds. They also have different maximum catalytic activities and tissue distributions, and as a consequence are important in diagnostic enzymology (Section 1.7.3).

Multienzyme complexes

Some enzymes that promote consecutive reactions in a metabolic pathway associate to form a multienzyme complex. Examples include fatty-acid synthase (EC 2:3:1:86) (seven catalytic centres), pyruvate dehydrogenase (EC 2:7:1:99) (three catalytic centres) and DNA polymerase (EC 2:7:7:7) (three catalytic centres). Multienzyme complexes have a number of advantages over individual enzymes, including a reduction in the transit time for the diffusion of the product of one enzyme to the catalytic site of the next, a reduction in the possibility of the product of one enzyme being acted upon by another enzyme not involved in the pathway, and the possibility of one enzyme activating an adjacent enzyme (Section 15.4.7).

Units of enzyme activity

Units of enzyme activity are expressed either in the SI units of katals (moles of substrate consumed or product formed per second) or international units (IU) (μmoles of substrate consumed or product formed per minute). Allied to activity units is specific activity that expresses the number of IU per mg protein or katals per kg protein (note: 60 international units per mg protein is equivalent to 1 katal (kg protein)$^{-1}$).

15.2 ANALYTICAL METHODS FOR THE STUDY OF ENZYME REACTIONS

15.2.1 General considerations

Enzyme assays are undertaken for a variety of reasons, but the two most common are:

- to determine the amount (or concentration or activity) of enzyme present in a particular preparation (this is particularly important in diagnostic enzymology, see Section 1.7.3),
- to gain an insight into the kinetic characteristics of the reaction and hence to determine a range of kinetic constants such as K_m, V_{max} and k_{cat}.

Analytical methods for enzyme assays may be classified as either continuous (kinetic) or discontinuous (fixed-time). Continuous methods monitor some property change (e.g. absorbance or fluorescence) in the reaction mixture, whereas discontinuous methods require samples to be withdrawn from the reaction mixture and analysed by some convenient technique. The inherent greater accuracy of continuous methods commends them whenever they are available.

Initial rates

When an enzyme is mixed with an excess of substrate there is an initial short period of time (a few hundred microseconds) during which intermediates leading to the formation of the product gradually build up (Fig. 15.1). This so-called pre-steady state requires special techniques for study and these are discussed in

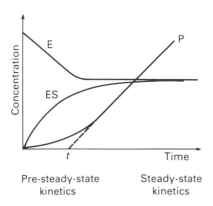

Fig. 15.1. Pre-steady-state progress curve for the interaction of an enzyme (E) with its substrate (S). P, product; t, induction time.

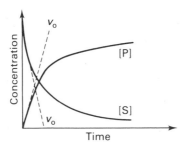

Fig. 15.2. Calculation of initial rate (v_0) from the time-dependent change in the concentration of substrate (S) and product (P) of an enzyme-catalysed reaction.

Section 15.2.3. After this pre-steady state, the reaction rate and the concentration of intermediates change relatively slowly with time and so-called steady-state kinetics exist. Measurement of the progress of the reaction during this phase gives the relationships shown in Fig. 15.2. Tangents drawn through the origin to the curves of substrate concentration and product concentration versus time allow the initial rate, v_0, to be calculated. This is the maximum rate for a given concentration of enzyme and substrate under the defined experimental conditions. Measurement of the initial rate of an enzyme-catalysed reaction is a prerequisite to a complete understanding of the mechanism by which the enzyme works, as well as to the estimation of the activity of an enzyme in a biological sample. Its numerical value is influenced by many factors, including substrate and enzyme concentration, pH, temperature and the presence of activators or inhibitors.

For simplicity, initial rates are sometimes determined experimentally on the basis of a single measurement of the amount of substrate consumed or product produced in a given time rather than by the tangent method. This approach is valid over only the short period of time when the reaction is proceeding effectively at a constant rate. This linear rate section comprises at the most the first 10% of the total possible change and clearly the error is smaller the earlier the rate is measured. In such cases, the initial rate is proportional either to the reciprocal of

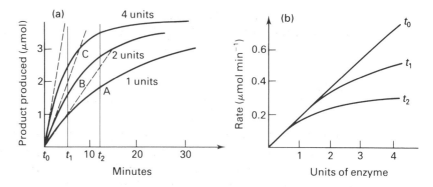

Fig. 15.3. The importance of measuring the initial rate in the assay of an enzyme. (a) Time-dependent variation in the concentration of products in the presence of (A)1, (B)2 and (C)4 units of enzyme; (b) variation of reaction rate with enzyme concentration using true initial rate (v_o) and two fixed time assays (t_1 and t_2).

the time to produce a fixed change (fixed-change assays) or to the amount of substrate reacted in a given time (fixed-time assays). The potential problem with fixed-time assays is illustrated in Fig. 15.3, which represents the effect of enzyme concentration on the progress of the reaction in the presence of a constant initial substrate concentration (Fig. 15.3a). Measurement of the rate of the reaction at time t_0 (by the tangent method) to give the true initial rate or at two fixed times, t_1 and t_2, gives the relationship between initial rate and enzyme concentration shown in Fig. 15.3b. It can be seen that only the tangent method gives the correct linear relationship. Since the correct determination of initial rate means that the observed changes in the concentration of substrate or product are relatively small, it is inherently more accurate to measure the increase in product concentration because the relative increase in its concentration is significantly larger than the corresponding decrease in substrate concentration.

15.2.2 Analytical methods for steady-state studies

Visible and ultraviolet spectrophotometric methods

Many substrates and products absorb light in the visible or ultraviolet region and the change in the absorbance during the reaction can be used as the basis for the enzyme assay. It is essential that the substrate and product do not absorb at the same wavelength and that the Beer–Lambert law (Section 12.4.1) is obeyed for the chosen analyte. A large number of common enzyme assays are based on the interconversion of NAD(P)$^+$ and NAD(P)H. Both of these nucleotides absorb at 260 nm but only the reduced form absorbs at 340 nm. Enzymes that do not involve this interconversion can be assayed by means of a coupled reaction, which involves two enzyme reactions linked by means of common intermediates. The assay of 6-phosphofructokinase (PFK) (EC 2:7:1:11) coupled to fructose-bisphosphatase aldolase (FBPA) (EC 4:1:2:13) and glyceraldehyde-3-phosphate dehydrogenase (G3PDH) (EC 1:2:1:12) illustrates the principle:

$$\text{D-fructose 6-phosphate} \quad \xrightarrow[\text{ATP} \quad \text{ADP}]{\text{PFK} \ + \ \text{Mg}^{2+}} \quad \text{D-fructose 1,6-bisphosphate}$$

FBPA

$$\text{1,3-bisphosphoglyceric acid} \quad \xleftarrow[\text{NADH} \quad \text{NAD}^+]{\text{G3PDH} \ + \ \text{Pi}} \quad \text{D-glyceraldehyde} \ + \ \text{glycerone} \\ \text{3-phosphate} \qquad \text{phosphate}$$

The assay mixture would contain D-fructose-6-phosphate, ATP, Mg^{2+}, FBPA, G3PDH, NAD^+ and P_i all in excess so that the reaction would go to completion and the rate of reduction of NAD^+ and the production of NADH, and hence the increase in absorbance at 340 nm, would be determined solely by the activity of PFK added to the reaction mixture in a known volume of the test enzyme preparation. In principle there is no limit to the number of reactions that can be coupled in this way provided that the enzyme under investigation is always present in limiting amounts.

The number of units of enzyme in the test preparation can be calculated by applying the Beer–Lambert law to calculate the amount of product formed per second:

$$\text{enzyme units (katal per cm}^3 \text{ test solution)} = \frac{\Delta E_{340}}{\varepsilon_\lambda} \times \frac{a}{1000} \times \frac{1000}{x}$$

where ΔE_{340} is the control-corrected change in the absorbance at 340 nm per second, a is the total volume (cm^3) of reaction mixture (generally about 3 cm^3) in a cuvette of 1 cm light path, x is the volume (mm^3) of test solution added to the reaction mixture, and ε_λ is the molar extinction coefficient for NADH at 340 nm ($6.3 \times 10^3 (\text{mol dm}^{-3})^{-1} \text{cm}^{-1}$). By dividing the above equation by the total concentration of protein in the test enzyme preparation, the specific activity (katal per kg) of the preparation can be calculated.

The scope of visible spectrophotometric enzyme assays can be extended by the use of synthetic substrates that release a coloured product. Many such artificial substrates are available commercially, particularly for the assay of hydrolytic enzymes. The favoured coloured products are phenolphthalein and p-nitrophenol, both of which are coloured in alkaline solution. An example is the assay of α-D-glucosidase (maltase) (EC 3:2:1:20):

p-nitrophenyl-α-D-glucopyranoside   D-glucose p-nitrophenol (yellow)

An extension of this approach is the use of synthetic dyes for the study of oxidoreductases. The oxidised and reduced forms of these dyes have different colours. Examples are the tetrazolium dyes, methylene blue, 2,6-dichlorophenol indophenol, and methyl and benzyl viologen (Table 1.8). Their use is dependent upon them having an appropriate redox potential (Section 1.5.1), relative to that of the substrate, so that the free energy change for the reaction is negative, allowing the reaction to proceed in the required direction.

Spectrofluorimetric methods

Fluorimetric enzyme assays have the significant practical advantage that they are highly sensitive and can therefore detect and measure enzymes at low concentrations. However, they are sensitive to traces of impurities in the enzyme preparation that can quench the emitted radiation. Additionally, some fluorescent compounds are unstable, especially in the presence of ultraviolet light. NAD(P)H is fluorescent and so enzymes utilising it can be assayed either by their absorption at 340 nm or by their fluorescence (primary wavelength 340 nm, reference wavelength 378 nm). Synthetic substrates that release a fluorescent product are also available for the assay of some enzymes. An example is the assay of β-D-glucuronidase (EC 3:2:1:31) using 4-methlyumbelliferyl-β-D-glucuronide as the substrate that releases the fluorescent product 4-methylumbelliferone.

Luminescence methods

Bioluminescence reactions are commonly used as the basis for an enzyme assay owing to their high sensitivity. The assay of luciferase is an example:

$$\text{luciferin} + \text{ATP} + O_2 \quad \underset{}{\overset{\text{luciferase}}{\rightleftharpoons}} \quad \text{oxyluciferin} + \text{AMP} + PP_i + CO_2 + \textit{light}$$

The assay can be used to assay ATP and enzymes that utilise ATP by means of coupled reactions. An example is the assay of malate dehydrogenase (MD) (EC 1:1:1:37). This coupled assay is based on the fact that bacterial luciferase uses reduced FMN to oxidise long-chain aliphatic aldehydes (RCHO):

$$(S)\text{-malate} + \text{NAD}^+ \quad \underset{}{\overset{\text{MD}}{\rightleftharpoons}} \quad \text{oxaloacetate} + \text{NADH} + H^+$$

$$\text{NADH} + H^+ + \text{FMN} \quad \underset{}{\overset{\text{oxidoreductase}}{\rightleftharpoons}} \quad \text{FMNH}_2 + \text{NAD}^+$$

$$\text{FMNH}_2 + \text{RCHO} + O_2 \quad \underset{}{\overset{\text{luciferase}}{\rightleftharpoons}} \quad \text{FMN} + \text{RCOOH} + H_2O + \textit{light}$$

The use of excess reagents would ensure that each reaction went to completion.

Immunochemical methods

Monoclonal antibodies raised to a particular enzyme can be used as a basis for a highly specific enzyme-linked immunosorbent assay (ELISA) for the enzyme. Such assays can distinguish between isoenzyme forms, which make them attractive for diagnostic purposes. An important clinical example is creatine kinase (CK). It is a dimer based on two different subunits, M and B. The MB isoenzyme is important in the diagnosis of myocardial infarction (heart attack) and an immunological assay is important in its assay. Further details of the assay of CK-MB are given in Section 1.7.3. The principles of this type of assay are discussed in Section 7.7.

Ion-selective and oxygen electrode methods

The availability of ion-selective electrodes (ISEs) and gas-sensing electrodes, such as those for the ammonium ion, oxygen, carbon dioxide and ammonia have allowed attractive methods to be developed for many enzyme assays in which these species are consumed or released. The methods are sensitive, reproducible and can be applied to very small volumes of test solution (Section 1.5.2).

Radioisotope methods

Although potentially very sensitive, radioisotope methods for enzyme assays are restricted to applications where it is possible to separate easily the radiolabelled forms of the substrate and product. It is most commonly applied to cases in which one of the products is a gas. The assay of glutamate decarboxylase (GD) is an example:

$$\text{HOOCCH}_2\text{CH(NH}_2)^{14}\text{COOH} \xrightleftharpoons{\text{GD}} {}^{14}\text{CO}_2 + \text{HOOCCH}_2\text{CH}_2\text{CH}_2\text{NH}_2$$

$$\text{L-glutamic acid} \qquad\qquad \gamma\text{-aminobutyric acid}$$

The $^{14}\text{CO}_2$ evolved is trapped in alkali and hence the rate of $^{14}\text{CO}_2$ evolution measured. In other cases not involving the evolution of a gas, the substrate and product can be separated by a solvent extraction technique but this does not lend itself to routine analysis. GD can also be assayed using a CO_2 electrode.

Practical considerations

Once the analytical method for a particular assay has been selected, a number of practical issues should be considered:

- All reactants should be of a high purity and all apparatus should be scrupulously clean.
- Variables such as pH, temperature and ionic strength should be controlled.
- All studies should include an appropriate control that is in all respects the same as the test assay but lacking either enzyme or substrate. Changes in the experimental parameter in the control lacking the test enzyme will give an assessment of the extent of the non-enzymatic reaction whereas changes in the control lacking added substrate will evaluate any background reaction in the enzyme preparation. It is worthwhile assaying the enzyme using different volumes of the test solution to confirm linearity between initial rate and enzyme concentration, thereby confirming the absence of activators or inhibitors in the preparation.
- Enzyme assays should be carried out with excess substrate (at least 10 K_m (see Section 15.3)).
- Kinetic studies should be carried out with substrate concentrations ranging from 0.1 to 10 K_m.
- Most assays are carried out at 30 °C but some are performed at 37 °C because of the physiological significance of the temperature.

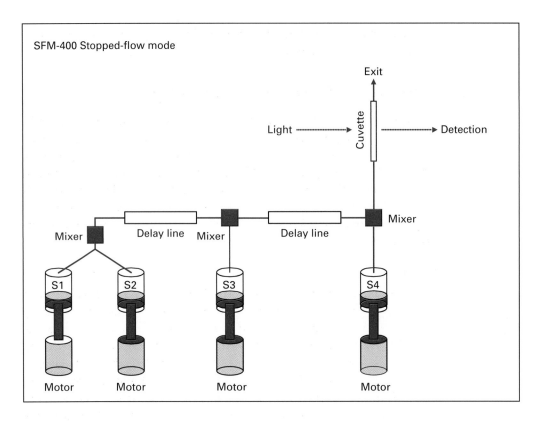

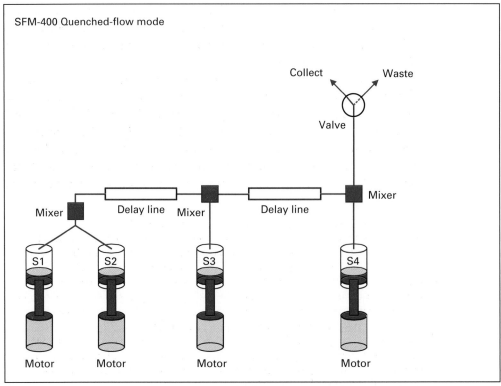

- the assay method should be appropriately calibrated and validated using the principles discussed in Section 1.6.5.

15.2.3 Analytical methods for pre-steady-state studies

The experimental techniques discussed in the previous section are not suitable for the study of the progress of enzyme reactions in the short period of time (commonly milliseconds) before steady-state conditions, with respect to the formation of enzyme–substrate complex, are established. Fig. 15.1 shows the progress curves for this pre-steady-state initial stage of an enzymatic reaction. The induction time t is related to the rate constants for the formation and dissociation of the enzyme–substrate (ES) complex. Two main types of method are available for the study of this pre-steady state.

Rapid mixing methods

In the continuous flow method, separate solutions of the enzyme and substrate are introduced from syringes, each of $10 \, cm^3$ maximum volume, into a mixing chamber typically of $100 \, mm^3$ capacity. The mixture is then pumped at a pre-selected speed through a narrow tube that is illuminated by a light source and monitored by a photomultiplier detector. Flow through the tube is fast, typically $10 \, m \, s^{-1}$, so that it is turbulent, thus ensuring that the solution is homogeneous. The precise flow time from the time of mixing to the observation point can be calculated from the known flow rate. By varying the flow rate the reaction time at the observation point can be varied, allowing the extent of reaction to be studied as a function of time. From these data the various rate constants can be calculated. The technique uses relatively small amounts of reactants and is limited only by the time required to mix the two reactants.

The stopped-flow method is a variant of the continuous-flow method in that shortly after the reactants emerge from the mixing chamber the flow is stopped and the detector triggered to continuously monitor the change in the experimental parameter such as absorbance or fluorescence (Fig. 15.4). Special flow cells are used together with a detector that allows readings to be taken 180° to the light source for absorbance, transmittance or circular dichroism measurements, or at 90° to the source for fluorescence, fluorescence anisotropy or light-scattering measurements.

Fig. 15.4. The Bio-Logic stopped-flow (top) and quenched-flow (bottom) apparatus. The reactants are placed in separate syringes each driven by a microprocessor-controlled stepping motor capable of delivering 0.01 to 10.00 $cm^3 \, min^{-1}$ with a minimum injection volume of 10–30 mm^3. The reactants are pre-mixed before they enter the delay line (variable volume between 25 and 1000 mm^3) and then the flow cell cuvette with a minimum dead time of 0.6 ms. The flow can be stopped at any predetermined time either by stopping the stepping motor or by closing the outlet from the reaction cuvette. The reaction can be studied by visible, ultraviolet, fluorescence or circular dichroism spectroscopy. The optical path length can be varied between 0.8 and 10 mm. In quench-flow mode the minimum ageing time is <2 ms. The quenching agent is added from the third or fourth syringe. (Reproduced by permission of BioLogic Science Instruments, France: website <www.bio-logic.info>.)

It is also possible to take measurements by mass spectrometry, X-ray scattering and conductivity. The attraction of the method is its conservation of reactants.

A variant of the stopped flow method is the quenching method. In this technique the reactants from the mixing chamber are treated with a quenching agent from a third syringe. The quenching agent, for example trichloroacetic acid, stops the reaction, which is then monitored by an appropriate analytical method for the build-up of intermediates. By varying the time between mixing the reactants and adding the quenching reagent, the kinetics of this build-up can be studied. A disadvantage of this approach is that it uses more reactants than the stopped-flow method, since the kinetic data are acquired from a series of studies rather than by following one reaction for a period of time. Both methods have difficulty in monitoring the first millisecond of reaction owing to the need to allow mixing to take place, but this problem can be partly solved by changing the pH or temperature in order to slow down the reaction. Both methods commonly use synthetic substrates that release a coloured product or give rise to a coloured acyl or phosphoryl intermediate.

Relaxation methods

The limitation of the stopped-flow method is the dead time during which the enzyme and substrate are mixed. In the relaxation methods an equilibrium mixture of the reactants is preformed and the position of equilibrium altered by a change in reaction conditions. The most common procedure for achieving this is the temperature jump technique in which the reaction temperature is raised rapidly by 5–10 deg.C by the discharge of a capacitor or infrared laser. The rate at which the reaction mixture adjusts to its new equilibrium (relaxation time τ, generally a few microseconds) is inversely related to the rate constants involved in the reaction. This return to equilibrium is monitored by one or more suitable spectrophotometric methods. The recorded data enables the number of intermediates to be deduced and the various rate constants calculated from the relaxation times.

These pre-steady-state techniques have shown that the enzyme and its substrate(s) associate very rapidly, with second-order rate constants for the formation of ES in the range 10^6–$10^8 (mol\,dm^{-3})^{-1}s^{-1}$ and first-order rate constants for the dissociation of ES in the range 10–$10^4 s^{-1}$. The association process is slower than that predicted by simple collision theory and confirms the need for the specific orientation of the substrate and enzyme, with subsequent conformational changes in the protein and probably the involvement of solvation processes.

The stopped-flow and quenching methods have also been used to study other biochemical processes that are kinetically fast and may involve transient intermediates. For example, the stopped-flow method has been applied to the study of protein folding, protein conformational changes and receptor–ligand binding, and the quenching method to the study of second-messenger studies.

15.2.4 Analytical methods for *in vivo* studies

In the extrapolation of *in vitro* kinetic data to the *in vivo* situation the assumption is made that intracellular compartments such as the cytosol and the mitochondrial matrix can be regarded as homogeneous bags of enzymes in which the individual enzyme, their substrates and products can diffuse freely. Support for this view originates from cell fractionation studies in which the great proportion of total cell proteins is released when cells are disrupted. However, there is now good evidence, obtained from studies with high voltage electron microscopy (HVEM), that mammalian cells contain an extensive network of interconnecting strands, termed the microtrabecular lattice (MTL), which appears to connect all the intracellular structures. Critics of the existence of the MTL have argued that such structures are artefacts, but there is increasing acceptance that MTL or closely related structures do represent a good approximation of the structure *in vivo*. The consequence of such a model is that previously regarded freely diffusing enzymes are more likely to be loosely bound to the MTL. Such a view gives rise to the concept of the wide existence of multienzyme complexes previously regarded as an exception to the norm. If these views are correct, then the concept arises of the channelling of products from one enzyme to the next (Section 15.4.7). Channelling could occur by a number of mechanisms including: the sequential covalent binding of intermediates to active sites; site-to-site transfer of non-covalently bound intermediates (so-called tight channelling), the transfer of intermediates in an unstirred aqueous layer and the prevention of diffusion of intermediates by electrostatic forces. It has been argued that channelling of metabolic intermediates within an organised enzyme complex could lead to increased flux (rate of utilisation of substrates) through the pathway and restriction of flux in competing pathways. Whether or not the loose association of enzymes will result in a metabolically significant change in the kinetic properties of these enzymes relative to the properties in free solution is still a matter of research.

The most successful analytical technique for studying enzymology in individual cells and in whole organisms is nuclear magnetic resonance spectroscopy (NMR). This non-invasive technique allows the measurement of steady-state metabolite concentrations and of metabolic flux using simple proton NMR, or the redistribution of a ^{13}C label among glycolytic intermediates or the use of ^{31}P NMR to measure ATP turnover and flux. Evidence for enzyme–enzyme interaction has been obtained by studying conformational changes in the enzyme protein. This approach requires the protein to be labelled in some appropriate way. One of the most attractive methods is to insert ^{19}F into the molecule. From an NMR point of view this is an excellent label, since it is an isotope that has a spin quantum number of $\frac{1}{2}$ and therefore has two spin states that are readily studied by NMR. The chemical shift change of the fluorine nucleus is large, making it very sensitive to its local environment in the protein. Moreover, its size is very similar to that of a proton, so that it is unlikely to modify the enzyme's structure. Since fluorine is very rare in biological systems, the NMR signal from the label can be interpreted unambiguously. By studying the relaxation times associated with the fluorine nucleus it is possible to detect restricted motion of the enzyme in a cell due to protein–protein aggregation.

A complementary approach to these NMR studies is that of genetic manipulation. Using molecular biology techniques, it is possible to delete, raise or lower the intracellular concentration of selected enzymes and to study the effect on enzyme kinetics and metabolic flux. The approach simply requires the availability of cDNA or a genomic clone for the selected enzyme, coupled with gene disruption and anti-sense RNA methodologies.

15.2.5 Analytical methods for substrate assays

Enzyme-based assays are very convenient methods for the estimation of the amount of substrate present in a biological sample. The principle of using excess enzyme (i.e. the substrate concentration should be less than the K_m (see Section 15.3)) and relating the substrate concentration in the test solution to the observed initial rate can be used. It is essential that the reaction goes to completion in a relatively short time. If the reaction is freely reversible, then it is necessary to change the experimental conditions, such as pH or by chemically trapping the product, so that the reaction does approach completion. Coupled reactions are commonly used in substrate assays and they have the attraction that they help in the displacement of reversible reactions. The sensitivity of this initial rate method to substrate assay depends upon the value of the molar extinction coefficient for the analyte being assayed and also on the K_m for the substrate. In practice these two factors place a constraint on the level of substrate that can be assayed. Several approaches are available to overcome this problem. The end-point technique avoids the measurement of initial rate by converting all the substrate to product and then computing the amount present by correlating it with the total change in parameter such as absorbance or fluorescence. The sensitivity of an assay can also be significantly increased by the technique of enzymatic cycling. In this method the substrate is regenerated by means of a coupled reaction and the total change in absorbance, etc., in a given time measured. Precalibration, using a range of substrate concentrations with all the other reactants in excess, allows the substrate concentration in a test solution to be computed. This method has a 10^4- to 10^5-fold increase in sensitivity relative to the end-point technique.

Enzyme-based assays are commonly used in clinical biochemistry to measure substrates in biological samples. For example, the three most common assays for serum glucose are those based on the use of hexokinase, glucose oxidase and glucose dehydrogenase. The first two are based on the coupled reaction technique:

- *Hexokinase method:* This couples the reaction to that of glucose-6-phosphate dehydrogenase and measures the absorbance at 340 nm due to NADH:

$$\text{D-glucose} + \text{ATP} \rightleftharpoons \text{D-glucose 6-phosphate} + \text{ADP}$$
$$\text{D-glucose 6-phosphate} + \text{NAD}^+ \rightleftharpoons \text{D-glucono-1,5-lactone 6-phosphate}$$
$$+ \text{NADH} + \text{H}^+$$

- *Glucose oxidase method:* This couples the reaction to peroxidase and measures the absorption of the oxidised dye in the visible region or uses an oxygen electrode to measure the oxygen consumption directly:

$$\text{D-glucose} + \text{H}_2\text{O} + \text{O}_2 \rightleftharpoons \text{D-gluconic acid} + \text{H}_2\text{O}_2$$
$$\text{H}_2\text{O}_2 + \text{dye}_\text{reduced} \rightleftharpoons \text{H}_2\text{O} + \text{dye}_\text{oxidised}$$

The glucose oxidase method uses β-D-glucose as substrate but blood glucose contains an equilibrium mixture of it and the α-isomer. Fortunately, preparations of glucose oxidase contain an isomerase that interconverts the two isomers thus allowing the assay of total D-glucose.

- *Glucose dehydrogenase method:* This requires no coupled reaction, but simply measures the increase in absorption at 340 nm:

$$\beta\text{-D-glucose} + NAD^+ \rightleftharpoons \text{D-glucono-1,5-lactone} + NADH + H^+$$

Other blood or urine substrates commonly assayed by enzyme-based techniques commonly used in clinical biochemistry include the following:

- *Creatinine:* This is used as an indicator of kidney function, and uses creatininase, creatine kinase, pyruvate kinase and lactate dehydrogenase:

$$creatinine + H_2O \rightleftharpoons creatine$$
$$creatine + ATP \rightleftharpoons phosphocreatine + ADP$$
$$ADP + phosphoenolpyruvate \rightleftharpoons ATP + pyruvate$$
$$pyruvate + NADH + H^+ \rightleftharpoons \text{L-lactate} + NAD^+$$

- *Cholesterol:* This is used as an indicator of atherosclerosis and susceptibility to coronary heart disease, uses cholesterol oxidase and peroxidase and measures the absorption in the visible region due to the oxidised dye:

$$cholesterol + O_2 \rightleftharpoons \text{4-cholesten-3-one} + H_2O_2$$
$$H_2O_2 + dye_{reduced} \rightleftharpoons H_2O + dye_{oxidised}$$

Any cholesterol ester in the sample is hydrolysed to free cholesterol by the inclusion of cholesterol esterase in the reaction mixture.

Biosensors, such as those for glucose and cholesterol (Section 1.5.2) are based on the above reactions and afford a simple means for the fast measurement of these substrates.

15.3 ENZYME STEADY-STATE KINETICS

15.3.1 Monosubstrate enzyme reactions

For many enzymes, the initial rate, v_o, varies hyperbolically with substrate concentration for a fixed concentration of enzyme (Fig. 15.5). The mathematical equation expressing this hyperbolic relationship between initial rate and substrate concentration is known as the Michaelis–Menten equation:

$$v_o = \frac{V_{max}\,[S]}{K_m + [S]} \tag{15.1}$$

where V_{max} is the limiting value of the initial rate when all the active sites are occupied, K_m is the Michaelis constant, and [S] is the substrate concentration. At low substrate concentrations the occupancy of the active sites on the enzyme molecules is low and the reaction rate is directly related to the number of sites

Example 1 ENZYMATIC ASSAY OF GLUCOSE

Question

The concentration of glucose in a test solution was assayed using hexokinase and glucose-6-phosphate dehydrogenase. These enzymes in the presence of NAD^+ and Mg^{2+} convert glucose to glucono-1,5-lactone-6-phosphate. If an excess of NAD^+ and enzymes is used, the equilibrium reaction is displaced to the right and essentially goes to completion. A $1.0\,cm^3$ portion of the test solution was taken and to it was added $1.0\,cm^3$ of a solution containing excess NAD^+, the two enzymes and $MgCl_2$. The change in absorption at 340 nm was measured in a 1 cm cuvette over a period of time. A maximum absorption change of 0.61 was observed. What was the original concentration of glucose in the test solution given that the molar extinction coefficient of NADH is $6.22 \times 10^3\,(mol\,dm^{-3})^{-1}\,cm^{-1}$ at 340 nm?

Answer

By using excess NAD^+ and the two linked enzymes, all the glucose in the test solution would be consumed and the absorption at 340 nm would be a measure of the amount of NADH produced. This is the only reactant or product that absorbs at 340 nm and as it is stoichiometrically related to the consumption of glucose, its concentration can be calculated.

Applying the Beer–Lambert law (Section 12.4.1, equation 12.5):

$$A = \varepsilon_\lambda c l$$
$$0.61 = 6.22 \times 10^3 \times c \times 1$$

Therefore

$$c = \frac{0.61}{6.22 \times 10^3 \times 1} = 9.807 \times 10^{-5}\,M$$

However, the original test solution was diluted 1:1 when the reagents were mixed so that the original concentration must have been twice this calculated value, making the original test solution of glucose $1.96 \times 10^{-4}\,M$.

occupied. This approximates to first-order kinetics in that the rate is proportional to substrate concentration. At high substrate concentrations effectively all of the active sites are occupied and the reaction becomes independent of the substrate concentration, since no more enzyme–substrate complex, ES, can be formed and zero-order or saturation kinetics are observed. Under these conditions the reaction rate is dependent upon the conversion of the enzyme substrate complex to products and the diffusion of the products from the enzyme.

It can be seen from equation 15.1, that when $v_o = 0.5\,V_{max}$, $K_m = [S]$. Thus K_m is numerically equal to the substrate concentration at which the initial rate is one-half of the maximum rate (Fig. 15.5) and has units of molarity. Values of K_m are usually in the range 10^{-2} to $10^{-5}\,M$ and are important because they enable the concentration of substrate required to saturate all of the active sites of the enzyme in an enzyme assay to be calculated. When $[S] \gg K_m$, equation 15.1 reduces to $v_o \approx V_{max}$, but a simple calculation reveals that when $[S] = 10\,V_{max}$, v_o is only 90% V_{max} and that when $[S] = 100 K_m$, $v_o = 99\%\,V_{max}$. Appreciation of this relationship is vital in enzyme assays.

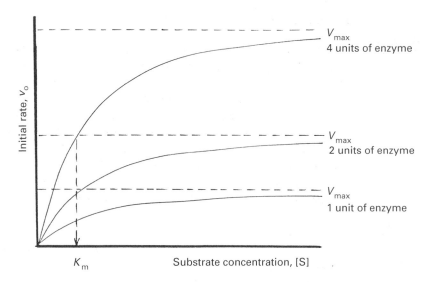

Fig. 15.5. The effect of substrate concentration on the initial rate of an enzyme-catalysed reaction in the presence of three different concentrations of enzyme. Doubling the enzyme concentration doubles the maximum initial rate, V_{max}, but has no effect on K_m.

As previously stated, enzyme-catalysed reactions proceed via the formation of an enzyme–substrate complex in which the substrate (S) is non-covalently bound to the active site of the enzyme (E). The formation of this complex for the majority of enzymes is rapid and reversible and is characterised by the dissociation constant, K_s, of the complex:

$$E + S \underset{k_{-1}}{\overset{k_{+1}}{\rightleftharpoons}} ES$$

where k_{+1} and k_{-1} are the rate constants for the forward and reverse reactions. At equilibrium, the rates of the forward and reverse reactions are equal and the law of mass action can be applied to the reversible process:

$$k_{+1}[E][S] = k_{-1}[ES]$$

hence:

$$K_s = \frac{[E][S]}{[ES]} = \frac{k_{-1}}{k_{+1}} = \frac{1}{K_a} \tag{15.2}$$

where K_a is the association (or affinity) constant.

It can be seen that when K_s is numerically large, the equilibrium is in favour of unbound E and S, i.e. of non-binding, whilst, when K_s is numerically small, the equilibrium is in favour of the formation of ES, i.e. of binding. Thus K_s is inversely proportional to the affinity of the enzyme for its substrate.

The conversion of ES to product (P) can be most simply represented by the irreversible equation:

$$\overset{k_{+2}}{\text{ES} \;\rightarrow\; \text{E} + \text{P}}$$

where k_{+2} is the first-order rate constant for the reaction.

In some cases the conversion of ES to E and P may involve several stages and may not necessarily be essentially irreversible. The rate constant k_{+2} is generally smaller than both k_{+1} and k_{-1} and in some cases very much smaller. In general, therefore, the conversion of ES to products is the rate-limiting step such that the concentration of ES is essentially constant but not necessarily the equilibrium concentration. Under these conditions the Michaelis constant, K_m, is given by:

$$K_m = \frac{k_{+2} + k_{-1}}{k_{+1}} = K_s + \frac{k_{+2}}{k_{+1}} \tag{15.3}$$

It is evident that, under these circumstances, K_m must be numerically larger than K_s and only when k_{+2} is very small do K_m and K_s approximately equal each other. The relationship between these two constants is further complicated by the fact that, for some enzyme reactions, two products are formed sequentially, each controlled by different rate constants:

$$\text{E} + \text{S} \;\rightleftharpoons\; \text{ES} \;\overset{k_{+2}}{\rightarrow}\; \text{P}_1 + \text{EA} \;\overset{k_{+3}}{\rightarrow}\; \text{E} + \text{P}_2$$

where P_1 and P_2 are products, and A is a metabolic product of S that is further metabolised to P_2.

In such circumstances it can be shown that:

$$K_m = K_s \frac{(k_{+3})}{(k_{+2} + k_{+3})} \tag{15.4}$$

so that K_m is numerically smaller than K_s. It is obvious therefore that care must be taken in the interpretation of the significance of K_m relative to K_s. Only when the complete reaction mechanism is known can the mathematical relationship between K_m and K_s be fully appreciated and any statement made about the relationship between K_m and the affinity of the enzyme for its substrate.

Although the Michaelis–Menten equation can be used to calculate K_m and V_{max}, its use is subject to error owing to the difficulty of experimentally measuring initial rates at high substrate concentrations and hence of extrapolating the hyperbolic curve to give an accurate value of V_{max}. Linear transformations of the Michaelis–Menten equation are therefore preferred. The most popular of these is the Lineweaver–Burk equation, obtained by taking the reciprocal of the Michaelis–Menten equation:

$$\frac{1}{v_o} = \frac{K_m}{V_{max}} \times \frac{1}{[S]} + \frac{1}{V_{max}} \tag{15.5}$$

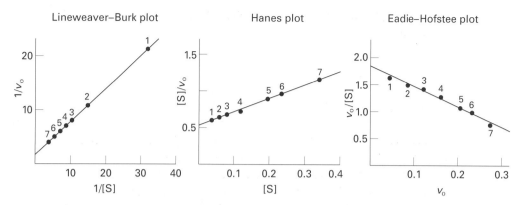

Fig. 15.6. Lineweaver–Burk, Hanes and Eadie–Hofstee plots for the same set of experimental data of the effect of substrate concentration, [S], on the initial rate, v_o of an enzyme-catalysed reaction.

A plot of $1/v_o$ against $1/[S]$ gives a straight line of slope K_m/V_{max}, with an intercept on the $1/v_o$ axis of $1/V_{max}$ and an intercept on the $1/[S]$ axis of $-1/K_m$. Alternative plots are based on the Hanes equation:

$$\frac{[S]}{v_o} = \frac{K_m}{V_{max}} + \frac{[S]}{V_{max}} \tag{15.6}$$

so that $[S]/v_o$ is plotted against $[S]$, and on the Eadie–Hofstee equation:

$$\frac{v_o}{[S]} = \frac{V_{max}}{K_m} - \frac{v_o}{K_m} \tag{15.7}$$

so that $v_o/[S]$ is plotted against v_o. The relative merits of the Lineweaver–Burk, Hanes and Eadie–Hofstee equations for the determination of K_m and V_{max} are illustrated in Fig. 15.6 using the same set of experimental values of v_o for a series of substrate concentrations (for further details, see Example 2).

It can be seen that the Lineweaver–Burk equation gives an unequal distribution of points and greater emphasis to the points at low substrate concentration that are subject to the greatest experimental error, whilst the Eadie–Hofstee equation and the Hanes equation give a better distribution of points. In the case of the Hanes plot, greater emphasis is placed on the experimental data at higher substrate concentrations and on balance it is the statistically preferred plot.

It is of course possible for two enzymes to have an affinity for the same substrate and, indeed, to have the same V_{max} value at a given enzyme concentration. If the two K_m values differ, however, the Michaelis–Menten plots will be different. This is shown in Fig. 15.7, which illustrates a concept that is important in the determination of the relative importance of branching in metabolic pathways. The same principle applies to the case where a given enzyme can act on two different substrates with different K_m values but the same or different V_{max} values. The reaction with the numerically smaller K_m value will be preferred at low substrate concentrations.

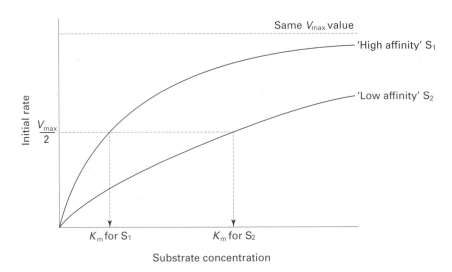

Fig. 15.7. The effect of the Michaelis constant, K_m, on the kinetic profile of an enzyme acting on two different substrates, S_1 and S_2. At low substrate concentrations the high affinity substrate will be the preferred substrate.

It is important to appreciate that, whilst K_m is a characteristic of an enzyme for its substrate and is independent of the amount of enzyme used for its experimental determination, this is not true of V_{max}. It has no absolute value but varies with the amount of enzyme used. This is illustrated in Fig. 15.5 and is discussed further in the Example 2. A valuable catalytic constant in addition to K_m and V_{max} is the turnover number, k_{cat}, defined as:

$$k_{cat} = \frac{V_{max}}{[E_t]} \qquad (15.8)$$

where $[E_t]$ is the total concentration of enzyme. The turnover number is the maximum number of moles of substrate that can be converted to product per mole of enzyme in unit time. It has units of reciprocal time in seconds. Its values range from 1 to $10^7\,s^{-1}$. Catalase has a turnover number of $4 \times 10^7\,s^{-1}$ and is one of the most efficient enzymes known. The catalytic potential of high turnover numbers can be realised only at high (saturating) substrate concentrations and this is seldom achieved under normal cellular conditions. An alternative constant, termed the specificity constant, defined as k_{cat}/K_m, is a measure of how efficiently an enzyme converts substrate to product at low substrate concentrations. It has units of $(mol\,dm^{-3})^{-1}s^{-1}$.

For a substrate to be converted to product, molecules of the substrate and of the enzyme must first collide by random diffusion and then combine in the correct orientation. Diffusion and collision have a theoretical limiting value of about $10^9(mol\,dm^{-3})^{-1}s^{-1}$ and yet many enzymes, including acetylcholine esterase, carbonic anhydrase, catalase, β-lactamase and triosephosphate isomerase, have specificity constants approaching this value, indicating that they have evolved to almost maximum kinetic efficiency. Since specificity constants

Example 2   **PRACTICAL ENZYME KINETICS**

Question

The enzyme α-D-glucosidase isolated from *Saccharomyces cerevisiae* was studied using the synthetic substrate *p*-nitrophenyl-α-D-glucopyranoside (PNPG), which is hydrolysed to release *p*-nitrophenol, which is yellow in alkaline solution (for further details, see Section 15.2.2). A 3 mM solution of PNPG was prepared and portions used to study the effect of substrate concentration on initial rate using a fixed volume of enzyme preparation. The total volume of each assay mixture was 10 cm^3. A 1 cm^3 sample of the reaction mixture was withdrawn after 2 min, placed in 4 cm^3 borate buffer, pH 9.0, to stop the reaction and develop the yellow colour. The change in absorbance at 400 nm was determined and used as a measure of the initial rate. The following results were obtained:

PNPG (cm^3)	0.1	0.2	0.3	0.4	0.6	0.8	1.2
Initial rate	0.055	0.094	0.130	0.157	0.196	0.230	0.270

What kinetic constants can be obtained from this data?

Answer

Subject to the calculation of the molar concentration of PNPG in each reaction mixture, it is possible to construct Lineweaver–Burk, Hanes and Eadie–Hofstee plots to obtain the values of K_m and V_{max}. The fact that a 1 cm^3 sample of the reaction mixture was used to measure the initial rate is not relevant to the calculation of [S]. Lineweaver–Burk, Hanes and Eadie–Hofstee plots derived from this data are shown in Fig. 15.6 in which v_o measurements are expressed simply as the increase in absorption at 400 nm. The plots give K_m values of approximately 0.2 mM and V_{max} values of approximately 0.4.

As pointed out in Section 15.3.1, V_{max} values can be expressed in a variety of units and their experimental value is dependent on a number of variables, particularly the concentration of enzyme. For comparative reasons, V_{max} is best expressed in terms of the number of moles of product formed in unit time. To do this, it is necessary to convert absorbance units to amount of product by means of a Beer–Lambert law plot. Data for such a plot in this experiment is given in Table A.

Table A

[PNP] (μM)	2.0	4.0	6.0	8.0	12.0	16.0	24.0
Absorbance (400 nm)	0.065	0.118	0.17	0.23	0.34	0.45	0.65

A plot of these data confirms that the Beer–Lambert law is held and enables the amount of product to be calculated. From this, v_o values in units of $\mu \text{mol min}^{-1}$ can be calculated. The data for the three linear plots are presented in Table B.

Table B

[S] (mM)	0.03	0.06	0.09	0.12	0.18	0.24	0.36
$v_o \, (\mu \text{mol min}^{-1})$	0.054	0.096	0.138	0.168	0.210	0.251	0.294
$1/[S] \, (\text{mM})^{-1}$	33.33	16.67	11.11	8.33	5.55	4.17	2.78
$1/v_o \, (\mu \text{mol min}^{-1})^{-1}$	18.52	10.42	7.25	5.95	4.76	3.98	3.40
$v_o/[S] \times 10^3 \, (\text{dm}^3 \text{min}^{-1})$	1.8	1.6	1.53	1.40	1.17	1.05	0.82
$[S]/v_o \times 10^{-3} (\text{min dm}^{-3})$	0.56	0.63	0.65	0.71	0.85	0.95	1.22

Example 2 (*Cont.*)

Data derived from the three linear plots are presented in Table C.

Table C

Plot	Regression coefficient	Slope	Intercept	K_m (mM)	V_{max} (μmol min^{-1})
Lineweaver–Burk	0.9997	0.499	1.91	0.26	0.52
Hanes	0.9970	1.990	0.489	0.25	0.50
Eadie–Hofstee	0.9930	−3.995	2.030	0.25	0.51

The agreement between the three plots for the values of K_m and V_{max} was good but the quality of the fitted regression line for the Lineweaver–Burk plot was noticeably better. However, the distribution of the experimental points along the line is the poorest for this plot (Fig. 15.6). The value for V_{max} indicates the amount of product released per minute, but of course this is for the chosen amount of enzyme and is for 10 cm^3 of reaction mixture. For V_{max} to have any absolute value, the amount of enzyme and the volume of reaction mixture have to be taken into account. The volume can be adjusted to 1 dm^3 giving a V_{max} of 51 μmol min^{-1}dm^{-3}, but it is only possible to correct for the enzyme amount if it was pure and of a known amount in molar terms. The enzyme is known to have a molecular mass of 68 kDa so, if there were 3 μg of pure enzyme in each 10 cm^3 reaction mixture, its molar concentration would be $4.4 \times 10^{-3}\,\mu$M. This allows the value of the turnover number k_{cat} to be calculated (see equation 15.8):

$$k_{cat} = V_{max}/[E_t] = 51\ \mu\text{mol min}^{-1}\text{dm}^{-3}/4.4 \times 10^{-3}\,\mu\text{mol dm}^{-3}$$
$$= 11 \times 10^3\,\text{min}^{-1}\text{ or } 1.8 \times 10^2\text{s}^{-1}$$

k_{cat} is a measure of the number of molecules of substrate (PNPG in this case) converted to product per second by the enzyme under the defined experimental conditions. The value of 1.8×10^2 is in the mid-range for the majority of enzymes. It is also possible to calculate the specificity constant that is a measure of the efficiency with which the enzyme converts substrate to product at low (K_m) substrate concentrations:

$$k_{cat}/K_m = 1.8 \times 10^2\text{s}^{-1}/0.25\ \text{mM} = 7.2 \times 10^3\,(\text{mM})^{-1}\text{s}^{-1}\text{ or } 7.2 \times 10^5\,(\text{mM})^{-1}\text{s}^{-1}$$

Note that the units of the specificity constant are that of a second-order rate constant, effectively for the conversion of E + S to E + P. Its value in this case is typical of many enzymes.

are a ratio of two other constants, enzymes with similar specificity constants can have widely different K_m values. As an example, catalase has a specificity constant of 4×10^7 (mol dm^{-3})$^{-1}$s^{-1} with a K_m of 1.1 M (very high), whilst fumarase has a specificity constant of 3.6×10^7 (M)$^{-1}$s^{-1} with a K_m of 2.5×10^{-5}M (very low). Multienzyme complexes overcome some of the diffusion and collision limitations to specificity constants. The product of one reaction is passed directly by a process called channelling to the active site of the next enzyme in the pathway

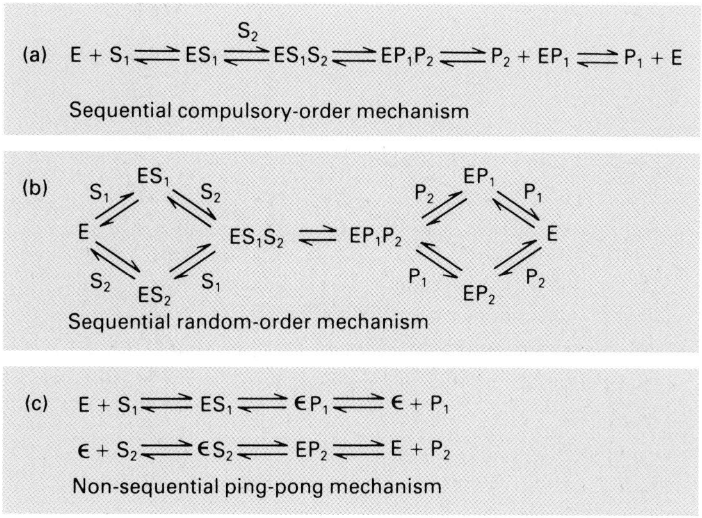

Fig. 15.8. Possible reaction mechanisms for bisubstrate reactions.

as a consequence of its juxtaposition in the complex, thereby eliminating diffusion limitations (Section 15.4.7).

15.3.2 Bisubstrate enzyme reactions

Bisubstrate reactions (Fig. 15.8) such as those catalysed by the transferases, kinases and dehydrogenases, in which two substrates S_1 and S_2 are converted to two products P_1 and P_2 (two substrate, two product, bi-bi, reactions), are inherently more complicated than monosubstrate reactions in that they may be as follows:

- *Sequential:* In this case both substrates bind at specific regions within the enzyme active site to give a ternary complex before the products are formed. Sequential reactions may be either compulsory ordered, in which case the two substrates bind in a definite sequence, or random ordered, in which case either substrate can bind first.
- *Non-sequential:* In this case one product is released before the second substrate is bound.

A compulsory-order and a random-order ternary complex mechanism both give non-parallel Lineweaver–Burk double reciprocal plots with a progressively smaller intercept on the $1/v_0$ axis as the concentration of fixed second substrate is increased (Fig. 15.8b).

An example of the non-sequential mechanism is a ping-pong reaction, which proceeds via a modified form of the enzyme (ε) that may take the form of an acylated enzyme. A ping-pong mechanism is indicated, but not confirmed, by a series of parallel lines in Lineweaver–Burk double reciprocal plots when the variation of initial rate with increasing concentration of one substrate is investigated in the

(a)

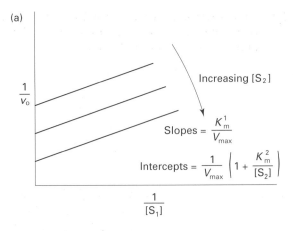

(b)

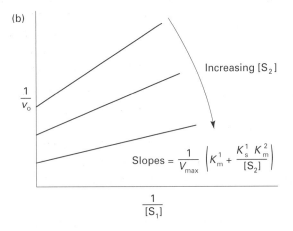

Fig. 15.9. Lineweaver–Burk plots for bisubstrate reactions. (a) For a ping-pong bi-bi mechanism, a series of parallel plots is obtained. (b) For a random or ordered bi-bi mechanism a series of plots that converge to the left of the x-axis is obtained. K_m^1 and K_m^2 are the Michaelis constants for substrates S_1 and S_2, respectively. K_s^1 is the dissociation constant for ES_1.

presence of a series of fixed concentrations of the second substrate. Double reciprocal plots give a progressively smaller intercept on the 1/[S] axis as the concentration of second substrate is increased (Fig. 15.8a).

In these bisubstrate reactions, V_{max} is defined as the maximum initial rate when both substrates are saturating, and the K_m for a particular substrate as the concentration of that substrate which gives $0.5 V_{max}$ when the other substrate is saturating. To determine these K_m values, the initial velocity is studied as a function of the concentration of one substrate at a series of fixed second substrate concentrations. A double reciprocal plot is made for each second substrate concentration, giving a series of straight lines called primary plots (Fig. 15.9). A secondary plot is then made

Table 15.1 **Patterns of product inhibition to distinguish sequential bisubstrate mechanisms for the conversion of two substrates, S_1 and S_2, to two products, P_1 and P_2**

Mechanism	Product	S_1 variable	S_2 variable
Ordered bi-bi	P_1	Mixed	Mixed
	P_2	Competitive	Mixed
Random bi-bi	P_1	Competitive	Competitive
	P_2	Competitive	Competitive

of the $1/v_0$ intercepts of the primary Lineweaver–Burk plots against the reciprocal of the second (fixed) substrate. This gives a straight line, slope K_m (for the second substrate)/V_{max} and intercept $1/V_{max}$. This study is then repeated reversing the roles of the two substrates. The principle of secondary plots is illustrated in Fig. 15.15.

The elucidation of the reaction mechanism associated with a particular bisubstrate reaction generally involves a study of the variation of the initial rate with the concentration of one substrate at a series of fixed concentrations of the second substrate, in the absence and presence of the two reaction products, and the application of a series of rules formulated by W. Cleland. Two of these rules are that:

- the intercept on the $1/v_0$ axis of double reciprocal plots is affected by an inhibitor only if it binds reversibly to an enzyme form other than that to which the variable substrate binds;
- the slope of double reciprocal plots is affected by an inhibitor that binds to the same enzyme form as the variable substrate or to an enzyme form that is connected by a series of reversible steps to that to which the variable substrate binds.

The consequence of the first rule is that, if characteristic competitive inhibition (Section 15.3.7) behaviour is observed, the inhibitor and the substrate whose concentration is being varied bind at the same site. The consequence of the second rule is that, if characteristic uncompetitive inhibition (Section 15.3.7) is observed, there must be no reversible link between the inhibitor and the substrate whose concentration is being varied (Table 15.1).

Studies applying these rules have, for example, revealed that lactate dehydrogenase operates via a compulsory-order mechanism in which the NAD^+ binds first whereas phosphoglycerate mutase from yeast or mammalian sources (but not plant), which interconverts 2-phospho-D-glycerate (2PG) and 3-phospho-D-glycerate (3PG), operates via a ping-pong mechanism involving 2,3-bisphospho-D-glycerate (BPG) as a primer and a phosphorylated enzyme intermediate:

$$E + BPG \rightleftharpoons E\text{--}P + 2PG$$
$$E\text{-}P + 3PG \rightleftharpoons E + BPG$$

Net reaction:

$$3PG \rightleftharpoons 2PG$$

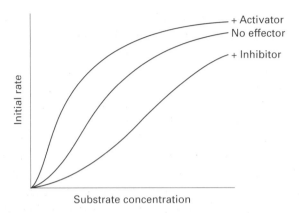

Fig. 15.10. Effect of activators and inhibitors on the sigmoidal kinetics of an enzyme subject to allosteric control.

15.3.3 **Oligomeric enzyme reactions**

A number of enzymes contain several protein subunits, which may be identical or different, and multiple catalytic sites. Such enzymes are said to be oligomeric and some do not display simple Michaelis–Menten kinetics, but give a sigmoidal relationship between initial rate and substrate concentration (Fig. 15.10). Such a curve is indicative of an allosteric enzyme, which is one whose catalytic activity is modified by conformational changes induced in the enzyme. In cases where these conformational changes are the result of the progressive binding of substrate molecules, the process is referred to as a homotropic effect. These conformational changes are initiated in one subunit but are transmitted to others, thereby altering the ease of binding of further substrate molecules. Progressive binding of the substrate molecules to the subunits is therefore said to be cooperative. This cooperativity may result in either increased (positive cooperativity) or decreased (negative cooperativity) activity towards the binding of further substrate molecules. Changes in catalytic activity towards the substrate may also be brought about by conformational changes induced by the binding of molecules other than the substrate at distinct allosteric binding sites on one or more subunit. Compounds that induce such changes are referred to as heterotropic effectors. They are commonly key metabolic intermediates such as ATP, ADP, AMP and P_i that, on binding to the allosteric site, change the conformation of the catalytic site. Heterotropic activators increase the catalytic activity of the enzyme, making the curve less sigmoidal and moving it to the left, whilst heterotropic inhibitors cause a decrease in activity, making the curve more sigmoidal and moving it to the right (Fig. 15.10). The diagnosis of cooperativity by use of the Lineweaver–Burk plot is shown in Fig. 15.14c. The operation of cooperative effects may be confirmed by a Hill plot, which is based on the equation:

$$\frac{\log v_o}{V_{max} - v_o} = h \log [S] + \log K \tag{15.9}$$

where h is the Hill constant or coefficient, and K is an overall binding constant related to the individual binding constants for n sites.

The Hill constant, which is equal to the slope of the plot, is a measure of the cooperativity between the sites such that: if $h = 1$, binding is non-cooperative and normal Michaelis–Menten kinetics exist; if $h > 1$, binding is positively cooperative; and if $h < 1$, binding is negatively cooperative. At very low substrate concentrations that are insufficient to fill more than one site and at high concentrations at which most of the binding sites are occupied, the slopes of Hill plots tend to a value of 1. The Hill coefficient is therefore taken from the linear central portion of the plot. One of the problems with Hill plots is the difficulty of estimating V_{max} accurately. It is sometimes argued that h is numerically equal to the number of binding sites, n, for the substrate. This is an oversimplification and very often h is not an integer. For example, h for the binding of oxygen to haemoglobin, for which the number of binding sites is known to be four, is 2.6. In practice, h can be taken to be a minimum estimate of the number of interacting binding sites as well as a measure of the cooperativity.

The Michaelis constant K_m is not used with allosteric enzymes. Instead, the term $S_{0.5}$, which is the substrate concentration required to produce 50% saturation of the enzyme, is used. It is important to appreciate that sigmoidal kinetics do not confirm the operation of allosteric effects because sigmoidicity may be the consequence of the enzyme preparation containing more than one enzyme capable of acting on the substrate. It is easy to establish the presence of more than one enzyme, as there will be a discrepancy between the amount of substrate consumed and the expected amount of product produced.

Models of allosterism

Several models have been proposed to interpret allosteric regulation. They are all based on the assumption that the allosteric enzyme consists of a number of subunits (protomers) each of which can bind substrate and exist in two conformations referred to as the R (relaxed) and T (tense) states. It is assumed that the substrate binds more tightly to the R form. One of the most successful models, proposed by Jacques Monod, Jeffries Wyman and Jean-Pierre Changeux, is the symmetry model. It assumes that conformational change between the R and T states is highly coupled so that all subunits must exist in the same conformation. Thus binding of substrate to a T state protomer, causing it to change conformation to the R state, will automatically switch the other protomers to the R form, thereby enhancing reactivity (Fig. 15.11). The alternative induced-fit or sequential model of Daniel Koshland does not assume the tightly coupled concept and hence allows protomers to exist in different conformations but in such a way that binding to one protomer enhances the reactivity of others. Conformational changes in a protein can be studied by spectroscopic and sedimentation techniques but X-ray crystallography gives the most clear-cut evidence. Thus the enzyme aspartate carbamoyltransferase, which catalyses the first step in pyrimidine biosynthesis in *Escherichia coli*, has been shown by crystallography to display many of the characteristics of the symmetry model. In this case, CTP acts as an allosteric activator and ATP as an allosteric inhibitor.

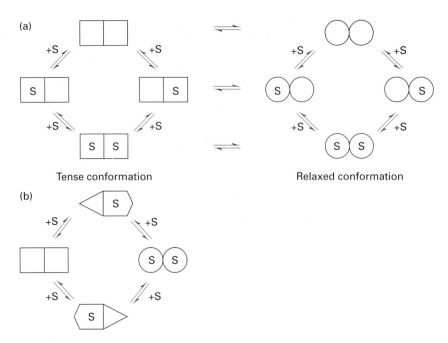

Fig. 15.11. Symmetry and sequential models of allosterism for a dimeric enzyme.
(a) Symmetry model. The enzyme is assumed to exist in two conformations T and R, which differ in their affinity for the substrate. Conformational changes within each subunit (protomer) are assumed to be tightly coupled so that each can exist only in the same conformation. The binding of the substrate disturbs the equilibrium between the T and R states in favour of the R state, giving a concerted structure change such that the symmetry of the enzyme is preserved. Note that the model cannot explain how binding of a substrate molecule to one protomer decreases the affinity of the other protomer for the substrate, i.e. negative cooperativity. (b) Sequential model. Substrate binding to one protomer induces a change in its conformation and a cooperative interaction with the neighbouring protomer such that its reactivity towards substrate binding may be either enhanced (positive cooperativity) or decreased (negative cooperativity). The structure of individual protomers changes sequentially. Unlike the symmetry model, the sequential model does not preserve the symmetry of the enzyme during substrate binding.

An example of an enzyme displaying allosteric regulation is 6-phosphofructo-kinase (PFK), the key regulatory enzyme of glycolysis:

$$\text{D-fructose-6-phosphate} + \text{ATP} \xrightleftharpoons[\quad]{\text{PFK}} \text{D-fructose 1,6-bisphosphate} + \text{ADP}$$

PFK is a tetramer in most organisms but exists as an octomer in yeasts. It can exist in two states consistent with the Koshland model (see below). Each subunit has a catalytic site and an allosteric inhibitor site for ATP. The catalytic site binds ATP in both the R and T states but the allosteric site binds only ATP in the T state. At low concentrations ATP is a substrate but at higher concentrations it acts as an inhibitor by binding to the T state and as a consequence reducing the affinity for the other substrate, fructose 6-phosphate, and reducing the rate of the glycolytic pathway. The enzyme is also inhibited by citrate and phosphoenol pyruvate but activated by ADP, P_i, AMP and fructose 2,6-bisphosphate. These activators preferentially bind to the R state thus releasing the ATP inhibition. The balance between activation and inhibition is determined by the relative availability of these effectors. These effects are readily rationalised in terms of cellular energy demands and the associated need for the glycolytic pathway to be activated or inhibited. The control of PFK activity is discussed further in Section 15.5.2.

15.3.4 Effect of enzyme concentration

It can be shown that for monosubstrate enzymatic reactions that obey simple Michaelis–Menten kinetics:

$$v_0 = \frac{k_{+2}[E][S]}{K_m + [S]}$$

and hence that

$$v_0 = \frac{k_{+2}[E]}{K_m/[S] + 1} \tag{15.10}$$

Thus, when the substrate concentration is very large, equation 15.10 reduces to $v_0 = k_{+2}[E]$, i.e. the initial rate is directly proportional to the enzyme concentration. This is the basis of the experimental determination of enzyme activity in a particular biological sample (Section 15.2). Fig. 15.3 illustrates the importance of the correct measurement of initial rate.

15.3.5 Effect of temperature

The initial rate of an enzyme reaction varies with temperature according to the Arrhenius equation:

$$\text{rate} = A\,e^{-E/RT} \tag{15.11}$$

where A is a constant known as the pre-exponential factor, which is related to the frequency with which molecules of the enzyme and substrate collide in the correct orientation to produce the enzyme–substrate complex, E is the activation energy ($J\,mol^{-1}$), R is the gas constant ($8.2\,J\,mol^{-1}\,K^{-1}$), and T is the absolute temperature (K). Thus a plot of the natural logarithm of the initial rate (or better k_{cat}) against the reciprocal of the absolute temperature allows the value of E to be determined. Equation 15.11 explains the sensitivity of enzyme reactions to temperature as the relationship between reaction rate and absolute temperature is exponential. The rate of most enzyme reactions approximately doubles for every 10 deg.C rise in temperature (Q_{10} value). At a temperature characteristic of the enzyme, and generally in the region 40–70°C, the enzyme is denatured and enzyme activity is lost. The activity displayed in this 40–70°C temperature range depends partly upon the equilibration time before the reaction is commenced. The so-called optimum temperature, at which the enzyme appears to have maximum activity, therefore arises from a mixture of thermal stability, temperature coefficient and incubation time

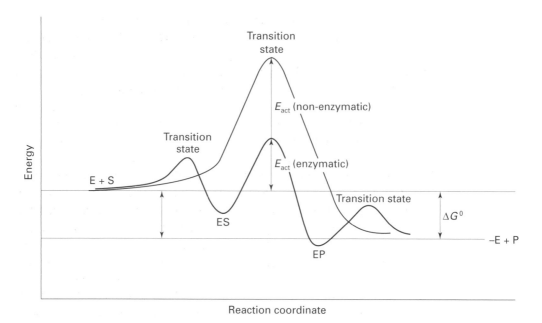

Fig. 15.12. Energy profile of a simple enzyme-catalysed reaction. The formation of ES and EP and the subsequent release of E + P proceeds via several transition states. The activation energy for the overall reaction is dictated by the initial free energy of E and S and the highest energy transition state. The non-enzyme-catalysed reaction proceeds via a higher energy transition state and hence the reaction has a higher activation energy than the enzyme-catalysed reaction.

and for this reason is not normally chosen for the study of enzyme activity. Enzyme assays are routinely carried out at 30 or 37 °C (Section 15.2). Interestingly, recent work with enzymes from mesophiles and thermophiles has indicated that some have a genuine temperature optimum in that above a certain temperature the enzyme becomes reversibly less active but not as a consequence of denaturation. The nature of the structural changes responsible for such observations has yet to be determined.

Enzymes work by facilitating the formation of the transition state, thereby decreasing the activation energy for the reaction relative to the non-enzyme catalysed reaction (Fig. 15.12). A decrease in the energy barrier of as little as 5.7 kJ mol^{-1}, equivalent in energy terms to a hydrogen bond, will result in a 10-fold increase in reaction rate. The energy barrier is, of course, lowered equally for both the forward and reverse reactions, so that the position of equilibrium is unchanged. As an extreme example of the efficiency of enzyme catalysis, the enzyme catalase decomposes hydrogen peroxide 10^{14} times faster than does the uncatalysed reaction! Fig. 15.12 shows a simple energy profile for the conversion of a substrate to products as a function of the reaction coordinate that measures the time-related progress of the reaction. The number of energy barriers in the profile will depend upon the number of kinetically important stages in the reactions. For the majority of enzyme-catalysed reactions the major energy barrier, which dictates the activation energy for the reaction and hence its rate, is the formation of one or more transition states, in which covalent bonds are being made and broken and which cannot be isolated. An example is shown in Figure 15.17. However, for a few enzymes, notably ATP synthase, the energy-requiring step is the initial binding of the substrate(s) and the subsequent release of the product(s).

Proof that enzymes function by facilitating the creation of the transition state has come from the development of transition state analogues, which mimic the structure of the transition state. For example, the transition state for the esterase hydrolysis of carboxylic acid esters is a tetrahedral intermediate that is mimicked by a phosphonate ester with similar substituents (Fig. 15.13). If a monoclonal anti-body is raised to an antigen consisting of the phosphonate ester as the hapten (Section 7.2.2), one of the antibodies raised will be complementary to the tetra-hedral phosphonate ester intermediate and will effectively behave as the active site of the esterase. Proof of this ability was confirmed by the ability of the antibody to convert the ester to products in the absence of esterase at an enhanced rate (by factor of up to 10^5) relative to the uncatalysed reaction. The success of these studies lay in using the optimum structures for R and R′. Antibodies with this ability to promote catalysis have been called catalytic antibodies or simply abzymes (antibodies as enzymes) or mabzymes (monoclonal antibodies as enzymes).

The thermodynamic constants ΔG^0, ΔH^0 and ΔS^0 for the binding of substrate to the enzyme can be calculated from a knowledge of the binding constant, K_a (= $1/K_s$). ΔG^0 can be obtained from the equation:

$$\Delta G^0 = -RT \ln K_a \tag{15.12}$$

If K_a is measured as a function of temperature, a plot of $\ln K_a$ versus $1/T$, known as the van't Hoff plot, will give a straight line of slope $-\Delta H^0/R$ with intercept on the y-axis of $\Delta S^0/R$, the relevant equation being:

$$\ln K_a = \frac{\Delta S^0}{R} - \frac{\Delta H^0}{RT} \tag{15.13}$$

Recent research has indicated that a small number of enzymes may operate by a mechanism that does not rely on the formation of a transition state. Work with the enzyme methylamine dehydrogenase, which promotes the cleavage of a C−H bond, has shown that the reaction is independent of temperature and hence is inconsistent with transition state theory. The observation is explained in terms of enzyme-catalysed quantum tunnelling. Under this mechanism, rather than overcoming the potential energy barrier the reaction proceeds through (hence 'tunnelling') the barrier at an energy level near to that of the ground state of the reactants. Concerted enzyme and substrate vibrations are coupled in such a way as to reduce the width and height of the potential energy barrier and facilitate the cleavage of the C−H bond by the process of quantum mechanical tunnelling. This phenomenon is known to occur with some chemical reactions but only at low temperatures. The fine detail of precisely how enzymes promote this process remains to be elucidated.

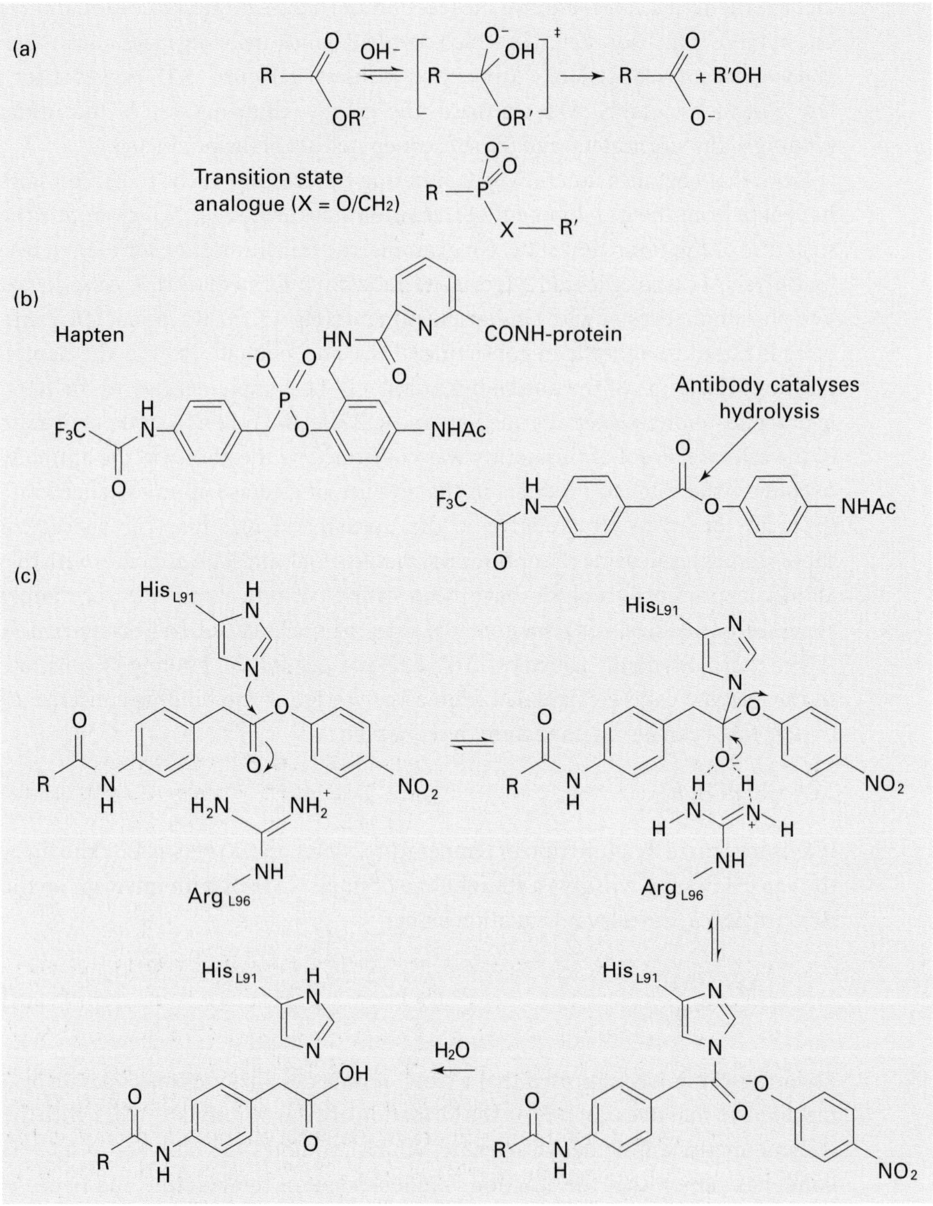

Fig. 15.13. Catalytic antibodies for ester hydrolysis. (a) The catalytic mechanism for ester hydrolysis involves a tetrahedral transition state. (b) The catalytic antibody is based on a hapten containing a tetrahedral organophosphorus compound resembling the ester transition state. The antibody raised against the hapten will contain a structural component complementary to the hapten and hence capable of binding an appropriate ester and facilitating the formation of the transition state. (c) The antibody 43C9 has been shown to promote ester hydrolysis by an acid-catalysed mechanism similar in principle to that of ribonuclease A (see Fig 15.17). (Reproduced from T. Bugg (2004), *An Introduction to Enzyme and Coenzyme Chemistry*, 2nd edn, by permission of Blackwell Science Limited.)

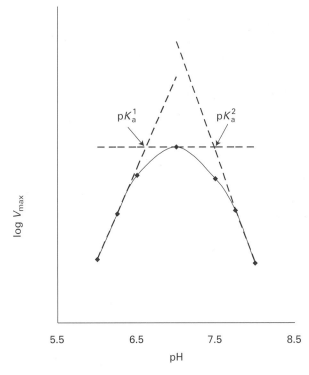

Fig. 15.14. The effect of pH on V_{max} of an enzyme-catalysed reaction involving two ionisable groups in the active site of the enzyme. The construction of tangents to the experimental line allows the pK_a values of the ionisable groups to be estimated.

15.3.6 Effect of pH

The state of ionisation of amino acid residues in the catalytic site of an enzyme is pH dependent. Since catalytic activity relies on a specific state of ionisation of these residues, enzyme activity is also pH dependent. As a consequence, plots of $\log K_m$ and $\log V_{max}$ (or better, k_{cat}) against pH are either bell shaped (indicating two important ionisable amino acid residues in the active site), giving a narrow pH optimum, or have a plateau (one important ionisable amino acid residue in the active site). In either case, the enzyme is generally studied at a pH at which its activity is maximal. By studying the variation of $\log K_m$ and $\log V_{max}$ with pH, it is possible to identify the pK_a values of key amino acid residues involved in the binding and catalytic processes (Fig. 15.14).

15.3.7 Effect of enzyme inhibitors

Irreversible inhibition

An enzyme inhibitor binds to an enzyme in such a way as to reduce the ability of the enzyme to either bind substrate and/or convert it to product. Irreversible inhibitors, such as the organophosphorus and organomercury compounds, cyanide, carbon monoxide and hydrogen sulphide, combine with the enzyme to form a covalent bond. The extent of their inhibition of the enzyme is dependent upon the reaction rate constant (and hence time) for covalent bond formation and upon the amount of inhibitor present. The effect of irreversible inhibitors, which cannot be removed by simple physical techniques such as dialysis, is to reduce the amount of enzyme available for reaction. The inhibition involves reactions with a functional group, such as hydroxyl or sulphydryl, or with a metal atom in the active site or a distinct allosteric site. Thus the organophosphorus compound, diisopropylphosphofluoridate, reacts with a serine group in the active site of esterases such as acetylcholinesterase, whilst the organomercury compound p-hydroxymercuribenzoate reacts with a cysteine group, in both cases resulting in covalent bond formation and enzyme inhibition. Such inhibitors are valuable in the study of enzyme active sites (Section 15.4.2).

Competitive reversible inhibition

Reversible inhibitors combine non-covalently with the enzyme and can therefore be readily removed by dialysis. Competitive reversible inhibitors combine at the same site as the substrate and must therefore be structurally related to the substrate. An example is the inhibition of succinate dehydrogenase by malonate:

CH$_2$COOH   CH$_2$COOH
| |
CH$_2$COOH   COOH

succinic acid (substrate)   malonic acid (inhibitor)

‖ succinate dehydrogenase   ‖

CHCOOH   no reaction
‖
CHCOOH

fumaric acid (product)

All types of reversible inhibitors are characterised by their dissociation constant K_i, called the inhibitor constant, which may relate to the dissociation of EI (K_{EI}) or of ESI (K_{ESI}), where I is the inhibitor. For competitive inhibition the following two equations can be written:

E + S $\rightleftharpoons$ ES $\rightarrow$ E + P

E + I $\rightleftharpoons$ EI $\rightarrow$ no reaction

Since the binding of both substrate and inhibitor involves the same site, the effect of a competitive reversible inhibitor can be overcome by increasing the substrate concentration. The result is that V_{max} is unaltered but the concentration of substrate required to achieve it is increased so that when $v_o = 0.5 V_{max}$ then:

$$[S] = \frac{K_m (1 + [I])}{K_i} \tag{15.14}$$

where [I] is the concentration of inhibitor.

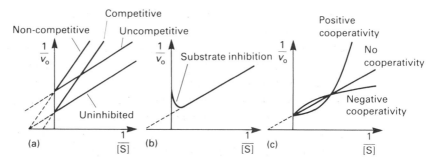

Fig. 15.15. Lineweaver–Burk plots showing (a) the effects of three types of reversible inhibitor, (b) substrate inhibition, and (c) homotropic cooperativity.

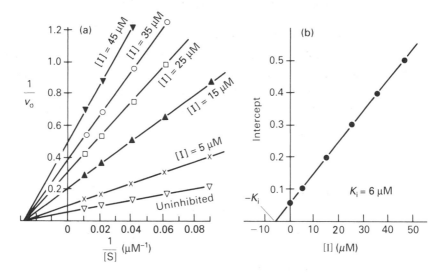

Fig. 15.16. (a) Primary Lineweaver–Burk plots showing the effect of a simple linear non-competitive inhibitor at a series of concentrations and (b) the corresponding secondary plot that enables the inhibitor constant K_i to be calculated.

It can be seen from equation 15.14 that K_i is equal to the concentration of inhibitor that apparently doubles the value of K_m. With this type of inhibition, K_i is equal to K_{EI} whilst K_{ESI} is infinite because no ESI is formed. In the presence of a competitive inhibitor, the Lineweaver–Burk equation (15.5) becomes:

$$\frac{1}{v_o} = \frac{K_m}{V_{max}} \times \frac{1}{[S]} \frac{(1+[I])}{(K_i)} + \frac{1}{V_{max}} \tag{15.15}$$

Application of this equation allows the diagnosis of competitive inhibition (Fig. 15.15a). The numerical value of K_i can be calculated from Lineweaver–Burk plots for the uninhibited and inhibited reactions. In practice, however, a more accurate value is obtained from a secondary plot (Fig. 15.16). The reaction is carried out for a range of substrate concentrations in the presence of a series of fixed inhibitor concentrations and a Lineweaver–Burk plot for each inhibitor concentration constructed. Secondary plots of the slope of the primary plot against the inhibitor concentration or of the apparent K_m, (K'_m) (which is equal to $K_m \{(1 + [I])/K_i\}$ and which can be calculated from the reciprocal of the negative intercept on the I/[S] axis) against inhibitor concentration, will both have intercepts on the inhibitor concentration axis, of $-K_i$. Sometimes it is possible for two molecules of inhibitor to bind at the active site. In these cases, although all the primary double reciprocal plots are linear, the secondary plot is parabolic. This is referred to as parabolic competitive inhibition to distinguish it from normal linear competitive inhibition.

Non-competitive reversible inhibition

A non-competitive reversible inhibitor combines at a site distinct from that for the substrate. Whilst the substrate can still bind to its catalytic site, resulting in the formation of a ternary complex ESI, the complex is unable to convert the substrate to product and is referred to as a dead-end complex. Since this inhibition involves a site distinct from the catalytic site, the inhibition cannot be overcome by increasing the substrate concentration. The consequence is that V_{max}, but not K_m, is reduced because the inhibitor does not affect the binding of substrate but it does reduce the amount of free ES that can proceed to the formation of product. With this type of inhibition, K_{EI} and K_{ESI} are identical and K_i is numerically equal to both of them. In this case the Lineweaver–Burk equation (15.5) becomes:

$$\frac{1}{v_o} = \frac{K_{m-}}{V_{max}} \times \frac{1}{[S]} + \frac{1}{V_{max}} \left(\frac{1 + [I]}{K_i} \right) \tag{15.16}$$

Once non-competitive inhibition has been diagnosed (Fig. 15.15a), the K_i value is best obtained from a secondary plot of either the slope of the primary plot or of $1/V'_{max}$ (which is equal to the intercept on the $1/v_o$ axis) against inhibitor concentration. Both secondary plots will have an intercept of $-K_i$ on the inhibitor concentration axis (Fig. 15.16).

Uncompetitive reversible inhibition

An uncompetitive reversible inhibitor can bind only to the ES complex and not to the free enzyme, so that inhibitor binding must be either at a site created by a conformational change induced by the binding of the substrate to the catalytic site or directly to the substrate molecule. The resulting ternary complex, ESI, is also a dead-end complex.

$$\begin{array}{ccc} E + S \rightleftharpoons ES & \longrightarrow & E + P \\ +I \big\| -I & & \\ ESI & \longrightarrow & \text{no reaction} \end{array}$$

As with non-competitive inhibition, the effect cannot be overcome by increasing the substrate concentration, but in this case both K_m and V_{max} are reduced by a factor of $(1 + [I])/K_i$. An inhibitor concentration equal to K_i will therefore halve the values of both K_m and V_{max}. With this type of inhibitor, K_{EI} is infinite because the inhibitor cannot bind to the free enzyme so K_i is equal to K_{ESI}. The Lineweaver–Burk equation (15.5) therefore becomes:

$$\frac{1}{v_0} = \left(\frac{K_m}{V_{max}} \times \frac{1}{[S]} + \frac{1}{V_{max}} \right) \left(\frac{1 + [I]}{K_i} \right) \tag{15.17}$$

The value of K_i is best obtained from a secondary plot of either $1/V'_{max}$ or $1/K'_m$ (which is equal to the intercept on the $1/[S]$ axis) against inhibitor concentration. Both secondary plots will have an intercept of $-K_i$ on the inhibitor concentration axis.

Mixed reversible inhibition

For some inhibitors either the ESI complex has some catalytic activity or the K_{EI} and K_{ESI} values are neither equal nor infinite. In such case so-called mixed inhibition kinetics are obtained. Mixed inhibition is characterised by a linear Lineweaver–Burk plot that does not fit any of the patterns shown in Fig. 15.15a. The plots for the uninhibited and inhibited reactions may intersect either above or below the $1/[S]$ axis. The associated K_i can be obtained from a secondary plot of the slope either of the primary plot or of $1/V_{max}$ for the primary plots against inhibitor concentration. In both cases the intercept on the inhibitor concentration axis is $-K_i$. Non-competitive inhibition may be regarded as a special case of mixed inhibition.

Substrate inhibition

A number of enzymes at high substrate concentration display substrate inhibition characterised by a decrease in initial rate with increased substrate concentration. The graphical diagnosis of this situation is shown in Fig. 15.15b. It is explicable in terms of the substrate acting as an uncompetitive inhibitor and forming a dead-end complex.

End-product inhibition

First enzymes in an unbranched metabolic pathway are commonly regulated by end-product inhibition. Here the final product of the pathway acts as an inhibitor of the first enzyme thus switching off the whole pathway when the final product begins to accumulate. The inhibition of aspartate carbamyltransferase by CTP in the CTP biosynthetic pathway is an example of this form of regulation. In branched pathways, product inhibition usually operates on the first enzyme after the branch point.

Applications of enzyme inhibition

The study of the classification and mechanism of enzyme inhibition is of importance in a number of respects:

- it gives an insight into the mechanisms by which enzymes promote their catalytic activity (Section 15.4.2),
- it gives an understanding of the possible ways by which metabolic activity may be controlled *in vivo*,

Table 15.2 Examples of enzyme inhibitors as therapeutic agents

Inhibitor	Enzyme	Application
Zidovudine (AZT), didanosine (ddI)	Reverse transcriptase	HIV therapy
Ritonavir, saquinavir	HIV protease	HIV therapy
Sulphonamides	Dihydrofolate synthase	Bacterial infections
Trimethoprim, methotrexate	Dihydrofolate reductase	Bacterial infections
Organophosphorus compounds	Cholinesterase	Insecticides
Celastatin	Dehydropeptidase-1	Enhancement of antibacterial action
Iproniazide	Monoamine oxidase	Mood control
Disulfiram	Aldehyde dehydrogenase	Treatment of alcoholism
Allopurinol	Xanthine oxidase	Treatment of gout
Mevinolin	Hydroxymethylglutaryl CoA reductase	Inhibition of cholesterol synthesis
Aspirin	Cyclo-oxygenase (COX-1 and COX-2)	Inhibition of prostaglandin and thromboxane synthesis

HIV, human immunodeficiency virus.

- it allows specific inhibitors to be synthesised and used as therapeutic agents to block key metabolic pathways underlying clinical conditions.

The use of enzyme inhibitors as therapeutic agents is of enormous commercial value. Examples of some such agents are given in Table 15.2. The HIV-1 protease inhibitors, such as ritonavir and saquinavir, were designed from knowledge of the active site of the aspartyl proteases of the pepsin class to which the HIV-1 protease belongs. The enzyme cleaves specific peptide bonds including -Phe-Pro- and -Tyr-Pro-. The two drugs were designed to resemble the tetrahedral transition state known to be involved in the catalytic mechanism of the enzyme. Both inhibitors contain bulky groups and a non-hydrolysable structure such that binding to the active site is possible but enzymatic cleavage is not, thus blocking the enzyme's action. The successful clinical use of the compounds relies on the fact that the drugs are sufficiently selective to be capable of binding to the HIV-1 protease but not the human aspartyl proteases, such as renin, involved in normal physiological functions.

15.4 ENZYME ACTIVE SITES AND CATALYTIC MECHANISMS

As previously pointed out, enzymes are characterised by their high specificity, catalytic activity and capacity for regulation. These properties must reflect the specific three-dimensional interaction between the enzyme and its substrate. A complete understanding of the way enzymes work must therefore include the elucidation of the mechanism underlying the binding of a substrate(s) to the enzyme catalytic site and the subsequent conversion of the substrate(s) to product(s). The mechanism must include details of the nature of the binding and catalytic sites, the nature of the intermediate enzyme–substrate complex(es), and the associated electronic and stereochemical events that result in the formation of the product. A wide range of strategies and analytical techniques has been adopted to gain such an understanding and brief experimental details and the relative merits of each will now be considered.

15.4.1 X-ray crystallographic studies

X-ray crystallography is capable of giving, either directly or indirectly, decisive information about the mechanism of enzyme action. It requires the enzyme to be purified and obtained in crystalline form – itself a difficult challenge (Section 8.4.5). X-ray diffraction patterns enable the position of each amino acid in the protein to be located and the details deduced of how the substrate binds and undergoes reaction. Such deductions are facilitated by the study of crystals grown in the presence and absence of the substrate, competitive inhibitor or effector molecules. The limitation of the technique is that X-ray diffraction provides details of the enzyme in a static, stable state; yet proteins are known to be highly flexible and dynamic in solution and capable of existing in multiple microconformations. Fortunately, all the evidence to date confirms the applicability of the X-ray data to the aqueous *in vivo* environment. Classic examples of the power of this approach come from studies of lysozyme, ribonuclease, hexokinase, a number of peptidases, phosphorylase and triosephosphate isomerase, all of which have revealed distinct binding clefts or pockets within the protein three-dimensional structure into which the substrate can fit, often in the process inducing a structural change or reorientation of specific amino acid residues to create the catalytic site. Such induced changes support the induced-fit theory of active sites rather than the earlier lock–key hypothesis, which visualised the binding site as being a permanent, integral feature of the enzyme. The juxtaposition of specific amino acid residues, within the induced site, to particular covalent bonds in the substrate molecule commonly favours the establishment of hydrogen bonding or electrostatic attractions between the enzyme and the substrate and the formation of the energetically favourable transition state required for reaction. Amino acid residues commonly found in active sites are therefore those with side-chains containing key functional groups such as those found in the side-chains of aspartic acid, glutamic acid, serine, cysteine, histidine, lysine and arginine.

As knowledge of protein structures and catalytic mechanisms has increased, computer programs have become available that enable the chemical and stereochemical conformations of the substrate(s) to be modelled and a prediction made of the three-dimensional structure of the enzyme that promotes the formation of product(s). This approach is now widely used in the pharmaceutical industry to identify 'lead' compounds for the development of new drugs.

15.4.2 Irreversible inhibitor and affinity label studies

Irreversible inhibitors act by forming a covalent bond with the enzyme (Section 15.3.7). By locating the site of the binding of the inhibitor, information can often be obtained about the identity of specific amino acids in the binding site. Thus cyanide binds to metal atoms that are important for the activity of some enzymes, whilst the organomercury compounds and iodoacetate react with sulphydryl groups of cysteine residues. The organophosphorus compounds, such as diiso-propylphospho-fluoridate, are powerful inhibitors of acetylcholinesterase and serine proteases by virtue of the covalent bond they form with a serine hydroxyl group in the active site. This specific labelling of amino acids in the active site can be exploited by using an analogue of the natural substrate that contains a reactive group that will form a covalent bond with the enzyme. An example is the use of bromoglycerone phosphate to inhibit triosephosphate isomerase:

$$O_3^{2-}POCH_2COCH_2Br + Enzyme\text{-}OH \longrightarrow Enz\text{-}O\text{-}CH_2COCH_2OPO_3^{2-}$$

| 3-bromoglycerone | triosephosphate | alkylated enzyme |
| phosphate | isomerase | |

A development of this approach is the use of photoaffinity labels that structurally resemble the substrate but which contain a functional group, such as azo (-N=N-), which on exposure to light is converted to a reactive functional group, such as a carbene or nitrene, which forms a covalent bond with a neighbouring functional group in the active site. It is common practice to tag the inhibitor or photoaffinity label with a radioisotope so that its location in the enzyme protein can easily be established experimentally.

15.4.3 Kinetic studies

Kinetic studies using a range of substrates and/or competitive inhibitors and the determination of the associated K_m, k_{cat} and K_i values allow correlations to be drawn between molecular structure and kinetic constants and hence deductions to be made about the structure of the active site. In the case of bisubstrate reactions, information about the reaction mechanism and substrate binding sequence can be also be deduced (Section 15.3.2). Further information about the structure of the active site can be gained by studying the influence of pH on the kinetic constants. Specifically, the effect of pH on K_m (i.e. on binding of E to S) and on V_{max} or k_{cat} (i.e. conversion of ES to products) is studied. Plots are then made of the variation of log K_m with pH and of log V_{max} or log k_{cat} with pH. The intersection of tangents drawn to the curves gives an indication of the pK_a values of ionisable groups involved in the active site (Fig. 15.14). These are then compared with the pK_a values of the ion-isable groups known to be in proteins. For example, pH sensitivity around the range 6–8 could reflect the importance of one or more imidazole side-chains of a histidine residue in the active site because of its known pK_a in this range.

15.4.4 Isotope-exchange studies

The replacement of the natural isotope of an atom in the substrate by a different isotope of the same element and the study of the impact of the isotope replacement on the observed rate of enzymatic reaction and its associated stereoselectivity often enable deductions to be made about the mechanism of the reaction. Two examples illustrate the principle. First, alcohol dehydrogenase (AD), which oxidises ethanol to ethanal using NAD^+:

$$CH_3CH_2OH + NAD^+ \overset{AD}{\rightleftharpoons} CH_3CHO + NADH + H^+$$

ethanol   ethanal

The two hydrogen atoms on the methylene ($-CH_2$) group of ethanol are chemically indistinguishable, but if one is replaced by a deuterium or tritium atom the carbon atom becomes a chiral centre and the resulting molecule can be identified as either R or S configuration according to the Cahn–Ingold–Prelog rule for defining the stereochemistry of asymmetric centres. Studies have shown that alcohol dehydrogenase exclusively removes the hydrogen atom in the proR configuration, i.e. (R) CH_3CHDOH always loses the D isotope in its conversion to ethanal but (S)-CH_3CHDOH retains it. Such a finding can be interpreted only in terms of the specific orientation of the ethanol molecule at the binding site such that the two hydrogen atoms are effectively not equivalent. All dehydrogenases have been shown to display this type of stereospecificity and can be classified as either A-side dehydrogenases (e.g. alcohol dehydrogenase, lactate dehydrogenase, malate dehydrogenase) or B-side dehydrogenases (e.g. glycerol-3-phosphate dehydrogenase, glucose dehydrogenase, glyceraldehyde-3-phosphate dehydrogenase). Interestingly, the class type is independent of the hydrogen acceptor being NAD^+ or $NADP^+$.

Secondly, esters may be hydrolysed by esterases that convert the ester to a mixture of acid and alcohol, simultaneously incorporating a molecule of water into the products:

$$RCOO*R' + H_2O \overset{esterase}{\longrightarrow} RCOOH + R'O*H$$

ester   acid   alcohol

In this reaction the oxygen atom identified as O* can be retained either in the acid or in the alcohol depending upon which side of the labelled oxygen atom the bond is broken, with water providing the second oxygen atom in the products. Labelling the oxygen atom in question as ^{18}O and studying, by mass spectrometry, its location after hydrolysis enables details to be drawn about the mechanism of the hydrolysis of the ester by the esterase. In practice, the labelled oxygen atom is found in the alcohol, which supports the view that the reaction mechanism involves initial attack by water, acting as a nucleophile, on the carbonyl carbon atom and the subsequent elimination of the R'O* group.

15.4.5 Spectrophotometric studies

NMR and Raman spectroscopy have both been used to deduce information about enzyme active sites. In the case of NMR, studies are confined to relatively small enzymes such as ribonuclease A. This single-chain protein contains four histidine

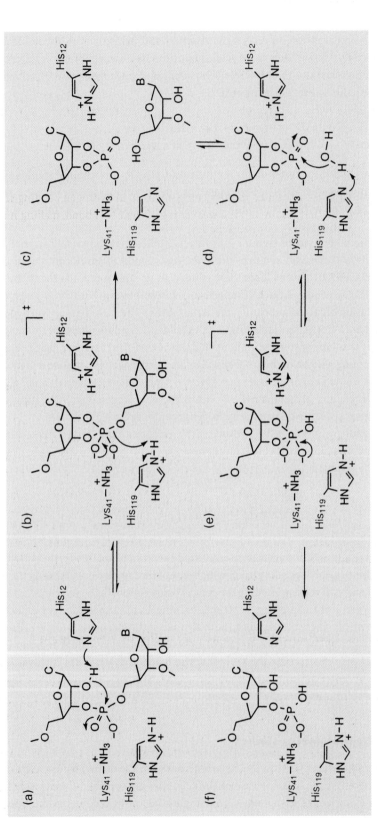

Fig. 15.17. Mechanism for the hydrolysis of RNA by ribonuclease A. (a) The RNA lies in a cleft of the ribonuclease such that the pyrimidine group, C, hydrogen bonds with Thr45. His12, acting as a base, removes a proton from the hydroxyl group, and the oxygen, acting as a nucleophile, attacks the phosphate group. (b) His119, acting as an acid, attacks the pentavalent phosphorus transition state cleaving the P–O link to the adjacent ribose group to form a cyclic phosphate diester on the first ribose group. (c) The 5′-OH product leaves the site. (d) A molecule of water attacks the cyclic phosphate diester that donates a proton to His119, acting as a base. (e) His12, acting as an acid, donates a proton to the second pentavalent phosphorus transition state to give the final 3′-phosphate product shown in (f). (Reproduced from T. Bugg (1997), *An Introduction to Enzyme and Coenzyme Chemistry*, by permission of Blackwell Science Limited.)

residues, two of which are implicated by pH/activity studies to be involved in enzymatic activity, one histidine being protonated, the other unprotonated. In this case, NMR studies were possible because the histidine protons gave signals quite distinct from the mass of the other protons in the enzyme. Changes in the NMR signal as a function of pH implicated the two histidine residues in positions 12 and 119. This deduction was confirmed by inhibition studies of ribonuclease A using iodoacetate. Iodoacetate does not normally react chemically with histidine but it did react with two histidine residues in ribonuclease A, thereby simultaneously indicating that these two particular histidine residues were more reactive than normal. This was attributed to their being involved in hydrogen bonding within the active site that resulted in the weakening of their N-H bond, making it more reactive towards iodoacetate (Fig. 15.17).

15.4.6 Site-directed mutagenesis studies

Advances in molecular biology, and particularly in the ability to clone genes and express them in a particular vector, have opened up the possibility of producing variants of the enzyme in which a particular amino acid residue, thought to be involved in substrate binding and catalysis, is replaced by another amino acid. By studying the impact of the replacement of an ionisable or nucleophilic amino acid with an unreactive one on the catalytic properties of the enzyme, conclusions can be drawn about the role of the amino acid residue that has been replaced. Thus in the case of ribonuclease A, discussed above, replacement of either His12 or His119 has a deleterious effect on the catalytic properties of the enzyme. In principle it is also possible to produce variants that are more active than the native enzyme. Such studies are based on knowledge of the protein structure, function and mechanism of course and assume that the impact of the single amino acid replacement is confined to the active site and has not affected other aspects of the enzyme's structure. This needs to be confirmed by complementary structural studies, for example spectroscopic techniques. This rational redesign approach has resulted in the generation of a superoxide dismutase with an enhanced activity relative to the native enzyme and an isocitrate dehydrogenase with specificity different from that of the native form.

15.4.7 Catalytic mechanisms – outcomes of studies on ribonuclease A

The application of the various strategies outlined above to a wide range of enzymes has enabled mechanisms to be deduced for many of them. Crystallographic and site-directed mutagenesis studies have been particularly successful in providing detailed information about the stereochemical and electronic events involved in substrate binding and product formation. Such studies emphasise the importance of conformational changes that occur in the enzyme. Equally important is the role of hydrogen bonding between the substrate and key amino acid residues in the binding and catalytic sites in facilitating 'activation' of the substrate and the lowering of the reaction activation energy barrier. Many of the mechanisms identified have other common features such as acid–base catalysis of the type well known in conventional organic chemistry. These findings are illustrated by studies on the enzyme ribonuclease A.

Ribonuclease A (RNase A)

RNase A is a small enzyme (molecular mass 13.68 kDa), consisting of only 124 amino acid residues including four histidine residues, which hydrolyses RNA, cleaving a ribose-phosphate ester bond attached to the ribose 5′ carbon, with a pyrimidine (cytosine or uracil) attached to the ribose in position 1′. The process has been shown to proceed via a 2′, 3′-phosphate cyclic diester that can be isolated and characterised. The evidence that allowed the mechanism of hydrolysis and the nature of the transition states to be deduced was obtained by application of a variety of strategies:

- pH-activity studies revealed a bell-shaped curve indicating the involvement of two histidine residues, one protonated and the other not, with pK_a values of 5.4 and 6.4, respectively.
- NMR studies gave signals for two protons from two histidine residues displaced from the remainder of the proton NMR signals (Section 15.4.5).
- Affinity labelling studies using iodoacetate indicated the involvement of His12 and His119. Similar studies using fluorodinitrobenzene indicated the involvement of Lys41 and possibly Lys7.
- Site-directed mutagenesis studies showed that Lys7, but not Lys41, could be replaced without loss of activity.
- Crystallographic studies revealed a cleft in the molecular structure into which the region of the RNA to be cleaved could bind. His12 and His119 were in close proximity but on opposite sides of the cleft. Lys7, Lys41 and Lys66 were in the same region as Asp121, which was adjacent to His119. It was deduced that the positively charged Lys residues would interact with the negatively charged phosphate groups of the RNA backbone and that Asp121, with its negative charge, would be involved in the transfer of a proton from water.
- Molecular modelling of the active site revealed that the pyrimidine group cytosine or uracil fits into the cleft in such a way as to form two hydrogen bonds with Thr45. Replacement of the pyrimidine by a purine (adenine or guanine) prohibited the formation of these bonds, thereby explaining the specificity for the pyrimidines.
- Model substrate studies showed that the enzyme cleaved a P-O ester bond attached to the ribose 5′-carbon and that the process proceeded via a 2′,3′-phosphate cyclic diester that could be isolated.

This evidence of the nature of the RNase A catalytic action enabled a probable catalytic mechanism to be deduced. It is summarised in Fig. 15.17. It is an example of acid–base catalysis that is common for hydrolase enzymes. Each of the two key histidine residues acts as both an acid and a base during the reaction sequence.

Confirmation of a pentavalent phosphoryl intermediate came from the fact that RNase A is competitively inhibited by uridine vanadate, in which the vanadium atom is pentavalent. The lack of a 2'-hydroxyl group in DNA (containing 2'-deoxyribose) prevents the formation of the pentavalent intermediates and thereby explains why RNase A does not hydrolyse DNA.

Multienzyme complexes

Studies on multienzyme complexes, including tryptophan synthase and carbamyl phosphate synthase, have demonstrated that the active site of one enzyme is coupled to that of the next enzyme in the metabolic sequence by means of allosteric conformational changes. The reaction products are channelled from one active site to the next by means of an intermolecular tunnel. In the case of tryptophan synthase, which is an $(\alpha\beta)_2$-complex in which the α- and β-subunits catalyse separate reactions, the tunnel is approximately 25 Å in length whereas that in carbamoyl phosphate synthase is approximately 100 Å long. (Note that angstroms are more commonly used for structural dimensions rather than the more correct nanometres.) The tunnels protect reactive intermediates from coming into contact with the external environment and reduce their transit time to the next active site. In the case of both enzymes the tunnels are formed prior to the binding of the initial substrates but with some other multienzyme complexes the tunnels are formed after the substrates bind to the active site.

15.5 **CONTROL OF ENZYME ACTIVITY**

15.5.1 **Control of the activity of individual enzymes**

The activity of an enzyme can be regulated in two ways:

- by alteration of the kinetic conditions under which existing enzyme is operating;
- by alteration of the amount of enzyme present either by promoting enzyme synthesis or enzyme degradation.

The latter option is inherently long-term and will be discussed later. In contrast, there are several mechanisms by which the activity of an enzyme can be altered almost instantaneously:

- *Product inhibition:*   Here the enzyme product acts as an inhibitor of the reaction so that, unless the product is removed by further metabolism, the reaction will cease. An example is the inhibition of hexokinase by glucose 6-phosphate. Hexokinase exists in four isoenzyme forms I, II, III and IV. The first three isoforms all have a low K_m for glucose (about 10–100 μM) and are inhibited by glucose 6-phosphate, whereas isoform IV has a higher K_m (10 mM) and is not inhibited by glucose 6-phosphate. Isoform IV is confined to the liver, where its higher K_m allows it to deal with high glucose concentrations following a carbohydrate-rich meal (see below). The other three isoforms are distributed widely and do not encounter such high glucose concentrations as those found in the liver. Thus their lower K_m values allow them to work optimally under their prevailing physiological conditions.

- *Allosteric regulation:*   Here a small molecule that may be a substrate, product or key metabolic intermediate such as ATP or AMP alters the conformation of the catalytic site as a result of its binding to an allosteric site (Section 15.3.3). A good example is the regulation of 6-phosphofructokinase discussed earlier.
- *Reversible covalent modification:*   This may involve adenylation of a tyrosine residue by ATP (e.g. glutamine synthase), the ADP-ribosylation of an arginine residue by NAD^+ (e.g. nitrogenase) but most frequently involves the phosphorylation of specific tyrosine, serine or threonine residues by a protein kinase. Most significantly, phosphorylation is reversible by the action of a phosphatase. Phosphorylation introduces the highly polar γ-phosphate group of ATP that is capable of inducing conformational changes in the enzyme structure such as to either activate or deactivate the enzyme.

Reversible covalent modification is quantitatively the most important of the three mechanisms. A very large number of protein kinases have been identified and shown to be of three basic types:

- *Receptor protein kinases:*   These are located on the cytoplasmic side of a cell membrane receptor that is activated as a result of the binding to an extracellular site of a hormone, neurotransmitter or other signalling ligand released by a distant cell. Ligand activation of the receptor most commonly results in the dimerisation of the receptor and the autophosphorylation of the latent protein kinase site. This autophosphorylation of the receptor protein activates the protein kinase site and simultaneously creates a binding site for a number of intracellular enzymes that have a key cell-signalling role, resulting in their phosphorylation and a resulting modification of their activity. This is discussed in detail in Section 16.5.3.
- *Non-receptor protein kinases:*   Members of this large group of kinases have vital roles in the control of cell differentiation, proliferation and death. The best studied are the Src family. They share a common structure and are all activated as a result of an initial dephosphorylation followed by phosphorylation by a receptor protein kinase of the type discussed above.
- *Second-messenger-coupled kinases:*   Members of this important group of kinases are activated or deactivated by second messengers released by an intracellular membrane-bound enzyme that is activated by a G-protein- coupled receptor. The second messenger may be cAMP, cyclic GMP (cGMP), Ca^{2+} or diacylglycerol (for further details, see the following section and Chapter 16). Examples include cAMP-dependent protein kinase involved in glycogenolysis, protein kinase C (activated by Ca^{2+} and diacylglycerol) involved in the phosphorylation of the epidermal growth factor (EGF) receptor, and Ca^{2+}/calmodulin protein kinases involved in the regulation of other kinases such as phosphorylase kinase.

A characteristic feature of many of these various kinases is that they are involved in a cascade of enzyme reactions such as glycogenolysis and glycogenesis, which will be discussed in the following section. Such cascades offer the opportunity for fine metabolic control and a large amplification of the original signal received by the membrane receptor.

15.5.2 Control of metabolic pathways

A large proportion of the thousands of enzymes in a cell are involved in the promotion of coordinated chemical pathways such as glycolysis, the citric acid cycle and the biosynthesis of fatty acids and steroids. Enzymes linked in a coordinated pathway are frequently clustered in one of three ways, namely:

- by being located in the same compartment of the cell,
- by being physically associated as a multienzyme complex such as that of the fatty acid synthase of *E. coli*,
- by being membrane bound, such as the enzymes of the electron transport system.

This clustering facilitates the transport of the product of one enzyme to the next enzyme in the pathway.

Identification of rate-controlling enzymes

The individual enzymes in a metabolic pathway combine to produce a given flow of substrates and of products through the pathway. This flow is referred to as the metabolic flux. Its value is determined by factors such as the availability of starting substrate and cofactors but above all by the activity of the individual enzymes. Studies have revealed that the enzymes in a given pathway do not all possess the same activity. As a consequence one, or at most a small number, with the lowest activity determine the overall flux through the pathway. In order to identify these rate-controlling enzymes three types of study need to be carried out:

- *in vitro* kinetic studies of each individual enzyme conducted under experimental condition as near as possible to those found *in vivo* and such that the enzyme is saturated with substrate (i.e. such that $[S] > 10K_m$),
- studies to determine whether or not each individual enzyme stage operates at or near equilibrium *in vivo*,
- studies to determine the flux control coefficient for each enzyme.

A reaction that is not at or near equilibrium, and which is therefore associated with a large free energy change, is potentially a rate-limiting enzyme, since the most probable reason for the non-establishment of equilibrium is the lack of adequate enzyme activity. To test for a non-equilibrium reaction it is necessary to analyse the concentration of each substrate and product *in vivo*. This is normally done by stopping all further reactions by denaturing the enzymes by the addition of a suitable denaturant to the *in vivo* test system and then analysing the analytes by a technique such as chromatography or NMR.

Table 15.3 Rate-controlling tests on the enzymes of the glycolytic pathway

Enzyme	Activity	Equilibrium	Flux control coefficient C
Hexokinase	Low	Non-	High
Phosphoglucomutase	High	Near	Low
6-Phosphofructokinase	Low	Non-	High
Fructose bisphosphatase aldolase	High	Near	Low
Triosephosphate isomerase	High	Near	Low
Glyceraldehyde-3-phosphate dehydrogenase	High	Near	Low
Phosphoglcerate kinase	High	Near	Low
Phosphoglycerate mutase	High	Near	Low
Enolase	High	Near	Low
Pyruvate kinase	Low	Non-	Medium

For each enzyme in the pathway it is possible to calculate a flux control coefficient, C, which measures the impact of a change in the activity of that enzyme in the cell, under the prevailing physiological conditions, on the flux of reactants through the whole pathway. Values for C can vary between 0 and 1. A flux control coefficient of 1 means that the flux through the pathway varies in proportion to the increase in the activity of the enzyme whereas a flux control coefficient of zero means that the flux is not influenced by changes in the activity of that enzyme. The sum of all C values for a given pathway is 1 so that the higher a given C value the greater is the impact of that enzyme on the flux through the pathway. These C values are therefore highest for the rate-determining enzymes.

The application of these three tests to the enzymes in the glycolytic pathway is illustrated in Table 15.3. The actual quantitative values for the three test parameters vary between cell types in a given organism and between cells of a given type in different organisms. It can be seen from Table 15.3 that in the glycolytic pathway three of the 10 enzymes involved in the conversion of glucose to pyruvate have a potential rate-limiting activity and do not achieve equilibrium but are associated with a large negative free energy change and are therefore effectively irreversible. The same three enzymes have the largest C values. Studies have revealed that all three enzymes are subject to various control mechanisms and all contribute to the control of flux through the glycolytic pathway.

Hexokinase exists in four isoenzyme forms, the first three of which are subject to inhibition by glucose 6-phosphate, the product of the reaction. Isoenzyme IV (also known as glucokinase) is not subject to this type of inhibition and has a higher K_m for glucose than have the other three forms. It is confined mainly to the liver, where it is able to metabolise high concentrations of glucose, the resulting glucose 6-phosphate being diverted to glycogen biosynthesis via glucose 1-phosphate. In some tissues the limiting activity of hexokinase is bypassed by the provision of glucose 6-phosphate from glycogen via glucose 1-phosphate.

The activity of pyruvate kinase is regulated allosterically, being inhibited by ATP and activated by AMP and fructose 1,6-bisphosphate. In muscle, pyruvate kinase is present in large amounts, hence minimising its rate-limiting constraint. The fact that pyruvate kinase is located at the end of the pathway makes it unlikely that it will have a major role in the regulatory control of glycolysis.

As discussed earlier (Section 15.3.3), 6-phosphofructokinase (PFK) is subject to allosteric control by a number of allosteric effectors that are related to the energy status of the cell. The principal activators are AMP and fructose 2,6-bisphosphate, whilst ATP is an activator at low concentrations but an inhibitor at higher concentrations (1 mM). AMP activates the enzyme by releasing it from the inhibitory control of ATP by binding to the R state, disturbing the equilibrium away from the T state that contains the ATP inhibitor site. The balance of control exerted by ATP and AMP is thus determined by their relative concentrations. This in turn is influenced by the enzyme adenylyl kinase, which catalyses the reaction:

$$2ADP \rightleftharpoons ATP + AMP$$

ATP is normally present in a cell at much higher concentrations than the other two nucleotides and, as a consequence, a small decrease in the concentration of ATP that is too small to relieve the inhibitory effect of ATP on PFK results in a proportionally much larger change in AMP concentration, which is normally only about 2% of that of ATP. This large percentage increase in the concentration of AMP allows it to exert a powerful activator effect on PFK, hence facilitating increased glycolytic flux.

Additional control of glycolytic flux by PFK is exerted by its involvement in a substrate cycle with the enzyme fructose bisphosphatase (FBP) that is part of the gluconeogenesis pathway from pyruvate to glucose (Fig. 15.18). Both reactions are strongly exergonic and essentially irreversible. Although AMP acts as a powerful activator of PFK, it acts as a potent inhibitor of FBP and hence plays a reciprocal role in the control of these opposing pathways. PFK converts D-fructose 6-phosphate to D-fructose 1,6-bisphosphate and simultaneously converts ATP to ADP, whilst FBP converts D-fructose 1,6-bisphosphate to D-fructose 6-phosphate and inorganic phosphate. The net result is apparently only the hydrolysis of ATP but in fact it results in a proportionally large increase in AMP concentration via adenylyl kinase. As discussed above, this produces a large increase in flux through the glycolytic pathway by the activation of PFK and inhibition of FBP. A two-fold increase in AMP concentration can increase the glycolytic flux by 200-fold. However, the regulatory importance of changes in AMP concentration is not confined to its stimulation of glycolytic flux. Equally important is the fact that decreases in AMP concentration result in the ATP inhibition of PFK activity becoming dominant, resulting in the virtual switching off of the glycolytic pathway and a concomitant increase in glycogen biosynthesis.

Although AMP is a significant regulator of the activity of PFK it is not the most potent activator of the enzyme. That role, at least in liver, is held by D-fructose 2,6-bisphosphate (F26BP) which is not an intermediate of glycolysis, although it is isomeric with fructose 1,6-bisphosphate, the product of PFK. F26BP activates PFK at concentrations as low as 1 μM. F26BP is part of another substrate cycle involving the enzymes phosphofructokinase-2 (PFK-2), which converts D-fructose

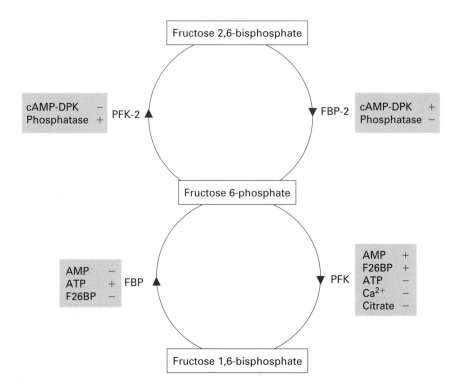

Fig. 15.18. Regulation of phosphofructokinase (PFK). Two substrate cycles each centred on fructose 6-phosphate are involved. Different enzymes promote the forward and reverse reactions of each cycle so that all reactions are exergonic (negative free energy changes). Each enzyme is subject to activation (+) or inhibition (−) either by allosteric effectors or by phosphorylation/dephosphorylation. The importance of each regulatory mechanism varies between organisms and between different tissues in a given organism. cAMP-DPK, cyclic-AMP-dependent protein kinase; F26BP, fructose 2,6-bisphosphate.

6-phosphate to D-fructose 2,6-bisphosphate, and fructose bisphosphatase-2 (FBP-2) that converts the bisphosphate back to the 6-phosphate. Interestingly, the two enzyme activities are located in different domains of the same dimeric protein. Both are subject to regulation by phosphorylation/dephosphorylation. FBP-2 is activated by phosphorylation and PFK-2 by dephosphorylation. Under cellular conditions in which the glucose concentration is high, PFK-2 is activated by dephosphorylation by an activated phosphatase thus increasing the concentration of F26BP, which in turn activates PFK and increases glycolytic flux. At the same time, FBP-2 is deactivated by dephosphorylation by the same phosphatase. When the glucose level is low, the cycle operates in reverse. The operation of this substrate cycle is the main mechanism that ensures that glycolysis and gluconeogenesis do not proceed *in vivo* at the same time.

Isoforms of PFK-2 and FBP-2 have been identified in different tissues. They differ in their affinity (K_s) for their substrates and in their sensitivity to regulation by phosphorylation/dephosphorylation. This rationalises the observation that the fine mechanistic detail for the control of PFK activity and hence of the regulation of glycolysis varies between different mammalian tissues.

In general, substrate cycles are an important means by which the activity of metabolic pathways is controlled. They operate at the expense of energy (ATP) and may simultaneously determine the relative importance of branch points in bidirectional pathways.

15.5.3 Signal amplification

The substrate cycles discussed above enable opposing pathways to be controlled and small changes in the concentration of ATP to be amplified in terms of concomitant changes in AMP, which is a key allosteric regulator of rate-limiting enzymes. This concept of amplification is important in the fine control of metabolic pathways and in the response of cells to hormone and neurotransmitter signals. Amplification is commonly achieved by a series of stages in which linked enzymes are themselves the substrate of a reaction, commonly based on phosphorylation or dephosphorylation, as a result of which the enzymes are either activated or deactivated. Such a series of reactions is referred to as a metabolic cascade and its merit is that it affords the opportunity for a large amplification of an original biochemical signal. The mobilisation of glycogen as glucose 1-phosphate by phosphorylase provides a good illustration of this principle. The components of this phosphorylase cascade are a membrane receptor that receives the original signal in the form of a hormone, neurotransmitter or similar, a G_s protein, adenylyl cyclase (also known as adenylate cyclase), cAMP-dependent protein kinase, phosphorylase kinase, phosphorylase and glycogen (Fig. 15.19). cAMP released from adenylyl cyclase, as a result of its activation by a G_s protein (see Section 16.5.2), activates cAMP-dependent protein kinase, which in its inactive form is a tetramer consisting of two regulatory (R) and two catalytic (C) subunits. Two cAMP molecules bind to each of the R subunits in a positively cooperative manner, causing them to dissociate:

$$R_2C_2 + 4cAMP \longrightarrow 2R\text{-}2cAMP + 2C$$
$$\text{inactive form} \qquad\qquad \text{active form}$$

The intracellular concentration of cAMP determines the proportion of cAMP-dependent protein kinase that is present in the active form. It is this form of the kinase that, in the presence of ATP, phosphorylates and thereby activates phosphorylase kinase:

$$\text{C unit}$$
$$\text{phosphorylase kinase} + ATP \longrightarrow \text{phosphorylated phosphorylase kinase} + ADP$$
$$\text{inactive} \qquad\qquad\qquad \text{active}$$

Phosphorylase kinase is a tetrameric protein with four different subunits, α, β, γ and δ. The γ-subunit contains the catalytic kinase site, the other three subunits having a regulatory role. The δ-subunit is calmodulin, a Ca^{2+}-binding protein

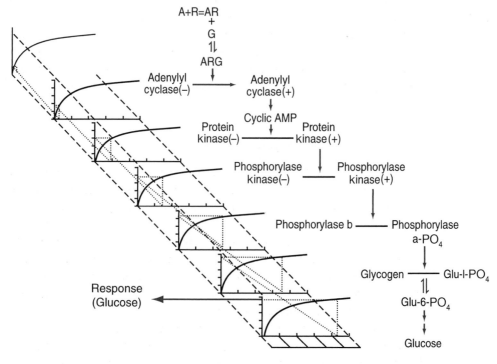

Fig. 15.19. A typical biochemical cascade showing the stages from the initial binding of the first messenger (A) to its cell-surface receptor, the resultant activation of a G-protein (G) by the AR complex, through the activation of adenylyl cyclase and the release of cAMP to the final cellular response, namely the release of glucose. Each step in the cascade is represented by a hyperbolic function. The initial low receptor occupancy triggers a sequence of progressively amplified responses so that the final release of glucose is nearly a maximal response. (Reproduced from T. Kenakin (1997), *Molecular Pharmacology: A Short Course*, by permission of Blackwell Science Limited.)

that contains two Ca^{2+}-binding sites. Phosphorylase kinase is activated by the phosphorylation of the α- and β-subunits and by the binding of two Ca^{2+} to the δ-subunit. The binding of Ca^{2+} to the δ-subunit promotes the autophosphorylation of the enzyme at a site different from that phosphorylated by cAMP-dependent kinase. The activated phosphorylase kinase activates phosphorylase b (a dimer) by the phosphorylation of Ser14 on each subunit, causing conformational changes and dimerisation to a tetramer to give phosphorylase a, which degrades glycogen to glucose 1-phosphate. Most interestingly, phosphorylase b can also be activated allosterically by AMP, two molecules of which are capable of inducing conformation changes to give phosphorylase a but by an induction mechanism different from that brought about by phosphorylation. ATP and glucose 6-phosphate can induce the reverse allosteric change, deactivating the enzyme.

At each step in the phosphorylase cascade there is amplification of at least 100-fold, moving the associated dose–response curve nearer the maximum (Fig. 15.19). Thus occupation of only a very small percentage of the membrane receptors is needed to produce a final metabolic response approaching the maximum. It is evident that the larger the number of components in the cascade, the greater is the potential for amplification.

The mobilisation of glycogen is reversed by glycogen synthase, which is inactivated by phosphorylation by phosphorylase kinase and activated by phosphoprotein phosphatase-1, which simultaneously inactivates phosphorylase kinase and glycogen phosphorylase a. Phosphoprotein phosphatase-1 is itself subject to control by phosphorylation/dephosphorylation.

15.5.4 **Long-term control of enzyme activity**

The forms of control of enzyme activity discussed so far are essentially short- to medium-term control in that they are exerted in a matter of seconds or a few minutes at the most. However, control can also be exerted on a longer time scale. Long-term control, exerted in hours, operates at the level of enzyme synthesis and degradation. Whereas many enzymes are synthesised at a virtually constant rate and are said to be constitutive enzymes, the synthesis of others is variable and is subject to the operation of control mechanisms at the level of gene transcription and translation. One of the best-studied examples is the induction of β-galactosidase and galactoside permease by lactose in *E. coli*. The expression of the *lac* operon is subject to control by a repressor protein produced by the repressor gene (the normal state) and an inducer, the presence of which causes the repressor to dissociate from the operator, allowing the transcription and subsequent translation of the *lac* genes. The lac repressor protein binds to the lac operator with a K_i of 10^{-13} M and a binding rate constant of $10^7 (M)^{-1} s^{-1}$. This rate constant is greater than that theoretically possible for a diffusion-controlled process and indicates that the process is facilitated in some way, possibly by DNA.

The metabolic degradation of enzymes is the same as that of other cellular proteins, including membrane receptors. It is a first-order process characterised by a half-life. The half-life of enzymes varies from a few hours to many days. Interestingly, enzymes that exert control over pathways have relatively short half-lives. The precise amino acid sequence of a protein is thought to influence its susceptibility to proteolytic degradation. N-terminal Leu, Phe, Asp, Lys and Arg, for example, appear to predispose the protein to rapid degradation. Proteins for proteolytic degradation are initially 'tagged' by a small protein (76 amino acid residues), called ubiquitin (Ub), which requires ATP and is able to form an enzyme-catalysed peptide-like bond with the C-terminal end of the protein to be degraded. Ubiquitin may either mono-ubiquitinate or poly-ubiquitinate a protein and the functional consequences vary. Mono-ubiquitination leads to the 'trafficking' of the protein, a process that is fundamental to the cycling of receptors (Section 16.6.2), whereas poly-ubiquitination leads to degradation. The interaction between ubiquitin and a protein involves a series of enzymes: ubiquitin-activating enzymes (E1s), ubiquitin-conjugating enzymes (E2s), ubiquitin protein ligases (E3s) and deubiquitylating enzymes (DUBs). The ubiquitin protein ligases play a key role in the whole process as they recognise the target protein. Results from the Human Genome Project provide evidence for the existence of several hundred of these E3 enzymes.

The poly-ubiquitinated protein is degraded by a multicatalytic complex based on a 20 S proteasome (the S stands for Svedberg, see Section 3.5.3). Proteasomes are multisubunit proteases with a cylindrical core that has a 'lid' at both ends. The catalytic sites are within the core cylinder. The 20 S proteasome consists of 14 α-subunits and 14 β-subunits arranged in four rings, each of seven units. The proteolytic activity is located in the β-subunits at five sites that lie in the core. Entry of the substrate protein into the cylindrical core is controlled by a number of activators and either may proceed sequentially, starting from one end of the protein, or may involve a 'hairpin' conformation of the protein entering the proteasome, allowing limited proteolysis of an internal segment. Proteolysis is ATP dependent and involves an additional 19 S proteasome that contains ATPase sites. This 19 S proteasome combines with the 20 S proteasome to form a 26 S proteasome that promotes the cleavage of the peptide bonds, with the concomitant hydrolysis of ATP. In addition to the proteasome route for enzyme degradation there is also a lysosomal route that does not require pre-ubiquitination of the enzyme.

The balance between enzyme *de novo* synthesis and proteolytic degradation coupled with the regulation of enzyme activity enables the amount and activity of enzymes present in a cell to be regulated to meet fluctuating cell and whole organism needs. There is growing evidence to indicate that ubiquitination/ deubiquitination is as important as phosphorylation/dephosphorylation for cellular homeostasis.

15.6 SUGGESTIONS FOR FURTHER READING

General texts

BUGG, T. (2004). *An Introduction to Enzyme and Coenzyme Chemistry*, 2nd edn. Blackwell Science, Oxford. (A readable text that emphasises the chemical principles underlying enzymology.)

FELL, D. (1997). *Understanding the Control of Metabolism*. Portland Press, London. (An authoritative coverage of this important topic in which the underlying mathematical concepts are carefully explained.)

Review articles

CHEN, R. (2001). Enzyme engineering: rational redesign versus directed evolution. *Trends in Biotechnology*, 19, 13–14.

CIECHANOVER, A. and BEN-SAADON, R. (2004). N-terminal ubiquitination: more protein substrates join in. *Trends in Cell Biology*, 14, 103–106.

DANIEL, R. M., DANSON, M. J. and EISENTHAL, R. (2001). The temperature optima of enzymes: a new perspective on an old phenomenon. *Trends in Biochemical Sciences*, 26, 223–225.

FÖSTER, A. and HILL, C. P. (2003). Proteasome degradation: enter the substrate. *Trends in Cell Biology*, 13, 550–553.

HUANG, H., HOLDEN, H. M. and RAUSHEL, F. M. (2001). Channeling of substrates and intermediates in enzyme-catalysed reactions. *Annual Reviews of Biochemistry*, 70, 149–180.

Chapter 16

Cell membrane receptors

16.1 RECEPTORS FOR CELL SIGNALLING

Cells within multicellular organisms need to be able to communicate with each other in order to coordinate essential functions such as growth and differentiation and to respond to changes in their external environment. Cells in physical contact with each other can interact by the exchange of small molecules via gap junctions but cells physically distant from each other, with the extreme examples being found in plants and animals, need an effective communication system. This is achieved by the release of ligand signalling molecules by the signalling cells and the specific recognition of these ligands by protein receptors either embedded within and spanning the cell membrane or located in the cytoplasm of the target cells. Most commonly the ligand is water soluble and therefore incapable of diffusing across the cell membrane. It therefore binds to a ligand-binding site exposed on the extracellular side of the receptor. The binding initiates a sequence of events, in many cases involving protein–protein interactions at the membrane interface, which result in the cellular response. Examples of such ligands include amines, amino acids, peptides and proteins. However, some ligands are lipid soluble and can diffuse freely across the membrane and bind to cytosolic receptors. The receptor–ligand complexes subsequently diffuse across the nuclear membrane and accumulate in the nucleus where they modulate DNA transcription. For this reason, the receptors are referred to as nuclear receptors. Examples of ligands acting in this way are steroid hormones (progesterone, oestrogen, testosterone) and non-steroid hormones (thyroxine and triiodothyronine).

A ligand acting on a cell membrane receptor is often referred to as a first messenger, since with many membrane receptors ligand binding does not directly result in the desired intracellular response. Rather, it results in the activation of the intracellular region of the receptor that then either:

- initiates a series of intracellular protein activation processes that climax in the cellular response, or
- interacts with a second membrane-bound protein that in turn promotes the generation or release from intracellular stores of one or more of a group of molecules including cAMP and Ca^{2+}, collectively called second messengers,

that diffuse to, and react with, various protein targets, modifying their activity and thereby stimulating the cellular response.

In both cases, a series of reactions, collectively referred to as a cascade, is involved in the transduction (linking) of the original signal received by the receptor to the eventual cellular response. One of the advantages of a cascade system is that it results in a large amplification of the cellular response relative to that which could possibly have been produced by the first messenger acting alone (for further details see Section 15.5.3). The signalling ligand has no other physiological function in addition to its role of promoting the formation of the active conformation of the receptor. With two of the three main classes of receptor, the receptor–ligand complex is internalised by endocytosis, causing the ligand to dissociate under the acidic conditions prevailing in the endocytic vesicles. The vacated receptor may be either recycled or degraded (Section 16.6.2).

16.2 QUANTITATIVE ASPECTS OF RECEPTOR–LIGAND BINDING

16.2.1 Dose–response curves

Pharmacological objectives

Much of the early work on the study of receptor–ligand binding was carried out on isolated tissue preparations and was aimed at the quantification and characterisation of the response as a function of the ligand concentration. The work was largely driven by the search for ligand blockers, which could mimic the binding of the physiological ligand but did not produce a cellular response. These ligand blockers had the potential for pharmacological exploitation. In the 1960s it was realised that if such blockers were sufficiently selective in their binding they might be able to distinguish between the various subclasses of the receptor that were believed to exist but which at the time had not been identified. The existence of subclasses of receptors would allow the development of blockers as therapeutic agents that would be tissue- and response-selective, thereby minimising undesirable side-effects. It was as a result of this approach that Sir James Black achieved his pioneering work on β-adrenergic and histamine H_2 receptors, which resulted respectively in the development of the blood pressure-lowering β-blocker propranolol and the gastric acid secretion H_2 receptor blocker cimetidine, used in the treatment of gastric and duodenal ulcers. As will be discussed in detail later, this approach to receptor classification, coupled with the newer technique of cloning and identification of encoding genes, has resulted in the identification of a plethora of receptor subtypes for most receptors.

Dose–response curves

The response of the membrane receptor to exposure to an increasing concentration (dose) of ligand is a curve that has three distinct regions:

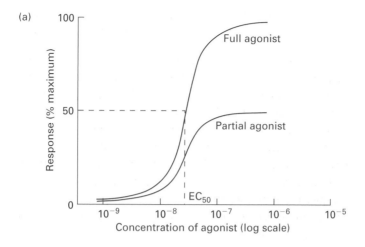

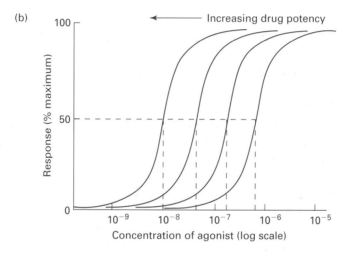

Fig. 16.1. Dose–response curves. (a) The biological effect (% maximum response) and the concentration of a full agonist are plotted on a logarithmic scale. An equipotent partial agonist has a lower efficacy than a full agonist – it cannot achieve the maximum response even when all available receptors are occupied. EC_{50} is the concentration of agonist that produces 50% maximum effect. (b) Dose–response curves for four full agonist drugs of different potencies but equal efficacy. (Reproduced from S. R. J. Maxwell and D. J. Webb (1999), Receptor functions. *Medicine*, **27**, 5–9, by permission of The Medicine Publishing Company.)

- an initial threshold below which little or no response is observed,
- a slope in which the response increases rapidly with increasing dose,
- a declining response with further increases in dose and a final maximum response.

Since such plots commonly span several hundred-fold variations in ligand concentration, they are best expressed in semilogarithmic form (Fig. 16.1).

Dose–response studies for a given receptor using ligands with a wide range of molecular structures have shown that receptors are capable of binding ligands other than the physiologically active ligand and that the response to such binding is variable. As a result of such studies, receptor ligands have been categorised as follows:

- *Full agonists:*   These ligands produce the same maximal response but differ in the dose required to achieve it (Figs. 16.1 and 16.2).
- *Partial agonists:*   These ligands produce only a partial response even when present in large excess such that all the receptors are occupied (Figs. 16.1 and 16.2).
- *Antagonists:*   These ligands produce no response. Three subclasses have been identified:
    - (i) *Competitive reversible antagonists:*   The antagonist competes with the agonist for the same binding site so that the effect of the antagonist can be overcome by increasing the concentration of agonist (Fig. 16.2).
    - (ii) *Non-competitive reversible antagonists:*   The antagonist binds at a different site on the receptor from that of the agonist so that the effect of the antagonist cannot be overcome by increasing the concentration of agonist.
    - (iii) *Irreversible competitive antagonists:*   The antagonist competes with the agonist for the same binding site but the antagonist forms a covalent bond with the binding site so that its effect cannot be overcome by increasing the concentration of agonist.

As a result of this classification of ligands, they can also be characterised by a number of parameters:

- *Intrinsic activity:*   This is a measure of the ability of an agonist to induce a response by the receptor. It is defined as the maximum response to the test agonist relative to the maximum response to a full agonist acting on the same receptors. All full agonists, by definition, have an intrinsic activity of 1 whereas partial agonists have an intrinsic activity of <1.
- *Efficacy (e):*   This is a measure of the inherent ability of an agonist to initiate a physiological response following binding to the receptor. The initiation of a response is linked to the ability of the agonist to promote the active conformational of the receptor. While all full agonists must have a high efficacy their efficacy values will not necessarily be equal, in fact values of e have no theoretical maximum value. Partial agonists have a low efficacy and antagonists have zero efficacy.
- *Potency:*   This is a measure of the concentration of agonist required to produce the maximum effect: the more potent the agonist, the smaller the concentration required. The potency of an agonist is related to the position of the sigmoidal curve on the log dose axis. It is expressed in a variety of forms including the effective dose or concentration for 50% maximal response, ED_{50} or EC_{50}. On a semilogarithmic plot, the value emerges as pED_{50} or pEC_{50} value (i.e. $-\log_{10} ED_{50}$). Thus an agonist with EC_{50} of 3×10^{-5} M would have a pEC_{50} of 4.8.
- *Affinity:*   This is a measure of the concentration of ligand required to produce 50% binding. This is the only parameter that can be used to characterise

(a)

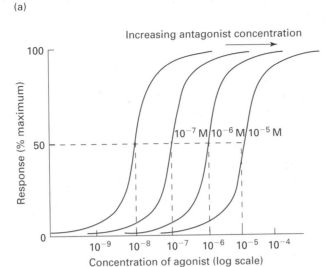

(b)

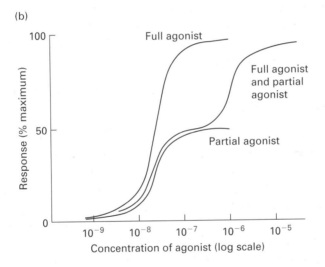

Fig.16.2. Receptor–ligand interactions. (a) In the presence of an antagonist, the dose–response curve of the full agonist is shifted to the right because the full agonist competes for receptor binding. The higher the concentration of antagonist, the greater is the shift. (b) In the presence of a partial agonist, the dose–response curve of the full agonist is shifted to the right. (Reproduced from S. R. J. Maxwell and D. J. Webb (1999), Receptor functions. *Medicine*, **27**, 5–9 by permission of The Medicine Publishing Company.)

antagonists. As will be shown in the following section, affinity is a reflection of both the rate of association of the ligand with the receptor and the rate of dissociation of the resulting complex. The rate of association is a reflection of the three-dimensional interaction between the two and the rate of dissociation a reflection of the strength of binding within the complex. Affinity can be expressed by an affinity or binding constant, K_a, but is more commonly expressed as a dissociation constant, K_d, of the receptor–ligand complex, where K_d is equal to the reciprocal of K_a.

- *Selectivity:*   This is a measure of the ability of an agonist to discriminate between receptor subtypes. This is particularly important from a therapeutic perspective.

Mechanisms of receptor activity

The existence of agonists and antagonists was originally explained by the two-state theory of receptors, also known as the del Castillo–Katz model. The model assumes that the occupied receptors can exist in two forms, one inactive (AR) and the other active (AR*) such that the two forms exist in equilibrium:

A	+	R	$\rightleftharpoons$	AR	$\rightleftharpoons$	AR*
agonist		vacant		occupied		occupied
		inactive		inactive		active
		receptor		receptor		receptor

It was envisaged that full agonists could readily induce conformational changes in R thereby creating the active R* state and displacing the equilibrium totally in favour of AR*, but partial agonists were less able to induce the change and hence could only partially displace the equilibrium. Antagonists could not induce the change at all. However, the discovery that some receptors are active even in the absence of agonists, and are said to possess constitutive activity, has led to the model being superseded by the conformational selection model. This model envisages that in the resting state (i.e. in the absence of any agonist) receptors exist as an equilibrium mixture of active (R*) and inactive (R) forms that can readily interconvert. The equilibrium may be predominantly in favour of the inactive state or such that a significant amount of the active state exists, thereby explaining the observed constitutive activity. According to this model, agonists preferentially bind to the R* state, thereby stabilising it and causing a concomitant displacement of the equilibrium, resulting in a greater proportion of the receptors being in the R* conformation. Similarly, partial agonists are capable of binding to both R and R* states, with variable preference for R* again resulting in an increase in the proportion of this conformation but smaller than that produced by full agonists. Support for this model has come from the identification of ligands that reduce the activity of receptors with constitutive activity. Since antagonists are believed to be unable to combine with the active state and do not produce any direct change in receptor activity, these ligands have been termed inverse agonists, since they have opposite or negative activity to that of agonists. They preferentially bind to the R state, stabilising it and displacing the equilibrium in its favour. Partial inverse agonists can bind to both states with a preference for the R state, thus decreasing the constitutive activity. Ligands with equal affinity for both states will not displace the equilibrium and are termed neutral antagonists. Most previously classified antagonists on re-evaluation against receptors possessing constitutive activity have been found to be inverse agonists, but of course it is only possible to undertake such a re-evaluation with receptors displaying constitutive activity and at present these remain a minority. However, the technique of plasmon-waveguide resonance spectroscopy (Section 16.3.2) has recently proved to be an effective technique for distinguishing between these various classes of ligand.

The conformational selection model assumes that the various forms of the receptor (R, R*, AR, AR*) are in equilibrium so their relative proportions will be determined by the values of the associated equilibrium constants:

$$
\begin{array}{ccc}
 & K_1 & \\
\text{(inactive)} \quad R & \rightleftharpoons & R^* \text{(active)} \\
+ & & + \\
L & & L \\
K_2 \;\Big\Updownarrow & & \Big\Updownarrow\; K_3 \\
\text{(inactive)} \quad LR & \rightleftharpoons & LR^* \text{(active)} \\
 & K_4 &
\end{array}
$$

The important feature of this model is that the role of the ligand (L) is to bind to a particular receptor conformation, thereby stabilising it and causing a displacement of the equilibrium between the two states of the receptor. It is evident that the two-state model is a limiting case of this model and arises when the values of K_1 and K_3 are very small. The model does not require the agonist to induce the active conformation of the receptor. In this respect, receptors displaying this type of behaviour are reflecting the symmetry model of allostery put forward by Monod, Wyman and Changeux rather than the induced fit model proposed by Koshland (Section 15.5, Fig. 15.11). Receptors with constitutive activity have been identified among ligand-gated ion-channel and G-protein-coupled receptors.

16.2.2 Receptor–ligand binding parameters

The general process of the binding of a ligand to a receptor is initiated by the diffusion of the ligand to the surface of the receptor protein. Here the ligand locates the binding site by a series of random collisions within the two dimensions of the receptor surface in the membrane. The initial binding with the site may involve amino acid residues that are not functionally part of the final binding site, which most commonly consists of a few specific amino acid residues. This final binding can be represented as follows:

$$
\text{R} \quad + \quad \text{L} \quad \underset{k_{-1}}{\overset{k_{+1}}{\rightleftharpoons}} \quad \text{RL} \tag{16.1}
$$

receptor   ligand   receptor–ligand
                                      complex

where k_{+1} is the association rate constant and k_{-1} is the dissociation rate constant.

Saturation studies

If under the conditions of the binding studies the total concentration of ligand is very much greater than that of receptor (so-called saturation conditions), changes in ligand concentration due to receptor binding can be ignored but changes in the free (unbound) receptor concentration cannot. Hence if:

$[R_t]$ is the total concentration of receptor that determines the maximum binding capacity

$[L]$ is the free ligand concentration

$[RL]$ is the concentration of receptor–ligand complex

then $[R_t]-[RL]$ is the concentration of free receptor.

At equilibrium, the forward and reverse reactions for ligand binding and dissociation (equation 16.1) will be equal:

$$k_{+1}([R_t]-[RL])[L] = k_{-1}[RL]$$

therefore

$$\frac{k_{-1}}{k_{+1}} = K_d = \frac{1}{K_a} = \frac{([R_t]-[RL])[L]}{[RL]} \tag{16.2}$$

where K_d is the dissociation constant for RL and K_a is the association or affinity constant. Rearranging gives:

$$[RL] = \frac{[L][R_t]}{K_d + [L]} \tag{16.3}$$

Determination of K_d

Equation 16.3 is of the form of a rectangular hyperbola that predicts that ligand binding will reach a limiting value as the ligand concentration is increased and therefore that receptor binding is a saturable process. The equation is of precisely the same form as equations 15.1 and 15.2, which define the binding of the substrate to its enzyme in terms of K_m and V_{max}. For the experimental determination of K_d, equation 16.3 is best converted to a linear form. Rearrangement of equation 16.3 gives the Scatchard equation (16.4):

$$\frac{[RL]}{[L]} = \frac{[R_t]}{K_d} - \frac{[RL]}{K_d} \tag{16.4a}$$

This equation predicts that a plot of $[RL]/[L]$ against $[RL]$ will be a straight line of slope $-1/K_d$, allowing K_d to be calculated. However, in many studies the relative molecular mass of the receptor protein is unknown so that the concentration term $[RL]$ cannot be calculated in molar terms. In such cases it is acceptable to express the extent of ligand binding in any convenient unit (B), e.g. pmoles $(10^6 \text{ cells})^{-1}$, pmoles $(\text{mg protein})^{-1}$ or more simply as a change in fluorescence (ΔF) under the defined experimental conditions. Since maximum binding (B_{max}) will occur when all the receptor sites are occupied, i.e. $[R_t] = B_{max}$, equation 16.4a can be written in the form:

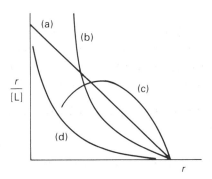

Fig. 16.3. Scatchard plot for (a) a single set of sites with no cooperativity, (b) two sets of sites with no cooperativity, (c) a single set of sites with positive cooperativity, and (d) a single set of sites with negative cooperativity.

$$\frac{B}{[L]} = \frac{B_{\text{max}}}{K_d} - \frac{B}{K_d} \tag{16.4b}$$

Hence a plot of $B/[L]$ against B will be a straight line, slope $-1/K_d$ and intercept on the y-axis of B_{max}/K_d (Fig. 16.3). In cases where the relative molecular mass of the receptor protein is known the Scatchard equation can be expressed in the form:

$$\frac{B}{[L]B_{\text{max}}} = \frac{n}{K_d} - \frac{B}{B_{\text{max}}K_d} \tag{16.5}$$

where n is the number of independent ligand-binding sites on the receptor.

The expression B/B_{max} is the number of moles of ligand bound to one mole of receptor. If this expression is defined as r, then:

$$\frac{r}{[L]} = \frac{n}{K_d} - \frac{r}{K_d} \tag{16.6}$$

In this case, a plot of $r/[L]$ against r will again be linear with a slope of $-1/K_d$ but in this case the intercept on the x-axis will be equal to the number of ligand-binding sites, n, on the receptor.

Alternative linear plots to the Scatchard plot are:
Lineweaver–Burk plot

$$\frac{1}{B} = \frac{1}{B_{\text{max}}} + \frac{K_d}{B_{\text{max}}} \times \frac{1}{[L]} \tag{16.7}$$

Hanes plot

$$\frac{[L]}{B} = \frac{K_d}{B_{\text{max}}} + \frac{[L]}{B_{\text{max}}} \tag{16.8}$$

In practice, Scatchard plots are most commonly carried out, although statistically they are prone to error, since the experimental variable B occurs in both the x and y terms so that linear regression of these plots overestimates both K_d and B_{max}. It can be seen from equation 16.2 that, when the receptor sites are half saturated, i.e. $B = B_{max}/2$, then $[L] = K_d$. This is analogous to $S = K_m$ when $v_o = V_{max}/2$ (Section 15.3.1). Hence K_d will have units of molarity.

The derivation of equation 16.2 is based on the assumption that there is a single set of homogeneous receptors and that there is no cooperativity between them in the binding of the ligand molecules. In practice, two other possibilities arise: first, that there are two distinct populations of receptors each with different binding constants; and, secondly, that there is cooperativity in binding within a single population. In both cases the Scatchard plot will be curvilinear (Fig. 16.3). If cooperativity is suspected, it should be confirmed by a Hill plot, which, in its non-kinetic form, is:

$$\log\left(\frac{Y}{1-Y}\right) = h \log [L] - \log K_d \tag{16.9}$$

or

$$\log\left(\frac{B}{B_{max} - B}\right) = h \log [L] - \log K_d$$

where Y is the fractional saturation of the binding sites (from 0 to 1) and h is the Hill constant.

For a receptor with multiple binding sites that function independently, $h = 1$, whereas, for a receptor with multiple sites that are interdependent, h is either >1 (positive cooperativity) or <1 (negative cooperativity). Scatchard plots that are biphasic due to ligand multivalence (i.e. multiple binding sites), rather than receptor cooperativity, are sometimes taken to indicate that the two extreme, and approximately linear, sections of the curvilinear plots represent high affinity (high bound:free ratio at low bound values) and low affinity (low bound:free ratio at high bound values) sites and that tangents drawn to these two sections of the curve can be used to calculate the associated K_d and B_{max} values. This is incorrect, and the correct values can only be obtained from the binding data by means of careful mathematical analysis, generally undertaken by the use of special computer programs, many of which are commercially available.

Competitive binding experiments

An alternative approach to that described above for the determination of K_d values for an experimental ligand is to use the ligand as a competitive inhibitor of a second ligand, normally the physiological agonist, whose K_d value is known. This will give rise to a K_i value for the experimental ligand but this will be numerically equal to its K_d value. The most common approach is to use the physiological agonist in radiolabelled form and to use a range of concentrations of the experimental ligand with a fixed concentration of the radiolabelled ligand. A plot is then made of the extent of binding of the radiolabelled ligand against the log of the experimental ligand concentration. An IC_{50} value (the concentration required to inhibit the binding of the physiological ligand by 50%) is then calculated for the experimental ligand. From knowledge of the IC_{50} value the K_i value is calculated using the Cheng–Prusoff equation:

$$K_i = \frac{IC_{50}}{\{1 + ([L]/K_d)\}} \tag{16.10}$$

Determination of rate constants

To determine the dissociation rate constant, k_{-1} (units: time^{-1}) some of the receptor–ligand complex (B_0) is allowed to form, usually using radiolabelled ligand. The availability of the unoccupied receptors to the ligand is then blocked by the addition of at least 100-fold excess of unlabelled agonist or competitive antagonist and the decrease in the extent of binding (B_t) monitored as a function of time. The rate of release of the radiolabelled ligand from its binding site is given by the expression:

$$\frac{dB_0}{dt} = -k_{-1}B_0$$

and the equation governing the release by the expression:

$$B_t = B_0 e^{-k_{-1}t}$$

hence:

$$\log B_t = \log B_0 - 2.303 k_{-1}t \tag{16.11}$$

Thus a plot of $\log B_t$ against time will give a straight line with a slope of $-2.303k_{-1}$, allowing k_{-1} to be estimated.

The association rate constant, k_{+1} (units: (mol dm^{-3})$^{-1}$ time^{-1}) is best estimated by the approach to equilibrium method, by which the extent of ligand binding is monitored continuously until equilibrium is reached under conditions that are such that $[L] \gg [R_t]$. (This gives pseudo first-order conditions rather than second order. Under these conditions, $[R_t]$ decreases with time but $[L]$ remains constant.) Ligand binding increases asymptotically such that:

$$\log\left(\frac{B_{eq}}{B_{eq} - B_t}\right) = 2.303(k_{+1}[L] + k_{-1})t \tag{16.12}$$

Thus a plot of $\log [B_{eq}/(B_{eq} - B_t)]$ against time will be linear, with a slope of $2.303(k_{+1}[L] + k_{-1})$, where B_{eq} and B_t are the ligand binding at equilibrium and time t respectively. From knowledge of k_{-1} (obtained by the method discussed above) and $[L]$, the value of k_{+1} can be calculated from the slope.

16.3 TECHNIQUES FOR THE STUDY OF RECEPTOR–LIGAND BINDING

16.3.1 Experimental design

General experimental problems

The rate and extent of receptor–ligand binding is influenced by such physical experimental variables as temperature, pH and ionic concentration. In addition, there are some physiological problems that need to be taken into account. For example, if intact cells are the source of the receptor, it is essential to minimise receptor trafficking influences (Section 16.6.2) as otherwise receptor numbers may change during the study. This problem can be avoided in a number of ways including:

- carrying out the study at lowered temperatures, usually about 5 °C, that minimise trafficking processes,
- including an inhibitor of trafficking, such as phenylarsine oxide, in the incubation mixture,
- using isolated receptors or membrane fragments rather than whole cells.

Historically, the most common method of monitoring the progress of receptor–ligand binding has been to use a radiolabelled ligand and to measure the radioactivity associated with the receptor fraction of the ligand. However, this technique does not easily allow the determination of rate constants and is uneconomical if a large range of ligands is being screened against orphan receptors, i.e. those whose natural agonist is unknown, for example from cloned gene lines. For such reasons, fluorimetric techniques have become increasingly popular and for similar reasons, miniaturised ligand-binding assays based on protein microarray technology have been developed (Sections 8.5 and 16.3.2).

Receptor preparations

Preparations of receptors for ligand-binding studies may either leave the membrane intact or involve the disruption of the membrane and the release of the receptor with or without membrane fragments, some of which could form vesicles with variable receptor orientation and control mechanisms. A further potential problem of membrane disruption is that the process may expose receptors previously not within the cell membrane, thereby resulting in an overestimation of the number of available receptors. Such receptors could have been undergoing endocytosis (Section 16.6.2) or synthesis and insertion into the membrane.

Membrane receptor proteins show no or very little ligand-binding properties in the absence of phospholipid, so that a purified receptor protein must be introduced into a phospholipid vesicle for binding study purposes. In practice, common receptor preparations include:

- tissue slices, usually 5–50 μm thick cut with a cryostat and adhered to a gelatin-coated glass slide,
- isolated cells, produced by either the mechanical or the enzymatic (collagenase or trypsin) disruption of the whole tissue,
- cultured cells (Chapter 2), taking care to ensure their lack of contamination,
- cell membrane preparations, obtained by the use of a variety of methods for cell disruption coupled with differential centrifugation,
- solubilised receptor preparations, obtained by the use of detergents as the membrane disruption agents and purified by affinity chromatography using a competitive antagonist as the immobilised ligand,

- recombinant receptors, obtained using cell lines transfected with cloned receptor genes, increasingly of human origin.

Tissue slices are best for the study of receptor distribution and number by auto-radiography or fluorescence spectroscopy, but the study of the kinetics of ligand binding in these preparations is complicated by the existence of diffusion barriers.

Isolated cells as a source of receptors are widely used for a wide range of bio-chemical studies including receptor post-translational modification, membrane insertion and downregulation, and the study of receptor–response coupling. However, binding studies using intact cells have a number of potential problems:

- the cells may contain enzymes capable of metabolising the experimental ligand thereby reducing its effective concentration,
- receptor trafficking (Section 16.6.2) and other cellular processes may affect receptor numbers and hence ligand binding,
- more than one type of cell may be present but the use of receptor gene cloning and expression in a specific cell line effectively overcomes this problem.

Cell membrane preparations are an experimentally useful source of receptors, but they lack the cytoplasmic components that may influence the regulation of ligand binding.

Recombinant receptors are increasingly being used for ligand binding studies, but care has to be taken to ensure that they have the same functional characteristics as the native receptor. It is particularly important to ensure that post-translational processes have been carried out and that, for example, the receptor protein has been correctly glycosylated.

Kinetic studies aimed at the determination of individual rate constants are best carried out using either isolated cells or the patch clamp technique (Section 16.3.2), since they avoid errors due to the diffusion of the ligand to the receptor. Studies of the number of receptors in intact tissue are best achieved by labelling the receptors with a radiolabel, preferably using an irreversible competitive antag-onist and applying the technique of quantitative autoradiography. An alternative approach is to label the receptors with a positron emitter (e.g. ^{11}C) and to apply the technique of positron emission tomography (PET).

Ligands

By far the most common technique for the study of ligand–receptor interaction is the use of a radiolabelled ligand with isotopes such as ^{3}H, ^{14}C, ^{32}P, ^{35}S and ^{135}I. Generally, a high specific activity (Section 14.1.6) ligand is used, as this minimises the problem of non-specific binding (see below). The most effective alternative to the use of radiolabelled ligands is the use of fluorescence spectroscopy. This is dis-cussed in Section 16.3.2.

For the study of ligand–receptor interactions that occur on a submillisecond timescale, special approaches need to be taken to deliver the ligand to the recep-tor (see stopped-flow and quench-flow methods in Section 15.2.3). One such approach is the use of so-called caged compounds. These possess no inherent ligand properties but, on laser flash photolysis with light of a specific wavelength, a protecting group masking a key functional group is instantaneously cleaved releasing the active ligand.

Experimental procedures

The general experimental approach for studying the kinetics of receptor–ligand binding is to incubate the receptor preparation with the ligand under defined conditions of temperature, pH and ionic concentration for a specific period of time that is sufficient to allow equilibrium to be attained. The importance of allowing the system to reach equilibrium cannot be overstated as equations 16.1–16.9 do not hold if equilibrium has not been attained. Using an appropriate analytical procedure, the bound and unbound forms of the ligand are then quantified. This quantification may necessitate the separation of the bound and unbound fractions. The study is then repeated for a series of ligand concentrations to cover 10–90% of maximum binding at a fixed receptor concentration. The binding data are then analysed using equations 16.4–16.9, often in the form of a computer program.

Historically, ligand binding studies have been carried out on a manual basis but recent advances in molecular biology, especially gene cloning, have opened up the need for fast, high throughput screening techniques for large numbers of orphan receptors of unknown function but of potential pharmacological value. Some of the approaches taken to solve this need are discussed later.

Non-specific binding

Irrespective of the analytical procedure chosen to separate the bound and free ligand, a general problem is the non-specific binding of the ligand to sites other than the specific ligand binding site(s). Such non-specific binding may involve the membrane lipids and other proteins either located in the membrane or released by the isolation procedure. The characteristic of non-specific binding is that it is non-saturable but is related approximately linearly to the total concentration of the ligand. Thus the observed ligand binding is the sum of the saturable (hyperbolic) specific binding to the receptor and the non-saturable (linear) binding to miscellaneous sites. The specific binding component is usually obtained indirectly by carrying out the binding studies in the presence of an excess of non-labelled ligand (agonist or antagonist) if a labelled ligand is being used to study binding. The presence of the excess unlabelled ligand will result in the specific binding sites not being available to the labelled ligand and hence its binding would be confined to non-specific sites (Fig. 16.4). In practice, a concentration of the competitive ligand of at least 1000 times its K_d must be used and confirmation that under the conditions of the experiment, non-specific binding was being studied would be sought by repeating the study using a range of different and structurally dissimilar competitive ligands that should give consistent estimates of the non-specific binding.

Separation of bound and free ligand

Binding studies based on the use of a radiolabelled ligand necessitate the separation of the receptor-bound and free ligand fractions. This can be achieved in a

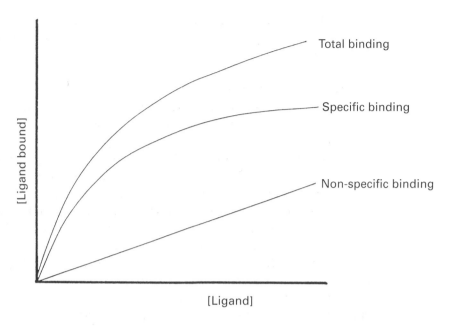

Fig. 16.4. Specific and non-specific binding of a ligand to a membrane receptor. Specific binding is normally hyperbolic and shows saturation. Non-specific binding is linear and is not readily saturated.

number of ways, the simplest of which is centrifugation. Care has to be taken to ensure that the pelleted ligand-bound fraction is washed free from unbound ligand and that in the washing process the dissociation of bound ligand from the receptor is minimised. Alternative methods include equilibrium dialysis and ultrafiltration.

16.3.2 Analytical procedures for the study of receptor–ligand binding

Procedures requiring the separation of bound and free fractions

Equilibrium dialysis   The receptor preparation and ligand, each in a buffer of the same pH and concentration, are placed in opposite halves of a dialysis cell. The cell, which generally has a total internal volume of about 3 cm³, is constructed of transparent plastic such as Perspex^R and unscrews into two halves, which are separated by a cellulose acetate or nitrate semipermeable membrane mounted on an inert mesh support. Many commercial variants of the cell are available, some consisting of banks of up to six cells. The temperature of the cell is thermostatically controlled and the cell is slowly rotated to help the system to reach equilibrium. The ligand molecules, which are small and diffusible, readily cross the membrane until their unbound concentration is the same on both sides (Fig. 16.5). The receptor protein is confined to one half of the cell. At equilibrium, samples are taken from each half of the cell and analysed for ligand. The sample from the receptor half of the cell will give the sum of the bound and unbound ligand concentrations,

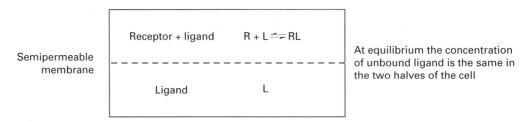

Semipermeable
membrane

Receptor + ligand $R + L \rightleftharpoons RL$

At equilibrium the concentration
of unbound ligand is the same in
the two halves of the cell

Ligand   L

Fig. 16.5. The study of receptor–ligand (R–L) binding by equilibrium dialysis.

whereas that in the other half will simply give the unbound ligand concentration, which will be the same as the unbound ligand concentration in the other half of the cell containing the receptor.

For reliable results the binding of both the ligand and protein to the semipermeable membrane must be minimal and the total ion concentration in each half of the cell equalised to minimise any possibility of a charge inequality on either side of the membrane affecting the distribution of ligand (Donnan effect). The limitations of the technique are the relatively long period of time it takes to establish equilibrium and the fact that it cannot be applied to cases where the ligand is a macromolecule such as insulin, since it will be unable to diffuse across the membrane.

Ultrafiltration   The receptor preparation and ligand in a buffered solution are contained in a thermostatically controlled cell (generally 1–3 cm³ capacity) containing a semipermeable membrane on an inert mesh support at its base. Since no diffusion across a membrane is required to establish equilibrium, attainment of equilibrium is rapid (a few minutes, but this should be checked experimentally). A small sample (100 mm³) is then forced across the membrane into a collection cup, either by application of a gas pressure to the mixture side or more simply by placing the cell in a low speed centrifuge and centrifuging at about 3000 *g* for a few minutes. By analysing the ultrafiltrate (representative of the unbound ligand concentration) and the reaction mixture (bound plus unbound ligand), the influence of ligand concentration on the extent of binding can be studied readily. The attraction of the method is its speed, but binding of the reactants to the semipermeable membrane must be checked and the volume of the ultrafiltrate kept to a minimum to minimise any possibility that the sampling procedure displaces the equilibrium. As with equilibrium dialysis, the method cannot be used to study the binding of macromolecular ligands.

Binding study techniques not requiring the separation of bound and free ligand fractions

Scintillation Proximity Assay™   In this technique the receptor within a membrane fragment is covalently attached to scintillant beads and the ligand is labelled with a weak β-particle emitter such as ³H or ¹²⁵I. The reactants are mixed in a photometric cuvette. When the ligand binds to the receptor the β-particles cause the scintillant to emit light that is detected by a photomultiplier and quantified, thereby allowing the bound ligand to be measured. Unbound ligand distant from the surface of the scintillant beads does not cause light emission, since the low energy β-particles emitted by the unbound ligand are absorbed by the surrounding reaction medium (see Section 14.2.2). Binding can be monitored continuously.

Fluorescence spectroscopy   Recently, the use of fluorescence-based techniques for the study of ligand–receptor binding has gained in popularity, as the techniques are ultrasensitive, avoid the need to separate bound and free ligand fractions and are capable of studying binding involving a few or even individual ligand molecules and single receptors. The general principles of fluorescence spectroscopy are discussed in Chapter 12. The methods are based on either the intrinsic fluorescence of the receptor protein or the fact that the ligand or the receptor protein is tagged with a suitable fluorescent marker (fluor). Tagging is generally achieved by chemical attachment to functional groups such as amines, thiols, carboxyls and alcohols. Commonly used fluors include fluorescein, rhodamine and the dye Fluo-3. Alternatively, the green fluorescent protein (GFP) of the jellyfish *Aequorea victoria* or the red fluorescent protein of *Discosoma striata* can be attached to receptor proteins by genetic engineering techniques without altering the normal function of the protein. The main advantage of using either of these two autofluorescent proteins is that no cofactors are required for fluorescence to occur, hence the study protocols are relatively simple. The intrinsic fluorescence of proteins is linked to the presence of tryptophan residues, which, being hydrophobic, are commonly folded within the internal core of the protein. In all cases the intensity of fluorescence, which may be due to a modification of an amino acid at the active site, not the tryptophan per se, is sensitive to the chemical environment of the fluor so that such small conformational changes induced by ligand binding may result in:

- an increase or a decrease in the intensity of the fluorescence (and hence the quantum yield, Q) owing to changes in quenching as a result of ligand binding;
- a change in the fluorescence spectrum, i.e. a move to a longer or shorter wavelength;
- a change in the fluorescence lifetime, T;
- a change in the sensitivity of the fluor to induction of fluorescence by plane-polarised light.

In the study of the binding of ligands to receptor proteins, measurements may be made on a steady-state (single measurement) basis or a time-resolved (multiple measurements over a period of time) basis most commonly by stopped-flow or quench-flow procedures (Section 15.2.3).

Steady-state fluorescence spectroscopy measurements are based on one of three physical effects:

- Changes in the spectroscopic properties (extinction coefficient, emission wavelength) of the fluor induced by changes in its microenvironment caused by ligand binding and/or an alteration of the diffusion of the receptor protein in the membrane as a direct result of ligand binding. Changes in the intensity of fluorescence (ΔF) are used as a measurement of the extent of ligand binding, studied as a function of ligand concentration and used in Scatchard or Lineweaver–Burk plots for the calculation of K_d values.

- The induction of fluorescence anisotropy (anisotropy is the directional variation in optical properties (in this case fluorescence) along perpendicular and parallel axes): in this technique fluorescence is induced by plane-polarised (blue) light. Molecules of the fluor orientated parallel to this plane of polarisation will be excited preferentially. However, if some of these molecules rotate after the absorption of the light but before the fluorescence has time to occur, some of the resulting fluorescence will be depolarised (i.e. no longer in one plane). The extent to which this occurs can be used to deduce information about the size, shape and flexibility of the protein carrying the fluor. It can also be used to monitor the binding of a ligand to the protein. The fluorescence intensity is measured parallel (i.e. in the same plane) to the absorbed plane-polarised light and at right angles to it. From the two measurements it is possible to calculate the degree of fluorescence depolarisation and hence the fluorescence anisotropy, both of which are expressed in terms of the difference between the fluorescence parallel to the absorbed plane-polarised light and that perpendicular to it, the difference being expressed as a function of the sum of the fluorescence in the two planes.

- The induction of fluorescence resonance energy transfer (FRET). This technique relies on the presence of two fluors (intrinsic or extrinsic) in distinct locations within the receptor protein such that the emission spectrum of one and the excitation spectrum of the other overlap. In such circumstances it is possible for the emission light of one fluor to be absorbed by the second and be emitted as part of its emission. This process is called resonance energy transfer and the extent to which it occurs is proportional to $1/R^6$, where R is the distance between the two fluors. Ligand binding to the receptor may induce conformational changes that cause R to change.

Time-resolved fluorescence spectroscopy (TRFS) is based on the use of a europium-linked fluor and allows the study of the lifetimes (milliseconds to minutes) of the excited states of the fluor. It can distinguish between free and bound ligand and can give valuable information on conformational changes in the protein induced by the binding of the ligand and on the process of dimerisation of receptor proteins (see Sections 16.5.2 and 16.5.3) both *in vivo* and *in vitro*. It is increasingly popular in the technique of high throughput screening for genomics and proteomics (Section 8.5).

One of the major limitations of many of the techniques commonly used to study receptor–ligand binding is that they can be used to study only the final equilibrium position and are therefore not suitable for studying the rate constants for the formation and dissociation of the receptor–ligand complex. This disadvantage, when coupled with the fact that many of the methods are also slow and not amenable to automation, makes them unattractive for routine, repetitive studies of the kinetics of receptor–ligand binding. Recent developments in gene cloning have opened up the possibility of cloned receptors, including those of unknown physiological function, being available to the pharmaceutical industry as potential targets for new therapeutic agents. This has stimulated the development of automated techniques for the study of biomolecular interactions without the use of fluorescent or radioisotope labels, with the consequence that dedicated instruments are now available commercially for these types of study, the four most important of which will now be discussed.

Flow cytometry   This is a technique for making measurements on individual cells as they flow passed an array of detectors. Most commonly the measurements are based on fluorescence using the principles discussed previously. The technique was originally developed to allow the separation of a mixed population of cells but has been adapted to allow the study of many aspects of receptor function, including receptor–ligand interactions on cell membrane surfaces. It has the great advantage that the measurements are made on individual cells at rates that can be as high as $10\,000\,s^{-1}$, which enables accurate kinetic binding data to be calculated. There are two basic designs of cytometer. In coaxial mixing mode, a process known as hydrodynamic focusing is used to deliver the reactants to the detection point in the cytometer. Separate streams of reactants are brought into coaxial flow by means of a flow nozzle as they enter the cytometer, which is essentially a flow cell. The streams of reactants through the cytometer are surrounded by a faster moving 'sheath' of buffered medium that ensures that the cells flow in single file and such that the flow is not turbulent. The reactants in the coaxial flow mix by diffusion. Alternatively, the reactants are delivered from syringes by computer-controlled stepping motors, similar to those used in the stopped-flow technique for the study of enzyme–substrate interactions (Section 15.2.3), into a mixing chamber and then delivered into the cytometer by an additional syringe and again the flow of mixed reactants through the cytometer is surrounded by a sheath of buffered medium. The cytometer contains one or more light sources, usually lasers of a given wavelength chosen to cause the probe attached to the ligand to fluoresce, arranged at 90° to the flow and focused on the flow of cells. A series of lenses, filters and photomultipliers allow the fluorescence and scattered light to be studied at 90° and 180° to the light source within 100 ms of mixing. Variation of the point of measurement allows the mixing time to be varied and variation of the concentration of the ligand allows kinetic data to be calculated. The technique has also been used to study receptor numbers, desensitisation, interaction with G-proteins and arrestins and internalisation. It is possible to divide the cell flow into droplets after their measurement and to collect cells of a given type by causing appropriate droplets to be electrostatically charged and deflected into a fraction collector. This forms the basis of the technique called fluorescence-activated cell sorting (FACS).

Surface plasmon resonance (SPR) spectroscopy   In this technique the receptor under study is immobilised to a sensor 'chip' surface, such as a hydrogel layer on a glass slide, via either biotin–avidin interactions or covalent coupling using amine or thiol reagents similar to those for in affinity chromatography (Section 11.8.2)

(Fig. 16.6a). A typical surface concentration of receptor of 1–5 ng mm^{-2} is used. The sensor chip forms one wall of a micro-flow cell so that an aqueous solution of the ligand can be pumped at a continuous, pulse-free rate across the surface of the immobilised receptor (Fig. 16.6b). This ensures that the concentration of ligand at the surface is maintained at a constant value, which can be varied by altering the concentration of the circulating ligand. Variables such as temperature, pH and ionic concentration are carefully controlled, as is the duration of exposure of the receptor to the ligand. Replacing the ligand solution by a buffer solution enables the dissociation of bound ligand to be studied.

The binding of the ligand to the receptor causes an increase in mass at the surface of the chip. Equally, dissociation of the ligand causes a reduction in mass at the surface. These mass changes in turn cause changes in the refractive index of the medium at the surface of the chip and it is this change in refractive index that is measured, since its value determines the propagation velocity of electromagnetic radiation in that medium. The measurement is based on a phenomenon called surface plasmon resonance (SPR) and on the principle of total internal reflection (TIR) of light. (Plasmon is a term for a collection of conduction electrons in a metal or semiconductor.) When polarised light is totally internally reflected at an interface separating two media with different refractive indices, the reflected beam leaks an electrical field, called an evanescent field wave, into the medium of lower refractive index (in this case the liquid containing the receptor) where it decays at an exponential rate and effectively only travels one wave length. If a thin layer of gold is placed at the interface between the two media, its electron cloud can be made to resonate (hence 'resonance' spectroscopy) by interaction with the plane-polarised component of the evanescent field wave. This SPR enhances the evanescent field wave (Fig. 16.6b) and simultaneously causes a decrease in the intensity of the reflected plane polarised light (Fig. 16.6b). The angle of the incident beam at which this SPR occurs depends on several factors, one of which is the refractive index into which the evanescent wave is propagated. As previously explained, binding of the ligand to the receptor causes a change in refractive index, hence monitoring the angle at which SPR occurs gives a continuous real-time record of receptor–ligand binding.

A wedge-shaped beam of plane-polarised light angled to the surface of the bound receptor is used (Fig. 16.6b) and an array of diode detectors monitors the reflected light. By continuously monitoring the SPR angle as a function of time and measuring the resonance signal (the 'sensorgram' in Fig. 16.6b,c), and by appropriate calibration, the measurements can be used to calculate binding constants and rate constants for the receptor–ligand interactions. The SPR angle is expressed in resonance units (RU) such that 1000 RU corresponds to a change in mass at the surface of the chip of about 1 ng mm^{-2}. The advantages of the technique are that it does not require the molecules to be fluorescent or radiolabelled, it can be used to study molecules as small as 100 Da and can be used with coloured or opaque solutions. In addition to enabling the kinetics of receptor–ligand interactions to be studied, the technique has also been used to study antibody–antigen and protein–protein interactions, identify DNA damage and cell signalling. It is extensively used in

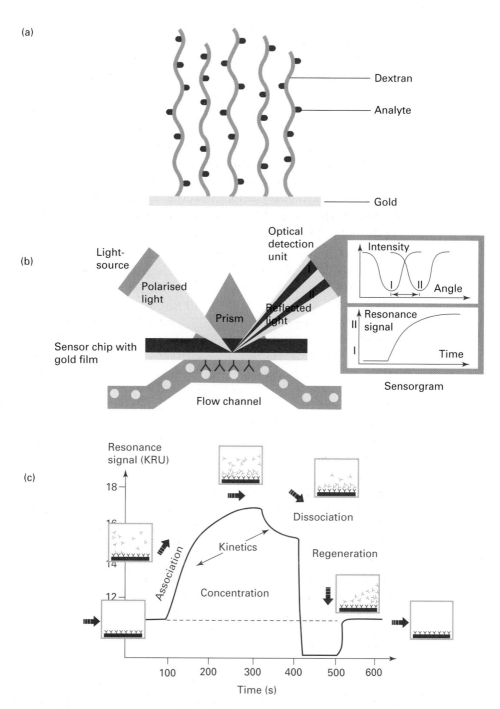

Fig. 16.6. The principles of surface plasmon resonance technology. (a) The sensor 'chip'
surface. (b) The flow channel and (insert) change in intensity of reflected light as a function
of angle of incidence of the light beam and change in resonance signal as a function of time.
(c) The sensorgram. (Reproduced by permission of Biacore AB, Uppsala, Sweden: website
<www.biacore.com>.)

proteomic research and in drug discovery and development. It is now possible to couple the technique to MALDI–TOF mass spectrometry (Section 8.5).

Plasmon-waveguide resonance (PWR) spectroscopy is closely related to SPR spectroscopy. In this technique the gold or silver layer is coated with a thicker layer of silica that behaves as a waveguide (a device for propagating electromagnetic radiation). The advantage of this is that the resonances from the metal can be induced by both *p*-polarised light, in which the electric vectors are polarised perpendicular to the resonator surface, and *s*-polarised light in which the electric vectors are polarised parallel to the resonator surface. This allows the anisotropic properties of the molecules near the surface of the silica layer to be studied and this in turn allows information about conformational changes induced in these molecules, for example as a consequence of ligand binding, to be deduced. It is more sensitive than SPR spectroscopy and can be used to study conformational changes in lipid bilayers. Thus a single lipid bilayer is deposited on the resonator surface and the receptor protein inserted from a detergent-solubilised solution. A solution containing the ligand is then passed over the layer, allowing the binding process to be studied. Such studies with G-protein-coupled receptors have shown that agonists, inverse agonists and antagonists can readily be distinguished by the conformational changes they induce in the membrane. Specifically, agonists and inverse agonists increase membrane thickness (agonists more so than inverse agonists) by causing an elongation of the receptor whereas antagonists cause no change (see Section 16.2.1).

Protein microarray technology   This approach to the study of receptor–ligand binding is based on the principle that assay systems that use a small amount of capture molecule (the ligand) and a small amount of target molecule (the receptor) can be more sensitive than systems that use a hundred times more material. In this miniaturisation approach, the ligand is immobilised onto a small area of a solid phase, commonly a derivatised glass slide. The resulting 'microspot' contains a high density (concentration) of ligand but a very small amount of it. It is then incubated with the receptor, commonly fluorescently tagged, resulting in the binding of some of the target molecules. Since the microspot covers a small area there is effectively no change in the concentration of the target molecules in the sample even if its concentration was low and the binding affinity was high. This is true provided that $<0.1K_d$ of the capture molecules are bound in the complex, where K_d is the dissociation constant for the complex. The capture–target complex is then quantified by fluorimetric methods and the procedure repeated for a series of increasing microspot sizes (increasing ligand concentration) but such that the density of the capture molecules is constant. If, after each incubation, excess receptor protein is washed away, the remaining complex can be analysed by surface-enhanced laser desorption and ionisation (SELDI) mass spectrometry. In practice, microspots are immobilised in rows on the solid support, allowing the simultaneous analysis of hundreds or even thousands of samples.

Patch clamping   This technique is of particular value in the study of kinetics and structure of receptors involved in the ligand or voltage-induced gating of ion

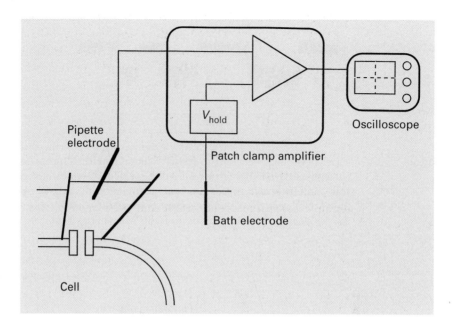

Fig. 16.7. Diagram for a patch clamp set-up in voltage mode. The potential between a bath electrode and a pipette electrode is compared with a reference potential V_{hold}. Current is injected via a feedback circuit until the two potentials are equal. Ion flow across the patch membrane is therefore represented by the required current injected to maintain V_{hold} across the two electrodes. (Reproduced by permission of A. Molleman, University of Hertfordshire.)

movements across the membrane. It involves the use of a glass micropipette with a tip internal diameter of the order of a few micrometres containing a Ag/AgCl electrode and Ringer's solution and, where appropriate, the ligand under study. The tip of the micropipette is brought into contact with the membrane of the cell and a slight vacuum applied. The tip forms a very high resistance seal (10^9 ohms, hence 'gigaohm' seal) with the membrane, thus isolating a patch of about 50 μm^2. The location of the tip is viewed through a microscope. The salt solution in the electrode is connected through the Ag/AgCl junction to a device that allows the simultaneous recording of current and the control of potential (voltage clamp) or vice versa (current clamp) over the patch of membrane (Fig. 16.7). The former option is used more frequently than the latter because the activity of many ion channels is dependent on the potential across the membrane. If the patch contains one or only a few ion channels, ionic currents through the individual channels can be recorded. The magnitude of these currents is of the order of a few picoamperes (10^{-12} A) and they last for a few microseconds. Single-channel traces show the characteristic irregular rectangular jumps representing transitions between the open and closed states of the ion channel (Fig. 16.8). One of the great powers of the technique is that many configurations are possible (Fig. 16.9) each having its distinct advantages depending upon the objectives of the study. Thus the outside-out patch is most convenient

Cell membrane receptors

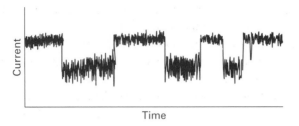

Fig. 16.8. An example of single-channel activity as it appears on the oscilloscope. The current level jumps between two average values as the channel opens (lower level) and closes (upper level). The current scale is of the order of a few picoamperes and the time scale in the range milliseconds to seconds, depending on the channel type. (Reproduced from A. Molleman (2003), *Patch Clamping: An Introductory Guide To Patch Clamp Electrophysiology*, p. 111, by permission of John Wiley and Sons Ltd.)

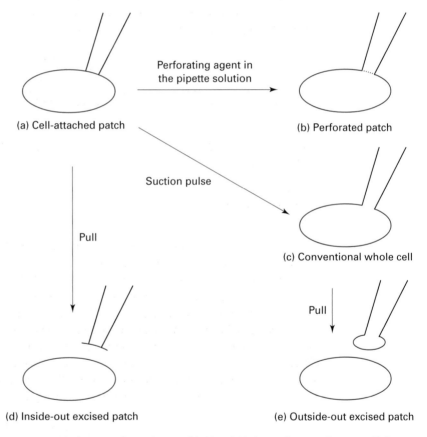

Fig. 16.9. Patch clamp configurations. In (b), (c) and (e) the medium on the extracellular side of the membrane under study can be changed during a recording. In configuration (d) the intracellular side can be manipulated. Configurations (a) and (b) leave the cytoplasm relatively intact. (Reproduced by permission of Areles Molleman, University of Hertfordshire.)

for the application of a range of ligands to the membrane. It is also possible to study the action of a single molecule in *situ*.

By studying the size and direction of the current as a function of ion concentration gradient, deductions can be made about the identity of the ions flowing through the channel. For example, a current of 1.0 pA through a channel for 1 ms is equivalent to the movement of about 7800 sodium ions per channel per millisecond. Patch clamp studies have revealed that the number of ion channels per cell membrane is low.

Example 1 ANALYSIS OF LIGAND BINDING DATA

Question

The extent of the binding of an agonist to its membrane-bound receptor on intact cells was studied as a function of ligand concentration in the absence and presence of a large excess of unlabelled competitive antagonist. In all cases the extent of total ligand binding was such that there was no significant change in the total ligand concentration. What quantitative information about the binding of the ligand to the receptor can be deduced from this data?

	[Ligand] (nM)							
	40	60	80	120	200	500	1000	2000
Total ligand bound (pmol $(10^6 \text{ cells})^{-1}$)	0.284	0.365	0.421	0.547	0.756	1.269	2.147	2.190
Ligand binding in presence of competitive antagonist (pmol $(10^6 \text{ cells})^{-1}$)	0.054	0.068	0.084	0.142	0.243	0.621	1.447	1.460

Answer

To address this problem it is first necessary to calculate the specific binding of the ligand to the receptor (B_s). The use of a large excess of unlabelled competitive antagonist enables the non-specific binding to be measured. The difference between this and the total binding gives the specific binding. Once this is known, various graphical options are open to evaluate the data. The simplest is a plot of the specific ligand binding as a function of the total ligand binding. More accurate methods are those based on linear plots such as a Scatchard plot (equation 16.4) and a Lineweaver–Burk plot (equation 16.7). In addition, it is possible to carry out a Hill plot (equation 16.9) to obtain an estimate of the Hill constant, h. The derived data for each of these three plots are shown in the following table:

	[Ligand](nM)							
	40	60	80	120	200	500	1000	2000
Total bound ligand (pmol $(10^6 \text{cells})^{-1}$)	0.284	0.365	0.421	0.547	0.756	1.269	2.147	2.190
Non-specific binding (B_{ns}) (pmol $(10^6 \text{ cells})^{-1}$)	0.054	0.068	0.084	0.142	0.243	0.621	1.447	1.460

Example 1 (*Cont.*)

	[Ligand](nM)							
	40	60	80	120	200	500	1000	2000
Specific binding (B_s) (pmol (10^6 cells)$^{-1}$)	0.230	0.297	0.337	0.405	0.513	0.648	0.700	0.730
$B_s/[L] \times 10^3$ (dm^3(10^6 cells)$^{-1}$)	5.75	4.95	4.21	3.37	2.56	1.30	0.70	0.43
$1/[B_s]$ (pmol (10^6 cells)$^{-1}$)	4.35	3.37	2.97	2.47	1.95	1.54	1.43	1.37
$1/[L]$ (nM)$^{-1}$	0.0250	0.0170	0.0125	0.0083	0.0050	0.0020	0.0010	0.0005
$(B_{max} - B_s)$ (pmol (10^6 cells)$^{-1}$)	0.52	0.45	0.413	0.345	0.237	0.102	0.050	0.020
$B_s/(B_{max} - B_s)$	0.44	0.66	0.816	1.174	2.164	6.35	14.00	36.50
log $B_s/(B_{max} - B_s)$	−0.356	−0.180	−0.088	0.070	0.335	0.803	1.146	1.562
log [L]	1.60	1.78	1.90	2.08	2.30	2.70	3.00	3.30

The hyperbolic plot allows an estimate to be made of the maximum ligand binding, B_{max}. It is approximately 0.75 pmol (10^6cells)$^{-1}$. An estimate can then be made of K_d by reading the value of [L] that gives a ligand binding value of $0.5 B_{max}$ (0.375 pmol (10^6 cells)$^{-1}$). It gives an approximate value for K_d of 100 nM.

A Scatchard plot obtained by regression analysis gives a correlation coefficient, r, of 0.996, B_{max} of 0.786 pmol (10^6 cells)$^{-1}$ and K_d of 97.3 nM. A Lineweaver–Burk plot gives a correlation coefficient, r, of 0.998, B_{max} of 0.746 pmol (10^6 cells)$^{-1}$ and K_d of 90.5 nM. Note that there is some variation between these three sets of calculated values and the ones given by the Lineweaver–Burk plot are more likely to be correct since, as previously pointed out, the Scatchard plot overestimates both values when the binding data are subjected to linear regression analysis.

The Hill plot based on a value of B_{max} of 0.75 pmol (10^6cells)$^{-1}$, gave a correlation coefficient of 0.998 and a value for the slope of 1.13. This is equal to the Hill constant, h.

16.3.3 Receptor–ligand binding data

K_d, k_{+1}, k_{-1} values and receptor numbers and occupancy

The K_d values observed for a variety of receptors binding to their physiological agonist are in the range 10^{-6} to 10^{-11} M, which is indicative of a higher affinity than is typical of enzymes for their substrates. The corresponding k_{+1} rate constants are in the range 10^5 to 10^8 (M)$^{-1}$min^{-1} and k_{-1} in the range 0.001–0.5 min^{-1}. Studies with G-protein-coupled receptors that form a tertiary complex (AR*G) have shown that the tertiary complex has a higher affinity for the ligand than has the binary complex (AR*). Receptor affinity for its agonist is also influenced by receptor interaction with various adaptor protein molecules present in the intracellular cell membrane. This is discussed more fully later.

It is relatively easy to calculate the number of receptors on cell membranes from binding data. The number is in the range 10^3–10^6 per cell. Although this may appear large, it actually represents a small fraction of the total membrane protein. This partly explains why receptor proteins are sometimes difficult to purify. From knowledge of receptor numbers and the K_d values for the ligand, it is possible to calculate the occupancy of these receptors under normal physiological concentrations of the agonist. In turn it is possible to calculate how the occupancy and the associated cellular response will respond to changes in the circulating concentration of the agonist. The percentage response change will be greater the lower the normal occupancy of the receptors. This is seen from the shape of the dose–response curve within the physiological range of the agonist concentration. It is clear that, if the normal occupancy is high, the response to change in agonist concentration is small. Under such conditions, the response is likely to be larger if the receptor–agonist binding is a positively cooperative process.

Binding studies have revealed that some agonists can stimulate the maximal response from the receptor preparation with only a small proportion of the receptors occupied. This has given rise to the concept of spare receptors, which are indistinguishable from the occupied receptors. It is believed that spare receptors maximise the sensitivity of the cell to the available agonist. However, to regard 'spare' receptors as being in excess of physiological requirement is misleading and in this sense the term is unfortunate. 'Spare' receptors are an intrinsic part of the cell's strategy to ensure a maximum response to a low dose of agonist and to facilitate speed in on–off responses. However, binding studies have also shown that the number of receptors in a membrane is time variable. The number is subject to upregulation or downregulation, depending upon the needs of the cell. Control of receptor numbers is exerted at a number of levels ranging from transcription and translation to endocytotic internalisation and subsequent degradation by ubiquitin-linked enzymes (Section 16.6.2). Some receptors can be shown by labelling studies to be recycled back into the membrane following endocytosis, the whole cycling time taking as little as a few minutes. The half-life of the insulin receptor is 9 h. Prolonged exposure of receptors to their ligand has been shown to result in desensitisation in some cases. The mechanism of this process is discussed later (Section 16.6.1).

Receptor subclasses

Binding studies using both agonists and antagonists have identified the heterogeneity of many membrane receptors. Classification of receptor subclasses based on such studies is not without ambiguity, and indeed controversy, and clearly identifies the need for such classification studies to be paralleled by those based on a gene cloning approach. As an example, this dual approach has confirmed the existence of over a dozen types of 5-HT (5-hydroxytryptamine or serotonin) receptor. An interesting feature of some receptor subclasses is that not only do they have different binding characteristics but they may also trigger opposing cellular responses. As an example, β-adrenergic receptors are activated by adrenaline and noradrenaline but there are three subclasses β_1, β_2 and β_3 with different amino acid composition, affinities for agonists and physiological responses. Thus β_1-adrenergic receptors mediate cardiac responses, β_2-adrenergic receptors are involved in skeletal and smooth muscle function, and β_3-adrenergic receptors are involved in metabolic responses. Subtype-selective synthetic agonists such as salbutamol readily discriminate between the three groups.

Receptor mobility

The ability of receptors to interact with other membrane-associated molecules, essential for the process of signal transduction, requires the receptor to diffuse freely within the two-dimensional lipid bilayer. This receptor mobility can be studied by the technique of fluorescence recovery after photobleaching (FRAP) that requires the receptor to be tagged with a fluor. Labelled receptors within a small circular region of the membrane ($1–10\ \mu m^2$) are then exposed to an intense attenuated laser beam that irreversibly bleaches the fluorescent receptors within the beam. The subsequent time-dependent increase in fluorescence within this bleached area, owing to diffusion into the area of non-bleached fluorescent receptor molecules, is then monitored, allowing the rate of diffusion of the receptors to be calculated. Such studies have revealed that a given receptor can traverse the whole surface of a cell in times ranging from 4 min to 7 h.

16.4　MOLECULAR STRUCTURE OF RECEPTORS

16.4.1　Molecular nature of the receptor

In principle, the study of the molecular nature of a receptor protein and its linkage to signal transduction is best carried out with the receptor embedded in the membrane. However, low expression levels and the presence of unrelated proteins within the membrane can complicate such studies. In spite of these difficulties, it is possible to study receptor proteins in their membrane environment either in the native state or by using purified receptor protein inserted into liposomes (artificial membrane structures) or giant unilamellar vesicles (diameter up to $100\ \mu m$). The techniques employed for such studies include the following:

- *Freeze-fracture electron microscopy:*　The procedure enables the oligomeric nature of the receptor in the membrane to be evaluated and an estimate made of the number and size of transmembrane α-helices.
- *Optical microscopy:*　Studies can be made of the rate of diffusion of individual receptor molecules in the fluid membrane.
- *Electron-spin resonance spectroscopy (ESR):*　Using a nitroxide spin label attached to a cysteine residue, studies can be made of the effective radius of the protein and its rotation in the membrane.
- *Anti-receptor antibodies:*　These have been used to study aspects of receptor biochemistry, including their cellular location and the location of binding

sites within the receptor. Anti-receptor antibodies can be raised using cell-bound or membrane-bound receptor protein, purified receptor protein or receptor protein produced by gene cloning. One of the problems associated with the use of anti-receptor antibodies is that they will certainly have more than one epitope, some of which may be located within the membrane or on the intracellular side of the membrane rather than simply on the ligand-binding side of the membrane. Thus anti-receptor antibodies may bind to sites other than the physiological ligand-binding site and may even trigger receptor aggregation owing to their large multivalent nature. The use of monovalent Fab antibody fragments (Section 7.1.2) may help to confirm whether or not the ligand-binding site is being studied.

It is possible to release the receptor from its membrane by treatment with detergents and to isolate the receptor by conventional techniques especially lectin affinity chromatography, affinity chromatography using an antagonist as the immobilised ligand, or hydrophobic interaction chromatography. The purified protein, in detergent solution, can then be studied by a number of techniques:

- *Analytical ultracentrifugation:*   The procedure of sedimentation equilibrium (see Section 3.5.3), which is independent of the shape of the protein, allows a study of the receptor's size and the stoichiometry and interaction between its subunits. The alternative procedure of sedimentation velocity allows an assessment of the purity of the preparation and an estimate of the relative molecular mass of the receptor, provided details of the receptor shape are available. However, the binding of detergent molecules to the protein can complicate the interpretation of the data.
- *Molecular exclusion chromatography:*   In principle this technique enables an estimate to be made of the relative molecular mass but the choice of calibration proteins is a potential problem.
- *Gel electrophoresis:*   using the Coomassie Brilliant Blue technique, an estimate of purity and the relative molecular mass of the receptor can be made.

Once purified, the receptor protein can be crystallised and its structure investigated by X-ray crystallography. However, it is far more common to undertake such studies on recombinant proteins. The crystal structure of a number of receptor proteins has been studied. Examples include the rhodopsin, glutamate, insulin and nicotinic acetylcholine receptors. The crystal structures have provided an understanding of the molecular mechanisms that are responsible for the physiological function of the receptors. The main limitations of crystallographic studies are the inherent difficulty of producing high quality crystals and the fact that the technique gives data only on the solid phase of the protein.

The main alternative to the X-ray crystallography is NMR spectroscopy especially multidimensional NMR by the COSY, NOESY and ROESY procedures (Section 13.4.1). The advantages of the NMR approach are that it can be applied to the receptor protein in solution and the fact that the more flexible parts of the protein give a stronger NMR signal thus making it ideal for the study of conformational changes induced by ligand binding. NMR studies of the rate of deuterium exchange in aqueous solution by receptor proteins have been particularly successful in showing that receptor proteins exist as a collection of many microconformations (a so-called protein assembly), some of which are energetically more favourable than others, and that there is constant motion between states with similar energies. These microconformations result from the folding and unfolding of specific small hydrophobic regions of the protein. Indirect evidence for this protein mobility comes from studies with G-protein-coupled receptors. It has been possible to immunoprecipitate complexes between the receptor and a G-protein in the absence of the receptor agonist, confirming that the receptor must be flipping spontaneously between inactive and active states. Binding of an agonist may induce structural changes that facilitate the formation of otherwise energetically less favourable states. Equally, different agonists for a given receptor may induce different states, thus rationalising differences in their efficacy.

16.4.2 Receptor-binding domains

The classical experimental strategies adopted for the study of the binding domain of receptor proteins are very similar to those used so successfully for the study of enzyme active sites. Affinity labelling (Section 15.4.2) has been adopted, with success, for the insulin receptor. The insulin receptor consists of two α-subunits (molecular mass 84 kDa) and two β-subunits (molecular mass 70 kDa) linked as a tetramer by disulphide bridges. Hydrophobicity studies (Section 8.4.3) revealed that only the two β-subunits span the membrane and protrude into the intracellular region. The two α-subunits are entirely on the outside of the membrane. In the study of the insulin-binding site, 4-azido-2-nitrophenyl-^{125}I-insulin was used as a photoaffinity label. Once the label was bound to the insulin receptor, the receptor–label complex was exposed to ultraviolet light, which converted the azido group to a nitrene that covalently attached itself to the binding site. The reagent was shown to be linked to an α-subunit. The N-terminal regions of the α-subunits are cysteine rich and contain a binding domain that has similarities to the ligand-binding site identified for the epidermal growth factor (EGF) receptor.

There are two modern approaches to the study of receptor-binding domains. The first is to study the receptor–ligand specificity by binding studies and to use computer-based molecular modelling analysis of the structure/specificity relationships to deduce the details of the binding domain. The second is to study the crystal structure of the receptor protein in the presence and absence of the physiological ligand. Both approaches can be complemented by site-directed mutagenesis studies that enable key amino acid residues in the binding domain to be identified. Such approaches to the study of the tyrosine kinase receptors have identified 20 subclasses that all have multiple extracellular domains containing common folds that may be cysteine rich, Ig like or fibronectin III like.

The realisation that receptor proteins have considerable mobility and are constantly flipping between different conformations means that the binding domain must be flexible rather than rigid and hence that the domain shape and size is to some extent determined by the ligand. This explains why, for some receptors, structurally diverse ligands can bind with similar ease.

Classification of cell surface receptors

The application of the various analytical approaches discussed above to the study of structure and size of receptor proteins coupled with studies of the type of transduction mechanism induced by the receptors, has lead to the identification of three main types of cell membrane receptors:

- *Ligand-gated ion-channel receptors:*   These are responsible for the selective movement of ions such as Na^+, K^+ and Cl^- across membranes. Binding of the agonist triggers the gating (opening) of the channel and the movement of ions across the membrane. This ion movement is a short-term, fast response that results in the propagation of a membrane potential wave. They may be excitatory and result in the depolarization of the cell (e.g. the nicotinic acetylcholine and ionotropic glutamate receptors), or directly or indirectly inhibitory (e.g. the γ-aminobutyric acid A ($GABA_A$) receptors, which stimulate chloride influx and thus result in the repolarisation of the cell). All receptors in this class consist of four or five homo- or heteromeric subunits. Responses produced by this class of receptors occur in fractions of a second.
- *G-protein-coupled receptors (GPCRs):*   Receptors in this class are linked to a G-protein that is trimeric. Receptor activation triggers its interaction with a G-protein, resulting in the exchange of GTP for GDP on one subunit that dissociates from the trimer causing the activation of an effector molecule such as adenylyl cyclase that is part of an intricate network of intracellular signalling pathways. Responses produced by GPCRs occur in a timescale of minutes.
- *Protein kinase receptors:*   These receptors all undergo agonist-stimulated autophosphorylation in the intracellular region. This activates the kinase activity towards intracellular proteins. The majority of activated receptor kinases catalyse the transfer of the γ-phosphate of ATP to the hydroxyl group of a tyrosine in the target protein. This phosphorylation process controls the activity of many vital cell processes. Members of a minor subgroup of protein kinase receptors transfer the phosphate group of ATP to a serine or threonine group rather than tyrosine. Examples of protein kinase receptors include the insulin receptor and the EGF receptor. Responses produced by protein kinase receptors occur over a timescale of minutes to hours.

Structural studies coupled with molecular cloning techniques have revealed that all cell membrane receptor proteins possess three distinct domains:

- *Extracellular domain:*   This protrudes from the external surface of the membrane and contains all or part of the ligand-binding site.
- *Transmembrane domain:*   This is inserted into the phospholipid bilayer of the membrane and may consist of several regions that loop repeatedly across the membrane. In some cases these loops form a channel for the 'gating' (hence

the channel may be open or closed) of ions across the membrane, whilst in other receptors the loops create part of the ligand-binding site.

● *Intracellular domain:*   This cytosolic region of the protein has to respond to the extracellular binding of the ligand to initiate the signal transduction process.

The existence of three domains within receptor proteins reflects their amphipathic nature. Each receptor protein has regions of 19–28 amino acid residues that are hydrophobic, consisting of non-polar side-chains, and other regions that are hydrophilic, consisting of polar and ionised side-chains. The hydrophobic regions, generally in the form of α-helices, are the transmembrane regions that are inserted into the non-polar, long-chain fatty acid portion of the phospholipid bilayer of the membrane. In contrast, the hydrophilic regions of the receptor are exposed on the outside and inside of the membrane where they interact with the aqueous, hydrophilic environment. The need for the hydrophobic region to span the membrane is so characteristic of receptors that it is possible to identify the membrane-spanning regions simply by inspecting the amino acid sequence of the protein. Superfamilies of receptor proteins can be recognised from the precise number of transmembrane regions each possess. Such multiple TM regions may be the consequence of the oligomeric nature of the receptor protein and in many cases the function of the receptor is linked to this oligomeric nature (see Section 8.4.3).

Receptor superfamilies

One-pass receptors (one transmembrane domain, 1TM)   Members of this group include the insulin receptor, the EGF receptor and the platelet-derived growth factor (PGDF) receptor, each of which has intrinsic protein kinase activity.

Two-pass receptors (2TM)   Members of this family have the involvement of ATP in common and as a consequence they are referred to as P2 receptors. There are two subtypes: P2X, which are ligand-gated ion-channels, and P2Y, which are G-protein coupled. In all cases there is one intracellular loop and the N- and C-terminal ends are located extracellularly.

Three-pass receptors (3TM)   These receptors are all ligand-gated ion channels involving excitatory amino acid neurotransmitters such as L-glutamate. The best-studied examples are the NMDA (*N*-methyl-D-aspartate) receptor and the AMPA (α-amino-3-hydroxy-5-methyl-4-isoxazole propionate) receptor. There is one intracellular and one extracellular loop. The N-terminal region is extracellular and the C-terminal region intracellular. All receptors in the class are homo- or heteropolymeric and require the binding of two agonist molecules for activation.

Four-pass receptors (4TM)   These receptors are also all ligand-gated ion channels related to the nicotinic acetylcholine receptor, serotonin receptor (5-HT$_3$), glycine receptor and the γ-aminobutyric acid (GABA$_A$ and GABA$_C$) receptors. In all cases the N- and C-terminal ends are located extracellularly. Only the TM2 region has α-helical structure.

Six-pass receptors (6TM)   This is currently a very small receptor family. Two examples, both of which are ligand-gated ion channels, are the inositol trisphosphate (IP_3)-activated receptor (present on the intracellular membrane) and the capsaicin-activated vanilloid receptor. Each receptor has three intracellular and two extracellular loops and both N- and C-terminal ends are extracellular.

Seven-pass receptors (7TM)   This is the largest and most diverse receptor superfamily. Many, but not all, are G-protein coupled. The range of first messengers involved with this family includes ions (Ca^{2+}), amino acids (glutamate), amines (catecholamines), purines (ATP), lipids (prostaglandins), peptide hormones (bradykinin), neuropeptides (tachykinins), kinins (interleukin-8) and glycoprotein hormones (thyroid-stimulating hormone, follicle-stimulating hormone). Each receptor has three extracellular and three intracellular loops. The N-terminal region is extracellular and the C-terminal region intracellular.

16.5 MECHANISMS OF SIGNAL TRANSDUCTION

16.5.1 Signal transduction through ligand-gated ion channels

Ligand-gated ion channels constitute one of the mechanisms for the control of the transmembrane movement of ions down their concentration gradient, resulting in a change in membrane potential. This control of ion movement is exerted on the basis of ion type (anion or cation), ion charge and ion size. Binding of the ligand to the resting state of the receptor induces a conformational change in the receptor protein, which results in the opening of the channel and the movement of ions. The channel remains open until either the ligand is removed or when, in the continued presence of the ligand, the receptor protein changes to its desensitised state, in which case the channel is closed. Since this mechanism of transduction is independent of any other membrane component or intracellular molecule, the cellular response to ligand binding is almost instantaneous. This class of membrane receptors includes numerous receptors that are involved in signal transmission between neurones, between glia and neurones, and between neurones and muscles.

Four superfamilies of ligand-gated ion channels, classified on the basis of the number of transmembrane segments within the subunits (2TM, 3TM, 4TM and 6TM), have been identified. The 4TM family has been the most thoroughly investigated and one of its major members is the excitatory nicotinic acetylcholine receptor (nAChR) found in large amounts in the eel and electric ray. Mammalian muscle nAChRs are located on the membrane of the postsynaptic cell adjacent to the synaptic neurone and are involved in muscle contraction. The snake venom toxin α-bungarotoxin binds irreversibly to the receptor, causing a block to the action of acetylcholine. The receptor has been shown to consist of five subunits of four types, α, β, γ and δ, with a stoichiometry of $\alpha_2\beta\gamma\delta$ and a molecular mass of 280 kDa. All of the five subunits span the membrane four times, mainly with α-helical structure, but with some β-structure. Each α-helical region has been designated TM1–TM4 and the experimental evidence from photoaffinity labelling studies and the production of point mutations supports the view that each of the TM2 regions of the five subunits lines the ion channel with the TM1 and TM3 regions, forming a scaffold to support the channel. Binding studies using native receptors and cloned receptors expressed in fibroblasts have provided evidence for the allosteric binding of two molecules of agonist with a Hill constant (Section 15.3.3) of about 2. Affinity labelling studies using competitive antagonists with a wide range of molecular structures have shown that the ligand-binding sites are in a cleft between two subunits. In both cases an α-subunit has the principal role in binding, with the γ- and δ-subunits playing a minor role. The first ligand molecule binds to the α_1-subunit that is in contact with the δ-subunit and the second molecule to α_2, which is in contact with the γ-subunit. Thus the two binding sites are not structurally identical. Genetically engineered variants of the five subunits structure have shown that the absence of the α-subunit results in the lack of binding of acetylcholine, thereby confirming the importance of this subunit. Mutagenicity and affinity labelling studies using irreversible competitive antagonists have demonstrated the importance to ligand binding of the A, B and C loops within the α-subunits and, in particular, a number of aromatic amino acid residues within these loops. Interestingly, there is high conservation of these residues within the known variants of nAChR.

Electron microscopic study of the nAChR on the *Torpedo torpedo* electric organ postsynaptic membrane has given an indication of the three-dimensional structure of the channel. It is funnel shaped, with a large proportion of the receptor outside the membrane protruding into the postsynaptic cleft. The channel is 25–30 Å wide at the entrance and only 6.4 Å wide at its narrowest point. Three rings of negatively charged amino acid residues, all on the four TM2 helices, line the narrow part of the channel and appear to determine its selectivity. The importance of these amino acid residues has been confirmed by mutagenicity studies.

Patch clamp studies of the nAChR have enabled the kinetics of channel opening to be evaluated. The whole process is kinetically complex but the essential features may be represented as follows:

$$A + R \rightleftharpoons AR + A \rightleftharpoons A_2R \rightleftharpoons A_2R^* \rightleftharpoons A_2R^{**}$$

Channel: closed   closed   closed   open   desensitised

where A is acetylcholine and R the receptor containing two binding sites for acetylcholine, one on each α-subunit.

Measurement of the numerous rate constants for these reversible processes has revealed that the rate constant for the opening of the channel is greater than the rate constants for the corresponding reverse process (i.e. the reversion to the closed conformation), for the dissociation of a ligand molecule from the closed conformation and for the transition from the open active state to the desensitised state. The consequence of this is that many opening and closing events of the channel occur before either the transition to the desensitised state or a molecule of ligand dissociates from the binding site. The mean channel open time for *Torpedo* nAChR is 3.0 ms and the mean closed time 94 µs within the bursts of opening and closing activity. The desensitised receptor (R**) eventually reverts to the closed resting state (R).

Desensitisation may be linked to phosphorylation. All five subunits contain amino acid residues located between the TM3 and TM4 regions that are potential sites for phosphorylation, and phosphorylation of the receptor has been shown to occur at two serine residues on each of the γ- and δ-subunits. Each phosphate group introduces two negatively charged oxygen atoms that could induce important conformational changes in the receptor structure and desensitisation. Mutagenesis studies of these serine residues have shown that their replacement by non-polar amino acids minimises the susceptibility of the receptor to acetylcholine-induced desensitisation. In contrast, replacement of the serine residues by glutamate, which contains negatively charged carboxyl groups, permanently desensitises the receptor. Such Glu and Ala substitutions are widely used as a technique in the study of protein kinases. This phosphorylation-induced modulation of receptor function is found in many other types of ion-transport proteins, indicating a common mechanism, but it is not clear whether or not phosphorylation is a prerequisite for receptor desensitisation (Section 16.6.1).

Structural studies similar to those carried out on the nAChR have been carried out on other ligand-gated ion-channels, in particular the $GABA_A$ and glycine receptors. These studies have provided evidence for commonality of channel structure and mechanism of ion selectivity. Consistent with this is the observation that there is considerable conservation of amino acid sequence in specific regions of the respective subunits. However, not all receptors linked to ion channels are directly ligand gated, but rather involve G-proteins as an intermediate between ligand binding and channel gating. An example is the cardiac muscarinic receptor linked to K^+ channels.

16.5.2 Signal transduction through G-protein-coupled receptors

Unlike receptors linked to ion channels of the nAChR type, in which agonist binding is linked directly to channel gating, most receptors require another protein to couple ligand binding to the transduction of the cellular response. In the case of the majority of the seven-pass superfamily (7TM) receptors (see below), the linkage is made by a family of membrane-associated proteins collectively known as G-proteins, so named because they bind GTP and GDP. It has been estimated that the human genome encodes for more than 1000 GPCRs, emphasising their considerable importance. With this group of receptors, the cellular response to agonist binding is linked to the formation of a ternary complex AR*G, although receptors with constitutive activity may act via the binary complex R*G (see Section 16.2.1).

7TM receptor structure

All GPCRs have a tertiary structure that consists of the seven transmembrane helices linked by alternating intracellular and extracellular loops with an

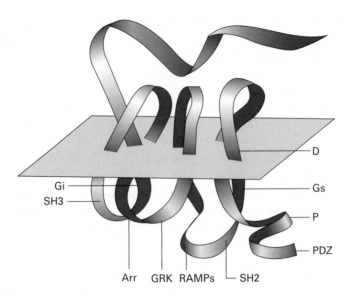

Fig. 16.10. Schematic diagram of a hypothetical G-protein-coupled receptor (GPCR). Labels denote general regions of interaction of the receptor with other cellular proteins including different G-proteins (G_i and G_s), PDZ, SH2- and SH3-domain proteins, receptor-activity-modifying proteins (RAMPs), arrestin (Arr), G-protein-coupled receptor kinase (GRK), sites for dimerisation with other GPCRs (D), and phosphorylation sites that lead to uncoupling and internalisation (P). Any one of these active processes could be considered a form of expression of efficacy. The figure is a general description of various loci for protein interactions, but does not represent accurate locations, as, in most cases, these are not well characterised. (Reproduced from T. Kenakin (2002), Efficacy at G-protein-coupled receptors. *Nature Reviews Drug Discovery*, **1**, 103–110, by permission of Macmillan Magazines Ltd.)

extracellular N-terminal end and an intracellular C-terminal region (Fig. 16.10). Although these receptors have this common 7TM structural feature, their ligand-binding domains vary considerably. For small agonists (e.g. adrenaline, histamine, dopamine, serotonin) the domain is partially embedded within the transmembrane helical structure, but for large agonists, including the neuropeptides and chemokines, the domain may span the extracellular loops or be located near the N-terminal region. This variability in the location of the binding domain emphasises that there must be several ways by which the agonist can stabilise the active conformation. The C-terminal region contains key proline-containing domains by which the active receptor couples with the G-protein.

GPCRs have been classified into three families:

- *Family A (also called class I):*   This is characterised by the presence of several conserved regions in the TM loops and the presence of a palmitolyated cysteine in the C-terminal tail. There is 15–20% homology between all the members. The family includes the rhodopsin, adrenergic, histamine, dopaminergic, muscarinic and tachykinin receptors. It is the largest group.

- *Family B (class II):* This is characterised by a long N-terminal tail containing six conserved cysteine residues linked by disulphide bridges and involved in ligand binding. The family includes the glucagon, calcitonin, secretin and parathyroid hormone receptors. They all activate adenylyl cyclase and couple through the same G_s-protein.
- *Family C (class III):* These members bind either glutamate or GABA or are involved in either Ca^{2+} metabolism or taste. Members include some of the metabotropic glutamate receptors (mGluR), of which eight have been identified and each shown to be distributed in specific regions of the brain. Binding of glutamate triggers the production of a second messenger that modulates the activity of the direct-gated (ionotropic) glutamate receptor. mGluRs contain an allosteric site that is a potential target for drugs involved in the treatment of Parkinson's disease (mGluR4), schizophrenia (mGluR5) and addiction (mGluR2).

There is considerable experimental evidence to indicate that GPCRs interact to form homo- and heterodimers and oligomers. In the case of the receptors in families B and C the evidence is that the functional activity of the receptors is linked to these forms, but in the case of family A receptors this link is less clear. The functional unit of both the mGluR1 and $GABA_B$ receptors in family C, for example, is a homodimer. X-ray crystallographic studies on the glutamate receptor have indicated that the dimer exists as a dynamic equilibrium between two conformations, one 'open' and the other 'closed', and that the role of glutamate is to stabilise the closed, active form. In contrast, the $GABA_B$ receptor is a heterodimer involving two receptors from family B.

The molecular activity and specificity of family B receptors is linked to the formation of both dimers and oligomers. In some cases the oligomeric association involves receptor–receptor interaction but in others it involves the association of the monomeric receptor with a member of a family of receptor activity-modifying proteins (RAMPs). Currently three RAMPs (RAMP1, 2 and 3) have been characterised and shown to be relatively small (RAMP1 is a 140 amino acid residue protein) with a single membrane-spanning domain, a large extracellular domain and a small intracellular domain. The RAMP–receptor heterodimers determine the specificity of the functional protein. Thus association of RAMP1 with calcitonin-receptor-like (CL) receptor gives a high affinity calcitonin gene-related peptide (CGRP) receptor whereas interaction of the CL receptor with either RAMP2 or 3 gives rise to an adrenomedullin receptor. Confocal microscopic evidence indicates that these heterodimers are formed in the endoplasmic reticulum and the Golgi apparatus and are retained during the processes of exocytosis to the membrane surface, ligand binding, endocytosis and ubiquitin-directed degradation (Section 16.6.2).

Receptor–signal transduction protein complexes

For the majority of the time GPCRs exist in the cell membrane as complexes with signal transduction proteins rather than as free floating proteins. These complexes are stabilised by scaffolding or adaptor proteins whose functions are similar but different in detail. Examples of the adaptor proteins include the multi-PDZ proteins, the Shank family of proteins and the Homer proteins. As their name implies, multi-PDZ proteins possess a number of PDZ (PSD-95, Dig and ZO-1/2) domains each of which can bind to the C-terminal region of different receptor and effector proteins involved in the transduction of a given signal. The resulting complex ensures speed and efficiency of the propagation of the signal, which is especially important in synaptic transmission. The Shank proteins possess several protein–protein interaction motifs including the SH2 (Src-homology domain 2) motif that recognises and binds tyrosine-phosphorylated sequences (this includes some receptors with intrinsic protein kinase activity (Section 16.5.3) and the SH3 (Src-homology domain 3) motif that recognises and binds sequences that are proline rich. GPCRs therefore possess domains capable of recognising and binding to these various motifs (Fig. 16.10). They also appear to possess an allosteric regulatory site. In the majority of cases the identity of the modulator is unknown but the site is a potential target for new therapeutic drugs.

G-protein structure

G-proteins are heterotrimeric, consisting of one of each of three subunits: α (40–45 kDa), β (36–40 kDa) and γ (8 kDa), which are loosely attached to the inner surface of the cellular membrane through lipophilic tails on the α- and γ-subunits. The β- and γ-subunits are firmly attached to each other but the linkage to the α-subunit is weaker. In addition to the binding site for the β-subunit, the α-subunit has a binding site for the C-terminal region of the receptor located near the N-terminal end and a guanine nucleotide-binding site that also possesses GTPase activity. Although the α-subunit contains the binding site for the receptor, binding occurs only when the α-subunit is bound to the $\beta\gamma$-dimer. Studies have revealed a very complex picture of the G-proteins. Twenty different α-subunits, 6 β-subunits and 12 γ-subunits have been identified. The potential number of different $G\alpha\beta\gamma$ functional trimers is therefore very large.

G-protein subgroups

Eight subgroups of G-proteins have been classified on the basis of their action. The five most important are as follows:

- the G_s subgroup that stimulates adenylyl cyclase,
- the G_i subgroup that inhibits adenylyl cyclase and activates some K^+ channels and phosphotidylinositol 4,5-bisphosphate (PIP$_2$) hydrolysis,
- the G_q subgroup that couples receptors to calcium mobilisation through phospholipase C$_\beta$, which generates the two second messengers inositol trisphosphate (IP$_3$) and diacylglycerol (DAG),
- the G_0 subgroup that reduces the probability of opening of some voltage-gated Ca^{2+} channels involved in neurotransmitter release,
- the G_t subgroup that stimulates phosphodiesterase following light stimulation of rhodopsin.

The study of G-protein transduction

Numerous methods have been used to study the structure of G-proteins and their interaction with receptors and intracellular effectors. Examples include the following:

- Use of analogues of GTP that bind to the α-subunit but are poorly hydrolysed, effectively leaving the α-subunit permanently active, e.g. [^{35}S]GTPγS.
- Use of bacterial toxins, such as cholera and pertussis toxin, which act by virtue of the fact that they are ADP-ribosyl transferases and stimulate the transfer of the ADP-ribose moiety of NAD^+ to the α-subunit of G-proteins. In practice ^{32}P-labelled NAD^+ is used.
- Use of N-ethylmaleimide as a reversible inhibitor of α-subunits, which it selectively alkylates.
- Use of photoaffinity labelling using analogues of GTP such as GTP-azidoanilide, which is converted to a nitrene by light and covalently labels the α-subunit.
- Use of antibodies raised to each subunit.
- Use of gene cloning and site-directed mutagenesis techniques and expression of the clones in *Xenopus* oocytes.
- Production of chimera receptors by genetic engineering techniques.
- Synthesis and use of a range of ligand analogues to identify the structural and kinetic features of receptor–ligand binding. The advent of combinatorial chemistry, which allows the simultaneous synthesis of a very large number of structurally related compounds, has increased the importance of this approach.

The G-protein cycle

Agonist binding to the receptor triggers a G-protein cycle (Fig. 16.11):

- In the normal resting state, the trimeric G-protein has a molecule of GDP bound to the α-subunit. At this stage the G-protein is not coupled to the receptor but is nearby.
- Agonist binds to the receptor to form the active receptor–agonist complex, concomitantly inducing a rapid conformational change in the TM6 helix of the receptor that activates the G-protein-binding site located in intracellular loops. The complex interacts by diffusion translocation with a G-protein–adaptor complex and binds to the α-subunit. Numerically there are more G-proteins than receptor proteins in the membrane.
- Binding of the receptor–agonist complex to the G-protein–adaptor complex induces a conformational change in the guanine nucleotide-binding site on the α-subunit, causing the dissociation of the GDP and the formation of a transient 'empty state'.
- GTP binding to the nucleotide-binding site on the α-subunit triggers a rapid conformational change in the α-subunit and subsequent dissociation of the GTPα subunit, leaving the G$\beta\gamma$-subunits as a dimer. Both the GTPα-subunit and the G$\beta\gamma$-dimer remain attached to the cell membrane.

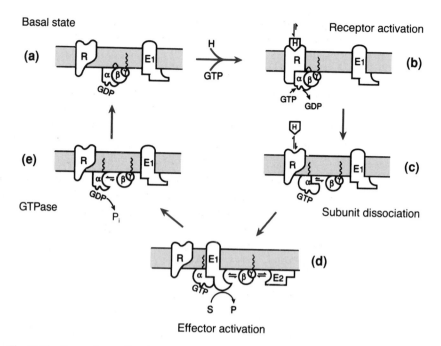

Fig. 16.11. G-protein-mediated transmembrane signal transduction. (a) The basal state consists of GDP tightly bound to the α-subunit of the heterotrimer. The receptor (R) is unoccupied and the effector (E₁), e.g. adenylyl cyclase, is inactive. (b) Ligand binding induces a conformational change, resulting in the replacement of GDP by GTP. (c) GTP binding causes the G-protein to dissociate from the receptor and the α-subunit–GTP complex (GTP$_\alpha$) to dissociate from the βγ-subunits. (d) The GTP$_\alpha$ complex binds to, and activates, the effector. The βγ-subunit complex may activate a second effector (E₂). (e) The GTPase activity of the α-subunit causes the hydrolysis of GTP to GDP and the deactivation of, and dissociation from, the effector. The GDP$_\alpha$ reassociates with the βγ-complex, returning the system to its basal state. (Reproduced from J. R. Hepler and A. G. Gilman (1992), G-Proteins. *Trends in Biochemical Sciences*, **17**, 383–389, by permission of Elsevier Science.)

- The GTPα-subunit and/or the Gβγ-dimer binds to an inactive effector molecule causing its activation or inhibition.
- Hydrolysis of GTP to GDP by the GTPase site of the α-subunit terminates the activation or inhibition by reversing the conformational change originally induced by the receptor–agonist complex. This facilitates the dissociation of the α-subunit from the effector and its reassociation with the Gβγ-dimer, thus completing the cycle.

Each G-protein cycle results in a very large amplification of the original signal.

A given G-protein may be activated by a large number of different receptors (referred to as G-protein promiscuity), whilst a given receptor may interact with different G-proteins and/or produce more than one response (referred to as receptor promiscuity). A receptor capable of activating more than one type of G-protein and hence of initiating more than one response is referred to as a pleiotropic receptor (meaning it has multiple phenotypic expressions). An example is the human calcitonin receptor, which can couple to G_i, G_s and G_q.

G-protein–effector coupling

It was originally believed that only the GTPα-subunit could interact with an effector but more recent research has shown that the Gβγ-dimer can also act as an independent transducer. Two important examples of the role of Gα-GTP as a transducer are the activation of adenylyl cyclase that converts ATP to the second messenger cAMP, and phospholipase C, which cleaves phosphatidylinositol 4,5-bisphosphate (PIP_2), a component of the cytoplasmic side of the cell membrane, to two second messengers, inositol 1,4,5-trisphosphate and diacylglycerol. Most examples of the transducer role of the Gβγ-dimer are linked to the activation of G_i and G_0. Examples include the activation of β-adrenergic receptor kinase (βARK), phospholipase A_2 and the K^+ channel GIRK (G-protein-activated inwardly rectifying potassium channel).

Regulation of G-protein transduction

The heterogeneity of G-proteins and the diversity of the responses they may induce via the transduction pathways offer a number of biochemical advantages, including amplification, control and specificity. Each Gα-GTP complex on binding, for example to adenylyl cyclase, may result in the synthesis or release of many molecules of second messenger, each of which may induce multiple responses (amplification) from the other components of the cascade system to which they are linked. Control is exerted at the level of the receptor by virtue of the fact that binding of the Gα-GTP complex to the receptor results in a decreased affinity by the receptor for the ligand (increased K_d), thus encouraging the release of the ligand, whilst hydrolysis of GTP to GDP reverses the affinity change. Control is also exerted by a group of over 20 proteins collectively called RGS (regulation of G-protein signalling) proteins that can be grouped into five subfamilies based on sequence homology. They all have the ability to bind to the Gα-GTP subunit at an RGS binding domain (Fig. 16.12), where they have two actions:

- they reduce the binding of the Gα-GTP to the effector,
- they act as GTPases, accelerating the hydrolysis of GTP to GDP by a factor of over 2000-fold.

Both actions result in the deactivation of the effector. This may allow the termination of the signal following removal of the stimulus or a redirection of a signal within a signalling network. There is evidence that specific RGS proteins regulate specific G-protein-coupled pathways. This specificity is determined by a combination of factors, including cell type-specific expression of RGS proteins, the intracellular localisation of the RGS proteins, the presence of domains other than the RGS domain that facilitate coupling to specific signalling pathways and the ability of some RGS proteins to act as effector antagonists that prevent a G-protein from coupling with its effector.

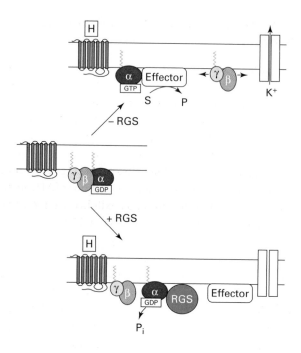

Fig. 16.12. Regulators of G-protein signalling (RGS) proteins negatively regulate
receptor-directed G-protein signalling. In the resting state (centre), cell surface receptors
for neurotransmitters and hormones are unoccupied by agonist, and G-proteins exist as
a GαβY heterotrimer with GDP bound to the α-subunit. Hormone agonists (H) binding
to the receptor (top) initiate guanosine nucleotide exchange, which facilitates GTP
binding to the Gα-subunit and the release of the GβY. The active Gα-subunit–GTP
complex and the GβY-dimer are free to regulate the activity of target effector proteins
such as certain ion channels or enzymes that convert substrate molecules (S) into
second-messenger products (P). Signalling is terminated as a result of the intrinsic
GTPase activity of the Gα-subunit. Most of the RGS proteins bind to the active Gα-
subunit–GTP complex (bottom) and greatly accelerate intrinsic Gα-subunit–GTPase
activity. GTP hydrolysis by the Gα-subunit terminates Gα-subunit–effector interactions
and promotes reassociation of the Gα-subunit–GDP complex with the GβY-dimer, which
blocks GβY-dimer signalling. (Reproduced from J. R. Hepler (1999), Emerging roles for
RGS proteins in cell signalling. *Trends in Pharmacological Sciences*, **20**, 376–382, by
permission of Elsevier Science.)

Recent evidence indicates that phosphorylation may be an important activation mechanism for GPCRs. It has been established for some years that phosphorylation is important in receptor desensitisation (Section 16.6.1), and endocytosis
(Section 16.6.2) but it appears that it may also be involved in coupling receptors to
specific signalling pathways. Research with the muscarinic M_3 receptor, for
example, has shown that it is phosphorylated by the enzyme casein kinase 1α at a
site distinct from that leading to desensitisation and that this phosphorylation is
essential for the activation of the extracellular-signal-regulated kinase 1 and 2
pathway (ERK-1 and 2).

16.5.3 **Signal transduction through receptors with intrinsic protein kinase activity**

It has been appreciated for over 20 years that phosphorylation coupled with dephosphorylation represents an important mechanism for the regulation of protein activity. A large number of intracellular kinases and phosphatases have been characterised and their regulatory action linked to conformational changes induced in the target protein as a result of the introduction or removal of a phosphate group. Phosphorylation can be studied by the use of ^{32}P-ATP. Control of protein activity by the kinase/phosphatase principle is found in a broad range of organisms, indicating its early evolution. It operates with the net consumption of ATP, but with the considerable gain in sensitivity, amplification and flexibility that more than compensate for the ATP consumed (for further details see Section 15.4).

More recently it has been shown that a large number of cell membrane receptors possess latent protein kinase activity that is activated by agonist binding. The transduction action of these receptors is linked to this kinase activity. Agonist binding induces the autophosphorylation of one or more tyrosine, serine or threonine residues within the intracellular region of the receptor protein and in the concomitant activation of the protein kinase activity of the intracellular domain of the receptor towards intracellular proteins. There are two main types of receptor kinase based on the specificity of the kinase.

Receptor tyrosine kinases

Twenty subclasses of receptor tyrosine kinases (RTKs) are known on the basis of their extra- and intracellular structures. Three of the best characterised are the EGF receptor, the insulin receptor and the PDGF receptor shown in Fig. 16.13. The majority of RTKs are single-chain, monomeric proteins in the absence of their agonist but dimerise on agonist binding. However, a few, including the insulin receptor, are dimeric but in all cases there is a single membrane-spanning domain within each monomer. There is evidence that, like G-protein-coupled receptors, the protein kinases interact with membrane-anchoring proteins of the Shank family type.

The agonist-binding site of the RTKs is located on the glycosylated extracellular region, whilst immediately after the transmembrane region there is the tyrosine kinase domain. Agonist binding causes a conformational change that allows the occupied receptors to recognise each other, resulting in their dimerisation. This is rapidly followed by the mutual cross-autophosphorylation of one to three tyrosine residues in the tyrosine kinase domains on each monomer, thus switching on their activity. The activated sites bind effectors, causing their phosphorylation and activation and the concomitant formation of receptor–signalling complexes. In this respect, therefore, these receptors resemble the G-protein-coupled receptors. These complexes are also stabilised by adaptor proteins but their identity is different from those associated with GPCRs. Examples include Gab-1, p85 and Grb2. The effectors and adaptors possess common binding domains for the tyrosine residues that have been phosphorylated by the kinase activities that may or may not be near

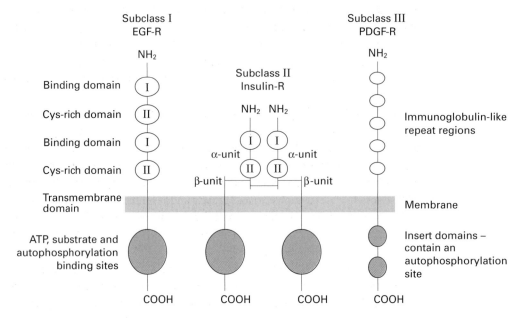

Fig. 16.13. Diagrammatic representation of three receptor tyrosine kinase subclasses. The EGF subclass contains two ligand-binding domains that are located in juxtaposition so that the ligand binds in a cleft between the two domains. The two cysteine-rich domains are both located near the membrane surface. On ligand binding, both the EGF and PDGF subclass receptors dimerise so that the intracellular tyrosine kinase domain possesses elevated activity and enhanced binding affinity relative to the monomeric forms. The insulin subclass receptors are effectively dimeric, but, as with the subclasses I and III, there is allosteric interaction between the two αβ halves of each receptor on ligand binding. The tyrosine kinase domains of the three subclasses show the greatest degree of homology between the three subclasses.

to the kinase active sites, including SH2 domains and phosphotyrosine-binding (PTB) domains. The effector may possess additional binding domains to which other effectors can bind. As a consequence of these additional domains the first effector is acting as an adaptor for the second effector, thereby enabling a web of signalling pathways with the potential for pathway branching to be established to meet prevailing cellular demands.

Receptor serine and threonine kinases

Complementary to the tyrosine kinase group of receptors is a second group of protein kinase receptors characterised by their ability to autophosphorylate serine and threonine residues in the intracellular domain of the receptor. These protein serine/threonine kinase receptors are specific for members of the transforming growth factor (TGF)-β superfamily that regulate growth, differentiation, migration and cell adhesion. They are classified into a number of subgroups on the basis of their structure, particularly their serine/threonine kinase domain. They are all single transmembrane receptors that, on binding of their ligand, form hetero-oligomeric complexes between subgroup types. This stimulates autophosphorylation and activation of the serine/threonine kinase activity towards other cytosolic proteins that are components of the transduction pathway. Some growth factor receptors lack kinase activity after dimerisation and autophosphorylation. In these cases they bind intracellular kinases and operate as a normal receptor kinase.

Like the GPCRs, receptor protein kinases stimulate numerous transduction pathways. The downstream members of these transduction pathways include the phospholipases and phosphoinositide kinases that are also involved in the G-protein transduction pathways. Among a number of effectors unique to the protein kinases is Ras, a membrane-bound guanosine-binding protein with intrinsic GTPase activity that is involved in cell growth and development in all eukaryotes.

Crucial to the control of transduction by receptor kinases is the existence of a group of protein phosphatases that can either deactivate or activate pathways by dephosphorylation. Phosphatases specific for tyrosine and others that act on serine and threonine as well as tyrosine have been identified. Some are purely cytoplasmic whilst others are receptor-like with a transmembrane domain. Most have two phosphatase domains, for reasons that are not clear, but their specificity may be linked to interaction between the two sites. The activity of the phosphatases appears to be linked to their own phosphorylation and a significant number have an SH2 domain for the receptor tyrosine kinases.

16.6 RECEPTOR DESENSITISATION AND TRAFFICKING

16.6.1 Receptor desensitisation

One of the characteristics of all of the three major groups of cell membrane receptors is that they display desensitisation characterised by a reduction or termination of the cellular response despite the continued presence of the agonist. However, from a kinetic perspective there are differences in the rate of onset of their desensitisation between the three classes. Thus, with ligand-gated ion channels, typified by the nAChR, desensitisation occurs within seconds of agonist activation whereas with GPCRs and protein kinase receptors desensitisation takes minutes and occasionally hours to occur. Such differences are a clear indication that different mechanisms are responsible for this loss of activity. In the case of the nAChR, the desensitised conformation of the receptor has a higher affinity for the agonist than has the active open channel conformation and this higher affinity alone is sufficient to drive the transition to the desensitised state but not before the ion channel has opened and closed many times. Removal of the agonist immediately reverses the desensitisation. It is known that some ligand-gated ion channels also undergo phosphorylation following activation and this too may facilitate desensitisation but by a kinetically slower route.

The kinetically slow onset of desensitisation of GPCRs and protein kinase receptors is believed to be linked to covalent modification of the receptor by phosphorylation at a site that is distinct from that of the autophosphorylation of the receptor that is an essential part of their activation. Postactivation phosphorylation of a tyrosine, serine or threonine residue in the intracellular region of the receptor introduces a polar phosphate group that can induce conformational changes deleterious to the normal functioning of the receptor. Studies with GPCRs have shown that phosphorylation by the second-messenger-activated kinases such as cAMP-dependent kinase and protein kinase A results in the uncoupling of the receptor from its G-protein. Phosphorylation can also be promoted by a family of seven serine/threonine GPCRs (GRK-1–7) that are capable of acting on agonist-occupied or constitutively active GPCRs. Phosphorylation of receptors has also been shown to trigger the internalisation (sequestration) and trafficking (recycling and degradation) of receptors. Internalisation may occur by a number of mechanisms, the most thoroughly understood of which is endocytosis.

16.6.2 Endocytosis and receptor trafficking

The internalisation and trafficking of receptors has been most thoroughly investigated using GPCRs, particularly the β_2-adrenergic receptor. Studies have revealed that the processes involve three stages:

- The recruitment of the receptors, normally with agonist bound to its binding site (agonist-dependent internalisation), but in some cases in the absence of bound agonist (agonist-independent internalisation), to discrete endocytic sites in the membrane. In the case of the agonist-dependent route, the receptor is phosphorylated by a GRK prior to internalisation.
- The internalisation of the receptors to form an early endosome or receptosome.
- The intracellular sorting of the endosome for either the subsequent recycling of the receptors or for their degradation following the fusion of the endosome with a lysosome.

Endocytosis is the process by which extracellular molecules and membrane proteins, including receptors, are taken up into the cell. The uptake process for receptors has been investigated using the fluorescence technique of tagging the receptor with green fluorescent protein or one of its several genetically modified variants (Section 16.3.1). In the case of G-protein-coupled receptors, after binding the ligand and G-protein, the receptors undergo ligand-dependent phosphorylation by a GRK and this stimulates interaction with one of the β-arrestin family of protein adaptor complexes. These cytosolic adaptors facilitate the disruption of the interaction of the receptors with G-proteins and the recruitment of the receptors into coated pits in the membrane where they link the receptor to a protein called clathrin via a second adaptor protein called AP-2. This protein interacts with phosphoinositides and promotes both the assembly of the coated pits and the recruitment of the activated receptors to them. A Tyr-X-Arg-Phe-region near the C-terminal region of the receptor binds to one end of AP-2, whilst the other end binds to the clathrin. Coated pits are regions in the membrane that are rich in clathrin, which is located on the cytoplasmic side of the membrane. The pits tend to accumulate in one area of the cell, a process known as patching, and eventually coalesce. Clathrin consists of three heavy chains and the light chains that can polymerise to form a polymeric cage-like structure or lattice that links to the C-terminal end of the receptor. The polymerisation of clathrin into the network involves the phosphorylation of the light chains at several sites, possibly involving different kinases. This phosphorylation is energy dependent and drives the whole endocytosis process. Ca^{2+} are involved in the stabilisation of the clathrin network. The polymeric clathrin network drives membrane deformation and the 'budding' of the coated pit to create an endocytic vesicle. Once the vesicle has formed, the clathrin coat is lost as a result of the action of one of the proteins of the heat shock protein family (hsp 70). The vesicles then fuse to form an early endosome or receptosome (Fig. 16.14). The formation of endosomes leaves the cytoplasmic region of the receptor exposed to the external environment. A number of adaptor molecules in addition to AP-1 and AP-2 have been identified and there is evidence that two of them, AP-3 and AP-4, may act independently of clathrin. The molecular details of the agonist-independent route of receptor internalisation are less well established. It appears that arrestins and GRKs are not required but that AP-2 and clathrin-coated pits are essential for the formation of an endosome.

Once the endosome is within the cell, the clathrin coat is depolymerised probably by hsp 70, with the concomitant hydrolysis of ATP. There are two possible fates for the receptors within the endosome:

- dephosphorylation followed by recycling to the membrane, thereby restoring a functional receptor;
- proteolysis resulting a net decrease in membrane receptor function, a process known as downregulation.

The pathways for endocytic sorting are determined by the operation of sorting signals. The main sorting signal appears to reside in the cytoplasmic region of the receptor itself. Thus, for the β_2-adrenergic receptor, a PDZ-binding domain in the C-terminal region interacts with a protein called ezrin–moesin-binding phosphoprotein 50 (EBP50), with the result that the receptor undergoes recycling, the process also involving arrestin and a protein known as N-ethylmaleimide-sensitive fusion protein (NSF) (Fig. 16.14). Chimeras of the receptor lacking the PDZ domain are directed to the degradative pathway. Receptors sorted for recycling are first dephosphorylated by an endosome-associated phosphatase and recycled back to the membrane via the Golgi complex. In the case of receptors directed to degradation the sorting signal again appears to reside in its C-terminal region. In these cases this region of the receptor interacts with a sorting protein called nexin 1, which promotes the fusion of the endosome with a lysosome, the resulting decrease in pH to 5.3 within the vesicle facilitating the downregulation of the receptor by proteolysis. There is evidence that this downregulation process is also dependent upon the ubiquitination of the receptor, a process that may include an active role for arrestin. Ubiquitin is known to 'tag' proteins for degradation, the process involving the action of a number of proteasomes (Section 15.5.4).

Much of the research on the mechanism of receptor endocytosis has been carried out using relatively few GPCRs and a few receptor protein kinases such as the

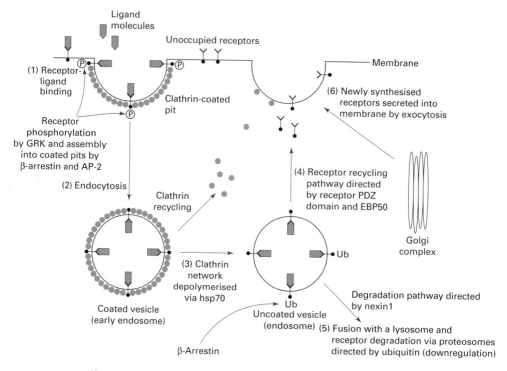

Fig. 16.14. Pathway of agonist-dependent G-protein-coupled receptor internalisation and endocytic sorting. (1) Occupied receptors are phosphorylated (Ⓟ) by a G-protein-coupled receptor kinase (GRK), leading to the recruitment of arrestins. Arrestins serve as adaptor proteins by linking phosphorylated receptors to components of the transport machinery such as clathrin and adaptor protein AP-2 and their recruitment to clathrin-coated pits. (2) The coated pit 'buds' into the cytoplasm aided by the clathrin, which forms a network, leading to the formation of an endosome. Note that the cytoplasmic domain of the receptor remains exposed to the cytoplasm following endocytosis. (3) The clathrin network is depolymerised and the clathrin recycled to the inner membrane. (4) The receptors are dephosphorylated and as a result of the interaction of EBP50 with a PDZ domain on the receptor, traffic back to the cell surface, resulting in functional resensitisation. Alternatively, (5) dephosphorylated receptors are tagged with ubiquitin (Ub) and enter the degradation pathway. Here they interact with nexin1, which promotes the fusion of the endosome with a lysosome and the degradation of the receptor by a number of proteasomes – a process known as downregulation. (6) The Golgi complex secretes newly synthesised receptor molecules to the outer membrane surface by exocytosis. The balance between receptor cycling, receptor degradation and receptor synthesis, and exocytosis determines the number of functionally active receptors on the membrane surface at any time.

epidermal growth factor receptor (EGR). It has yet to be established just how universal the clathrin-linked endocytotic pathway is among the large number of other receptors and various cell types. What is very clear is that the expression, regulation and desensitisation of receptors are dependent on numerous protein–protein interactions, many of which occur at the plasma membrane interface, that each cause crucial conformational changes in the receptor, and/or their regulators such as to couple receptor activity to current cellular and whole organism demands. It is equally evident that reversible multisite phosphorylation plays a vital role in the regulation of the activity of receptors and their effectors.

The temporal variation in the number of cell surface receptors available for ligand binding is the net result of receptor trafficking and of new receptor synthesis, which takes place in the rough endoplasmic reticulum. A leader sequence in the protein results in its recognition and transport to the Golgi complex where it is glycosylated, packaged into coated vesicles and inserted into the membrane by exocytosis, in which clathrin plays a vital role. The balance between receptor synthesis, recycling and degradation is subject to various control mechanisms so that free receptor availability in the outer membrane meets current physiological needs. Temporal variations in cell membrane receptor numbers are also of significance in the clinical response to chronic drug administration that leads to the downregulation of receptor numbers, and also in neurodegenerative conditions in which the release of the physiological agonist is deficient, resulting in upregulation of receptor numbers.

16.7 SUGGESTIONS FOR FURTHER READING

General

FORMAN, J. C. AND JOHANSEN, T. (ed.) (2002). *Textbook of Receptor Pharmacology*, 2nd edn. CRC Press, New York. (An authoritative coverage of receptors covering their molecular biology, quantitative aspects of ligand binding and signal transduction systems. Contains some problems for students to solve.)

HARDING, S. E. and CHOUDHRY, B. Z. (ed.) (2001). *Protein–Ligand Interactions: Structure and Spectroscopy*, Oxford University Press, Oxford. (Particularly valuable for the coverage of the applications of various spectroscopic techniques to the study of receptor structure and ligand binding.)

MOLLEMAN, A. (2003). *Patch Clamping: An Introductory Guide to Patch Clamp Electrophysiology*. Wiley, Chichester. (A self-contained guide covering the relevant membrane biophysics, experimental design, data analysis and technical concerns relating to patch clamping.)

Review articles

DEVI, L. A. (2001). Heterodimerization of G-protein-coupled receptors: pharmacology, signalling and trafficking. *Trends in Pharmacological Sciences*, **22**, 532–537.

GUREVICH, V. V. and GUREVICH, E. V. (2004). The molecular acrobatics of arrestin activation. *Trends in Pharmacological Sciences*, **25**, 105–111.

HOVIUS, R., VALLOTTON, P., WOHLAND, T. AND VOGEL, H. (2000). Fluorescence techniques: shedding light on ligand–receptor interactions. *Trends in Biochemical Sciences*, **21**, 266–272.

KALLAL, L. AND BENOVIC, J. L. (2000). Using green fluorescent protein to study G-protein-coupled receptor localization and trafficking. *Trends in Pharmacological Sciences*, **21**, 175–180.

KENAKIN, T. (2003). Ligand-selective receptor conformations revisited: the promise and the problem. *Trends in Pharmacological Sciences*, **24**, 346–354.

MARCHESE, A., CHEN, C., KIM, Y.-M. and BENOVIC, J. L. (2003). The ins and outs of G-protein-coupled receptor trafficking. *Trends in Biochemical Sciences*, **28**, 369–376.

MEYER, T. and TERUEL, M. N. (2003). Fluorescence imaging of signalling networks. *Trends in Cell Biology*, **13**, 101–106.

MORFIS, M., CHRISTOPOULOS, A. and SEXTON, P. M. (2003). RAMPs: 5 years on, where to now? *Trends in Pharmacological Sciences*, **24**, 596–601.

NEDLELKOV, D. and NELSON, R. W. (2003). Surface plasmon resonance mass spectrometry: recent progress and outlook. *Trends in Biotechnology*, **21**, 301–305.

ROBERTSON, A. D. (2002). Intramolecular interactions at protein surfaces and their impact on protein function. *Trends in Biochemical Sciences*, **27**, 521–526.

ROBINSON, M. S. (2004). Adaptable adaptors for coated vesicles. *Trends in Cell Biology*, **14**, 167–174.

SKLAR, L. A., EDWARDS, B. S., GRAVES, S. W., NOLAN, J. P. and PROSSNITZ, E. R. (2002). Flow cytometric analysis of ligand–receptor interactions and molecular assemblies. *Annual Reviews of Biophysics and Molecular Structures*, **31**, 98–119.

STRANGE, P. G. (2002). Mechanisms of inverse agonism at G-protein-coupled receptors. *Trends in Pharmacological Sciences*, **23**, 89–95.

TOLLIN, G., SALAMON, Z. and HRUBY, V. J. (2003). Techniques: plasmon-waveguide resonance (PWR) spectroscopy as a tool to study ligand–GPCR interactions. *Trends in Pharmacological Sciences*, **24**, 655–659.

Useful websites

G-proteins

<www.gpcr.org>
<www.cis.upenn.edu/~krice/receptor.html>

Receptor endocytosis

<www.cytochemistry.net/cell-biology/recend.htm>
<cellbio.utmb.edu/cellbio/recend.htm>

Techniques

<www.biochem.arizona.edu/tollin/cpwr/principl.htm>

Index